BROWSE'S INTRODUCTION TO
The Investigation and Management of Surgical Disease

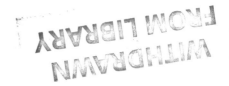

BROWSE'S INTRODUCTION TO
The Investigation and Management of Surgical Disease

Norman L. Browse KT MD FRCS FRCP
Professor of Surgery, Emeritus, University of London, UK
Honorary Consulting Surgeon, St Thomas' Hospital, London, UK
Past-President, Royal College of Surgeons of England, London, UK

John Black MD FRCS
Consultant Surgeon, Worcester Royal Hospital, UK
President, Royal College of Surgeons of England, London, UK

Kevin G. Burnand MS FRCS MBBS
Professor of Vascular Surgery, Emeritus, and Former Chairman
of the Academic Department of Surgery and Anaesthesia in the
Cardiovascular Division of King's College at the St Thomas' Campus,
London, UK
Honorary Consultant Surgeon, Guy's and St Thomas'
NHS Foundation Trust, London, UK

Steven A. Corbett BSc PhD FRCS FRCS (Tr&Orth)
Consultant Orthopaedic Surgeon, Guy's and St Thomas'
NHS Foundation Trust, London, UK

William E. G. Thomas MS FRCS
Consultant Surgeon, Sheffield Teaching Hospitals NHS Foundation Trust;
Honorary Senior Lecturer in Surgery, University of Sheffield, UK
Vice President and Member of Council, Royal College of
Surgeons of England, London, UK

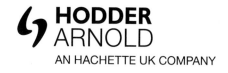
HODDER
ARNOLD
AN HACHETTE UK COMPANY

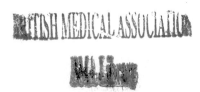

First published in Great Britain in 2010 by
Hodder Arnold, an imprint of Hodder Education, an Hachette UK company,
338 Euston Road, London NW1 3BH

http://www.hoddereducation.co.uk

British Library Cataloguing in Publication Data
A catalogue record for this book is available from the British Library

Library of Congress Cataloging-in-Publication Data
A catalog record for this book is available from the Library of Congress

ISBN-13   978-0-340-94574-2
ISBN-13 [ISE]   978-0-340-94693-0 (International Students' Edition, restricted territorial availability)

1 2 3 4 5 6 7 8 9 10

Commissioning Editor: Joanna Koster
Project Editor: Sarah Penny
Production Controller: Kate Harris
Cover Design: Amina Dudhia
Indexer: Laurence Errington

Typeset in 10/12 Pts, Minion by MPS Limited, A Macmillan Company
Printed and bound in India

What do you think about this book? Or any other Hodder Arnold title?
Please visit our website: www.hoddereducation.com

Dedication

To the better care of our patients

INSTRUCTIONS FOR COMPANION WEBSITE

This book has a companion website available at: **http://www.hodderplus.com/browsesintroductions.** To access the image library included on the website, please register using the following access details: Serial number: jxpz475ak9wr. Once you have registered, you will not need the serial number but can log in using the username and password that you will create during registration.

Contents

Contributors

Diane L. Back MBBS BSc Hons FRCS Ed Orth, Consultant Trauma and Orthopaedic Surgeon, Guy's and St Thomas' NHS Foundation Trust, London

Sabapathy P. Balsubramanian MBBS MS OMI FRCSEd, Consultant Senior Lecturer, Sheffield University and Sheffield Teaching Hospitals NHS Foundation Trust, Sheffield

Timothy J.P. Batchelor BSc MSc FRCS(CTh), Consultant Thoracic Surgeon, University Hospitals Bristol NHS Foundation Trust, Bristol

Christopher P. Chilton FRCS, Consultant Urological Surgeon, Department of Urology, Derby City General Hospital, Derby

Jeremy Collyer FRCS (omfs) FDS, Consultant Oral & Maxillofacial Surgeon, Department of Maxillofacial Surgery, Queen Victoria Hospital, East Grinstead

Thomas Ember MBBS MRCS FRCS (Tr and Orth), Consultant Orthopaedic Surgeon, Department of Orthopaedics, Guy's and St Thomas' Hospital, London

Ruth McKee BSc MBChB FRCS MD, Consultant Colorectal Surgeon, Glasgow Royal Infirmary, Glasgow

Bijan Modarai PhD FRCS, Clinical Lecturer in Vascular Surgery, King's College London; and Academic Department of Surgery, St Thomas' Hospital, London

Pari-Naz Mohanna MBBS BSc MD FRCS(plast), Consultant Plastic and Reconstructive Surgeon, Guy's & St Thomas' Hospital, London

Chris Munsch ChM FRCS (C/Th), Consultant Cardiac Surgeon, Yorkshire Heart Centre, Leeds

Hari L. Ratan BMedSci BMBS DM FRCS(Urol), Consultant Urological Surgeon, Department of Urology, Royal Derby Hospital, Derby

David Ross MD FRCS (Plast), Consultant Plastic & Reconstructive Surgeon, Guy's & St Thomas' Hospital, London

Benedict T. Sherwood BMedSci BMBS DM FRCS(Urol), Specialist Registrar in Urology, Nottingham City Hospital, Nottingham

Sam Singh MA MRCS MSc FRCS (Orth), Consultant Orthopaedic Surgeon, Guy's and St Thomas' NHS Foundation trust, London

Matthew Waltham MB BChir MA PhD FRCS, Senior Lecturer and Honorary Consultant Vascular Surgeon, King's College London/Guy's and St Thomas' NHS Foundation Trust, London

Preface

In 1980, two years after publishing the first edition of an 'An Introduction to the Symptoms and Signs of Surgical Disease' I suggested to Mr. Paul Price, the Managing Director of Edward Arnold's, that there would be a demand for a companion volume about investigation and management. However, I also said that I could not write it because my time was fully occupied with other tasks and because methods of investigation and treatment were advancing and changing so rapidly, that such a book would require many specialist authors and need revising every 5 years.

The notion lay dormant but not forgotten until in 2004 when, having persuaded three eminent general surgeons to help me produce the 4th edition of 'An Introduction to the Symptoms and Signs of Surgical Disease', I resurrected the idea and suggested to them that they might write a similarly styled companion volume about Investigation and Management.

This new book is, therefore, intended to be a companion to 'Symptoms and Signs'. It has been written and edited by the same co-authors, Mr. John Black, Prof. Kevin Burnand, Mr. William Thomas plus an orthopaedic surgeon Mr. Steven Corbett aided by a number of their specialist friends – Miss Diane Back, Mr. Sam Singh, Mr. Tom Ember, Mr. Andrew Brown, Mr. Christopher Munsch, Miss Ruth McKee and Mr Christopher Chilton.

My role has been to edit the whole text and ensure that it matches the pragmatic and repetitive style of 'Symptoms and Signs', which was intentionally designed in 1978 to inculcate into students' minds how to think about history taking and clinical examination. I hope this book does the same for investigation and management.

There are no clinical pictures or detailed clinical descriptions because they are in the companion volume but the important clinical features of each condition, called 'clinical diagnostic indicators', are summarised to emphasise that the first and most important method of investigation is the elucidation of a problem's history and its physical signs.

Investigations are becoming more and more complex and sophisticated. Their interpretation relies heavily upon the expertise of those who conduct them e.g. the radiologists and the biochemists. Although the clinician often has to consult these experts before deciding which test is the most appropriate and will provide the most relevant information the student should know how the tests are performed, and be able to interpret the results. Therefore, there are as many pictures of investigations – simple and advanced – as there are clinical pictures in the companion volume.

Similarly, management is also becoming more complicated. Surgical techniques are being replaced by less invasive and alternative methods. Nevertheless the student must know the basic forms and objectives of surgical treatments and more importantly their results and effects – good and bad. The text therefore contains simple drawings of operations, not confusing intra operative photographs, because this is not a textbook of operative surgery.

Because the book is what I call an introductory 'teach' book rather than a textbook to the investigation and management of surgical disease it does not contain any references. We believe that each student should search the literature themselves for the sources that support the facts figures and opinions we have expressed.

Sadly the bedside experience gained by undergraduate clinical students has so seriously diminished over the last fifteen years that this book's companion on symptoms and signs is now used by those sitting higher diplomas as well as undergraduates. Whilst we hope that this book will be equally useful to students at all levels we have not combined the two books because we believe that putting them together into a large tome might diminish the fundamental importance and distract the student from concentrating on learning about proper history taking and the techniques of clinical examination. Caring for a patient falls in to two phases – this book is part two and should be read after reading its companion.

Acknowledgments

The editors would like to thank Tarun Sabharwal, Renato Dourado and Gerald Carr-White for their images; as well as Kate Burnand for her artworks that were kindly contributed to the book.

Kevin Burnand would also like to thank Monica Brennan and Pat Webb, Secretaries at the Department of Academic Surgery, Kings College at the St Thomas' Campus, London, UK.

1

Principles and methods of investigation

William E. G. Thomas

This book has been written to accompany Browse's *Introduction to the Symptoms and Signs of Surgical Disease* and follows a similar format.

Once the symptoms and signs of a complaint (i.e. the problems) have been elicited, it is often necessary to employ special investigations to arrive at a definite diagnosis and prescribe the correct management.

Chapters 1 and 2 set out the approach to investigation and management used throughout the book.

Students should note that the term 'management' when used in an exam question embraces the initial history and clinical examination as well as the relevant investigations and appropriate treatment, but in this book it is used to describe everything that is done after taking the patient's history and completing the examination.

This chapter discusses the underlying principles, limitations, contraindications and complications of the many methods of investigation now available.

You must have a sound reason for ordering an investigation. Unnecessary investigations are a waste of resources and may put the patient to valueless inconvenience or suffering. There is a tendency, because of today's attitude towards medical litigation, to over investigate patients. This is not sound clinical practice. Investigations that are not clinically relevant or safe can lead to the misinterpretation of results and so be misleading. You should always ask yourself what you are seeking to learn from any particular investigation and be able to define its role in the care of your patient.

BLOOD TESTS

- Haematology
- Coagulation
- Biochemistry
- Microbiology
- Serology

Many blood tests, such as a full blood count, may be regarded as routine and required of most surgical patients, but others are specific and should only be undertaken when there are clear clinical indications, such as thyroid function tests. Avoid the tendency to consider many blood tests as being routine just because they are easy to perform.

If you keep in mind the principle of only ordering relevant investigations, this tendency should diminish.

Haematology

The **full blood count** is nowadays performed by automated methods. Modern analysers are available in almost all hospitals and by using electrical impedance or light-scatter flow cytometry provide the information given in Table 1.1. Normal values may vary from laboratory to laboratory depending on the method of measurement. Although these variations may be small, it is important to know the normal range of the laboratory in which the test was carried out before interpreting any

Table 1.1
Normal ranges for a full blood count

Haemoglobin	
Male	13.0–16.5 g/dL
Female	11.0–14.5 g/dL
Platelet count	$150–400 \times 10^9$/L
White blood cell count	$4–10 \times 10^9$/L
Neutrophils	$1.7–6.5 \times 10^9$/L
Lymphocytes	$1.0–3.0 \times 10^9$/L
Monocytes	$0.25–1.0 \times 10^9$/L
Eosinophils	$0.04–0.5 \times 10^9$/L
Basophils	$0–0.1 \times 10^9$/L

particular result. Most laboratories include their normal ranges alongside each individual result and highlight any result that is outside their normal range (Table 1.1).

The **microscopical examination** of a film (smear) of blood can provide information on morphological changes in the shape of the red blood cells (sickle cells, reticulocytes, etc.), the white blood cells and the platelets.

A **reticulocyte count** (immature erythrocytes) may be requested in patients who have been shown to be anaemic to provide information about bone marrow activity and its ability to respond to a state of anaemia, such as may follow blood loss, haemolysis or treatment with iron, vitamin B12 or folates.

The findings and results of a routine blood test determine the need for more specific haematological investigations. Tables 1.2 and 1.3 present some of the more common indications for ordering additional specific tests.

At times the many tests set out in Tables 1.2 and 1.3 fail to expose the underlying haematological problem and it becomes necessary to study the source of the blood cells – the bone marrow.

Bone marrow can be aspirated or a core of marrow trephined from the pelvic bones and sternum.

Table 1.4 lists the abnormalities revealed by routine blood tests that may have to be investigated further by a bone marrow biopsy.

Coagulation tests

A patient's coagulation status should be assessed when there is

- a known or suspected intrinsic bleeding disorder because of:
  - □ family history
  - □ excess bleeding after surgery or dental extractions
  - □ easy bruising

Table 1.2
Additional blood tests required to elucidate the cause of a microcytic anaemia

To detect an underlying iron deficiency

Serum iron – sensitive to diurnal variation, non-specific

Serum ferritin – reflects iron storage, i.e. diminished in iron depletion and increased in iron overload
Interpretation difficult in chronic disease as it can be raised or normal if patient is also iron deficient

Serum transferrin – iron-transporting protein, raised in iron deficiency and low in iron overload and chronic disease

Serum transferrin saturation – raised in iron overload and is a marker for haemochromatosis

To detect an underlying haemoglobinopathy

Haemoglobin electrophoresis – α or β chain abnormalities

α-thalassaemia – abnormalities 1–4 of the α-globin genes

β-thalassaemia – homozygous (transfusion dependent) or heterozygous (mild microcytic anaemia)

Sickle-cell anaemia – sickle-shaped red blood cells seen in the peripheral blood, homozygous (HbSS) or heterozygous (HbSC, HbSβ)

To detect the possibility of an underlying chronic disease

For example chronic infection, renal disease, rheumatoid arthritis, malignancies etc.

Erythrocyte sedimentation rate (ESR) raised

C-reactive protein (CRP) raised

Serum transferrin saturation – raised or normal

Need for more specific tests dependent upon clinical picture

For example, rheumatoid factor, renal function tests. etc.

Table 1.3
Additional blood tests required to elucidate the cause of a macrocytic anaemia (suggestive of deficiency of vitamin B12 or folate, liver disease, alcoholism, hypothyroidism, pregnancy, marrow failure or drug induced
May also reflect reticulocytosis following blood loss or haemolysis

Reduced serum vitamin B12 or folate levels

Liver function tests

Thyroid function tests

Pregancy test

Tests for haemolysis

Reticulocyte count

Plasma haptoglobin

Coombs tests – direct antiglobulin test (positive in autoimmune haemolysis or incompatible transfusions)

Lactic dehydrogenase and unconjugated bilirubin

Table 1.4
Abnormalities revealed by routine blood tests that may need to be followed by a bone marrow biopsy

Severe cytopenia: primary (anaemia, neutropenia, thrombocytopenia) or secondary (toxic substances, chemotherapy, radiotherapy, drugs)

Immature precursors in the blood (leuco-erythroblastic picture)

Abnormal cells (leukaemia, lymphoma, myeloma, megakaryocyte hyperplasia in thrombocytopenic purpura, erythroid hyperplasia in haemolysis)

Paraprotein in blood (or urine)

- □ spontaneous haemarthrosis, epistaxis, unexplained haematuria
- □ unexplained primary menorrhagia
- the patient is on anticoagulant drugs, e.g. warfarin
- the patient has a condition that can potentially affect the clotting cascade, e.g. jaundice/liver failure

- the patient has received a large quantity of transfused blood.

Routine coagulation tests include:
- **prothrombin time** (international normalized ratio (INR) – usually presented as a ratio based on the prothrombin time). The prothrombin time is increased in:
  - □ vitamin K deficiency
  - □ liver disease
  - □ warfarin therapy (it is insensitive in heparin therapy)
  - □ hypofibrinogenaemia
  - □ massive blood transfusions
  - □ disseminated intravascular coagulation (DIC), accompanied by:
    - raised fibrin degradation products (FDP)
    - reduced fibrinogen levels
    - reduced platelet count
    - raised D-dimer (produced by fibrinolysis)
- **activated partial thromboplastin time** (APTT). The APTT is increased in:
  - □ vitamin K deficiency
  - □ liver disease
  - □ warfarin therapy
  - □ heparin therapy (may be used to monitor heparin therapy other than low-molecular-weight heparin therapy which generally does not require monitoring and does not affect the APTT)
  - □ DIC
  - □ antiphospholipid antibodies
  - □ Von Willebrand's disease
  - □ deficiency of clotting factors VIII, IX, XI, XII
- **plasma fibrinogen**
- **fibrin degradation products in DIC and DVT, PE**
- **thrombin clotting time.**

Some special tests may be indicated by the results of the above routine tests, such as:
- **individual coagulation factor assays**
- **von Willebrand factor assay**
- **platelet function tests**
  - □ platelet aggregation studies
  - □ heparin-associated antibodies
- **bleeding time:** very operator dependent with wide laboratory variation.

At the opposite end of the clotting scale there are patients who exhibit an increased clotting/thrombotic tendency. It is important to exclude a thrombotic tendency in any patient with a history of a venous thromboembolic episode, especially if it was not associated with a known predisposing factor.

A thrombotic tendency should be investigated in all patients who:

- present with spontaneous thrombosis (especially if young)
- have a particularly extensive or severe thrombotic episode
- have a family history of thrombosis
- develop a thrombosis in an unusual site (e.g. spontaneous mesenteric venous thrombosis in the absence of gastrointestinal disease)

because these patients may have

- a **factor V Leiden** gene mutation (activated protein C resistance)
- a deficiency of **antithrombin III**
- a deficiency of **protein C** or **protein S**.

Patients in whom these tests prove positive may need to receive long-term/often life-long oral anti-coagulation therapy.

Biochemistry

This term refers to the chemical analysis of the constituents of any of the bodily fluids, not just the blood. Quantitative data can provide useful information on the function of organs such as the liver, kidneys and thyroid. Different biochemical patterns can indicate different disease processes, but it is important to define, as accurately as possible, what the objectives are for each biochemical analysis in order to utilize the information appropriately. Biochemical tests are not only valuable for diagnosis but are also useful in monitoring the response to treatment. As with haematological investigations, it is important to be familiar with each laboratory's normal ranges.

Before embarking on any biochemical test it is vital to ensure that optimal conditions exist at the time of sampling in order to be able to interpret the results. For example, certain tests require that the patient has been fasting for 6–8 hours, e.g. glucose tolerance tests and serum lipid levels, while in some patients fasting may actually elevate the levels of bilirubin and urate. Some blood tests are more accurate when the blood is taken without the venous congestion caused by the application of a tourniquet. Certain dynamic endocrine tests require the sampling to follow a complex timetabled protocol.

Once the sample had been obtained it is vital that it is placed in the correct specimen tube, with or without the correct anticoagulant, e.g.

- lithium heparin for most routine biochemical analyses
- EDTA for most haematological cell counts
- sodium citrate for coagulation studies
- a capped syringe with no additives kept at 4°C for pH or blood gas analysis.

Most laboratories produce a handbook with the tube requirements and normal values for that particular laboratory. Thus there are many factors that can cause results to vary which must be taken into account when interpreting the results. Some of the causes of these long- and short-term variables are presented in Table 1.5.

It is neither practical nor sensible to itemize all the possible variations or the normal ranges for all biochemical tests because the interpretation of all results must take into consideration the clinical state of the patient and any potential causes of biological variation.

Table 1.5
Some of the causes of variation of haematological and biochemical tests

Short term	Long term
Posture	Age
Exercise	Sex
Circadian rhythm	Nationality/race
Food	Altitude
Smoking	Season, e.g. sunlight and vitamin D
Alcohol intake	
Medication	Obesity
Trauma/shock/surgery	Malnutrition
External environment, e.g. heat	Menstrual cycle
	Pregnancy

If a result is not consistent with the patient's clinical state or their suspected condition, repeat the test.

Certain blood biochemistry results need to be interpreted together with simultaneous urine biochemistry results, e.g. calcium excretion (see 'Urine tests' below).

If there is any doubt as to the appropriate requirements for a particular test, advice should be sought from the laboratory staff.

Table 1.6 presents the normal ranges of some of the more common biochemical blood analyses. Although these test results are presented quantitatively, they are usually interpreted qualitatively by pattern recognition. However, in certain cases the actual quantitative result can be used to modify or change treatment.

Fluids other than blood and urine can be subjected to biochemical analysis. For example, if the amylase level of fluid draining from the abdomen following pancreatic surgery is markedly higher than the serum amylase level there may be a pancreatic fistula.

Microbiology

Microbiological investigations can be applied to any body fluid, discharge, pus or culture swab, but the microbiological investigation of blood usually involves blood cultures together with serological tests and serum assays. Urine microbiology is considered on page 8.

Sputum, pus, surgical drainage fluid, bronchial lavage, cerebrospinal fluid and any organ discharge can be subjected to microscopy, culture and antibiotic sensitivity tests.

- **Gram staining** provides a quick and easy assessment of any fluid and may provide a presumptive diagnosis of any organism involved as well as demonstrating the presence or absence of inflammatory cells. In cases where more specific organisms are being sought, special techniques may be used such as:
- **Ziehl–Neelsen staining** for mycobacterium
- **calcofluor white wet preparations** for fungi
- **electron microscopy** for viruses
- **fluorescent antibody techniques** using specific monoclonal antibodies against the antigens of microbes such as herpes simplex and chlamydia

- **latex agglutination,** e.g. for capsular antigens from *Streptococcus pneumoniae*
- **gene probes** to detect specific gene sequences, e.g. for methicillin-resistant *Staphylococcus aureus* (MRSA).

Any organisms isolated can be tested for antibiotic sensitivity but you must provide adequate clinical

Table 1.6
Normal ranges for some of the commonly performed biochemical blood analyses

Sodium	130–145 mmol/L
Potassium	3.5–5.0 mmol/L
Chloride	96–106 mmol/L
Bicarbonate	20–30 mmol/L
Urea	2.0–8.0 mmol/L
Creatinine	50–120 μmol/L
Glucose	4–8 mmol/L
Calcium	2.02–2.66 mmol/L
Phosphate	0.8–1.6 mmol/L
Total protein	65–80 g/L
Albumin	30–50 g/L
Globulin	20–35 g/L
Bilirubin	2–14 μmol/L
Alkaline phosphatase	60–300 U/L
Alanine aminotransferase	10–30 U/L
Aspartate aminotransferase	10–35 U/L
γ-Glutamyl transpeptidase	5–50 U/L
Lactate dehydrogenase	
Amylase	36–128 IU/L
C-reactive protein	0–5 mg/L
Arterial blood gases	
pH	7.35–7.42
PaO_2	10.5–13.5 kPa
$PaCO_2$	4.5–6.0 kPa
Bicarbonate	20–30 mmol/L
Base excess	−3 to +3
Cholesterol	<5.0 mmol/L
Triglycerides	<2.0 mmol/L

information on the laboratory request form, especially whether the patient has received antibiotics in the recent past.

With the emergence of resistant strains, it is becoming increasingly important to know the susceptibility of an organism to particular antibiotics. This can be measured in mg/L of the antibiotic. Reports usually indicate whether a microbe is susceptible, or resistant to a variety of antibiotic agents. If requested, and clinically important, the **mean inhibitory concentration** (MIC) may be given. The techniques used for sensitivity testing include agar gel and liquid dilution tests, disc diffusion tests and the E test, which uses graded strips of antibiotics and can provide quantitative data.

Microscopy and Gram staining can yield results within minutes of the specimen reaching the laboratory. The results of preliminary culture may not be available for 24 hours or, for anaerobic cultures, 48 hours. Antibiotic sensitivity should be available within 24–48 hours.

Blood cultures should be undertaken in any situation in which bacteraemia or septicaemia is suspected. Strict guidelines should be followed if the maximum results are to be achieved. The following principles should be applied.

- The blood should be withdrawn through a new uncontaminated venepuncture site using an aseptic technique.
- A minimum of 20–30 mL of blood should be obtained as the microbe count may be as low as 1 microbe/mL.
- The blood should be divided and placed, as soon as possible, in an anaerobic and an aerobic culture bottle (10 mL to each bottle).
- As any bacteraemia can be transient and intermittent, three sets of both bottles should be taken over a 24-hour period and if possible during fever spikes.
- Whenever possible samples should be withdrawn before starting antibiotic therapy.
- If a fungal infection is suspected, advice should be obtained from the laboratory staff about any special techniques and incubation periods that may be required.

Many laboratories are now using automated blood culture machines, which often yield evidence of bacterial growth within 6–8 hours. Gram staining of the fluid in the positive bottles will often identify the microbe involved but culture and antibiotic sensitivity take at least 12–24 hours. You should be notified if the result is positive within 24 hours but the final result on negative cultures is not issued for 5–10 days.

Serology tests

Serological tests for detecting circulating antigens or antibodies are of value in situations when the causative organism may not be cultured or when organism growth and isolation prove difficult. This is particularly relevant for viral infections in conditions such as rheumatic heart disease, HIV and hepatitis. Other helpful tests include:

- enzyme-linked immunosorbent assays (ELISAs)
- latex agglutination
- fluorescent antibody techniques.

These tests may detect circulating antigens (e.g. hepatitis B, invasive candidiosis), antibodies (e.g. HIV) and, by using monoclonal antibodies, other specific microbial antigens. It is always wise to discuss the clinical situation with the laboratory staff to avoid inappropriate requests and to warn the laboratory of the specimen's impending arrival.

Serum assays may be used to monitor blood levels of aminoglycosides antibiotics, especially in those patients with suspect or deteriorating renal function. It may be advisable to monitor the blood levels of other antibiotics to demonstrate that adequate therapeutic levels are being achieved. For example, in cases of bacterial endocarditis it is advisable to maintain a blood level eight times the mean bactericidal concentration (MBC).

Tumour markers

Some clinical circumstances, such as the presence of an undiagnosed abdominal mass or swelling, indicate the need to search for serum tumour markers or other serum markers. Such markers vary in their nature and may be antigens, proteins, enzymes, hormones, autoantibodies and chemicals. Table 1.7 lists several serum markers and the diseases that their presence may indicate and which may also help in monitoring the effect of treatment.

Table 1.7
Serum markers

Carcinoembryonic antigen	Colorectal cancer
Alpha-fetoprotein	Hepatoma
	Testicular tumours
Lactate dehydrogenase	Testicular tumours
CA125	Ovarian cancer
CA19–9	Pancreatic cancer
Prostate-specific antigen	Prostatic cancer
Autoantibodies	Cirrhosis of the liver
Smooth muscle antibodies	Chronic active hepatitis
Anti-mitochondrial antibodies	Primary biliary cirrhosis
β-Human chorionic gonadotrophin	Pregnancy
	Testicular tumours
	Ovarian cancer
	Hydatidiform mole
Thyroglobulin	Thyroid cancer

URINE TESTS

As with blood tests, there are routine urine investigations and those that are more specific and only ordered when there is a clear indication based on clinical grounds. Specimens of urine are often contaminated so obtain a **mid-stream sample** whenever possible.

- Biochemistry
- Microscopy
- Microbiology

Biochemistry

Routine urinary biochemistry tests are no longer performed in a laboratory because **'dipstick' analysis** is easy to perform in the ward, outpatients and office. Chemosensitive dipstick analysis can indicate the presence of microscopic haematuria, multichemical dipstick analysis can reveal the presence of:

- glucose
- bilirubin
- ketones
- specific gravity/density
- blood
- pH
- protein
- urobilinogen
- leucocyte esterase (white cell test)
- nitrites (indicating infection).

The results of routine dipstick analysis and/or a patient's clinical history and examination may indicate the need for a specific laboratory biochemical analysis, e.g. the urinary sodium concentration and osmolarity may be informative in patients with oliguria.

Twenty-four-hour urinary collections may be needed for the measurement of:

- calcium excretion in hyperparathyroidism, and to exclude familial hypocalciuric hypercalcaemia (2.5–7.5 mmol)
- vanyllymandelic acid excretion (VMA) for phaeochromocytomas ($<35\,\mu$mol)
- 5-hydroxy-indole-acetic acid (5HIAA) for carcinoid syndrome (15–88 μmol)
- urinary amylase for acute pancreatitis (this may remain elevated longer than the serum amylase after an acute attack: see Chapter 17)
- myoglobin in the urine for muscle damage after a crush injury or muscle ischaemia
- protein content (0.05 g)
- sodium (up to 200 mmol)
- potassium (60–80 mmol)
- urea (410 mmol).

Microscopy

This is an essential investigation in any patient with a suspected urinary tract infection or with symptoms and signs suggestive of urinary tract disease. Microscopy may reveal:

- **red blood cells**: dysmorphic red cells and red cell casts may indicate glomerular bleeding caused by:
  - acute glomerulonephritis
  - systemic lupus erythematosis (SLE)
  - polyarteritis nodosa
  - Goodpasture's syndrome
  - Henoch–Schönlein purpura

■ **white blood cells**: which suggest infection
■ **organisms**: which should be identified by culture and sensitivities
■ **casts**: coarse granular casts often indicate parenchymal renal disease
■ **abnormal cells**: urinary cytology is invaluable in confirming transitional cell carcinomas within the urinary tract, especially when cystoscopy is negative (see below).

Culture

Whenever urinary dipstick analysis or the clinical picture suggests a urinary infection, then routine culture and sensitivities should be undertaken. Adequate information must be provided on the request form, especially whether the patient has received antibiotics in the recent past. Microscopy and Gram staining can yield results within minutes of the specimen reaching the laboratory. Any cultured microbial growth should be subjected to antibiotic sensitivity studies. Preliminary culture results may take 24 or even 48 hours if anaerobic organisms are present.

Catheter-related sepsis is often related to microbial colonization of an indwelling urinary catheter. In the past, the only way of distinguishing between true catheter colonization and clinically insignificant contamination was by removing the catheter and culturing the tip. An endoluminal brush technique, passing a nylon brush down the lumen of the catheter to its tip and then culturing the brush end, can avoid the unnecessary removal on non-colonized catheters.

CELL AND TISSUE PATHOLOGY INVESTIGATIONS

■ Cytology
■ Histology

The clinician must decide and the pathologist be told the purpose of any investigation including the clinical question that is being asked. This will not only determine the most appropriate specimen to send to the pathology laboratory, but also focus the pathologist's attention on the main clinical issue. Adequate clinical information is essential to help the pathologist interpret the relevance of any

information that can be gleaned from the examination of a cellular or tissue specimen. This approach reduces unnecessary investigations.

Cytology

Cytology is the study of cell morphology in tissue samples. It can be used to confirm malignancy or infection.

Although a cytological examination may provide a cellular diagnosis, it rarely provides information about the structure of a lesion. This limits its value, for example, in lymphadenopathy, where the structure of the node may be as important clinically as the cytological changes. Discussion with the pathologist about the appropriateness or otherwise of cytological examination as opposed to histological examination may save valuable time and resources.

Specimens for cytological examination may be obtained by the following methods:

■ **exfoliation**, from epithelium and endothelium, e.g.
  □ touch preparations, e.g. Paget's disease of the nipple
  □ scrapings, e.g. skin and cervical lesions
  □ brush sampling, e.g. during bronchoscopy and gastrointestinal (GI) and genitourinary (GU) tract endoscopy
■ **fine needle aspiration** from breast, thyroid, soft tissue masses (Fig 1.1)
  □ clinically guided
  □ radiologically guided by ultrasound, CT scanning and mammography
■ **from body fluids** such as ascitic, pleural, and cerebrospinal fluid, sputum, urine, discharges, fistula output.

Fluid samples have to be spun down and the deposit smeared on to a slide. Touch, brush and fine needle aspiration sample preparations can be immediately smeared on to slides and air-dried or placed into an appropriate transport medium and spun down later. It is wise to leave the slide preparation to the cytopathology laboratory staff, as the better the preparation the more accurate the interpretation. Standard techniques such as the Papanicolaou stain with or without haematoxylin/eosin or Giemsa are used for routine microscopy,

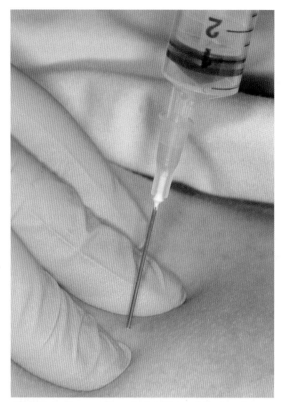

FIGURE 1.1 Fine needle aspiration biopsy. A fine needle aspiration being performed on a breast lump using a 21 gauge needle and a 10-mL syringe

but special stains may be more appropriate depending on the initial appearances, e.g. immunoperoxidase staining for melanoma or neuroendocrine tumours.

The reporting of the abnormalities seen in cytology specimens and their clinical interpretation should be unambiguous. For example, in the case of breast biopsies they should be reported as:

- inadequate   C1
- benign   C2
- probably benign   C3
- suspicious for malignancy   C4
- diagnostic of malignancy   C5

Similarly, thyroid specimens should be reported as:

- non-diagnostic – unsuitable for
  diagnosis   Thy1
- non-neoplastic, i.e. consistent with
  nodular goitre   Thy2
- all follicullar lesions   Thy3

(because it is usually possible to distinguish between follicular neoplasia and a colloid nodule, but histological confirmation of capsular or vascular invasion is needed to distinguish between a follicular carcinoma and a follicular adenoma: see Chapter 13)

- abnormal, suspicious of malignancy   Thy4
- diagnostic of malignancy – papillary,
  medullary, anaplastic   Thy5
- lymphocytes – it is usually impossible to distinguish cytologically between Hashimoto's thyroiditis and thyroid lymphoma.

These examples are given to stress the importance of a close liaison between the clinician and the cytopathologist working together within a multi-disciplinary team.

Histology

The histological examination of a piece of tissue allows the examination not only of its cells but also the nature and structure of the tissues around it.

Tissue samples can be obtained by means of:

- **needle biopsy**, e.g. with the Trucut needle (Fig 1.2) or core biopsy gun
- **punch biopsy**, e.g. of dermatological lesions
- **endoscopic biopsy**, e.g. at gastroscopy, bronchoscopy, colonoscopy
- **incisional biopsy**, the surgical removal of a piece of a lesion
- **excisional biopsy**, the surgical removal of an entire lesion
- **surgically excised operative specimens**: clips or ligatures should be attached to surgical specimens to identify their *in vivo* anatomical position.

Specimens should be cut up by the pathologist not by the surgeon, unless it is necessary for an intraoperative decision.

The samples the pathologist takes from the specimen are fixed, embedded in paraffin, sliced and then stained. Some of the commonly used stains are presented in Table 1.8.

The histological examination of an operative specimen can establish a formal diagnosis and confirm the adequacy of the therapeutic surgical procedure. In many cases an excision biopsy will both establish

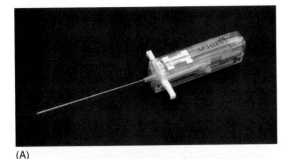

(A)

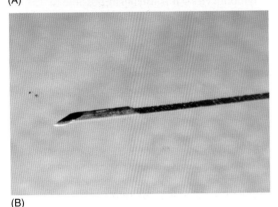

(B)

FIGURE 1.2   The Trucut biopsy technique. (A) A Trucut needle provides a core of tissue for histological analysis. It can be used freehand or under ultrasound guidance. (B) The needle

Table 1.8
Some tissue stains in common use

Haematoxylin and eosin (HE) – routine histological use

Papanicolaou with/without HE or Giemsa – cytology

Periodic acid–Schiff – glycogen

Van Giesen and Verhoff – collagen and elastin

Perl's ferric ferrocyanide – iron (haemosiderin)

Congo red – amyloid

the diagnosis and be adequate treatment, e.g. gastrointestinal polypectomy, skin lesions, many breast lumps and inflammatory conditions; but sometimes an excision biopsy will merely yield the diagnosis and indicate what further treatment is necessary.

Microscopical examination of surgically excised specimens of cancer will often provide information from which an accurate staging can be deduced. Staging of any condition, which may also require the radiological assessment of the presence of any distant metastatic spread, provides important data about prognosis and may also indicate whether further therapy is required.

Most staging systems are based on the **T**umour, **N**ode and **M**etastasis (**TNM**), classification adapted for each of the organs concerned, e.g. breast, colorectal (modified Dukes' staging), lung, ovary, bladder and prostate.

Special staging classifications also exist for conditions such as lymphoma and melanoma. These are discussed in greater detail in the relevant chapters.

Special histological techniques

Frozen section is used when a surgeon needs urgent pathological information during an operation. This can be provided by the histological examination of an instantly frozen piece of tissue taken during the operation. The need for this service is diminishing as a result of better preoperative diagnosis and as staging improves but when needed should be arranged before the operation in consultation with the pathologist.

Frozen section is indicated when there is a need:

- for intraoperative confirmation of the diagnosis, e.g. carcinoma of the pancreas when not confirmed preoperatively
- to confirm metastatic spread and guide the decision whether or not to proceed with the operation, e.g. lymph node biopsy in bronchial carcinoma
- to assess tissue margin status in cancer operations, e.g. skin cancer excisions and stapling gun tissue 'doughnuts' in oesophageal and rectal cancer
- to confirm the nature of excised tissue, e.g. parathyroidectomy.

Enzyme histochemistry is used for:

- leukaemia/lymphoma classification
- muscle biopsies.

Immunofluorescence (monoclonal antibody plus an indicator), e.g.

- immunoglobulin, complement, fibrinogen
- immunoenzyme – immunoperoxidase
  - □ membrane antigens
  - □ nuclear components
  - □ cytoplasmic components
  - □ infective agents – viral and bacterial
  - □ amyloid,

Electron microscopy (ultrastructure) is used for:

- childhood malignancies, e.g. neuroblastoma
- mesothelioma
- some viral diseases.

ENDOSCOPIC TECHNIQUES

Technological advances now allow the endoscopic examination of all body cavities and almost all organs, often in previously inaccessible areas. Endoscopes may be introduced through natural orifices into the stomach, colon, bronchi, urinary bladder and ureters, and nose, throat and larynx. Other forms of endoscopy require access via small incisions, e.g. laparoscopy, arthroscopy, thoracoscopy and mediastinoscopy. Endoscopic techniques may also be used during open operations, e.g. choledochoscopy during cholecystectomy.

Most of these techniques utilize flexible endoscopes that depend on flexible fibreoptics. Others such as routine laparoscopy, thoracoscopy, arthroscopy and sigmoidoscopy are usually performed with rigid scopes but use fibreoptic light sources.

In many cases an endoscopic technique can be used for both sampling and treatment, e.g.

- biopsy, polypectomy
- tumour ablation/fulguration/resection
- endoscopic papillotomy/sphincterotomy
- stenting
- insertion of feeding tubes (percutaneous endoscopic gastrostomy (PEG)) (Fig 1.3)
- arthroscopic menisectomy
- transurethral resection of bladder tumours and the prostate
- laparoscopic and thoracoscopic operations.

The application of endoscopic surgical procedures is expanding all the time. Their application to specific problems and diseases is described in the relevant chapters.

Rigid endoscopes consist of a central collection of rod lenses which transmit light from the image to an eyepiece and provide a magnified view of the organ being observed. Endoscopes are available with different angles of view. Laparoscopes are available with angles of view of 0, 30 and 45 degrees and cystoscopes and sinoscopes can have a viewing angle of up to 120 degrees. Surrounding the lens system is a sheath of fibreoptic glass fibres that transmit

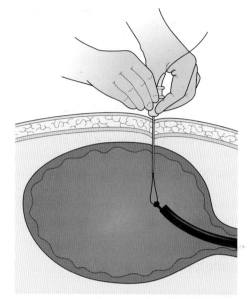

FIGURE 1.3 Percutaneous endoscopic gastrostomy (PEG). A thread attached to a PEG tube is inserted into the stomach percutaneously, then grasped via an endoscope so that the PEG tube can be pulled into the stomach

light from the light source to illuminate the cavity or organ under view.

Flexible endoscopes contain a bundle of flexible fibreoptic fibres that transmit the image either to an eyepiece or to a microchip video-camera from where the image is transmitted electronically to a television monitor/screen. Illumination is provided from an intense light source, and the light is transmitted via adjacent optical fibres included within the sheath of the scope. Certain endoscopes require the inside of the organ (e.g. stomach, colon) to be inflated to achieve a complete view. Others require fluid irrigation (e.g. urinary bladder, bile duct).

Most endoscopes have a working channel through which instruments can be passed such as biopsy forceps, diathermy snares, Dormia baskets, stents and balloon catheters. Most flexible endoscopes are controlled by rotating levers that allow the tip to be manipulated up and down, right and left. Additional manipulation can be achieved by rotating the whole scope, a manoeuvre which is particularly valuable during the insertion of a colonoscope and during endoscopic retrograde cholangiopancreatography (ERCP) (see below). Most endoscopes are end viewing except for the cannulating duodenoscope used for ERCP, which is side-viewing.

Oesophago-gastro-duodenoscopy

Flexible endoscopic examination of the oesophagus, stomach and duodenum using an end-viewing scope is now the examination of choice for most conditions affecting these organs. It allows accurate diagnosis of peptic ulceration, hiatus hernia, reflux oesophagitis, polyps, malignancy, strictures and oesophageal varices (see Chapter 18). The technique can be used therapeutically for stricture dilatation, tumour ablation (photodynamic and laser therapy), stenting of tumours, injection of varices and other haemostatic procedures. It can also be used to place feeding tubes.

Endoscopic retrograde cholangiopancreatography

This procedure requires the use of a side-viewing endoscope to facilitate cannulation of the ampulla of Vater and the bile and pancreatic ducts (which should be cannulated separately and selectively) for the injection of an X-ray contrast medium (see Chapter 18). If stones are found in the bile duct an endoscopic sphincterotomy can be performed using a diathermy sphincterotome and the stones removed with a balloon catheter or Dormia basket (Fig 1.4). If an obstructing tumour is encountered, a plastic stent or an expandable metal stent can be inserted. However, it is important to consider future treatment options before inserting a stent that may preclude further forms of treatment. Very occasionally, pancreatic duct stenting is used to treat chronic pancreatitis. The intrabiliary pressure can be measured with a fine manometry cannula in cases of suspected biliary dyskinesia.

Small bowel enteroscopy

This is a developing technique that uses a very long endoscope passed down into the small bowel with the assistance of peristalsis. It is not in routine use and is still being evaluated. It takes a considerable time to advance the scope down into the small bowel and, even then, very rarely provides a complete view of the bowel. It may be useful in patients with repeated undiagnosed GI bleeding.

Colonoscopy

Colonoscopy and flexible sigmoidoscopy can provide an excellent view of the whole colon following appropriate and adequate bowel preparation. In patients with a tortuous or rigid bowel, the full extent of the examination may be limited.

This investigation is, to a degree, operator dependent but experienced colonoscopists are usually able to reach the caecum and even enter the terminal ileum. Some endoscopists like to confirm this with an ileal biopsy. Colonoscopy also permits a range of treatment options such as diathermy snare polypectomy, 'hot biopsy' excision of small polyps, endscopic submucosal excision of sessile polyps (after elevation of the polyp by the submucosal injection of an adrenalin-containing fluid), balloon dilatation of strictures and stent insertion. It is the investigation of choice when looking for the source of bleeding such as angiodysplasia. Perforation of the bowel is a significant risk with all these procedures.

Laparoscopy

Diagnostic laparoscopy has been used for years by gynaecologists but its use has become increasingly popular with general surgeons over the last two decades. Open insertion (Hassan technique) has become increasingly utilized but the creation of an initial pneumoperitoneum by means of a Veress needle still remains popular with some surgeons. This latter technique requires the potentially hazardous blind introduction of both the Veress needle and the first trocar. To avoid serious damage both must be aimed away from the main retroperitoneal vessels – the inferior vena cava and the aorta.

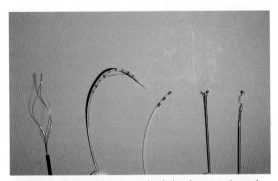

FIGURE 1.4 Endoscopic retrograde cholangiopancreatography (ERCP) instrumentation. Some of the instruments that can be used through an endoscope: a Dormia basket, a sphicterotome, a cannula, biopsy graspers and a biopsy brush

Although the majority of laparoscopic procedures are now therapeutic operations, diagnostic laparoscopy is still a valuable investigation for the staging of tumours, biopsy of peritoneal or liver metastases and the assessment of pelvic pathology, especially in young female patients with lower abdominal pain (see Chapter 17). Operative procedures are considered in the relevant chapters.

Cystoscopy

Rigid cystoscopy for diagnostic and some therapeutic procedures has been in use for many decades. The introduction of **flexible cystoscopes** has further expanded the investigative and therapeutic potential so that currently almost 90 per cent of urological procedures are performed endoscopically.

It is possible to obtain a safe and painless view of the whole of the lower urinary tract in both male and female patients within an hour or so of presentation, in the outpatient department, using local anaesthesia, and to take biopsies, resect small bladder tumours, visualize the upper urinary tracts radiologically, catheterize the ureters and insert or remove stents.

Formal transurethral endoscopic resection of large tumours and prostatectomy using diathermy loops, snares, knives or roller-balls still require general anaesthesia.

Small calibre **ureteroscopes** now make it possible to visualize the lumen of the ureter and the entire upper urinary tract and use laser lithotripsy, ultrasonic probes and fine basket catheters for the extraction of ureteric stones. When a retrograde approach is impossible or not appropriate, the antegrade puncture under radiological control allows direct nephroscopy and visualization of the proximal intrarenal collecting system. The use of techniques that fragment stones allows the removal of large calculi by this route.

Bronchoscopy

Fibreoptic bronchoscopy, which has almost completely replaced the rigid bronchoscope, provides an excellent view of the tracheobronchial tree. Insufflation is not required as the lumen is permanently open. The flexible bronchoscope can be passed transorally or transnasally and can be used for diagnosis and treatment. Some endoscopists still prefer to use a rigid instrument for the removal of foreign bodies and the endobronchial laser treatment of tumours, even though these procedures can now be satisfactorily performed with a flexible endoscope. Bronchoscopy is invaluable in evaluating the significance of symptoms such a haemoptysis, persistent cough and unexplained stridor. It is also useful for following up radiological abnormalities such as lung collapse, consolidation, lung masses and even diffuse interstitial lung disease. The therapeutic applications include biopsy, bronchial lavage to remove excessive secretions, laser therapy to resect or debulk endobronchial tumours, and the insertion of stents (see Chapter 14).

Bronchoscopy can be used to facilitate endotracheal intubation in patients who are difficult to intubate because of a retrosternal goitre or cervical spine immobility. Bleeding is a worrying complication as it can obscure the view and be difficult to treat because of the instrument's narrow suction channel. It is wise to obtain a clotting screen before subjecting a patient to a bronchoscopy.

Bronchoscopy may occasionally cause a minor deterioration of respiratory function, a slight fever or pneumonia. These problems require active treatment but are usually short lived.

Thoracoscopy

Thoracoscopy allows intrathoracic diagnostic and therapeutic procedures to be carried out without having to resort to open thoracotomy. It is performed through either a lateral or prone approach. The lateral approach provides a better view of the lungs while the prone approach gives a better view of the mediastinum and for performing operative procedures on the sympathetic chain. The procedure is facilitated by the anaesthetist using a double lumen endotracheal tube, which enables the lungs to be selectively collapsed. This means that insufflation is not an absolute requirement, but many thoracoscopists prefer to use a low pressure insufflation up to a maximum pressure of 5 mmHg. The technique allows direct pleural biopsies and lung biopsy. The potential use for operative procedures such as sympathectomy, splanchnicectomy, oesophageal myotomy and bullae resection is growing.

Major endoscopic surgical procedures such as oesophagectomy and pulmonary resection are still being evaluated and are discussed in the appropriate chapters.

Arthroscopy

Arthroscopy is now a routine part of the investigation of most joints but care must be undertaken in deep-seated and/or very small joints as damage may be caused both to adjacent neurovascular structures while entering the joint and to the articular structures within the joint. Arthroscopy provides an excellent view of any intra-articular disease process and, as with other endoscopic techniques, enables therapeutic procedures to be carried out.

Arthroscopes are rigid endoscopes usually with a 30-degree lens. The most commonly used instrument has a diameter of 4 mm. Smaller endoscopes are available for the more distal joints of the upper and lower limbs. Fluid irrigation is required to distend the joint, and a wide range of instruments such as probes, intra-articular scissors, graspers, basket forceps, bone burrs and cautery have been designed to facilitate surgical procedures such as:

- biopsy
- synovectomy
- chondroplasty
- removal of loose bodies
- meniscectomy
- ligament repairs
- treatment of osteochondritis dissecans
- drainage of septic arthritis
- removal of osteoarthritic debris.

Diagnostic arthroscopy and the above operative procedures are routinely carried out in the knee, ankle, shoulder, elbow and wrist. Hip arthroscopy is still under evaluation.

IMAGING TECHNIQUES

- Ultrasound (US)
- X-rays
- Computerized tomography (CT)
- Magnetic resonance imaging (MRI)
- Positron emission tomography (PET)
- Radionuclide scanning

Ultrasound

The Principles of US are as follows.

- Ultrasound scanning (Fig 1.5) depends upon the varying ability of different body tissues to absorb sound.
- When an ultrasonic wave strikes an interface between tissues with different acoustic impedance, some of the waves are reflected and can be detected by a receiver in line with the generator transmitting the waves.
- This echo can be displayed on an oscilloscope as a non-dimensional wave (an **A scan**) or if a sweeping beam is used, a two-dimensional black and white picture can be constructed (a **B scan**).
- The density of the image reflects the amplitude of the reflected wave and produces a picture with varying shades of grey (greyscale ultrasound).
- Ultrasound is non-invasive and carries no radiation risk and is therefore safe.
- Its spatial resolution depends upon the frequency of the exploring ultrasound wave. High frequency ultrasound can be used to monitor the progression of certain pathological processes, e.g. pancreatic cysts and arterial disease, as it can measure changes in size of less than 1mm

Ultrasound scanning can be used to direct biopsy needles.

Intraoperative, laparoscopic or endoluminal ultrasound scanning can be used to stage pancreatic cancer and reveal small hidden tumours.

Ultrasonic blood flow detection utilizes the Doppler principle. The change in the frequency of an ultrasound wave reflected from a moving red cell is directly related to the rate of movement of the cell.

Duplex scanning, which combines the production of an image with flow measurement, is achieved by using pulsed or continuous ultrasound waves and the Doppler principle. The rate and direction of flow can be colour coded.

X-rays

X-rays have been in clinical use since their discovery by Roentgen in 1895. They are presented to the

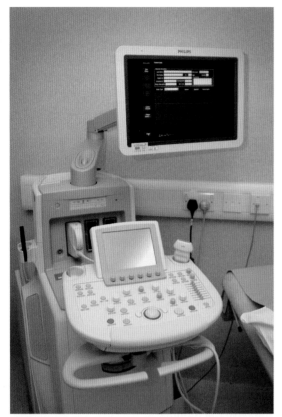

(A)

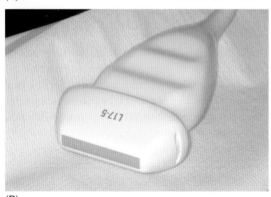

(B)

FIGURE 1.5 An ultrasound generator (A) and probe (B) are often used as the first-line investigation of several organs including the breast, neck, abdomen and scrotum

physician as a black and white image on a celluloid film or on a television screen.

Before attempting to interpret any X-ray, it is essential to establish the following facts by routinely asking these questions.

■ **On whom and when was the X-ray performed?**
   □ Is the patient name on the film the same as your patient's name?
   □ Is the film dated?
   □ Is it one of a series of films? Are the others available?

■ **What is the relationship between the position of the patient and the source of the X-rays?**
   There are three common X-ray views:
   □ posteroanterior view
   □ anteroposterior view
   □ lateral views (left or right)
   and three common patient positions:
   □ erect
   □ supine
   □ decubitus (lying on one side, right or left).

■ **Has a contrast medium been used?**
   □ Check its nature and purpose.
   □ Is a control film available?

The examination of any X-ray must be methodical and comprehensive. A quick glance and a spot diagnosis is a common cause of mistakes. Always begin with the sequence of questions described above before examining the details of the structures revealed on the X-ray film.

The questions you should memorize and always ask about a plain chest X-ray, a plain abdominal X-ray and X-rays of bones are set out in Revision panels 1–3.

Plain X-rays of the chest and abdomen should not be ordered automatically but should be undertaken with a specific diagnostic question in mind.

X-RAY INVESTIGATIONS USING RADIO-OPAQUE CONTRAST MEDIA

The barium meal

This investigation, which has been used to study the upper gastrointestinal tract for many years, has now been almost entirely replaced by gastroscopy.

The current universal contrast medium is *barium sulphate* dissolved in water.

The *water-soluble iodine-containing contrast media* (e.g. Gastrografin) are of value when a perforation or anastomotic leak is suspected. However, their use is contraindicated if there is any danger of pulmonary aspiration during swallowing and in dehydrated infants because of their high osmolarity and hygroscopic characteristics.

Double contrast techniques distend the stomach with air or carbon dioxide to increase mucosal definition. Air can be introduced directly into the stomach via a nasogastric tube, but more commonly the patient is given effervescent tablets (e.g. sodium bicarbonate, tartaric acid or calcium carbonate) which react with the gastric contents to produce carbon dioxide.

Buscopan 20 mg or *glucagon* 0.1–0.5 mg is sometimes given intravenously to relax the stomach or duodenal wall. For the opposite effect, intravenous *metoclopramide* (Maxolon) 20 mg may be given to increase peristalsis and speed the passage of barium.

The barium enema

Although this investigation has largely been superseded by endoscopy it is still needed when colonoscopy fails, usually because of a tortuous sigmoid colon or severe diverticular disease.

Adequate preliminary bowel preparation is essential, i.e. a low-residue diet for 48 hours followed by an aperient (e.g. Picolax) 24 hours prior to X-ray, and often by a pre-X-ray washout.

The contrast medium, a *25 per cent barium sulphate and water mixture*, is administered though a rectal catheter by gravity from a height of about 4 feet (120 cm). If double contrast films are required, air is introduced via the rectal tube once the barium has reached the splenic flexure.

Colonic spasm can be diminished by giving intravenous Buscopan (20 mg).

The biliary tract

Oral cholecystography and intravenous cholangiography have been superseded by ultrasound scanning and MRI scanning (see Chapter 18).

Endoscopic retrograde cholangiopancreatography

This method of displaying the biliary tree and pancreatic duct requires the introduction of a side-viewing duodenoscope into the second part of the duodenum, and cannulation of the ampulla of Vater by a highly skilled endoscopist. Although good views can be achieved of both the common bile duct and the pancreatic duct for purely diagnostic purposes, the endoscopic aspects of this investigation have almost been replaced by MRI scanning of the biliary and pancreatic ducts (MRCP). But the technique and approach of ERCP is invaluable for both stone retrieval and the stenting of malignant strictures.

Complications, especially after therapeutic manoeuvres, include acute pancreatitis (which can be fatal), perforation and bleeding.

Percutaneous transhepatic cholangiography

This investigation involves a percutaneous puncture of the liver and a dilated intrahepatic bile duct (often assisted by ultrasound scanning) followed by the injection of a radio-opaque contrast medium into the dilated intrahepatic system to outline the whole biliary tree. This approach to the bile ducts may also be used therapeutically to insert stents through malignant lesions.

Its complications include bleeding (it is essential to check the clotting screen before percutaneous transhepatic cholangiography (PTC)), cholangitis and biliary peritonitis.

The intraoperative cholangiogram

Direct cannulation of the cystic duct may be undertaken during both open and laparoscopic surgery.

X-rays are taken after injecting 3 mL, 6 mL and then 10 mL of 25 per cent Hypaque. Although this is usually watched with an image intensifier, it is important to obtain a hard copy for postoperative review and medico-legal reasons.

The biliary tree is considered normal if:

- the diameter of the duct is 10–12 mm or less
- there are no filling defects or strictures
- the intrahepatic biliary tree has a normal configuration
- the lower end of the common bile duct has a symmetrical taper end
- there is free flow of contrast medium into the duodenum.

The value of post-exploratory on-table 'T'-tube cholangiography is limited if the contrast medium fails to pass into the duodenum – something that often follows manipulation of the lower end of the duct. Sphincter spasm can be diminished by giving intravenous Buscopan or glucagon.

If the bile duct has been explored and a T-tube inserted, a T-tube cholangiogram should be obtained at the end of the operation and on subsequent days to ensure that there are no remaining stones.

Intravenous urogram

The intravenous urogram is used to display the anatomy of the urine-collecting system. It relies on the ability of the kidneys to excrete the contrast medium, so will fail if renal function is depressed.

After 24 hours of fluid restriction, a plain abdominal film is taken. The patient is then given 20–40 mL of contrast medium intravenously.

The contrast media in common use include:

- Conray (meglumine iothalamate)
- Hypaque (sodium diatrizoate)
- Renografin (methylglucamine diatrizoate).

A compression band placed just above the symphysis pubis may be used to hold the contrast in the kidneys and give clearer definition of the upper renal tracts. This technique should not be used in cases of urinary tract obstruction, calculi, impaired renal function or when an aortic aneurysm is present.

Films are taken 5 and 15 minutes after the injection, then after the compression is released, and then up to 2 hours or more later if there is an element of hold-up. Tomography may be valuable in delineating renal pathology.

ULTRASOUND AND X-RAY INVESTIGATIONS OF THE BLOOD VESSELS

Duplex scan

This technique combines B-mode scanning with information about the rate of blood flow derived using the Doppler principle. It superimposes information about blood flow velocity at a specific site on a real-time B-mode image. In a blood vessel the blood moves at different velocities depending on its position within the vessel (centre or side) and whether or not there is turbulence. In a normal vessel the range of velocities is narrow, whereas a stenosis produces a wide range of velocities, the maximum velocity being where the blood flows through the

centre of a stenotic segment. In the printed image the velocity is colour coded (see Chapter 11).

Arteriography

Detailed X-ray images of the arteries are obtained after the direct injection of an X-ray contrast medium.

The contrast media in common use include:

- Hypaque (sodium diatrizoate)
- Urografin (mixture of sodium and methylglucamine diatrizoate)
- Angiografin (meglumine amidotrizoate)
- Conray (meglumine iothalamate)
- Triosil (meglumine metrizoate)
- Renografin (methylglucamine diatrizoate).

Arteries are punctured using the **Seldinger technique**. The artery is first punctured with a hollow needle. A guide wire is then passed through the needle and then a catheter is passed over the guide wire. The position of the catheter can be adjusted for distal (to the puncture site) or proximal injections. Selective vessel catheterization is possible using preshaped radio-opaque catheters.

The contrast medium is injected as quickly as possible and a series of films taken using an automatic film changer.

Digital subtraction techniques after either venous or arterial injection are now in common use.

With digital enhancement, new catheters and improving technology, excellent quality images of the branches of the aorta can be achieved by free flush injections within the aorta or even injections into the large central veins (**intravenous digitally enhanced arteriography**).

CT angiography provides good images of blood vessels after the intravenous contrast.

Phlebography

Most phlebograms are performed to delineate the veins of the lower limbs and to detect deep vein thrombosis.

The procedure begins by placing narrow inflatable cuffs around the ankle and just below the knee but not inflated. A butterfly needle is inserted into a vein on the foot, a procedure made easier with the lower leg dependent. The cuffs are then inflated to 80 mmHg to occlude the superficial veins, and up to 50 mL of a low osmolar contrast medium, such as Niopam 300, is injected.

The legs are screened during the injection and anteroposterior (AP), internal and external rotation films taken. Good views should be obtained of the deep veins and any incompetent perforators.

When the below-knee cuffs are released good images can be obtained of the femoral and iliac veins and vena cava.

MR venography is becoming popular and can provide good images of the veins.

Lymphangiography

Lymphangiograpy is no longer used to detect metastases or primary disease in lymph glands but is an important diagnostic investigation in the management of complex cases of lymphoedema.

A 0.5-mL aliquot of 2.5 per cent patent blue violet dye is injected into the subcutaneous tissues of the toe web spaces to colour the lymph in the collecting lymphatics and make them visible.

A transverse incision is made on the dorsum of the foot, under local anaesthetic, to expose a suitable lymphatic vessel. A very fine needle is introduced into the vessel and an oily medium such as ultrafluid Lipiodol, at 7 mL/hour is infused using a special pump. No more than 10 mL of Lipiodol should be injected into each limb. Greater volumes will reach the lungs via the thoracic duct and may cause pulmonary oil embolism.

A water-soluble contrast medium should not be used because it diffuses out through the walls of the lymphatics.

OTHER SCANNING TECHNIQUES
Computerized tomography scanning

The principles behind CT scanning (Fig 1.6) are as follows.

- The patient is placed in the centre of a cluster of X-ray tubes that rotate around them.
- A computer integrates the multiple X-ray images to produce a series of three-dimensional images.
- The images are usually reconstructed in an axial plane.
- More recent helical/spiral CT scanning involves the patient being moved through the gantry

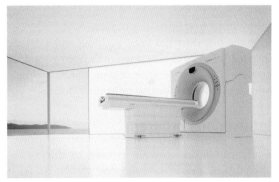

FIGURE 1.6   A computerized tomography scanner. (Image courtesy of Siemens)

while the X-ray tube rotates continuously following a helical path.
- A CT image is a matrix of pixels each having a greyscale intensity representing the X-ray attenuation value of the tissues, e.g.
  - fat and gas have negative attenuation values and are black
  - bone has a high attenuation value and is white
  - intravenous contrast medium can artificially increase local attenuation.
- The dose of irradiation is high and where possible CT scanning should be avoided in younger patients and women of childbearing age.
- Artefacts can be produced by barium, metallic clips and stents.

Magnetic resonance image scanning

The principles of MRI scanning (Fig 1.7) are as follows.

- The patient is placed in a powerful magnetic field in which all the protons of the abundant hydrogen nuclei in the body become aligned.
- Pulsed frequency radiowaves are transmitted into the patient to cause the alignment of the protons to change.
- When the radiowaves are turned off the protons return to their neutral position, emitting their own radiowave signals, which are picked up by a receiver coil. These signals are used to generate an image which depends not only on the proton density but on the way the protons resonate in their local environment.

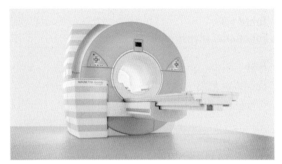

FIGURE 1.7 A magnetic resonance imaging scanner. (Image courtesy of Siemens)

- The image comprises an array of pixels, as in CT scanning, but there is greater contrast resolution with MRI than with CT and images can be acquired not only in the axial plane but in the coronal, sagittal or oblique planes.
- The natural contrast of MRI can be increased with contrast agents such as intravenous chelated gadolinium compounds, e.g. Gd-DTPA (diethylene-triaminepenta-acetate).
- MRI does not use any ionizing radiation and is therefore safe.
- MRI should be avoided in any patients with metal clips, stents, pacemakers, cochlear implants and some prosthetic heart valves.
- MRI scanning in the form of MRCP has almost replaced diagnostic ERCP (see above).

Positron emission tomography

The principles of PET scanning are as follows.

- A positron is a positively charged electron which is emitted by a decaying short-lived radioactive tracer isotope.
- The isotope is incorporated into a metabolically active molecule such as *fluorodeoxyglucose* (FDG) which is injected intravenously.
- When the molecule becomes concentrated in an area of interest it emits positrons that travel up to a few millimetres and then collide with an electron producing a couple of 'annihilation (gamma) photons' that are detected by a scintillation counter in the scanner.
- A PET scan can reveal a cancer, the stage of a cancer and demonstrate if chemotherapy is working.

Radionuclide scanning

The principles behind radionuclide scanning are as follows.

- Radionuclide imaging is based on the radioactive auto-emissions of a quantity of radioactive material after it has been administered to the patient.
- The radioactive material is administered as a radiopharmaceutical agent that has been chosen to follow a specific metabolic pathway, e.g. radio-iodine and thyroid uptake.
- Scintillation scans can demonstrate the outline of an organ and assess the extent to which it is functioning by means of indicating areas of abnormally low or abnormally high uptake.
- Imaging depends upon the measurement of the quantity of g-photons emitted from sites of radioactivity. This is done with a gamma-camera with four fundamental processes:
  - □ collimation (a multichannelling device to allow spatial resolution)
  - □ scintillation detection
  - □ electronic signal processing
  - □ display of information.

The following forms of radionuclide scanning are in common use.

Liver

- ^{99m}Tc-labelled sulphur colloid for reticuloendothelial scanning
- ^{75}Se-labelled methionine in liver cell tumours
- ^{67}Ga citrate for liver abscesses or tumour location
- ^{111}Indium-labelled white blood cells for foci of infection
- ^{99m}Tc-labelled butyl-imino-diacetic acid (BIDA) for excretion

Small bowel

- ^{99m}Tc pertechnetate for Meckel's diverticulum
- ^{51}Cr-labelled red blood cells for assessing blood loss
- ^{57}Co-labelled vitamin B12 for the Schilling test

Thyroid

- ^{131}I to search for metastases from differentiated thyroid carcinoma and for therapy

Parathyroid

▨ ^{201}Tl thallous chloride/^{99m}Tc pertechnetate subtraction scan

Adrenal glands

▨ ^{75}Se 6-selenomethylnorcholesterol for the cortex
▨ ^{123}I or ^{131}I meta-iodobenzylguanidine (m-IBG) for the medulla

Kidneys

▨ ^{99m}Tc-labelled DTPA
▨ ^{99m}Tc-labelled dimercaptosuccinic acid (DMSA)

Lungs

▨ Ventilation/perfusion scanning for pulmonary embolism
▨ ^{99m}Tc-labelled microaggregates of albumin for perfusion
▨ ^{81m}Kr gas for ventilation studies (xenon can be used)

Bone

▨ ^{99m}Tc-labelled hydroxymethylene diphosphonate (HDP)

Lymphatics

▨ ^{99m}Tc-labelled Rhenium sulphur colloid.

FUNCTIONAL INVESTIGATIONS

These form a very heterogeneous group of investigations mostly undertaken in a surgical physiology laboratory. They are not easy to classify and a comprehensive review of them all is not practical. More detailed coverage of some of these investigations, their indications and value as they relate to the investigation and treatment of specific conditions will appear in the appropriate chapters.

A summary of some of the more valuable functional investigations and their indications is presented in Table 1.9 with the intention of providing an insight as to the wide variety of functional investigations that are available. Discussion with the physiology laboratory staff is essential before ordering any of these investigations.

Table 1.9
Functional investigations

Test	Indications
Secretion tests	
Acid secretion	Recurrent peptic ulceration (not commonly performed)
Pancreatic secretion	Chronic pancreatitis or other pancreatic conditions
Breath tests	
^{13}C or ^{14}C urea test	Presence of *Helicobacter pylori*
Manometry	
Oesophageal	Oesophageal dysmotility
Biliary	Sphincter of Oddi dysfunction
Anal	Hirschsprung's disease
	Anal incontinence
Urethral	Bladder neck dysfunction
pH monitoring	
24-hour ambulatory	Gastro-oesophageal reflux
Transit studies	
Oesophagus	Oesophageal dysmotility
Stomach	Disordered gastric emptying
Bowel	Slow transit constipation
Urodynamics	
Uroflowmetry	Prostatism
Cystometry	Detrusor instability
Pressure/flow studies	Urinary obstruction and incontinance
Electrophysiology	
Anal	Problems with defaecation
Urological	Problems with micturition
Nerve conduction	Painful hand (carpal tunnel syndrome)

2

Principles and methods of management

John Black

Doctors with the qualifications that entitle them to be called 'surgeons' manage a wide variety of diseases that have one common feature – they could be treated by a physical manual method – a surgical operation. In fact, the majority of patients seen by surgeons are not advised to have an operation, and 'surgical' treatment now includes a multitude of methods or techniques.

The management of surgical patients can be divided into five categories:

- none (masterly inactivity)
- modification of lifestyle
- diet
- drugs
- interventions.

Surgical patients require support to help them withstand the effects of their disease and to give them the best chance of obtaining a successful outcome from any surgical intervention.

NO TREATMENT (MASTERLY INACTIVITY)

Many patients do not require treatment if:

- Their problem/disease is insignificant and will not interfere with their present or future health (e.g. a harmless skin lesion such as a Campbell de Morgan spot needs no treatment).
- The natural history of the condition is that it will resolve spontaneously without any interference or risk of complications (e.g. a hydrocele in a neonate).
- The risk of treatment is greater than the risks associated with the disease or its complications (e.g. a small direct inguinal hernia in a frail elderly man can usually be ignored).

Note that when you advise that no treatment is necessary, it is vital to reassure the patient who may be surprised, disappointed or even aggrieved at your opinion.

MODIFICATION OF LIFESTYLE

Some diseases are a consequence of the patient's lifestyle and are best managed by appropriate lifestyle modification. A good example is the role of smoking in peripheral vascular disease. Many of those suffering from mild intermittent claudication have a good chance of losing their symptoms if they stop smoking and lose weight.

On other occasions when even though the illness is not caused directly by the patient's lifestyle their symptoms may be alleviated by a different approach to life. Mild osteoarthritis of a knee joint might only be symptomatic with certain activity such as ski-ing. Giving up the triggering factor might be all that is needed to manage the problem, even in the long term.

DIET

Diet may be a specific treatment for some surgical conditions, e.g. increasing the intake of fibre for diverticular disease.

Diet may be part of treatment, such as a low-fat regimen to reduce the symptoms of gall stones prior to definitive surgery or to reduce symptoms in a patient in whom surgery is not appropriate.

Maintenance of nutrition is an important part of the support of all surgical patients especially those with temporary or permanent intestinal failure and who cannot be fed via the gut.

DRUGS

Drugs are used very frequently in the management of surgical conditions. Their indications, employment and complications are described in detail in the relevant subsequent chapters.

Drug treatment may be:

- **therapeutic**, i.e. the use of a specific drug to treat a specific disease, e.g. triple therapy to eradicate peptic ulcer disease, or
- **prophylactic**, to prevent disease. This may be *long term*, e.g. antibiotics given to prevent bacterial endocarditis in patients with prosthetic heart valves, or given on a *one-off single course* basis, e.g. the single peri-operative dose of an antibiotic given to reduce the incidence of postoperative infection, and be administered by various routes as discussed below.

Topical

The drug/agent is applied directly to the diseased area by means of a cream, ointment, or spray.

Local

A drug can be introduced into a body cavity if when given by any other route it would not penetrate into the cavity and reach an effective concentration. High concentrations can be achieved by intracavity injections with doses that would be toxic if given systemically (e.g. the injection of a steroid into an arthritic joint)

Enteral

- By mouth – as a liquid, tablet or capsule. Drugs that irritate the stomach can be coated or enclosed in a capsule to delay their absorption until they reach the small bowel.
- Per rectum – by suppository or enema.

Systemic

A drug can be introduced by intramuscular or intravenous injection. Systemic administration is necessary if:

- the drug is not absorbed, or inadequately absorbed from the gut
- the drug is degraded by gastric acid
- there is no gut available. (The patient may be unable to swallow or the gut may be diseased or absent.)

- high concentrations are needed immediately, as with anaesthetic agents.

INTERVENTIONS

The methods of applying the wide variety of treatment procedures available for patients with surgical disease may be divided into six categories; some overlap each other and many are often combined together:

- general medical care
- antitumour medication
- radiotherapy
- image-guided interventions
- endoscopic interventions
- surgical interventions.

GENERAL MEDICAL CARE

General medical interventions encompass a wide variety of treatments administered by surgeons, physicians and a wide range of the professions allied to medicine, usually supportive but sometimes definitive. For example, physiotherapy, which may provide specific curative treatment for postoperative atelectasis, may also help build muscle power and remove the need for surgery on an unstable knee.

Palliative care

Despite using all the surgical and oncological treatments available there will always be patients whose disease, usually cancer, is either incurable on presentation, fails to respond to treatment, or relapses after apparently curative treatment. The specialty of palliative care medicine has developed to manage these patients and also many other patients with incurable symptoms from non-malignant diseases.

The principles of palliative care are listed below.

- Always be truthful and open with the patient and their relatives and persuade the patient and their family to be similarly truthful with you.
- Treat your patient's disease to the best of your ability. Use pharmacological and oncological measures and occasionally surgical techniques to relieve symptoms.
- Relieve pain, using every technique available.
- Aim to obtain for your patient as normal a life as possible.

The 'mercy killing' fallacy There is a misconception among the general public and the media that palliation by giving massive doses of analgesics with sedative side-effects shortens life and in some way 'mercy kills' the patient. Nothing could be further from the truth. All experienced clinicians have seen patients with incurable cancer in a pitiable condition caused by severe symptoms, begging for death. But, if their symptoms can be relieved without harmful side-effects, something that may require massive doses of drugs, their wellbeing may be transformed, they may begin to feel hungry, start to take an interest in life again, and live longer.

Unfortunately, the doses needed to relieve severe symptoms may have side-effects such as respiratory depression, which, in a poorly nourished or immuno-deficient patient, may precipitate the onset of a fatal pneumonia. Before starting such palliative treatment the clinician must discuss the balance between its advantages and its risks with the patient, their family and nursing colleagues.

ANTITUMOUR MEDICATION

The wide use of drugs in the treatment of surgical disease is mentioned above, but of particular relevance to the surgeon and mentioned here as a special form of intervention are the drugs given as an adjunct to, or sometimes for, the primary treatment of malignant disease. These are usually defined as *oncological* treatments because they are targeted specifically at malignant tumours. The systemic side-effects and potential dangers can be as great as those associated with surgical procedures. There should be no doubt that most oncology and chemotherapeutic treatments are major interventions.

Oncological treatments may be:

- **curative**, where it is hoped to achieve cure
- **adjunctive**, where the medication is given in addition to surgery, usually afterwards (Treatment given before a definitive procedure is referred to as **neo-adjunctive**.)
- **palliative**, to prolong life or relieve symptoms when a cure cannot be achieved

Oncology treatments fall into four main categories: chemotherapy, hormone manipulation, immunotherapy and radiotherapy.

Chemotherapy

Cancer chemotherapy is the use of cytotoxic agents to treat malignant tumours. The drugs work by inhibiting cell division, and, like radiotherapy, work better on cells that are dividing rapidly. The drugs must be delivered to the malignant cells, and this requires that the cells have an adequate circulation. Large tumours tend to have necrotic centres, and so are best treated by surgery. The most effective role of chemotherapy is therefore to treat small volume tumours, and so in the surgical setting it is usually used as adjunctive treatment.

Chemotherapy was introduced after it was accidentally observed during the 1914–1918 Great War that horses which waded through mud soaked in mustard gas lost hair from the areas exposed to the toxic agent. It was reasoned that if mustard gas could stop hair growing on horses it might stop the growth of tumours. Such an effect was subsequently confirmed, and after considerable refinement modern cancer chemotherapy resulted.

There are many cytotoxic drugs available, with new ones appearing regularly. Each attacks different parts of the mitotic cycle. It has been found that combinations of drugs are significantly more effective than single agents. Their use is described in more detail in the relevant chapters.

The organs particularly sensitive to chemotherapeutic drugs are the gut and the bone marrow. Side-effects are usual and significant (Table 2.1).

The aim of treatment is to cause maximum damage to the cancerous cells and minimize the adverse effects on adjacent normal cells and the patient as a whole. The total dosage must therefore be strictly controlled and given in carefully timed cycles to allow the bone marrow time to recover between each dose. As most of these drugs have to be given intravenously it is customary to insert an indwelling, subcutaneously tunnelled, non-irritant catheter into a neck vein, such as the widely used Hickman catheter.

Hormone manipulation

Two of the solid cancers commonly treated by surgeons are usually hormone sensitive: carcinoma of the breast, which is often sensitive to oestrogen and progesterone, and carcinoma of the prostate, which may be sensitive to androgens.

Table 2.1
Side-effects of chemotherapy for cancer

Bone marrow damage leading to immunosuppression (this may be life-threatening from overwhelming infection)

Nausea and vomiting (a direct effect on the vomiting centre)

Hair loss, usually temporary (after recovery the hair is of different character, often curly)

Sterility, usually temporary (caused by toxic effects on the ovarian and testicular germ cells)

Organ damage specific to individual agents and organs (e.g. cardiotoxicity)

Chemotherapy-induced lymphoma (a late effect)

There are drugs available that eliminate or block the effect of the hormones that stimulate these tumours. This form of treatment is discussed in Chapters 15 and 19.

Immunotherapy

The purpose of cancer immunotherapy is to stimulate the patient's own immune system to kill the cancer cells by attacking their surface antigens. This can be done *actively* with a vaccine that stimulates the immune system to produce antibodies against the malignant cells, or *passively* by giving synthetic monoclonal antibodies.

Many of these forms of treatment are, to date, largely experimental, but two monoclonal antibodies are in clinical use:

▩ bevacizumab, for advanced colon cancer
▩ trastuzumab (Herceptin), for HER2 positive breast carcinoma.

RADIOTHERAPY

Radiotherapy is the application of ionizing radiation to kill malignant cells. It works by damaging the cells' DNA. Unfortunately, oxygen is needed for its maximum effect so the hypoxic cells in the centre of a tumour, or in a necrotic area, are relatively resistant. This means that radiotherapy is often more effective on small and rapidly growing cancers. Adding oxygen in a hyperbaric chamber is logical, but difficult.

Tissues vary widely in their susceptibility to radiotherapy. The most sensitive are those with the most rapid turnover of cells – the bone marrow and the mucosa of the gastrointestinal tract.

Death from massive accidental irradiation is usually caused by pancytopenia and intestinal failure.

Radiotherapy may be administered by:

▩ **external beam radiation**, which employs high energy X-rays generated in a linear accelerator
▩ **brachytherapy**, which is local treatment given by insertion of a radioactive substance into or near to the tumour
▩ **radioisotope therapy**, for tumour cells that assimilate a particular isotope. The best example of this is the use of 131-iodine in the treatment of follicular carcinoma of the thyroid (see Chapter 13).

External beam radiotherapy

This is aimed at the tumour and sometimes its field of lymphatic drainage but unavoidably irradiates normal surrounding tissue. To compensate for variable patient and physical factors between treatments and allow any irradiated surrounding normal tissue to recover, the dose is fractionated (given in multiple sessions). The patient is placed in the same position, using a variety of supports and moulds, for each session of treatment. To assist with this the skin may be marked with small tattoos. To minimize the risk of damage to adjacent normal tissue the angle of delivery is varied, with the tumour always at the intersecting point of the different angles. This is the same principle used with tomography.

Brachytherapy

This is the (usually temporary) insertion of radioactive material into or close to a tumour. The radioactive material may be placed in:

▩ an external mould, for superficial lesions on the skin
▩ wires, inserted with image guidance, for interstitial treatment
▩ seeds for intracavity brachytherapy. This is principally used for gynaecological malignancies.

Table 2.2
Side-effects of radiotherapy

Damage to skin – an initial severe sun-burn effect and long-term pigmentation, capillary dilatation and loss of sweating

Rarely necrosis and ulceration can develop

Damage to epithelial surfaces – sometimes severe in the upper respiratory tract and bowel

Swelling and oedema of tissues adjacent to the tumour

Damage to other organs

- the ovaries during pelvic radiation
- brachial plexus when treating axillary lymph nodes
- the heart when treating the breast and chest wall
- salivary glands when irradiating the neck
- late radiation-induced malignant tumours in radiated fields

Side-effects of radiotherapy

Treatment is painless. Low or moderate doses have little or no side-effects, but side-effects are common with high doses (Table 2.2).

Each area of the body has a maximum dose that it can tolerate. This means that radiotherapy can only rarely be repeated to the same area.

IMAGE-GUIDED INTERVENTIONS

Image-guided interventions are used with increasing frequency as techniques and technology improve. Team working between radiologists and surgeons is essential. All image-guided interventions need the following.

- **A method of imaging**. This can be
  - optical (light)
  - X-rays
  - ultrasound
  - CT (computerized tomography)
  - MRI (magnetic resonance imaging)
  - PET (positron emission tomography).
- **A real-time display** for the operator(s).

- **Three-dimensional** definition of the target, known as stereotaxis, first used 100 years ago for studies of the animal brain.
- **A treatment method/technique**, of which there are very many including:
  - insertion of a drainage tube – as in dealing with an abdominal abscess
  - placement of biopsy needles or forceps
  - placement of a balloon – as used in angioplasty
  - catheter embolization – as used to reduce the bulk of a renal carcinoma
  - stenting – the insertion of a prosthetic rigid tube through a stenosis to maintain patency, or to replace an abnormally dilated organ to prevent rupture. The technique is widely used for coronary artery occlusions and may be combined with the local administration of a drug by using eluting stents, which release appropriate agents on a long-term basis.
  - external acoustic pulsation – used to fragment urinary tract calculi in the technique of extracorporeal shock wave lithotripsy (ESWL)
  - radioactivity – as in brachytherapy
  - laser and cryotherapy – as used to ablate liver metastases.

ENDOSCOPIC INTERVENTIONS

Endoscopic procedures are used to treat those disease processes that can be reached with the appropriate instruments inserted through natural orifices. These instruments may be *rigid*, using a system of lenses, or *flexible*, using fibreoptics.

The major advantage of flexible instruments is that the patient rarely requires the general or regional anaesthetic sedation which rigid instruments usually need. The range of procedures possible with flexible instruments is limited when compared with rigid instruments, but technical ingenuity is closing this gap.

A very wide range of procedures may be performed, using either direct vision through a telescope, or increasingly these days by using a television monitor. The television camera may be attached to a telescope, or it may be incorporated into the tip of the endoscope. Therapeutic uses include:

- dilatation – for oesophageal and urethral strictures

- destruction – the use of diathermy or laser to destroy colonic polyps or obliterate tumours of the oesophagus
- resection – transurethral resection of the prostate or bladder tumours
- extraction – removal of foreign bodies and calculi
- sclerotherapy – where a sclerosing agent is injected into or around a lesion to obliterate it and stop bleeding. This technique is used for bleeding peptic ulcers and oesophageal varices
- injection of foam to improve valve function.

SURGICAL INTERVENTIONS

Surgical procedures are the surgeon's *raison d'être*, and their indications, use and complications are described in subsequent chapters.

There are two main methods of carrying out surgery.

Traditional open surgery

An incision is made in the skin to expose the abnormality so that it can be examined, dissected out, removed or bypassed. The whole procedure is performed manually under direct vision.

Minimal access surgery

Minimal access surgery requires a cavity in which to operate. This may be a natural cavity or one created artificially as in extraperitoneal renal surgery. A number of small (5–10 mm) skin incisions are required. A telescope is inserted and the surgeon sees and works via a television picture on a screen using long thin instruments. Various instruments and telescopes have been available for many years, but a breakthrough came in the 1980s with the invention of small colour-accurate television cameras. Previously, because the surgeon had to hold a telescope to one eye, he had only one hand available to manoeuvre the instruments. Once the operative field could be displayed on a television monitor, both hands, and those of the assistants, could be used. Indeed the view and access is usually better than with open surgery as it does not depend on the size of the entry wound. This is a particular advantage in the fat patient.

Thoracoscopy This is used in the staging of lung cancer, pleurodesis and increasingly for pulmonary surgery. The sympathetic chain can be destroyed through a thoroscope and the oesophagus mobilized.

Laparoscopy can be used to perform virtually every abdominal operation. Cholecystectomy is now rarely performed by open surgery and the use of laparoscopic techniques for hernia repair, appendicectomy and colorectal resections is steadily increasing.

Arthroscopy is now the routine approach for most procedures on the knee and other joints.

Endovascular minimally invasive surgery is now being used to repair cardiac valves and treat peripheral vascular problems.

Many percutaneous techniques are being developed which gain access through spaces **artificially created** between subcutaneous planes, e.g. for procedures such as sentinel axillary lymph node biopsy.

Note that **natural orifice transluminal endoscopic surgery** is a refinement of abdominal laparoscopic surgery. The instruments are inserted through a natural orifice and entry to the peritoneal cavity obtained by puncture of the wall of the organ entered. There are therefore no external scars. Three routes of entry are available:

- the mouth, puncturing the wall of the stomach
- the vagina, entering through a fornix
- the anus, with access though the colon.

Sophisticated, largely flexible instruments are required, and special techniques needed for the safe closure of the puncture wound in the wall of the organ of entry. These techniques are experimental and it is impossible to predict how they will develop.

The advantages and disadvantages of minimal access surgery are set out in Table 2.3.

PREOPERATIVE ASSESSMENT OF THE SURGICAL PATIENT

A full medical and drug history must be taken from all patients before surgery, except in dire emergency. The purpose is to alert the anaesthetist and surgeon to any problems likely to arise from concomitant medical illness or treatment. Particular issues arise if there is a history of the following.

Table 2.3
Advantages and disadvantages of minimal access surgery

Advantages of minimal access surgery	Disadvantages of minimal access surgery
Less trauma on the way to the target organ	Specific complications in gaining access such as those with the induction of pneumoperitoneum
Less postoperative pain	May take longer with consequent increased risk of certain complications
Better appearance with no big scar	
More rapid recovery	Theoretically higher risk, e.g. converts hernia repair into an abdominal operation
Improved access in many cases	
Technically easier for many procedures, e.g. appendectomy	May unjustifiably extend the indications for surgery if seen as a lesser procedure
May be used in the less fit patient because of lower risk	Requires equipment and facilities
Reduced blood contamination of theatre staff so less risk of blood-borne virus infections	

Diabetes

Ideally this should be controlled before admission. In general, no precautions are necessary if the condition is diet controlled but those on oral hypoglycaemic drugs should discontinue them and be given insulin if required.

Insulin-dependent diabetics should not be on long-acting preparations.

The complication to be avoided at all costs is hypoglycaemia and its associated unconsciousness, which may be fatal. This is prevented by giving intravenous glucose, and erring on the side of a high rather than a low blood sugar.

Myocardial infarction

If an operation is performed shortly after a patient has had a myocardial infarct there is a significant chance of a further infarct, which is quite likely to be fatal. This risk is greatest shortly after the original infarct, but persists for at least 6 months. *Elective surgery is thus contraindicated within 6 months of a proven myocardial infarction.* Unavoidable essential emergency surgery earlier than this carries an added risk.

Obesity

Obesity increases the incidence of almost every postoperative complication. Patients frequently lack insight

into this effect of their obesity and wrongly believe they are being denied surgery for unjustifiable reasons.

Coagulopathy

Coagulopathy, particularly that associated with obstructive jaundice, should be corrected, usually with vitamin K.

Chronic obstructive airways disease

Such patients may do better if given elective postoperative ventilation.

Haemoglobinopathies

Sickle cell anaemia and other haemoglobinopathies provide major problems for the anaesthetist. It is vital to maintain high concentrations of oxygen.

American Society of Anesthesiologists grading

Operative risk caused by co-morbidity is often graded using a scale produced by the American Society of Anesthesiologists (**ASA grade**). There are six levels, with the risk of death increasing as the grade increases (Table 2.4). These gradings are imprecise and leave room for interpretation, but the ASA system is widely used.

Table 2.4
The American Society of Anesthesiologists grading system

Grade	Description
I	Normal healthy patient
II	Mild systemic disease
III	Severe systemic disease, not incapacitating
IV	Severe systemic disease that is a threat to life
V	Moribund, will not survive without operation
VI	Brain dead, awaiting organ donation

PREVENTION OF DEEP VEIN THROMBOSIS AND PULMONARY EMBOLISM

Deep vein thrombosis (DVT) leading to pulmonary embolism (PE) is a major risk for all surgical patients, not just those having operations but all those admitted to hospital for non-operative treatment. The process usually starts in the calf veins as a response to three factors know as Virchow's triad:

- stasis in the veins
- damage to the venous endothelium, produced by immobility
- hypercoagulability of the blood, a normal response to any form of injury such as an operation or acute illness.

The natural history and ubiquity of the condition first became apparent in the 1970s when the radioactive iodine-labelled fibrinogen test became available and it became possible to detect and follow the progress of subclinical DVT. Half of the thromboses begin during the operation. The rest develop in the following 5 days while the hypercoagulable state persists.

The incidence of DVT varies with the type of surgery and the health of the patient. For example, almost half of patients undergoing a major open abdominal procedure, such as a hemicolectomy, develop isotopically detectable thrombosis in their calf veins, as do virtually 100 per cent of those patients having a total hip replacement.

The principal risk factors for DVT are:

- increasing age
- malignant disease
- major operations
- history of a previous DVT or PE.

Oestrogen therapy is a risk factor for thromboembolism. Oestrogens are commonly taken by fit women in the form of oral contraceptives and postmenopausal HRT. The complex epidemiological studies required to assess which groups of patients may have an increased risk of DVT and PE after surgery have not been performed and so it is very difficult to decide an individual patient's risk.

The current consensus view is:

- The contraceptive pill is a low to negligible risk factor. It should be stopped before elective surgery but, if this is not possible, prophylaxis should be stepped up one level. (It has been argued that the risk of an unwanted pregnancy following stopping the pill is greater than the risk of a DVT!).
- Hormone replacement therapy does not increase normal oestrogen levels; it replaces something that is lacking. There should therefore be no increased risk and it need not be stopped before surgery.

There are two consequences of peri-operative DVT:

- **pulmonary embolism**, which may be fatal
- **the post-thrombotic syndrome**, which takes many years to appear but is a cause of chronic morbidity.

The current risk of fatal PE after an operation is difficult to establish because of the universal use of prophylaxis and the belief that a new clinical trial with an untreated control group would be unethical. In the untreated control groups of the first major trials on elective general surgical patients performed in the 1970s, the incidence of fatal PE ranged from 0.7 to 3.4 per cent.

The risk is much higher in emergency patients and in those who have been seriously ill and/or immobile in bed before operation.

Table 2.5
A simple protocol for the prevention of deep vein thrombosis and pulmonary embolism

Patient	Surgery	Regimen
Low risk	Day-case minor surgery	Anti-embolism stockings during surgery
Low risk	Overnight stay	Anti-embolism stockings during surgery and for a week afterwards
Medium risk	Intermediate/major surgery, short stay	Stockings as above plus low molecular weight heparin
High risk	Major inpatient surgery, long stay	Stockings as above plus low molecular weight heparin Consider intermittent pneumatic calf compression during surgery and afterwards
Very high risk	Major inpatient surgery, long stay with previous DVT/PE	Consider full anticoagulation

Prophylaxis

There are two methods of prophylaxis – mechanical and pharmacological. Mechanical methods aim to overcome stasis and to a certain extent prevent changes in the venous endothelium. Pharmacological methods endeavour to counteract hypercoagulability. Many trials have demonstrated the efficacy of both methods.

Mechanical methods include the following.

- **Graduated compression stockings.** These are moderately effective and easy to introduce and manage. They should be donned before operation and ideally worn for a week or so afterwards.
- **Intermittent calf compression.** Pneumatic intermittent calf compression is applied with inflatable leggings. The method is effective but cumbersome and cannot be used when the operation is on the leg.

Pharmacological methods aim to inhibit thrombosis at the beginning of the clotting cascade (Factors X to Xa) not the coagulation at its end (prothrombin to thrombin), which would lead to increased bleeding during and after surgery.

Low molecular weight semi-synthetic heparins are the principal agents. They must be given by daily injection and it is important to give the first dose an hour or so before surgery commences.

It is impossible to overemphasize the importance of a surgical unit having a rigorous policy based on simple protocols to prevent thromboembolic disease (Table 2.5). It is better to treat some patients unnecessarily as part of a blanket regimen than have someone die of an avoidable PE.

Prophylactic measures are much more likely to reach every patient at risk if they are applied to all, i.e. every patient in short-stay areas should wear stockings and all inpatients should receive high-level prophylaxis.

Full anticoagulation should be considered for patients who have a history of a previous major life-threatening PE provided the operation is not itself associated with a high risk of bleeding.

WOUND HEALING

Wound healing is a remarkably efficient process. When the edges of a clean incised wound are approximated, there are histological signs of healing within an hour. However, the scar does not achieve its final full strength for 6 months, longer in specialized tissues such as bone. There are four stages.

1. The edges of a wound rapidly become covered with a thin layer of clotted blood. If they lie close together without tension or compression, this layer helps stick the edges of the wound together.

The first principle of surgical wound closure is to achieve these conditions.

2. An inflammatory reaction develops. (Note that inflammation is a distinct pathological process quite separate from, though usually associated with, the changes that accompany infection.)
3. Macrophages and fibroblasts pass into the layer of clotted blood between the wound edges and begin to lay down collagen.
4. As the collagen matures and cross-links the scar gains in strength.

Wound closure

Wounds may be opposed by sutures, staples or, in the skin, adhesive strips and adhesives.

In deep tissues, it is best to use absorbable suture material. Reliable synthetic materials have superseded catgut (made from the submucosa of sheep small intestine) but they must maintain their strength until healing is complete. Abdominal wall closure requires a material that keeps its full strength for at least three months.

In the skin, monofilament interrupted non-absorbable sutures give good results, provided they are removed early enough to avoid leaving scars at their entry and exit points either side of the main wound.

Longitudinal subcuticular sutures should be non-absorbable and removed. Absorbable material often causes scar reddening and tenderness.

Causes of failure to heal

Many factors other than the obvious mechanical ones may interfere with the healing process. These include immunosuppression, infection and starvation. The cells in a healing wound need oxygen and nutrition, without these essential factors the process of healing may fail and the wound break down. Although this may be a minor problem in a superficial wound, it may be fatal if it occurs in an intestinal anastomosis.

Scars

All scars tend to shrink, and this must be born in mind when fashioning anastomoses, which must have an adequate lumen. Epithelia and endothelia heal to each other quite readily. This can be seen in every patient who has an external stoma or when bowel is used to substitute for ureter or bladder.

In the skin, scars may become **hypertrophic** or **keloid**. A hypertrophic scar is thickened, but the scar tissue remains between the edges of the original wound and tends to regress. Keloid scars become heaped up and extend beyond the original margins. Their management involves excision followed by local steroid injections to try to suppress the overgrowth and local invasion. Results are poor (see Chapter 5).

COMPLICATIONS THAT FOLLOW OPERATIONS

No surgical procedure (open or endoscopic) is free from complications. It is essential to balance the risk of complications against the purpose and value of the procedure.

As a rule, the more major the surgery the greater the risk of serious and life-threatening complications. Such complications must be considered against the threat to life and well being by the disease to be treated.

The most serious complications after surgery are seen in elderly people undergoing emergency procedures when, without operation, death would have been inevitable. At the other end of the scale, minor cosmetic procedures should not be undertaken if they have any significant risks.

Complications may be early or late, and be related to the operation site or be general.

EARLY POSTOPERATIVE COMPLICATIONS

Early postoperative complications are listed in Table 2.6.

Pain

Pain occurs after most operations as any reader who has undergone surgery will remember. After minor and intermediate procedures it is of short duration, but after major surgery it interferes with coughing, causes anxiety and confusion and stops the patient returning to their normal lifestyle. It is normally managed by the anaesthetist, or a specialized team.

Table 2.6
Postoperative complications

At the operation site

Early	Late
Pain	Pain
Vomiting	Scarring
Haemorrhage	Wound failure
Haematoma	Recurrence of condition
Wound infection	
Pyrexia	
Damage to other organs	
Dehiscence/disruption	
Wound dehiscence	

Systemic

Early	Late
Deep vein thrombosis	Psychosis
Pulmonary embolism	Fatigue
Urinary retention	
Atelectasis and chest infection	
Cardiac problems	
Mental confusion	

The regional blocks, e.g. epidural anaesthesia, which are effective and frequently used to relieve pain have their own complications, such as immobility and delay of the return of gut function.

Opiates in adequate doses are also effective, but it is an unfortunate fact that a dose adequate to relieve pain almost invariably induces nausea and vomiting.

Postoperative vomiting

Postoperative vomiting is common, and poorly understood. It is traditionally blamed on the anaesthetic, but the nature of the surgery clearly plays a role. It is more frequent after some operations than others, and is capricious. Patients who have repeated anaesthetics with the same agent may have no problems on one occasion and vomit profusely another time.

Vomiting after an abdominal operation may indicate a mechanical problem such as an early intestinal obstruction and should always be taken seriously.

Haemorrhage

Haemorrhage may be **primary**, where the bleeding is intraoperative and has not been controlled; or **secondary**, sometimes called reactionary, where the bleeding was controlled during the operation but recurs in the early postoperative phase when the blood pressure returns to normal.

The management of significant post-operation haemorrhage is most likely to require surgical intervention, once blood coagulation has been checked and any haematological defect corrected.

Haematoma

A haematoma is most likely to develop in the wound but may lead to extensive discoloration around it as the blood tracks along tissue planes. It may be treated conservatively, but it is better to evacuate large collections of blood clot to avoid the risk of the clot becoming infected. The insertion of closed suction drainage systems into cavities that cannot be obliterated after surgery reduces the incidence of haematomata.

Wound infection

Wound infection is covered in detail in Chapter 3.

Postoperative pyrexia

Postoperative pyrexia is common, and not always of significance.

- The patient should be assessed generally. If there is an associated tachycardia the fever is more likely to indicate a significant problem.
- A transient rise in temperature is common after most operations mainly caused by the inflammatory element of wound healing.

Particular attention should be given to the following.

- The chest in the early postoperative phase. There may be atelectasis and basal pneumonia.
- The operative site. There may be evidence of a major problem such as an anastomotic leak.

- If nothing else is found, consider the possibility of a DVT.
- Wound infection is not usually seen until a few days after surgery. If it is responsible for the pyrexia there will be clear signs of inflammation in the wound.
- A swinging fever after seven to ten days may indicate an internal abscess.

The investigation of a postoperative pyrexia should include:

- a blood leucocyte count; a minimal elevation may not be significant
- a chest X-ray
- an ultrasound or CT scan of the abdomen
- a duplex ultrasound scan of the legs if DVT is suspected.

Damage to other organs

This is specific to each operation. An example is hoarseness after thyroid surgery caused by temporary or permanent damage to a recurrent laryngeal nerve.

Disruption

Disruption at the site of the operation will usually be obvious, e.g. dislocation of a joint replacement or the breakdown of an anastomosis.

External intestinal fistula

The development of an external intestinal fistula is a serious complication of an abdominal bowel resection. If an anastomosis breaks down because of poor technique, ischaemia or failure to heal, leaking bowel content may cause generalized peritonitis. When the anastomosis has been walled off with omentum the leakage will be confined until it finds its way out through the wound or, if a drain has been placed, through the drain site.

A faecal fistula after a colonic resection may have few systemic consequences, but a small bowel fistula loses large volumes of fluid and electrolytes (see Chapters 18 and 19). The reduction of the absorption of fluid in the small bowel can lead to severe dehydration and starvation.

Patients with an intestinal fistula need the **lost extracellular fluid replaced**, i.e. the output of the fistula plus the patient's normal physiological requirements, and also need **feeding**, usually parenterally.

Fistulae will usually close spontaneously unless there is residual disease, distal obstruction or epithelialization of the tract. Nevertheless further surgery is often needed in many cases.

Wound dehiscence

This may be superficial or deep. It is commonly associated with infection, failure to heal because of immunosuppression, or necrosis of wound edges. Management is usually conservative with serial dressings, accepting delayed healing.

Abdominal wall dehiscence

Abdominal wall dehiscence after laparotomy is a very serious complication with a mortality rate in severely ill patients as high as 50 per cent.

Before it occurs, large volumes of *pink stained serous fluid* leak through the skin. The entire wound then gives way, and loops of small bowel appear.

The patient should be returned to the operating theatre immediately for resuture of the wound, which is never easy.

Prevention Do not let it happen. With modern mass suture techniques and modern suture materials, abdominal wound dehiscence is preventable, even in the immunosuppressed patient.

Deep vein thrombosis

DVT is only rarely clinically obvious in the surgical patient. Its prevention is discussed on page 28. If suspected as a cause of postoperative pyrexia it should be investigated by:

- estimation of D-dimer. A high level indicates the presence of fibrin degradation products in the circulation, but venous thrombosis is only one of several causes. However a negative D-dimer means that DVT is unlikely.
- duplex ultrasound scanning of the leg veins
- phlebography.

Treatment is by immediate anticoagulation with heparin followed by warfarin for a period of 3–6 months.

Table 2.7
Management of postoperative pulmonary embolism

Suspect the condition if there is:

acute dyspnoea

pleuritic chest pain

haemoptysis

Treat *immediately* with:

intravenous heparin, then warfarin

oxygen

analgesia

Confirm diagnosis with:

ECG looking for signs of right heart strain

isotope ventilation/perfusion scan

CT pulmonary angiography

If no clinical improvement:

thrombolysis with streptokinase or urokinase via a right atrial catheter

surgical thrombectomy only in extremis

Pulmonary embolism

PE is a life threatening postoperative emergency. Its management is described in Table 2.7.

Retention of urine

This is dealt with in Chapter 20.

Atelectasis and chest infection

Pulmonary complications are common after chest and abdominal surgery, when breathing is painful and hence impaired. The patient becomes uncomfortable and sometimes breathless. There may be a fever, and low oxygen saturation. A chest X-ray will show areas of collapsed lung.

Treatment is vigorous physiotherapy, with adequate analgesia to reduce the pain at the operation site. Antibiotics are indicated if there is evidence of pneumonia such as a raised leucocyte count and high fever. Any sputum should be cultured.

Infection and atelectasis are more common and tend to be worse in patients who smoke or who are known to have chest disease before surgery. If the situation deteriorates the patient may require assisted ventilation.

Cardiac problems

Cardiac dysfunction, usually an arrhythmia, is much more common in those with known ischaemic heart disease and should be treated in the appropriate way.

Mental confusion

Confusion is common in older patients after major surgery. It usually begins a few days after operation, at a time when intravenous infusions, invasive monitors and catheters have been discontinued. The patient should be checked for occult chest infection or urinary infection. Deprivation of sleep is a contributing factor.

Once the patient has a normal fluid intake and diet it generally remits. Patients rarely remember their behaviour when they were confused.

Patients who are dependent on alcohol often become confused when access is restricted.

LATE POSTOPERATIVE COMPLICATIONS

Late postoperative complications are listed in Table 2.6.

Pain

Wound pain that develops weeks or months after an operation is specific to the procedure. A common cause is entrapment of segmental nerves in scar tissue, e.g. chronic groin pain after a hernia repair and post-thoracotomy pain. Alternatively, it may arise from a divided nerve, e.g. limb phantom pain after an amputation.

Scarring

All incisions leave scars. The patient may be dissatisfied with the best result that can be achieved, whereas others are proud of their battle honours. Hypertrophic and keloid scars are discussed on page 30 and in Chapter 5.

Wound failure

Scars can give way after apparently healing satisfactorily. In the abdomen late wound failure is revealed when an **incisional hernia** appears, usually within a year but sometimes much later. Factors likely to lead to this unsatisfactory outcome include obesity, wound infection, immunosuppression and any condition that raises the intraperitoneal pressure such as a chronic cough (see Chapter 16).

Recurrence of the original condition

An operation may fail to achieve its object. A hernia may recur or a joint may continue to be painful.

Psychosis

Patients may undergo a subtle personality change or show features of mild dementia, particularly after cardiac bypass surgery. Sometimes this is only obvious to the spouse and close family members. It may be caused by cell debris coming from the bypass system causing cerebral micro-infarcts. It may occur following other major surgery or trauma, and be caused by fat micro-emboli.

Fatigue

Patients feel tired after surgery. This lasts for a period depending on the severity of the operation. It is part of the metabolic response to trauma – surgery is controlled trauma. It is not psychological for there is demonstrable muscle weakness, lack of coordination, deterioration of cognitive function and biochemical abnormalities such as impairment of the complement system.

Patients should be told to expect these vague symptoms and their likely duration. It may take 3 months before a patient feels completely recovered after a major operation. There is no treatment of proven efficacy but reducing surgical trauma by employing minimally invasive techniques makes recovery significantly more rapid. After open removal of the gall bladder the usual time to complete recovery is about 2 months. After the same operation done laparoscopically, full function usually returns in 3 weeks.

METHODS OF MONITORING THE SURGICAL PATIENT

Patients undergoing an operation, or being treated for an acute illness not requiring primary surgery, require support to maintain their metabolic and cardiovascular equilibrium in order to promote healing and recovery. Various forms of monitoring are required to plan and maintain this support (Table 2.8).

Urinary catheter

The urinary catheter provides a basic but essential measurement of a patient's fluid balance and has become ubiquitous in all major surgical procedures. It not only allows measurement of the urinary output but in the early postoperative phase avoids patients having to suffer the discomfort of getting out of bed to pass urine. It also prevents postoperative retention, but may of course only delay it until the time comes to remove the catheter.

The urethral route is usually used but the suprapubic route may be better for males with symptoms suggestive of lower urinary tract obstruction. Urethral catheterization is not without complications.

- **Infection**. A catheter is a potential route for the entry of infection, particularly in the immunocompromised patient liable to hospital infections such as MRSA (methicillin-resistant *Staphylococcus aureus*).
- **Urethral stricture**. This risk has been much reduced by the use of catheters made of silicone.
- **Haematuria** from balloon trauma – particularly when there are coagulation problems.
- **Blockage**. This is not infrequent so the first thing to do when a patient appears to be anuric is to check the patency of the catheter.

Table 2.8
Methods used to monitor the acutely ill surgical patient

Urinary catheter
Central venous pressure catheter
Pulse oximetry
Measurement of cardiac output

Central venous pressure

Measurement of the central venous pressure (CVP) is fundamental to perioperative monitoring and intensive care. It reflects venous return and hence gives a basic guide to the adequacy of circulating volume replacement. The catheter is inserted into the subclavian or internal jugular vein in the neck, and advanced into the superior vena cava where the pressure is approximately equal to the right atrial pressure.

The *Seldinger* technique is employed:

1. A needle is inserted into the vein, often facilitated by ultrasound guidance.
2. A guide wire is passed through the needle into the vein and the needle removed.
3. The catheter is then passed over the guide wire, sometimes after the passage of a dilator.

The insertion of a CVP catheter is not a minor procedure and major complications may occur which are occasionally fatal (Table 2.9). *Infection in or around a CVP catheter is dangerous.* Full sterile techniques must be employed during its insertion, and the catheter connected to a closed system. Infection is more likely if the catheter is used to give parenteral nutrition. Remember:

- Sepsis should be suspected if the patient gives any of the general indications of infection such as fever, tachycardia or leucocytosis.
- Whenever a CVP line is removed, send the tip for culture.
- When a patient has positive blood cultures and a CVP line, the latter is highly likely to be the source of the infection.
- If in doubt about the source of the sepsis remove any intravenous lines and obtain access to the circulation via another vein.

Pulse oximetry

The pulse oximeter is a non-invasive method of determining oxygen saturation The device is essentially a colorimeter. It works by shining light of two wavelengths whose absorption changes with the colour of the arterial blood.

It is entirely safe and widely used because it allows continuous monitoring of both the pulse rate and arterial oxygenation and so gives an indication

Table 2.9
Complications of central venous catheterization

Immediate

Pneumothorax and haemothorax

Arterial cannulation

Damage to the brachial plexus

Pericardial tamponade

Late

Thrombosis

Infection

Fracture and migration of the catheter

of tissue perfusion. It is widely used as its sensor can be clipped on to a digit or an ear lobe. *It has no value in diagnosing the cause of a change in oxygenation, but alerts the clinician that something is wrong.*

Measurement of cardiac output

One of the principal objects of peri/postoperative and intensive care is to maintain tissue perfusion. Cardiac output indicates how well the heart is performing this function, and its accurate measurement is fundamental to cardiovascular assessment. There are two commonly used methods of measurement, one invasive and the other non-invasive.

The **Swan–Ganz catheter** is inserted as for a CVP line but then passed through the right side of the heart and wedged into a pulmonary artery to record the **pulmonary capillary wedge pressure.** The catheter incorporates a thermocouple, and by introducing a small volume of cold fluid through its tip and measuring the temperature of the blood a known distance away, it is possible to calculate the **cardiac output**.

The technique is falling out of favour because during its insertion the catheter may rupture the pulmonary artery and cause fatal cardiac tamponade. *There is also no evidence that its routine use improves patient survival.* It is being superseded by less invasive methods.

Ultrasound methods employ the Doppler effect to measure arterial blood flow. Because the oesophagus is closely related to the descending aorta, a probe passed orally can be positioned adjacent to it. Although the method measures **aortic blood flow**, this can be used to calculate the **cardiac output** with reasonable accuracy and no risk.

There are other methods of measuring cardiac output under development, but the Swan–Ganz catheter and the oesophageal Doppler are the current methods the student is most likely to see used.

METHODS OF SUPPORT AFTER AN OPERATION

Monitoring and management are different concepts, although sometimes confused! You do not treat a patient by taking multiple physiological measurements: you collect the data to select the correct management (Table 2.10).

Fluid balance

To maintain optimum body function, any fluid lost must be replaced with the same volume of the same composition. This is the fundamental (and simple) principle of maintaining fluid balance.

A patient losing more fluid than has been taken in is said to be in *negative fluid balance*. When more fluid has been given than has been lost the patient is in *positive fluid balance*.

The calculation of fluid balance must always include an estimate of the body's insensible loss. This is the fluid lost through the skin by sweating

and from the lungs during respiration. It has to be estimated/guessed but is usually assumed to be between 0.5 and 1.0 L per 24 hours.

Tables 2.11 and 2.12 set out the normal distribution of body fluids and electrolytes.

In addition to the insensible loss and the measurable losses of fluid in the urine and faeces, surgical patients lose fluid in two main ways:

- loss of circulating whole blood volume by:
  - haemorrhage, when whole blood is lost
  - burns, when plasma colloids are lost
- loss of extracellular fluid by:
  - vomiting
  - diarrhoea
  - sequestration into the bowel lumen when distended by obstruction or paralysis as in peritonitis
  - external loss via a fistula.

Extracellular fluid depletion is commonly referred to as *dehydration*, a well-established but highly inappropriate term because it actually means just loss of water. Pure water loss is not seen in surgical practice.

The extracellular fluid volume in the average adult is only 15 L, and when a significant amount

Table 2.10
Methods for providing support to the surgical patient

Fluid balance
Acid/base balance
Nutrition
Blood transfusion
Pharmacological and mechanical support for the
 Heart
 Respiration
 Kidneys
 Liver
 Cerebrum

Table 2.11
Summary of the normal distribution of body fluid

Two-thirds of body mass is water
Two-thirds of body water is inside cells
Extracellular fluid volume is about 15 L

Table 2.12
The normal distribution of body electrolytes

Normal osmolarity of body fluids is 300 mOsmol/L
The body has 4000 mmol of sodium, mostly in the *extracellular* compartment at a concentration of around 140 mmol/L
The body contains very nearly 4000 mmol of potassium, nearly all *intracellular*
Only about 60 mmol of potassium is in the extracellular compartment, at a concentration of around 4 mmol/L

of it is lost without immediate replacement the extracellular compartment shrinks, leading to the characteristic clinical features of:

- shrivelling of the skin and subcutaneous tissue, noticeable on the back of the hands
- dry mucous membranes, seen in the mouth and tongue
- thirst and headache
- oliguria, caused by increased antidiuretic hormone (ADH) and aldosterone output
- tachycardia
- hypotension
- a low CVP.

A traditional analogy is that between a plum and prune, which is in fact a reasonable comparison, although a more contemporary equivalent might be the difference between a fresh and a sun-dried tomato! The colloquial expression 'dry as a crisp' is also to the point.

Fluid replacement

Table 2.13 sets out the principles of the treatment of fluid loss.

Table 2.13
Principles of the treatment of fluid loss

Decide on clinical grounds which fluid has been lost

Replace this fluid intravenously:

blood with blood

colloid with plasma expander

extracellular fluid with isotonic electrolytes

Monitor the response by:

- clinical assessment – the patient will feel and look better
- routine measurement of pulse rate and blood pressure
- a rise in CVP towards normal
- restoration of urine output

A normal individual of about 70–80 kG (11–12 stones) requires about 2–3 L of fluid a day if they are having nothing by mouth. Most of this will be replaced as isotonic 5% dextrose (2 L), and half a litre of normal saline will provide enough salt.

The rate at which fluid is given must be tailored to the patient. A patient severely depleted of fluid because of an intestinal obstruction may need many litres of crystalloid to restore their fluid balance. A previously fit young patient can be given this over a few hours but an elderly patient with impaired myocardial function should be rehydrated slowly and delicately to avoid the development of right heart strain and even heart failure (a complication revealed by an abnormally high CVP).

Electrolyte replacement

Potassium depletion Most of the body's potassium is inside cells, but potassium depletion is common in surgical patients because potassium is lost by vomiting, the aspiration of gastric secretions and diarrhoea. In addition, when there is significant extracellular fluid depletion, the accompanying aldosterone response leads to an increased urinary loss of potassium.

As only 2 per cent of body potassium is in the extracellular fluid and circulation, measurement of serum potassium is not a good guide to potassium status. The basic principle of management of potassium depletion is to give no more than 50–100 mmol each day, depending on the size of the patient, together with their other fluid and electrolyte needs – unless there is evidence of renal failure.

Acid/base balance The body is very sensitive to changes in pH beyond the normal range of 7.36 to 7.44, principally because of the widespread enzyme dysfunction that occurs outside this range. There must therefore be a balance between the gains and losses of acid and base.

Acids are gained from carbon dioxide, production from protein metabolism, loss of bicarbonate in the urine and faeces, and by the ingestion of acids in food. Acids are used in the metabolism of some organic anions and are lost in the urine. An abnormal loss of hydrogen ions occurs with vomiting.

Acid/base balance is assessed by analysis of arterial blood gases. The instruments currently in use measure pH and the partial pressure of oxygen and carbon dioxide. By using the Henderson–Hasselbach equation, a calculation is made of the base excess.

Acidosis and alkalosis may be metabolic or respiratory in origin, usually the former in the surgical patient. Analysis and treatment of acid/base imbalance are complex and not considered further in this text.

Nutrition

Patients with surgical disease often become malnourished because of lack of food intake and an increased catabolism. This is known to affect wound healing and to suppress the immune response, but it is surprisingly difficult to demonstrate its effect on outcome. However it is good practice to maintain the nutrition of a surgical patient who cannot eat normally.

There is no simple method of assessing malnutrition other than weight loss and a fall in serum albumin concentration, but it is usually clinically obvious when starvation has occurred. If the patient is unable to eat normally other routes for nutrition must be sought, and it is a matter of clinical judgement when to do so. There is one clear indication, the loss of nutrition through an external fistula.

Feeding may be *enteral*, where the gut is used, or *parenteral*, where nutrient solutions are given intravenously.

Enteral feeding

In the patient unable to eat normally, access to the gut has to be achieved by other means. Sometimes the gut itself is normal but the patient cannot swallow, as with a patient undergoing mechanical ventilation. On other occasions there will be obstruction or injury to the upper gastrointestinal tract. Access to the small bowel with a fine bore tube may be:

- nasogastric
- nasojejunal, with X-ray guidance during placement
- by percutaneous gastrostomy
- by percutaneous gastrostomy inserted with endoscopic guidance (PEG)
- by jejunostomy, usually at time of surgery.

Various isotonic liquid diets are available containing balanced proportions of protein, fat and carbohydrate, with vitamins and trace elements. There are three common complications of enteral feeding:

- loss of appetite
- bloating
- diarrhoea.

Parenteral feeding

Parenteral feeding is required when the intestine cannot absorb food, either because a significant length of it has been removed, it has been short-circuited or it has lost function.

Total parenteral nutrition (TPN) is given intravenously either through a peripheral catheter that is changed regularly or through a long-term central catheter. Commercially available solutions include appropriate amounts of amino acids, lipids and glucose, with vitamins and trace elements. The complications include:

- problems with the access catheter, as listed for CVP lines (Table 2.9)
- infection: feeding solutions make a good culture medium for bacteria
- metabolic problems: particularly electrolyte and acid/base imbalance and impairment of liver function.

Enteral feeding is to be preferred to parenteral feeding whenever possible because:

- it is simpler
- there is much less risk of metabolic complications
- there is no risk of catheter infection
- for reasons that are poorly understood the same amount of food substitute given enterally is more effective than the same amount given parenterally.

The significant problems and complications listed above associated with parenteral feeding have been overcome in specialized units. Intravenous lines made with non-irritant silicone material can function for many years if infection is avoided by rigorous aseptic regimens. Throughout the world many patients who have lost all or most of their small intestine survive at home with long-term domiciliary TPN.

Blood transfusion

Blood transfusion became possible once the ABO blood grouping system was understood, and is now routine in the treatment of trauma. Many forms of major surgical intervention would not be feasible without it. It is however not without its risks and

Table 2.14
Complications of blood transfusion

Haemolytic reaction, due to mismatch or error

Febrile reaction, usually transient and mild

Acute lung injury, causing acute respiratory distress syndrome

Bacterial infection (rare)

Transmission of HIV or hepatitis

complications, and with the advent of blood-borne virus diseases is best avoided whenever possible.

Blood for transfusion is, except in dire emergency, cross-matched with the serum of the recipient patient. As well as the ABO and Rhesus antigens there are numerous other rare red cell antigens that may lead to progressive immunization in those receiving repeated transfusions.

Surgical patients usually require blood to replace lost red cells and circulating volume. In the western world, donated blood is separated into a wide variety of blood products – plasma, platelets, albumin and clotting factors – which are used to treat a wide variety of haematological diseases. The blood usually available to the surgeon consists of red cells and plasma only. As blood is also anticoagulated with citrate for storage, it is not surprising that surgical patients given blood bank-processed blood are at risk of developing impaired coagulation, which then has to be treated with the very factors that were removed from the blood after donation.

The complications of blood transfusion are many, but they are nearly all preventable and must be set against the need for red cell and volume replacement (Table 2.14).

Management of a transfusion reaction

A reaction during a blood transfusion is not a rare event. The patient may become acutely ill before the cause is obvious, with a variety of symptoms including distress, confusion and oddly enough backache. There may be tachycardia, hypotension and fever. The appropriate action is:

1. Stop the transfusion immediately and change the giving set – the transfusion may be incompatible.

2. Check for signs of respiratory distress and consider the need for ventilation.
3. Give a synthetic plasma expander.
4. Take blood cultures and give an adequate dose of a broad-spectrum antibiotic in case the problem is a bacteraemia.
5. Check coagulation – intravascular coagulation may have begun.

On most occasions the reaction is mild and settles rapidly, but it is best to be prepared for serious consequences.

Problems of massive transfusion

Sometimes surgical patients require a massive transfusion to keep them alive – defined as a replacement of at least one normal circulating blood volume. This can cause the following problems.

Hypothermia Despite attempts to warm the transfused blood, which has been stored in the refrigerator, the patient may become cold. This slows coagulation, which is a chemical process. Warming blankets are essential, and all infused fluids should be warmed to as near body temperature as possible.

Citrate toxicity Citrates chelate calcium in the circulation and this can lead to hypocalcaemia which must be corrected.

Transient hyperkalaemia Intracellular potassium leaks out of the transfused red blood cells during storage. Paradoxically the end result of massive transfusion is usually hypokalaemia, as during recovery potassium re-enters the red cells.

Coagulopathy This is caused by dilution of the patient's platelets and clotting factors and is compounded by hypothermia. It should be assessed clinically by measuring the platelet count and clotting times. Treatment is to give platelets, fresh frozen plasma and cryoprecipitate.

Ways of reducing the need for blood transfusion

An oxygen-carrying synthetic substance is the Holy Grail, but the search has not yet been successful. Use synthetic plasma expander colloids instead of blood whenever possible (1 litre maximum).

Table 2.15
Principles of treatment of organ failure

Failing system	Monitoring	Management
Circulation	Electrocardiogram	Inotropes
	Central venous pressure	Treat arrythmias
	Cardiac output	Reduce circulatory loading
Breathing	Pulse oximetry	Continuous positive airway pressure (CPAP)
	Arterial blood gases	Intubation and ventilation
Kidneys	Urine output	Restrict fluids and potassium
	Urine osmolarity	Haemofiltration
	Serum electrolytes and creatinine	Haemodialysis
Liver	Liver function tests	Enteral or parenteral nutrition
	Coagulopathy	Correct coagulation with plasma proteins
Brain	Confusion and unconsciousness	Correct acid/base imbalance
	Fitting	Anticonvulsants

Autologous transfusion Before elective surgery collect units of the patient's own blood for use if required.

Use 'cell-savers' Blood in the operative field can be sucked out, anticoagulated, filtered in special systems and reinfused. Clotting factors are lost and coagulopathy remains a problem. This technique cannot be used in contaminated fields.

Organ support

Organ support is carried out in the intensive care unit. There are various definitions of what constitutes intensive care but the concept implies either artificial ventilation or the need to treat failure of another major organ. An important and probably the key factor for success is adequate staffing – one nurse for each patient at all times.

Most hospitals also have a high dependency unit, where acutely ill patients may be monitored intensively but have no facilities for mechanical organ support.

As this is not a textbook of intensive care medicine it does not give a detailed account of the management of major organ failure, but the principles are summarized in Table 2.15.

Prognosis

Two **scoring systems** are used to estimate the prognosis. They are also helpful in deciding whether increasing the level of support is likely to be successful.

- **APACHE II** (Acute Physiology and Chronic Health Evaluation, second version) assesses the severity of disease based on age, medical history, and 12 current physiological measurements varying from simple pulse rate to arterial pH.
- **POSSUM** (Physiological and Operative Severity Score for the enUmeration of Mortality and morbidity) is used in the assessment of postoperative patients but also takes into account the severity of the surgery performed.

TRANSPLANT SURGERY

Organ transplantation has become a routine procedure in the last 40 years since the development of immunosuppressive drugs that prevent rejection. Only the general principles of this vast topic will be discussed here.

An **autograft** is the transfer of an organ from one part of an individual to another and although it uses the same surgical techniques is not really transplantation in the commonly used sense of the term.

An **allograft** is the transfer of tissue from one member of a species to another individual of the same species. Nearly all human transplants are allografts.

A **xenograft** is the transfer of tissues from one species to another. Perfused (living) xenografts are rarely used but dead and preserved tissue transplants such as the pig heart valve and porcine skin are used extensively.

Vascular anastomosis was developed in the early years of the twentieth century. The other major advance that made human allografts worthwhile was the introduction of immunosuppressive drugs such as:

- steroids
- azathioprine
- cyclosporine
- tacrolimus.

There are many other drugs, with more under development, including polyclonal and monoclonal antibodies.

The success of allograft transplantation depends on finding an organ from a donor with a tissue type similar to that of the recipient. Two methods of assessing this are employed:

- simple ABO compatibility as for blood transfusion
- HLA (human leucocyte antigen) compatibility.

The organ transplant most likely to succeed is one between identical twins, who are isogeneic. Such a situation is rare but the transplanted organ will not be rejected once the technical problems have been solved.

Organ donors may be:

- **Living and preferably related**. This gives the best technical conditions and, as HLA typing is genetic, the best chance of long-term graft survival. Ethical problems are considerable, as there is a risk to the healthy donor.
- **Cadaveric**. The donor has been declared brain-dead using standard criteria. Organ support is continued until the organs have been removed by the transplant team.
- **Donors after cardiac arrest**. This is the least satisfactory group as non-perfused organs deteriorate rapidly at body temperature. The organ must be removed in haste, which also may lead to technical problems. It does not matter with some tissue transplants, such as the cornea of the eye.

Transplants may be:

- **Orthotopic**. After the recipient's failing organ has been removed, the transplant is put into the same place, e.g. heart and most liver transplants.
- **Heterotopic**. The donated organ is placed in a different place. This may be because it is not necessary to remove the failing organ(s). Kidney transplants are almost invariably placed in one of the recipient's iliac fossae as it is technically a much simpler operation.
- **Auxiliary**. The organ failure is not complete and the transplanted organ is placed orthotopically to boost function.

The main difficulties of managing patients who have had transplants are:

- **Technical**. Organ transplantation is complex, with multiple vessel anastomoses each of which might fail.
- **Immunosuppression**. This leads to poor healing and poor resistance to infection.
- **Rejection**. This can be acute.

The indications, methods and success for the organ transplants in clinical use are described later in the relevant chapters.

3

Bacterial and viral infections

John Black

Infection impacts upon surgical practice in two main ways. First, many of the conditions treated by the surgeon are caused by infection, commonly bacterial but occasionally with other organisms. Second, safe surgical treatment is only possible if peri-operative infection is eliminated or controlled. It is nowadays taken for granted that operations are carried out in a clean environment rendered so by sterilization. However, as many infections come from organisms carried by the patient, infection remains a constant risk.

Antibiotics are used frequently in the treatment and prevention of infections, but their very wide use and often abuse has resulted in the emergence of resistant strains of bacteria that cause major problems, particularly in the hospital environment.

This chapter discusses the general principles of the investigation of infection in the surgical patient, particularly in the per-operative period, and the principles of management of those infections. Other specific infections are dealt with later in the appropriate chapters.

Virus infections rarely require surgical treatment, but patients suffering from conditions such as viral hepatitis and human immunodeficiency virus (HIV) present special problems, which are discussed below.

ANTISEPSIS AND STERILIZATION

Surgeons aim to carry out surgical operations in an environment free of bacteria. This may be achieved by:

- **asepsis:** the concept of eliminating all bacteria from instruments and everything that might enter the operative area
- **antisepsis:** the concept of reducing the number of bacteria, hopefully to zero by the use of antibacterial chemicals.

Lister carried out the first clean operations at the end of the eighteenth century. Although bacteria were known to exist at that time, following the work of Pasteur some years earlier, Lister did not believe that bacteria caused infection and used phenol, an antiseptic, on purely empirical grounds.

In practice, the distinction between asepsis and antisepsis is not important, and it is usual to combine both approaches.

Although it is always desirable to eliminate any bacteria before and during surgery, the intensity of the measures employed depends upon the type of operation contemplated, e.g. any infection after a heart valve or joint replacement can be a disaster, whereas the level of asepsis/antisepsis required for drainage of an abscess is less exacting. In the emergency setting the patient may already be infected with endogenous organisms.

PRECAUTIONS BEFORE AN OPERATION

Many wound infections are caused by the patient's own skin flora and many methods are used to reduce this source of contamination before operation. Evidence of their efficacy is largely lacking, but it is reasonable to allow the patient a bath or shower before surgery to achieve at least social cleanliness. Any obvious infection, such as infected acne, or any dirty areas such as material accumulated in the umbilicus, should be eliminated. If these simple methods fail, an operation may have to be postponed.

Bathing or showering with colourful antiseptic solutions before surgery is sometimes used, but there is no evidence that it has any effect on the rate of wound infection.

Shaving body hair is traditional. It is certainly neater if the area to be incised is cleared of hair. It also makes the removal of adhesive dressings less uncomfortable for the patient. There is some evidence that shaving a few hours before an operation increases the incidence of wound infection, probably by liberating otherwise hidden skin flora from hair follicles. If shaving is to be employed it should be done at the last possible moment or 1 or 2 days before the surgery.

PRECAUTIONS IN THE OPERATING THEATRE

The patient

Painting the skin adjacent to the operation site with an antiseptic solutions is routine, usually chlorhexidine or povidone/iodine. The area around the incision is then isolated with sterile drapes made of linen or disposable material. There is little evidence that this plays any part in reducing infection but it helps the operating team to concentrate their activities within the operative 'sterile field' and keeps the rest of the patient free of blood and body fluids.

The environment

The modern operating theatre is air-conditioned and kept scrupulously clean. Laminar airflow is used for various forms of surgery, particularly involving the implantation of synthetic materials such as artificial joints and heart valves. The air flowing over the operative field is filtered free of all particles. The maximum benefit of laminar flow systems is seen with operations where the consequence of infection is potentially disastrous and the infecting organisms come from the theatre environment, not from the patient.

The operating team

The members of the surgical team should wash their hands and scrub their nails using antiseptic solutions according to local protocol, and wear sterilized clothing and rubber gloves. Facemasks are widely used but there is no evidence that they reduce the risk of infection. They do however have a protective function for the surgeon.

Instruments and endoscopes

There are three main methods for sterilizing instruments and endoscopes:

- heat
- chemicals
- radiation.

The aim is to eliminate bacterial spores as well as bacteria.

Heat is applied in an **autoclave** filled with high-pressure steam. Usually the process is carried out at a central site, away from the theatre suite.

The most effective of the **chemical methods** is prolonged soaking in **gluteraldehyde**, but the solution is toxic and requires special facilities for its use. It is often the preferred method for delicate endoscopes.

Radiation with gamma-rays is highly effective but is not available in most hospitals. Its main use is to sterilize pre-packed mass-produced disposable items such as meshes for hernia repair and artificial joints.

There are many other methods of sterilization but a full discussion of their merits is beyond the scope of this book.

WOUND INFECTION

Wound infection almost invariably occurs *during* the operation when tissues are exposed and tissue planes opened and separated. In most cases the organisms come from the patient, either from the organ being operated upon or the skin. Other contaminating bacteria come from the theatre environment or personnel. Bacteria usually enter a wound directly, but it is possible for a wound to become infected by haematogenous spread with organisms coming from infected invasive monitoring and intravenous lines.

A wide variety of organisms may be involved. It is often possible to deduce the source of infection from the type of bacteria isolated, e.g. a coliform bacillus in a wound will suggest the gut as the likely source, particularly after abdominal surgery.

The precise definition of a wound infection is surprisingly difficult as wounds may become inflamed without infection. For most purposes, including the measurement of wound infection rates, a wound is declared infected if, after an operation, it discharges pus or bacteria are isolated from an exudate.

Risk factors that influence the incidence of wound infection after surgery

Contamination

The risks of wound infection after an operation depend upon the field through which the operation is being performed.

The site of the incision may be:

- *Clean*. Elective surgery through a clean field, e.g. the repair of a groin hernia, carries an infection risk of the order of 1 per cent. Nevertheless, the consequences may be significant if implanted synthetic materials become infected and have to be removed.
- *Clean then contaminated*. A clean wound may become contaminated by an intra-operative procedure that opens a contaminated area, e.g. opening a deep abscess or opening a viscus. A good example is cholecystectomy. The gall bladder is part of the gut and in 40 per cent of the gall bladders that contain gall stones the bile contains bacteria. The risk of wound infection after operating through a clean wound that becomes contaminated is 5–10 per cent.
- *Contaminated*. If the operative field contains bacteria at the time of surgery, as in an operation for appendicitis, the chance of infection is 10–20 per cent.
- *Dirty*. If the operative field contains pus or bowel content at the time of surgery the risk of postoperative infection is at least 50 per cent.

Obesity
Fat is a good culture medium for bacteria.

Diabetes

Immunosuppression caused by disease or chemotherapy

Heavy blood loss during the operation

Foreign bodies in the wound

Postoperative haematoma

Blood clot is a good culture medium. This risk can be reduced by the use of closed suction wound drainage.

ANTIBIOTIC PROPHYLAXIS AGAINST WOUND INFECTION

Prophylaxis with antibiotics is used when the risk of wound infection is high or when the consequences of infection are very serious. The basic principles guiding the use of prophylactic antibiotics are set out in Table 3.1.

The most effective way to give a prophylactic antibiotic is intravenously at the induction of the anaesthetic. Only in long procedures will it be necessary to give more than one dose. There is no advantage in continuing prophylactic antibiotics after the operation.

The illogical and indiscriminate use of antibiotics is a major factor in the induction of resistant strains of bacteria. The choice of antibiotic depends on the surgery and the likely infecting organisms. For example, with bowel surgery it is vital to include an agent such as metronidazole, which is active against anaerobic organisms.

The penetration of the antibiotic into the tissues must also be considered.

There is good evidence for the use of antibiotic prophylaxis against wound infection. Its incidence can be reduced to one-tenth. It is however important to appreciate that this is prophylaxis not treatment and it must be confined to the operative period.

Table 3.1
Principles for antibiotic prophylaxis against wound infection

The antibiotic prophylaxis must be given peri-operatively because infection occurs during the operation

There is no advantage (and potential disadvantages) in continuing antibiotic cover after the operation

The antibiotic chosen must be effective against the expected contaminating organism

MANAGEMENT OF WOUND INFECTION

- **Suspect the diagnosis** if there is an otherwise unexplained postoperative fever or leucocytosis.
- **Inspect the wound regularly** for the signs of inflammation described by Celsus in AD 30, namely **heat, redness, swelling and pain**.
- Whenever possible **collect any pus or exudate** and take a wound swab **for bacterial culture and sensitivity**.
- Only if the patient is systemically ill, or the consequences of infection serious, should antibiotics be started blindly. Otherwise await identification of the organism and then give an antibiotic to which it is sensitive.
- An exception to this is rapidly spreading erythema and tenderness around a wound, signs which indicate a streptococcal infection. In this event there will be no exudate or pus formation and usually a negative wound swab, so treatment with **penicillin** in adequate doses should be started at once.
- **Drain** small abscesses by removing one or more of the skin sutures.

With major wound infection a drastic but effective measure is to return the patient to the operating theatre and **lay the wound open** down to the deep fascia. The wound may subsequently be allowed to granulate or may be re-sutured once it is clean.

Synthetic material in the wound may act as a nidus of infection which will not drain fully and will not be penetrated by antibiotics. It may be necessary to **remove all synthetic material** before the infection will resolve, and this may result in failure of the operation, e.g. a hernia repair.

ABSCESSES

An abscess is defined as a discrete collection of pus usually surrounded by granulation tissue. To occur it is necessary to have an infection with an organism, such as *Staphylococcus aureus*, which produces toxins that cause local tissue necrosis which then liquefies – the pus. Pus contains bacteria, dead tissue and protein-rich inflammatory exudate. The wall of an abscess is not a definite layer but consists of inflamed compressed surrounding tissue. As the compression increases there is more ischaemic necrosis, which makes the abscess bigger. If the abscess is superficial, it will enlarge until it meets the skin. The skin is more resistant than subcutaneous fat but if it slowly undergoes necrosis, a dark area appears through which the abscess will eventually burst. This process is known as '*pointing*' (see Chapter 5).

Natural history of an abscess

An abscess may:

- **burst**, either externally, or internally into a hollow viscus or a serous cavity
- **become chronic**
- **resolve** spontaneously.

The likelihood of each event depends upon the infecting organism and the situation of the abscess. A superficial abscess such as one in an infected sebaceous cyst is likely to 'point' and burst through the skin. An intra-abdominal abscess such as an appendix abscess may burst into the adjacent right colon or through the overlying abdominal wall. Rapid resolution of the symptoms and signs follows rupture.

A small abscess in the abdomen may be observed to resolve on serial scanning.

The correct management of an abscess is to drain it (Table 3.2).

Table 3.2
General principles of management of an abscess

Remember, the core of an abscess is dead and not perfused with blood; therefore, antibiotics will not penetrate into it

Antibiotics may be needed if there is septicaemic toxicity

An external abscess may be allowed to point before drainage

An internal abscess needs to be localized with ultrasound or computed tomography scanning

There are three definitive treatments:

- surgical drainage, externally but sometimes into a hollow viscus

- serial aspiration, often with image guidance

- image-guided continuous drainage, by inserting a catheter for continued drainage and aspiration until the cavity obliterates

The management of the many specific varieties of abscess is discussed in the appropriate chapters. With the advent of safe image guidance and ultrasound scanning, abdominal and other internal abscesses are now more often drained by an interventional radiologist than a surgeon.

SEPTIC SHOCK

Septic shock is a state of profound tissue hypoperfusion and failure of oxygen delivery brought about by severe infection and septicaemia. It has a mortality of around 50 per cent and is more likely to occur in elderly and immunocompromised patients.

Investigation
Clinical diagnostic indicators
For the diagnosis of septic shock there must be:

- evidence of circulating bacteria, usually confirmed by a positive blood culture (virtually any human pathogen may be responsible)
- persistent and refractory hypotension.

There will also be tachycardia and hyperventilation.

A feature of septic shock is arterial vasodilatation. The patient may feel warm and have bounding pulses yet be *hypotensive.*

The clinical end result is often multi-organ failure, i.e.

- **acute renal failure** caused by tubular necrosis
- **acute lung injury** leading to adult respiratory distress syndrome (ARDS)
- **deteriorating liver function**
- **gastrointestinal tract damage**, allowing translocation of bacteria into the blood stream which adds to the septic burden
- **encephalopathy**, manifest as confusion.

Blood tests
Paradoxically although there may be fever and a raised leucocyte count, both of these may be low because the sepsis overwhelms the immune system.

The pathophysiology of septic shock is complex. There is an exaggerated inflammatory response brought about by inflammatory mediators released by bacteria. These include cytokines such as tumour necrosis factor (TNF), interleukins and many others. The complement system is activated. The inflammatory cytokines usually induce disseminated intravascular coagulopathy.

Management

The treatment of septic shock is set out in Table 3.3.

Table 3.3
Treatment of septic shock

Early recognition based on clinical suspicion

Adequate and immediate intravenous antibiotics

Vigorous resuscitation with replacement of circulating volume

Identification of the source of sepsis, usually clinically

Definitive treatment of the source of sepsis, which must be carried out as soon as resuscitation has been achieved

Support for failing organs

TETANUS

Tetanus is caused by *Clostridium tetani*, a Gram-positive, spore-forming, anaerobic organism found everywhere, particularly in soil. It produces a neurotoxin that prevents the release of inhibitory neurotransmitters that cause muscle spasm.

Tetanus is a rare disease in the UK, but not in the developing world. It has been virtually eradicated by immunization of the population with tetanus toxoid.

Investigation
Clinical diagnostic indicators
The clinical features of facial muscle spasm producing the 'risus sardonicus' and back spasms producing opisthotonos are diagnostic. Death is caused by respiratory failure.

The neurological complications appear several weeks after the patient sustains a wound. Diagnosis is clinical and difficult, as few doctors have seen a case. The original contaminated entry wound, the clue to suspecting the diagnosis, has usually been dealt with satisfactorily weeks before.

Management

The treatment of tetanus includes:

- **Drug-induced muscle paralysis to allow long-term ventilation** if the respiratory muscles are paralysed, until the toxin is eliminated. This may take a few of months, and has its own complications, particularly in older people. The mortality is around 40 per cent.
- **Wound excision**. Any dead tissue in the wound should be excised followed by delayed closure.
- **Penicillin**. Although *Clostridium tetani* is sensitive to penicillin, it has no effect on the neurological complications that are caused by neurotoxins.
- **Passive immunization**. Any un-immunized patient who sustains a high-risk wound should be passively immunized by giving, classically, antitetanus serum raised in horses, but nowadays immunoglobulin.

GAS GANGRENE

The pathogens causing gas gangrene are *Clostridium welchii* from soil or *Clostridium perfringens* found in normal gut flora. These anaerobic organisms produce toxins that cause necrosis and liquefaction of any ischaemic or poorly perfused tissues and a distinctive foul-smelling gas consisting mostly of nitrogen, with a small amount of hydrogen.

Investigation

Clinical diagnostic indicators

A clostridial infection occurs where there is dead tissue and often some degree of immunocompromise, e.g. the stump of a diabetic after an amputation.

There are the usual signs of wound infection but the patient is disproportionately ill. Septic shock is common. There may be evidence of gas in the tissues, manifest as a crackling sensation in the affected tissues when the area is palpated (surgical emphysema).

Microbiology

Clostridium welchii or *Clostridium perfringens* may be cultured from excised tissue or wound exudates.

These organisms may also be seen on a fresh microscopic specimen of the dead tissues.

Imaging

Gas may be seen in the soft tissues as radiolucent areas on X-rays (Fig 3.1).

Management

Penicillin Clostridial organisms are sensitive to penicillin, which should be given as prophylaxis in any situation where anaerobic infection is possible. In established cases the principles of treatment are to give high doses of **intravenous benzypenicillin**.

All dead tissue should be removed, at whatever cost. This may require a major limb amputation or massive debridement.

Hyperbaric oxygen, given in a national centre in an appropriate chamber, to increase tissue oxygen perfusion and palliate the effect of the clostridial toxins, may have a role.

Mortality is high. Most patients with gas gangrene die, whatever is done. This emphasizes the importance of prophylaxis (Table 3.4).

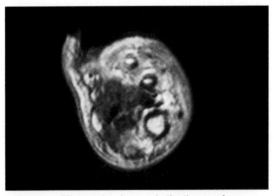

FIGURE 3.1   CT scan showing gas in the tissues of gas gangrene (dark area)

Table 3.4
Management of gas gangrene

Give prophylactic penicillin where there is any risk. If it does occur:

- give high-dose penicillin
- cut out all dead tissue
- consider hyperbaric oxygen

INTERSTITIAL INFECTIONS

There are a number of infections of the skin and subcutaneous tissues that have in common the involvement of a streptococcus and the ability to spread diffusely without becoming walled off to form an abscess.

Streptococcal cellulitis (erysipelas)

Investigation

Clinical diagnostic indicators

This pure streptococcal infection of the skin and subcutaneous tissues is characterized by redness, heat and tenderness (see Chapter 5 and *Symptoms and Signs*). A raised edge of the inflamed area caused by oedema of the subcutis is a reliable diagnostic feature. The entry site is rarely seen.

Erysipelas is the old name for streptococcal cellulitis.

Microbiology

There is rarely any exudate to culture but blood should be taken for culture. There may be no growth as the organisms may not have reached the circulation.

Management

Intravenous benzylpenicillin, to which streptococci are sensitive, should be commenced as soon as possible. Extension or regression of the infection may be monitored by marking the edge of the inflamed area.

Streptococcal cellulitis usually responds rapidly to penicillin.

SYNERGISTIC GANGRENE

This is a serious condition with a high mortality. There is infection with a streptococcus combined with an anaerobic organism such as a bacteroides.

The incidence is higher in those immunocompromised by conditions such as cancer, HIV infection, diabetes or immunosuppressive drugs. The combined infection produces toxins that cause tissue necrosis, which in turn acts as a culture medium for the responsible bacteria. The streptococci then flourish and spread, leading to a rapid advance of the process along tissue planes. A characteristic feature is necrosis of the fascia, usually with sparing of the underlying muscle (Fig 3.2). There is sometimes an obvious cause, such as local trauma or an infected wound, but sometimes the aetiology is obscure.

The condition has numerous synonyms:

- **Fournier's gangrene**, when the condition arises in the scrotum
- **Meleney's gangrene**
- **necrotizing fasciitis**
- **hospital gangrene**
- **'flesh-eating bugs'** (tabloid press).

The prognosis is poor and the mortality as high as 80 per cent, not surprising in an unfit population. The survivors tend to be young with a clearly defined and treatable cause.

Investigation

Clinical diagnostic indicators

Diagnosis is initially clinical. The patient is always very unwell, with signs of septicaemia. The local signs are a dusky erythema of the skin, which may turn purple and become blotchy. The underlying necrosis of fascia and muscle is always much more widespread than the skin changes suggest.

Microbiology

Investigation should include serial blood cultures.

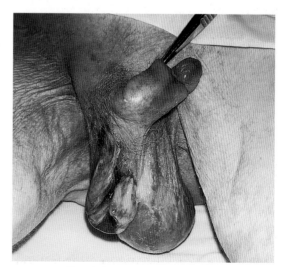

FIGURE 3.2 Fournier's gangrene of the scrotal skin and penis

Management

The treatment is similar to that for gas gangrene, given above (Table 3.4), namely:

- **High doses of the appropriate antibiotics**, always including penicillin to cover streptococci, and metronidazole to cover anaerobic organisms.
- **Total surgical excision of the necrotic areas**. This may be impossible if the process is extensive. Such patients invariably die. Large areas of skin may have to be removed, and survivors may need extensive tissue reconstruction. Failing to excise all dead tissue inevitably leads to further spread of the infection.
- **Hyperbaric oxygen** may have a role for patients who have had a surgical excision. It increases tissue viability and reduces the likelihood of further necrosis.

ACQUIRED HOSPITAL INFECTIONS

Two varieties of infection are found almost exclusively in hospitals because of the extensive use and abuse of antibiotic therapy over the past 50 years. Methicillin-resistant *Staphylococcus aureus* (MRSA) is a strain of staphylococcus that has developed resistance to most antibiotics, and has prospered by natural selection. *Clostridium difficile* is an organism, sometimes carried in the normal gut, which becomes a dangerous pathogen when broad-spectrum antibiotics alter the balance of the flora in the intestine.

METHICILLIN-RESISTANT STAPHYLOCOCCUS AUREUS

When penicillin, the first antibiotic of the beta-lactam group, was introduced in the 1940s it was found to be dramatically effective against infections caused by *Staphyloccoccus aureus*, but even then there were some strains of the organism that had the ability to produce beta-lactamase, an enzyme which destroys penicillin. These gradually became predominant and widespread as penicillin was overprescribed.

In the 1960s methicillin, a new beta-lactam antibiotic that was not destroyed by the enzyme, was introduced. Unfortunately there were some strains of staphylococcus that were resistant to methicillin and these also became widespread, particularly in environments where penicillin and methicillin were being widely used, i.e. hospitals.

Methicillin requires parenteral administration and has been replaced by flucloxacillin, which is well absorbed when taken orally. However, the term methicillin-resistant *Staphylococcus aureus* (MRSA) has persisted. *It is now used to describe any* Staphylococcus aureus *resistant to a beta-lactam antibiotic* ('multiple resistance').

Staphylococcus aureus is found in the nostrils and on the skin of approximately a quarter of the population. Patients bring it into hospital with them and many hospital staff are carriers. The organisms are transferred very easily from staff to patient and from patient to patient, usually by hand contact. In the population outside hospitals, only 2–3 per cent of nasal and skin staphylococci are resistant to methicillin, but in hospital staff resistance rates have been reported of 10 per cent.

Most patients with MSRA are therefore *colonized* by it rather than infected by it and it is only pathogenic in certain circumstances. MSRA *infections* are found in patients with the risk factors set out in Table 3.5.

The site of infection may be anywhere in the body. It has been argued that most of the morbidity in patients with MSRA infection is related

---

Table 3.5
Risk factors for methicillin-resistant *Staphylococcus aureus* infection in hospital patients

Immunosuppression

Burns

Open wounds

Surgical drains

Urinary catheter

Invasive monitoring

Admission to an intensive care unit

Increasing age

Previous or prolonged hospital stay

Antibiotic treatment, particularly when prolonged

to the underlying condition that introduces the risk of infection by what are normally commensal organisms. However, those studies that have been adjusted for the underlying disease present convincing evidence that MRSA infection alone increases mortality and prolongs hospital stay.

Diagnosis of MRSA infection

This is usually made on routine culture of the infected area. There should always be suspicion of an MRSA infection if any of the risk factors are present.

Treatment of MRSA infection in a patient

Various antibiotics are available. Vancomycin and ticoplanin are glycopeptide antibiotics that require parenteral administration. Both have toxic side-effects. Regrettably, resistance to these drugs has been seen and new agents and regimens are under development.

Treatment of MRSA in an institution

- **Isolate infected patients**, using barrier-nursing techniques with gowns and masks.
- **Transfer any infected patient to their home** at the earliest opportunity, if practicable, or to a specialized unit with isolation facilities.
- **Seek the source of the infection** by obtaining nasal swabs from the staff. Those infected may be treated with topical mupirocin and should be excluded from the hospital until they are shown to be clear of MRSA.
- **Educate hospital staff** in the importance of hygiene and hand washing after every patient contact.
- **Consider screening patients before admission.**

Prevention of MRSA infection

Although MRSA is endemic in large hospitals in Europe and North America, its incidence is much lower in those institutions which have:

- **single rooms** for patients
- **washing facilities beside every patient** and in every examination and treatment area

- **high standards of cleaning** of carpets, furniture and fabrics
- **lower occupancy rates** that allow time for rooms to be properly cleaned between patients.

The student will realize that the implementation of many of these measures requires the application of an ever vigilant and unrelenting clinical discipline.

CLOSTRIDIUM DIFFICILE

C. difficile is an anaerobic toxin-producing spore-forming organism found in about 2 per cent of healthy individuals in the community. It is found in the faeces of about 20 per cent of hospital inpatients, very few of whom have symptoms. The spores are omnipresent in the hospital environment and spread by hand contact. When antibiotics are given, the normal bowel flora alters in a way that favours *C. difficile* proliferation. About one in 200 inpatients develop symptoms of severe diarrhoea, with the incidence being higher in elderly people (Table 3.6).

The antibiotic-induced bowel disease caused by *C. difficile* is commonly called **pseudomembranous colitis** (PMC) because of the macroscopic and microscopic appearance of the exudate found in many cases. Koch's postulates proving *C. difficile* to be the causative agent were first fulfilled in 1977. The condition existed before that and was attributed to staphylococcal infection.

The mortality is significant, up to 30 per cent, although it is difficult to separate it from that associated with the underlying condition, as with MRSA. The most dangerous complication is *toxic*

Table 3.6
Diagnosis of *Clostridium difficile* infection

Clinical, with a high index of suspicion in those who develop diarrhoea and have a history of exposure to antibiotics

Repeated testing of faeces for the two toxins A and B

Direct culture is difficult (hence the name) and rarely necessary

Flexible sigmoidoscopy with biopsy is occasionally useful

Table 3.7
Treatment of *Clostridium difficile* infection

Withdraw the causative antibiotic, replacing it with another if necessary

Replace fluid and electrolyte losses

Isolate the patient

Treat with the appropriate antibiotics:

- First line – metronidazole

- Second line – vancomycin (given orally)

Look out for relapses requiring treatment

Be aware of the risk of toxic megacolon

---

megacolon, which is treated in the same way as when caused by other diseases (see Chapter 19).

The symptoms are diarrhoea, abdominal pain and, in half the cases, fever. There will always be a history of having taken antibiotics. The condition is particularly associated with broad-spectrum agents but has been connected with almost every antibiotic, including paradoxically some of those used to treat it. It is particularly common after treatment with lincomycin and clindamycin and has led to these agents being used only rarely. The interval between the administration of the antibiotic and the onset of symptoms is usually about a week, but can be shorter or much longer.

The treatment of *C. difficile* infection is set out in Table 3.7.

Prevention of *Clostridium difficile* infection

C. difficile infection is an antibiotic-related disease and will be less likely to occur if there is sensible and appropriate use of antibiotics, in particular stopping them after a standard course of treatment has been completed.

To develop the disease the gut must contain the spores. Most patients ingest these when in hospital. Isolate and barrier – nurse sufferers, with safe disposal of their faeces and proper cleaning of their environment.

Its frequency would be reduced and its spread curtailed if hospitals had single rooms, good washing facilities for its staff and high standards of domestic hygiene with adequate time for cleaning between patient discharge and the next admission.

BLOOD-BORNE VIRUS INFECTIONS

HUMAN IMMUNODEFICIENCY VIRUS

HIV is the cause of acquired immune deficiency syndrome (AIDS). It is a retrovirus that, by various mechanisms, attacks cell-mediated immunity. The virus is active in the circulation and in seminal fluid.

The highest risk of transmission is from a transfusion with infected blood. Many sufferers from haemophilia who were given frequent blood transfusions died of this disease before it was properly recognized and infected blood and blood products eliminated.

At least one-quarter of children born to infected mothers acquire the disease at birth. In developed countries these methods of transmission have been virtually eliminated.

The two other routes of infection are from needle sharing by abusers of intravenous drugs, and by sexual intercourse. Anal intercourse carries a much higher risk of transmission than vaginal intercourse. The risk from the latter is increased by violence and the co-existence of other sexually transmitted infections. Further discussion of the epidemiology, treatment and prevention of AIDS is beyond the scope of this book. There is no cure or vaccine for HIV infection, but with modern treatment the interval between the infection and the development of AIDS can be prolonged.

HIV infection compromises the immune response and is a risk factor for all infections.

AIDS presents to the surgeon in many and varied ways and should be suspected in any patient in any of the risk groups. The manifestations fall into three main areas:

- **Common infections which become refractory or recurrent** after treatment, e.g. tuberculosis. The commonest type of surgery required in the UK for patients with AIDS is for perianal sepsis, accounting for one-quarter of all operations on those with the HIV infection.

- **Unusual infections** particularly associated with AIDS, e.g. oesophageal candidiasis.
- **AIDS-related tumours**, principally lymphomas and occasionally the classical Kaposi sarcoma.

HEPATITIS

Approximately 2 per cent of the population carry one of the various hepatitis viruses. The surgical importance lies in the risk that the surgeon may acquire the infection from an infected patient.

Hepatitis B antigen is found in the blood and body fluids of all carriers. The infection is spread by sexual intercourse, sharing needles by drug abusers, and at birth from an infected mother to her child. Immunization is available and effective.

Hepatitis C was known previously as non-A non-B hepatitis and is spread in a similar manner to hepatitis B. There is currently no vaccine available.

There are other varieties of viral hepatitis some of which only proliferate in the presence of hepatitis B infection.

Transmission of HIV and hepatitis to members of the surgical team

This risk can be summarized as:

- surgeon to patient – rarely if ever
- patient to surgeon – significant, depending on the patient's infection.

Transmission of a blood-borne virus from a patient to a surgeon or any other member of the operating team requires a blood contaminated 'sharp' or 'needlestick' injury. 'Sharp' injury includes stabs with scalpels, cuts from broken glass and injuries from bone spicules and teeth.

There is no risk from inhalation or skin-to-skin contact, but the mucous membranes of the mouth or eyes are vulnerable. The surgeon may have a skin abrasion that has not been noticed which introduces a risk. The chances of transmission vary with the virus (Table 3.8).

It should be remembered that the hepatitis and HIV status of the patient will not be known in most cases. Clearly the risks to operating staff will vary with the demography of the local population but,

Table 3.8
Risk of hepatitis and human immunodeficiency virus (HIV) transmission following a sharp or needlestick injury

Hepatitis B: 1 in 3
Hepatitis C: 1 in 30
HIV: 1 in 300

nevertheless, the risk of contracting these diseases can never be discounted entirely.

General safety measures against virus infections

- **Screening and immunization** of operating theatre staff against the disease. This is currently available only for hepatis B.
- **General hygiene** avoiding contact with blood and removing spilt blood rapidly.
- **Universal use of gowns, gloves and other physical barriers**.
- **Occlusive dressings** over minor wounds and abrasions.

Specific precautions in the operating theatre

- Dispose of 'sharps' immediately into strong containers.
- Avoid handling anything sharp – use instruments.
- Modify surgical technique so that suture needles are touched only by instruments and not by the fingers. This may not be possible in open abdominal surgery.
- Use blunt needles whenever possible, e.g. when closing the abdomen.
- Stop using sharp-edged instruments whenever possible; for example make incisions with diathermy and use stapling devices on bowel and skin.
- Embrace laparoscopic and other endoscopic techniques where, once the serous cavity is entered, there is a barrier between the surgeon and the surgical site.
- Cover the mouth and eyes. Masks do not reduce patient infections but they do reduce the risk to the surgical team of virus infection.

Action to be taken after an accidental needlestick or sharp injury

After a significant incident, it may be appropriate to test the patient for HIV and hepatitis status so as to assess the degree of risk. Where the patient is known to carry the virus the measures available are:

- **passive immunization** with immunoglobulin (for hepatitis B)
- **post-exposure prophylaxis**: immunization for hepatitis B, antiretroviral drugs for HIV.

Remember to file an official accident report.

It should not need to be stated that the best way for the surgeon to avoid the small but potentially catastrophic risk of acquiring an incurable virus disease from a patient in the operating theatre is scrupulous care and good surgical technique.

4

General and facial appearances

Bijan Modarai and Kevin G. Burnand

Most of the chapters in this book begin with a list of the problems caused by diseases in a single anatomical or physiological system, but the problems that patients complain of related to their general and facial appearance are caused by a wide variety of diseases in many systems and so they are presented separately.

CHANGES IN THE COLOUR OF THE SKIN

Patients may complain about their skin being pale, florid (red), blue or yellow. These changes may also be noted by others. The common causes of these problems are anaemia, polycythaemia, cyanosis and jaundice.

ANAEMIA

This condition can be defined as a reduction in the circulating red blood cell (RBC) mass causing a reduction in the concentration of haemoglobin (Hb) per unit volume (g/dL) below the accepted normal range for the age and gender of the patient.

Anaemia is defined by a low haemoglobin (<13.5 g/dL in men and <11.5 g/dL in women). The common causes of anaemia are listed in Table 4.1.

Investigation
Diagnostic clinical indicators

A thorough history is invaluable in attempting to identify the underlying cause of anaemia. The condition may present with **fatigue, breathlessness** and **vasovagal episodes**. The source of blood loss may be identified by enquiring about the passing of fresh blood per rectum, dark stools, indigestion and weight loss (e.g. peptic ulcer) and menstrual losses.

The patient's dietary habits (e.g. vegan) are also important. Any exposure to paints and solvents

Table 4.1
The common causes of anaemia

Blood loss

Haemorrhage: acute and chronic

Excessive destruction of red cells caused by:

Congenital red cell defects: spherocytosis, elliptocytosis, haemoglobinopathies, thalassaemias, acanthocytosis

Acquired red cell defects: metabolic disorders in the red cell (e.g. vitamin B12/folate/iron deficiency), thermal injury, drugs (e.g. quinine, penicillin)

External insults: infections (e.g. malaria), chemicals (e.g. lead, naphthalene, sulphonamides, nitrofurantoin), traumatic (e.g. prosthetic heart valve)

Splenic sequestration

Immune mechanisms: transfusion reactions, cold agglutinin syndrome (e.g. viral pneumonia), autoantibodies (e.g. leukaemia, lymphoma, idiopathic)

Disseminated intravascular coagulation: septicaemia, malignancy

Defective production of red cells caused by:

Deficiency of essential factors: iron deficiency (e.g. negative iron balance, pregnancy), folate deficiency (dietary, malabsorption, alcohol excess, anticonvulsant drugs, pregnancy, malignancy), vitamin B12 deficiency (e.g. intrinsic factor deficiency-pernicious anaemia, post gastrectomy, dietary, tapeworm infestation)

Impaired haemoglobin synthesis: primary sideroblastic anaemia, thalassaemia

Invasion of the bone marrow: leukaemia, fibrosis, secondary carcinoma

Endocrine abnormalities: hypothyroidism, hypopituitarism, hypoadrenalism

should be documented. A detailed drug history is important because drugs such as chloromycetin and cytotoxics can cause aplastic anaemia. A sore tongue may indicate folate deficiency while paraesthesia is associated with pernicious anaemia. Finally, it is important to know of any family history of anaemia.

The patient may be wasted and malnourished. There may be evidence of shortness of breath on minimal exertion and tachycardia or heart failure may indicate profound anaemia. The conjunctivae and palmar creases of the hands may appear pale with 'spoon-shaped' nails (koilonychia). The tongue may appear smooth and red. Patients with a haemolytic anaemia may appear mildly jaundiced. The abdomen should be examined for presence of hepatomegaly, splenomegaly (leukaemia and lymphoma) or a tumour mass. A pelvic and rectal examination may show blood or a tumour.

Blood tests

Plasma haematinics should be measured; these include **serum iron, serum ferritin, the total iron binding capacity, B12 and folate**. The **mean RBC volume (MCV)** is measured (normal is 80–96 fL) and can be used to classify the cause of the anaemia.

A blood film can also be useful for diagnosing the type of anaemia. In iron deficiency anaemia the red cells are hypochromic and a variety of cell sizes are seen on the blood film (poikilocytosis). Target cells are present in liver disease and thalassaemia. Haemoglobin electrophoresis is required to confirm the diagnosis of sickle cell anaemia (Fig 4.1).

A **Schilling test** determines whether B12 deficiency is the result of malabsorption from the terminal ileum or caused by the lack of intrinsic factor. An oral dose of radioactive B12 is given and the proportion excreted in the urine is measured before and after the administration of intrinsic factor. A lack of intrinsic factor (pernicious anaemia) is likely to be responsible for the anaemia if isotope uptake is enhanced by its addition.

Iron deficiency anaemia without an obvious source for blood loss should lead to a careful examination of the **gastrointestinal tract**. This may involve testing for faecal occult blood, gastroscopy and colonoscopy. A small bowel capsule biopsy, endoscopy or computed tomography (CT) angiography

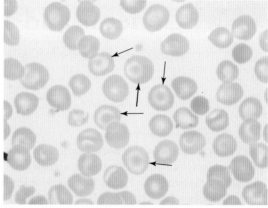

(A)

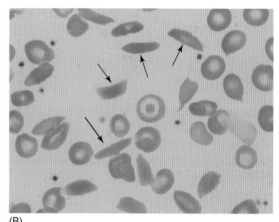

(B)

FIGURE 4.1 (A) The 'target cells' that are diagnostic of thalasaemia. (B) The distorted red cells, 'sickle cells', found in sickle-cell anaemia

may be required to identify the source of blood loss (see Chapter 18).

Management

Iron deficiency anaemia Oral iron supplements of **ferrous sulphate** should be given to patients with an iron deficiency anaemia (200 mg twice a day). The haemoglobin level will usually increase by 1 g/dL/week. Supplemental iron should be continued for at least 3 months after the haemoglobin level has returned to normal to ensure that the body's iron stores are completely replenished.

Anaemia secondary to chronic disease This is partly the result of a failure of erythropoietin production. **Recombinant erythropoietin** can be effective in restoring the haemoglobin level and is used extensively for patients with renal failure.

Blood transfusion should be avoided if at all possible until the cause of anaemia has been established (see page 55). Depending on the patient's symptoms (e.g. anaemia precipitating heart failure) and the underlying cause of the anaemia, blood is not usually given if the haemoglobin level is above 8 g/dL. **Packed red cells** are the transfusion product of choice.

Patients with **sickle-cell disease** who are symptomless and have a stable haemoglobin level do not require treatment. Red cell **exchange transfusions** should be considered when patients develop complications related to sickle cell disease or before anaesthesia. A painful sickle 'crisis' is best managed by warming the patient as well as giving oxygen, intravenous fluids and antibiotics.

Patients with **haemolytic anaemia** can be given high doses of **oral prednisolone**. This may be effective but a **splenectomy** is often eventually required.

Aplastic anaemia may be treated by blood and platelet transfusions. **Immunosuppresion** with high doses of steroids or cyclosporine may be effective. In severe cases a bone **marrow transplant** may be necessary.

POLYCYTHAEMIA

Polycythaemia is an increase in the red blood cell count, the haematocrit and the haemoglobin.

True polycythaemia occurs when there is an increase in the red cell mass. A decrease in plasma volume can lead to a relative polycythaemia.

Polycythaemia rubera vera is a myeloproliferative disorder which causes uncontrolled production of red cells by the bone marrow.

The causes of polycythaemia are listed in Table 4.2.

Investigation
Diagnostic clinical indicators
The patient typically has a **plethoric appearance**.

The sequelae of polycythaemia rubera vera include hypertension, gout, arterial and venous thrombosis. Splenomegaly and lymphadenopathy may be associated features and malignancy may develop.

Conditions associated with an increased production of erythropoietin can lead to a 'secondary' polycythaemia.

Table 4.2
The causes of polycythaemia

Relative polycythaemia
- Pyrexia
- Vomiting
- Diarrhoea

Primary polycythaemia
- Polycythaemia rubera vera

Secondary polycythaemia
- Acclimatization to high altitude
- Respiratory diseases, e.g. chronic obstructive pulmonary disease
- Cyanotic heart disease, e.g. Eisenmenger's syndrome
- Erythropoietin secreting tumours, e.g. hepatoma, carcinoma of kidney
- Increased erythropoietin from kidney, e.g. renal cysts, pyonephrosis

Blood tests
The red blood cell count, haematocrit and haemoglobin and uric acid are raised.

A high platelet count, white cell count and alkaline phosphatase suggest polycythaemia rubera vera rather than a secondary cause.

Management
The main aim is to reduce blood viscosity and prevent thrombosis and stroke.

Venesection is used to reduce the blood viscosity, which is in turn measured by a reduction in packed cell volume.

The patient may be given **aspirin** or anticoagulated with **warfarin** to prevent or treat thrombosis.

Cytotoxic drugs such as **hydroxyurea** can be used to suppress erythropoiesis and are required if malignancy develops.

CYANOSIS

The term cyanosis refers to a blue-purple discoloration of the skin caused either by deoxygenation of the central arterial blood (central cyanosis) or a stagnant flow of blood in the extremities caused by peripheral vasoconstriction (peripheral cyanosis).

The causes of cyanosis are listed in Table 4.3.

Investigation

Diagnostic clinical indicators

Central cyanosis affects the lips and tongue and the patient's peripheries are usually warm. Peripheral cyanosis occurs when the fingertips and toes are blue and cold but the lips and tongue are pink.

It is important to seek for any of the above predisposing conditions that may make the patient susceptible to cyanosis and exclude any exposure to drugs (e.g. methaemoglobin) and cold (e.g. Raynaud's phenomenon).

The examination should elicit if the patient is short of breath, has any signs of clubbing, cardiac murmurs or heart failure (e.g. ankle/feet swelling, chest crepitations, raised jugular venous pressure).

Blood tests

These should include **pulse oximetry**, which shows an oxygen saturation (SaO_2) of <85 per cent. The oxygen saturation will not increase in response to oxygen therapy if cardiac pathology is the cause of cyanosis. The oxygen saturation will usually improve, however, if lung disease is responsible.

Arterial blood gas analysis is usually normal in patients with peripheral cyanosis but demonstrates hypoxia (PaO_2 <8 kPa) with a low SaO_2 in central cyanosis. A full blood count may indicate a profound anaemia or polycythaemia.

Methaemoglobinaemia can mimic cyanosis and should be excluded.

Bacteriology

A sputum sample should be sent if the patient presents with an infective exacerbation of chronic obstructive airways disease (COAD).

Electrocardiography

An **ECG** may indicate ischaemia, arrythmias, hypertrophy of the ventricle or right heart strain (e.g. a possible pulmonary embolism).

Imaging

A **chest X-ray** may show an enlarged heart and fluid in the lung fields (heart failure).

Management

First secure and maintain the airway, breathing and circulation. **Endotracheal intubation** may be required. Subsequent management is treatment of the underlying cause.

Central cyanosis **Diuretics and vasodilators** such as glyceryl trinitrate may be indicated for heart failure. Anaemic patients and those in shock may require **blood transfusion**. Congentital cardiac disease and cardiac valvular disease can be treated by either open surgery or percutaneous intervention.

Table 4.3
The causes of cyanosis

Peripheral cyanosis

Peripheral arterial disease (e.g. claudication, rest pain)

Vasoconstriction (e.g. hypothermia, Raynaud's phenomenon, acrocyanosis)

Venous thrombosis (e.g. phlegmasia cerulea dolens)

Acute left ventricular failure

Hypovolaemic shock

Central cyanosis

Respiratory disease

Chronic obstructive pulmonary disease (COPD)

Pulmonary embolism

Asthma

Airway obstruction

Laryngeal trauma

Foreign body in the airway

Tracheal stenosis

Bronchial carcinoma

Carcinoma of the trachea

Trauma (e.g. pneumothorax or lung injury)

Cardiac disease

Cardiac valve disease

Congenital heart disease with right to left blood shunting (e.g. patent ductus arteriosus, tetralogy of Fallot, transposition, pulmonary atresia)

Peripheral cyanosis Patients with Raynaud's phenomenon should keep their peripheries warm. Vasodilators (e.g. calcium channel antagonists) are of limited value (see Chapter 11).

JAUNDICE

Jaundice is caused by an excess of bile pigments in the plasma. Jaundice is clinically suspected when there is yellow discoloration of the skin and sclera. Other diagnostic indicators include pale stools and dark urine. Obstructive jaundice may be accompanied by itching. Abdominal pain indicates gallstones. A history of weight loss suggests an underlying malignancy of the pancreas.

Table 4.4
The main causes of jaundice

Prehepatic

Increased haemolysis: thalassaemia, spherocytosis, sickle cell disease

Malaria

Crigler–Najjar syndrome

Gilbert's syndrome

Rhesus incompatibility

Hepatic

Viral hepatitis

Alcoholic hepatitis

Primary biliary cirrhosis

Toxic drugs (e.g. paracetamol overdose, isoniazid, pyrazinamide, rifampicin, halothane, sulfonylureas, phenothiazines, methyldopa, barbiturates)

Haemochromatosis

Post hepatic

Gallstones

Pancreatic malignancy compressing bile duct

Bile duct malignancies

Metastatic lymphadenopathy (e.g. porta hepatis lymph nodes)

Chronic pancreatitis

Bile duct strictures

Choledochal cysts

Enquiries should include a history of blood transfusions, recent foreign travel, sexual contacts, daily alcohol consumption and drug ingestion.

The main causes of jaundice are listed in Table 4.4.

The investigation and management of jaundice caused by disease in the alimentary tract is fully discussed in Chapter 18.

WASTING

CACHEXIA

Cachexia is the term used to describe a generalized wasting caused by excessive weight loss, lipolysis and muscle atrophy. The common causes are listed in Table 4.5.

Investigation

Diagnostic clinical indicators

The amount and time course of weight loss and dietary intake should be documented. Associated symptoms include weakness, lethargy and any symptoms related to the underlying malignancy or infection.

Table 4.5
The common causes of cachexia

Carcinoma (e.g. stomach, oesophagus, pancreas, ovary, melanoma, secondaries)

Tuberculosis

AIDS

Mesenteric ischaemia

Diabetes

Thyrotoxicosis

Severe cardiorespiratory disease

Malabsorption syndromes

Crohn's disease

Radiation bowel disease

Gastrointestinal fistula

Renal failure

Anorexia nervosa

Motor neurone disease

Kwashiokor

The most common causes are malignant disease and chronic infections that produce a catabolic state. Clubbing of the fingernails and lymphadenopathy may indicate a tumour.

The specific signs of the many diseases listed in Table 4.5 may be present.

Blood tests

The plasma albumin concentration is decreased. The blood sugar, white cell count, thyroid function tests, erythrocyte sedimentation rate (ESR) and C-reactive protein should be measured.

Tumour markers such as CEA, CA125 and CA19-9 should be requested.

Imaging

A **chest X-ray** and **CT scan of chest and abdomen** may reveal an occult malignancy of the lung, stomach, oesophagus or pancreas. **Endoscopy** of upper and lower GI tract and **mesenteric angiography** may be helpful.

Management

The underlying cause must be treated but this may require an operation on a malnourished patient. Such patients are more susceptible to complications after surgery, chemotherapy and radiotherapy.

Aggressive **nutritional supplementation** before any intervention can reduce the associated risks (see page 56). Patients may require **dietary advice**, supplemental **nasogastric feeding** or even **parenteral nutrition** if food cannot be given through the gastrointestinal tract. In patients with an obstruction of the upper gastrointestinal tract (e.g. oesophageal or mouth cancer) a **percutaneous endoscopic gastrostomy** can be used for nutritional supplementation.

Corticosteroids can help with weakness, anorexia and are anti-emetic.

Prokinetics like **metoclopramide** can improve nausea and the early satiety that patients with gastroparesis can experience.

MULTIPLE SWOLLEN GLANDS

LYMPHADENOPATHY

This term refers to enlarged lymph nodes found in any anatomical site. The causes of lymphadenopathy, whether generalized or localized, are listed in Table 4.6.

Investigation

Diagnostic clinical indicators

The history should indicate whether there are symptoms suggestive of an infection or malignancy at a particular site. Constitutional symptoms such as fatigue, night sweats or weight loss may be present. The patient's current or recent medication may have caused lymphadenopathy. Details of foreign travel, sexual activity and intravenous drug abuse should be recorded

The finding of palpable lymph nodes (as large as 1.5 cm) may be normal in pre-pubertal children. In adults lymph nodes greater than 1 cm diameter are considered abnormal. Generalized lymphadenopathy refers to enlargement of lymph nodes in two or more non-contiguous areas.

Tender, warm nodes beneath reddened skin suggests lymphadenitis. A careful examination of the territory drained by the nodes should be carried out to ascertain the source of the infection.

Non-tender, firm/hard and matted (connected together) lymph nodes suggests malignancy.

The differential diagnosis of both single and multiple lumps includes lipomata and neurofibromata.

Blood tests

A **full blood count** may show a raised white blood cell (WBC) count in the presence of infection or anaemia secondary to malignancy. The **C-reactive protein and the ESR** are often raised in infection and malignancy. **Liver and renal function tests** may be abnormal and indicate systemic disorder. **Viral titres** (e.g. HIV, Epstein–Barr) should be measured. An autoantibody screen is helpful to diagnose systemic lupus erythematosus or rheumatoid arthritis.

A **Mantoux test** is indicated to exclude tuberculosis. A **Kveim test** is required if sarcoidosis is suspected.

Imaging

A **chest X-ray** will show mediastinal lymphadenopathy in sarcoidosis and may show evidence of a primary or secondary malignancy or tuberculosis.

Ultrasound examination of the enlarged lymph node may distinguish malignant lymphadenopathy from a benign aetiology.

A CT scan of the chest, abdomen and pelvis may reveal the distribution of enlarged nodes, as well as

Table 4.6
The causes of lymphadenopathy

Generalized

Infective

Viral upper respiratory tract infections

Infectious mononucleosis (Epstein–Barr virus)

Measles

HIV

Cytomegalovirus

Tuberculosis

Syphilis

Typhoid fever

Toxoplasmosis

Primary neoplastic (e.g. lymphomas, leukaemias)

Secondary neoplastic (e.g. bronchus, stomach, breast)

Autoimmune (e.g. systemic lupus erythematosis, rheumatoid arthritis)

Storage disorders

Gaucher's disease

Niemann Pick disease

Drugs

Phenytoin

Allopurinol

Cephalosporins

Sulfonamides

Miscellaneous

Histiocytoses

Localized

Cervical

Upper respiratory tract infections

Infectious mononucleosis

Toxoplasmosis

Tuberculosis

Leukaemia

Lymphoma

Local skin infections

Supraclavicular

Lung cancer

Lymphoma

Gastrointestinal cancer

Axillary

Lymphoma

Infections

Breast cancer

Melanoma

Mediastinal

Lymphoma

Leukaemia

Tuberculosis

Sarcoidosis

Inguinal

Infections of leg or foot (e.g. ulcer, athletes foot)

Sexually transmitted diseases (e.g. herpes simplex, gonococcus)

Lymphoma

Pelvic malignancy

Melanoma and other skin cancers

any malignancy. It is an important staging tool for lymphoma.

Tissue biopsy

An **excisional biopsy** is indicated if a lymphoma is suspected, as it allows the architecture of the enlarged node to be assessed accurately.

Fine needle aspiration is indicated if secondary malignancy is suspected.

Management

Treatment of a lymphoma is by chemotherapy and/or radiotherapy. In cases where secondary malignant deposits are the cause of lymphadenopathy, resection of the primary tumour with radiotherapy and/or chemotherapy is the treatment of choice. If the primary tumour is disseminated and resection not thought to be curative then the patient will need palliative care (see page 22).

Patients with leukaemia are given chemotherapy.

Infected lymph nodes are treated by drainage of the abscess and antibiotics (see page 46).

PRURITIS (ITCHING) AND EXCORIATION

Itching of the skin excites the urge to scratch. Patients may present complaining of the itching or with the problems caused by their involuntary excoriation.

Itching may be caused by many conditions some of which are listed in Table 4.7.

Investigation

Diagnostic clinical indicators

It is important to distinguish the systemic causes of pruritis from a skin disorder. A thorough history should include time of onset of symptoms, severity, relationship to activities (e.g. hot/cold, bathing).

The skin should be examined closely for excoriation, signs of chronic itching, nodules and lichen simplex.

Signs of liver disease (jaundice, gynaecomastia, ascites, spider naevi) may be present. The patient may be uraemic. Both hypothyroidism and hyperthyroidism can cause pruritis. A malignant process may be indicated by the presence of lymphadenopathy, weight loss and icthyosis.

Blood tests

The **full blood count** may be abnormal, indicating polycythaemia, iron deficiency anaemia or haematological malignancy.

Liver function tests may show an elevated bilirubin and alkaline phosphatase if pruritis is hepatic in origin.

Urea and creatinine are elevated in renal failure.

Thyroid-stimulating hormone (TSH) and **thyroxine** levels may be abnormal.

Hepatitis and **HIV serology** should be measured.

Stools should be sent for faecal **occult blood testing** (gastrointestinal malignancy) and microscoped for parasites.

Imaging

Chest X-ray should be carried out to exclude lung pathology (e.g. mediastinal lymphadenopathy or hilar lymphadenopathy).

An **ultrasound scan** of the abdomen should be carried out if liver/biliary pathology is suspected.

Table 4.7
Some of the causes of itching

Dermatological causes

Scabies

Insect bites

Eczema/dermatitis

Lichen planus

Urticaria

Dermatitis herpertiformis

Pemphigoid

Systemic causes

HIV infection/AIDS

Thyrotoxicosis

Diabetes

Parasites (e.g. hookworms)

Sarcoidosis

Drugs (e.g. morphine)

Cholestasis

Obstructive jaundice

Primary biliary cirrhosis

Hepatitis C

Primary sclerosing cholangitis

Malignant disease

Lymphoma

Leukaemia

Carcinoid syndrome

Gastrointestinal malignancies

Myeloma

Haematological conditions

Polycythaemia rubera vera

Iron deficiency anaemia

Essential thrombocythaemia

Chronic renal failure (especially if on haemodialysis)

Management

The patient should be encouraged to wear **light clothing** and **avoid the heat**. **Antihistamines** are of limited benefit if there is an underlying systemic cause for pruritis.

Pruritis secondary to renal failure responds well to ultraviolet therapy and topical **tacrolimus** ointment.

For cholestatic pruritis, **cholestyramine** has some effect but treatment with **rifampicin** and opioid antagonists such as **naloxone** may be required.

5HT blockers (e.g. **mirtazapine**) may provide relief for cancer patients. Tricyclic antidepressants may also be effective.

Relief of biliary obstruction by placing a stent is effective.

Pruritis can be an independent indicator of a poor prognosis in patients with renal disease and malignancy.

CHANGES IN FACIAL APPEARANCE

SCLERODERMA

Investigation

Diagnostic clinical indicators

Scleroderma makes the skin thick, shiny and tight. These changes may be visible in the hands, face and feet. The tightening of the skin of the face makes the mouth small and tight (microstomia).

Other skin changes in diffuse scleroderma (systemic sclerosis) include skin ulcers, vitiligo, dry eyes and mouth (Sjögren's syndrome) and Raynaud's phenomenon. A limited form of scleroderma is known as the CREST (calcinosis, Raynaud's phenomenon, oesophageal problems, scleroderma, telangiectases) syndrome. It consists of calcinosis, Raynaud's phenomenon, oesophageal dysmotility and telangiectasia.

The diffuse and more malignant form of scleroderma, also known as systemic sclerosis, can involve many organs and cause pulmonary fibrosis, pulmonary hypertension, renal failure, primary biliary cirrhosis and pericardial effusions.

Blood tests

The clinical diagnosis may be confirmed by detecting raised levels of **autoantibodies**. In over 97 per cent of patients the anti-nuclear antibody is positive.

Urine testing may show proteinuria.

Imaging

A **chest X-ray** may reveal pulmonary fibrosis (Fig 4.2). **Hand X-rays** may show deposits of calcium at the fingertips (Fig 4.3). A **barium swallow** may demonstrate oesophageal dysmotility.

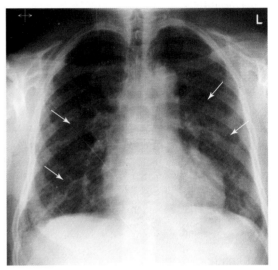

FIGURE 4.2 An X-ray of the diffuse pulmonary fibrosis that may develop in scleroderma

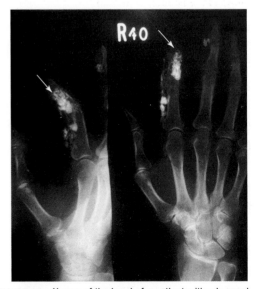

FIGURE 4.3 X-rays of the hand of a patient with advanced scleroderma and the CREST syndrome showing extensive deposits of calcium in the soft tissues of the index finger

Management

There is no definitive treatment for scleroderma.

Immunosuppresants such as **cyclophosphamide** and **methotrexate** can be effective in its early phase.

Raynaud's phenomenon can be managed by keeping the extremities warm, avoiding exposure to cold weather and using **vasodilator drugs** such as calcium channel blockers. Severe digital ulceration may respond to courses of **intravenous prostacyclin**.

Prognosis Scleroderma that is only manifest as cutaneous changes is the milder form and carries a better prognosis. If there is systemic involvement, only 50 per cent survive 10 years.

MYXOEDEMA

The myxoedematous (hypothyroid) patient appears overweight and mentally sluggish. The hair and skin often appear dry. There may be non-pitting oedema of the extremities.

The causes of myxoedema are listed in Table 4.8.

Investigation

Diagnostic clinical indicators

Symptoms include lethargy, weight gain, intolerance of cold, constipation, depression, hoarse voice and in severe cases cognitive impairment or dementia. A goitre may be palpable. Other signs include bradycardia, dry skin, hair loss and slowly relaxing reflexes. Signs of congestive cardiac failure may be present. Severe myxoedema can lead to coma.

Blood tests

Typically the **serum thyroxine** (T4) is low. The **TSH** is raised very occasionally, but is low or normal if pituitary dysfunction has led to myxoedema. The

---

Table 4.8
The causes of myxoedema

Primary autoimmune myxoedema

Post thyroidectomy

Post radioiodine treatment

Secondary to drugs (e.g. lithium, amiodarone)

Iodine deficiency

---

blood **cholesterol** and **triglycerides** are usually raised.

Electrocardiography

An **ECG** may show a sinus bradycardia and a prolonged QT interval.

Management

The treatment of myxoedema is by **oral thyroxine**. Patients in hypothermic coma should be treated with intravenous thyroxine.

ACROMEGALY

Acromegaly usually presents after the age of 30 and is caused by excess secretion of growth hormone by a pituitary tumour.

Investigation

Diagnostic clinical indicators

The patient may have noticed a change in their appearance and a change in the quality of their voice. A large face and jaw (macrognathism) is usually apparent (see *Symptoms and Signs*).

The soft tissues of the face, nose, lips and tongue are enlarged. The skin is oily and coarse with prominent supraorbital ridges, a large tongue (macroglossia), a deep voice and spade-like hands. Comparing old photographs with the patient's current appearance may be useful.

Patients can develop hypertension, diabetes mellitus, left ventricular hypertrophy and cardiomyopathy.

Blood tests

Growth hormone levels are raised. An oral **glucose tolerance test** should be carried out measuring both the glucose and growth hormone levels over 2 hours after an infusion of glucose. Growth hormone is suppressed by glucose in normal individuals but not in acromegalics. Diabetes develops in over a quarter of acromegalics and **hyperprolactinaemia** is also common.

Imaging

The pituitary fossa is imaged using **magnetic resonance imaging (MRI)** to discover if it is enlarged by a tumour (Fig 4.4).

The visual fields should be tested as bitemporal field loss may be present.

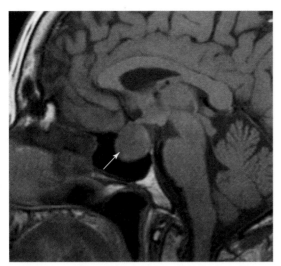

FIGURE 4.4   A sagittal T1 MRI image of the enlarged pituitary fossa of a patient with acromegaly

Management

Left untreated the prognosis for the patient is poor. Most patients die from heart failure. **Transsphenoidal surgery** to remove the pituitary tumour is now the treatment of choice and is successful in over 70 per cent of cases.

External beam radiotherapy to destroy the tumour is another option in older patients or in those in whom surgery has failed.

Somatostatin analogues such as **octreotide** can be used as an adjunct for cases resistant to surgical treatment or radiotherapy, or for short-term disease control.

DOWN'S SYNDROME

This is a congenital abnormality resulting from the presence of an extra chromosome 21 (trisomy 21), which causes mental retardation and floppiness. It is associated with advanced maternal age. The risk of having a child with Down's syndrome in a mother age 45 is 1200 fold higher than in a child born to a mother 10 years younger.

Investigation
Diagnostic clinical indicators
The characteristic facial appearance results from the outer ends of the palpaberal fissures slanting upwards and prominent epicanthic folds (see

Symptoms and Signs). The face is flattened and the tongue protrudes. A transverse palmar crease and clinodactyly may also be present. The patient has a short stature. There may be a co-existing squint and a congenital cardiac defect.

Thyroid function tests should be ordered to exclude myxoedema, and the visual acuity should be tested.

Amniocentesis and chromosome studies

Down's syndrome can be diagnosed pre-natally on amniotic fluid samples obtained by amniocentesis. The diagnosis can be confirmed post-natally with cytogenetic studies.

Imaging
A **cervical X-ray** is required to exclude atlantoaxial instability. **Echocardiography** will delineate any congenital cardiac abnormalities.

Management

There are many anomalies associated with Down's syndrome. A multidisciplinary approach is essential.

Surgical care may involve the correction of gastrointestinal pathology including pyloric stenosis, Hirschprung's disease, duodenal atresia, tracheo-oesophageal fistula, megacolon or an imperforate anus (see Chapters 18 and 19).

The airway may pose a challenge to the anaesthetist (e.g. in the presence of atlantoaxial instability).

Other surgical interventions can include **adenotonsillectomy** (to alleviate sleep apnoea), extraction of **congenital cataracts** and correction of cardiac defects.

Up to 20 per cent of patients with Down's syndrome develop **hypothyroidism**. Other medical problems include diabetes, seizures, otitis media and hearing loss. The mortality from this condition is greatest in the first year of life but a relatively high proportion of patients are now surviving into adulthood.

CUSHING'S SYNDROME

This is a syndrome caused by an excess of adrenal glucocorticoids (e.g. cortisol). The underlying causes are listed in Table 4.9.

Table 4.9
The causes of Cushing's syndrome

Adrenal adenoma

Adrenal hyperplasia

Steroid therapy

Adrenocorticotrophic hormone (ACTH) producing tumour of pituitary gland (Cushing's disease)

Ectopic ACTH production (e.g. small cell tumour of the lung)

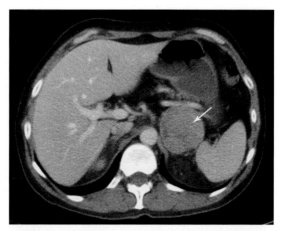

FIGURE 4.5   Computed tomography of an adrenal tumour

Investigation
Diagnostic clinical indicators

Weight gain, irregular menses, hirsutism and impotence are common symptoms.

The patient puts weight on the face, neck and trunk. The face may appear 'moon shaped'. The arms and legs stay thin. Striae develop, especially over the abdomen where the skin becomes stretched. There is excessive fat laid down over the trunk and a 'buffalo hump' may be present.

Hypertension, hyperglycaemia and osteoporosis are often detected.

Function tests

An overnight **dexamethasone suppression test** should be carried out. Dexamethasone is a synthetic steroid that is similar to cortisol. It reduces adrenocorticotrophic hormone (ACTH) release in normal individuals; therefore, administration of dexamethasone should lead to a reduction in cortisol levels. Cortisol levels remain unchanged after administration of dexamethasone in a patient with Cushing's syndrome.

Imaging

Abdominal CT is the best investigation to demonstrate adrenal tumours (Fig 4.5). **MRI of the pituitary fossa** may show a pituitary tumour (Fig 4.4).

Management

Surgery can be used to treat adrenal adenomata by either open or laparoscopic excision of the affected adrenal gland (**adrenalectomy**).

Pituitary tumours can be treated by either excision via a transnasal approach or external beam radiotherapy.

ACTH production by ectopic tissue not suitable for surgical removal can be treated with agents such as **metyrapone** that inhibit steroid synthesis.

FACIAL AND HEAD APPEARANCES

FACIAL NERVE PALSY

This presents with an inability to use the muscles of facial expression and speak clearly. The damage may lie in the upper or lower motor neurones of the nerves.

The underlying causes are listed in Table 4.10.

Investigation
Diagnostic clinical indicators

The facial weakness may have been preceded by earache or it may have developed rapidly without a cause (Bell's palsy). There may be a history of trauma. Chewing food and speaking may be difficult. The anterior part of the tongue may lose the power of taste. The corner of the mouth usually sags.

The eye may become irritated and dry as a consequence of an inability to close the eyelids. The eyelids may not oppose and there is inability to wrinkle the forehead. (The ability to wrinkle the

Table 4.10
The causes of facial nerve palsy

Local

Idiopathic (Bell's palsy)

Infection

    Herpes zoster – Ramsay Hunt syndrome

    HIV

    Meningitis

    Leprosy

    Tuberculosis

    Polio

    Lyme disease

Sarcoidosis

Metabolic

    Diabetes mellitus

    Hyperthyroidism

Guillan Barré syndrome

Neoplastic

    Parotid tumours

    Cholesteatomas

Trauma

    Temporal bone fracture/facial trauma

    Trauma to the skull base

    Forceps delivery

    Barotrauma (diving)

Central

Stroke

Neoplastic

    Acoustic neuroma

    Brain tumour

Multiple sclerosis

Otitis media

Myasthenia gravis

Brain abscess

Subdural haematoma

forehead is preserved if an upper motor neurone lesion is the cause.)

A red, herpetiform vesicular rash will be seen in the mouth or on the ear in cases of Ramsay Hunt syndrome.

A lumbar puncture and analysis of cerebrospinal fluid may aid diagnosis in atypical cases.

Blood tests
A full blood count, ESR, Lyme titre and antibody levels for varicella zoster may be helpful.

Imaging
A **CT scan** is useful in cases where a stroke is suspected and an **MRI scan** should be obtained for suspected brain, head and neck tumours.

Function studies
Electromyography and **nerve conduction** studies delineate the extent of injury to the facial nerve and can predict the time to recovery.

Management
The use of **steroids** for Bell's palsy is controversial but there is some evidence that they have a beneficial effect.

Antiviral agents such as **acyclovir** are sometimes given, as the cause of Bell's palsy is likely to be viral. The same agents are advocated for Ramsay Hunt syndrome.

Eye care is of paramount importance and lubricants should be regularly administered and eye shields prescribed to protect the eye from injury.

Prognosis Approximately 75 per cent of patients with Bell's palsy recover completely within 3 weeks. Less than 10 per cent develop a recurrent palsy.

HORNER'S SYNDROME
This clinical syndrome is caused by the interruption of sympathetic nerve supply to the head and neck.

The underlying causes of Horner's syndrome are listed in Table 4.11.

Investigation
Diagnostic clinical indicators
The eye cannot be completely opened on the affected side. There is an absence of sweating on one side of the face. Ipsilateral pain in the head, neck or face may also be experienced especially when it is the result of carotid artery dissection.

Table 4.11
The causes of Horner's syndrome

Injury to the lower roots of the brachial plexus

Malignancy, e.g. apical lung tumour, cervical malignancy (e.g. thyroid)

Injury to the base of neck resulting in high cervical cord lesion

Brain pathology: tumour, posterior inferior cerebellar artery thrombosis

Cervical sympathectomy (iatrogenic damage to stellate ganglion)

Aneurysm and dissection of the carotid artery and aortic arch

Spinal cord lesions: syringomyelia, tumours

The pupil on the affected side is small (miosis) with drooping of the eyelid (ptosis) and absence of sweating of the cheek on the same side (anhidrosis), which often appears pink and is warm.

The **differential diagnoses** of Horner's syndrome include:

▨ simple ptosis secondary to an oculomotor lesion
▨ Argyll Robertson pupil
▨ Holmes–Adie syndrome
▨ senile miosis
▨ drugs causing miosis (e.g. opioids and antipsychotics such as haloperidol).

The cocaine drop test

The cocaine drop test can be used to confirm the diagnosis. Cocaine blocks the reuptake of noradrenaline, which causes dilatation of a normal pupil. The pupil does not dilate in Horner's syndrome. This test is rarely required as the diagnosis is usually clear-cut.

Imaging

A **chest X-ray** or preferably a **CT scan** might show a tumour in the apex of the lung or a widened mediastinum in the presence of an aortic arch aneurysm.

A CT scan of the head may demonstrate cerebral pathology.

CT angiography of the head and neck is required if an aneurysm or dissection of the carotid artery or aortic arch is suspected (Fig 4.6).

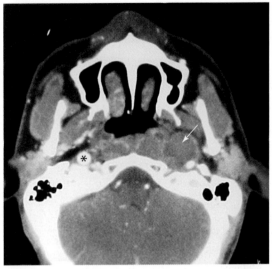

FIGURE 4.6 Computed tomography angiography of carotid dissection. The lumen of the left carotid artery is compressed by the large mass of blood in the anterior aspect of the split artery wall. As the mass does not contain contrast medium it is no longer in communication with the lumen of the artery or has clotted.
*normal carotid artery.

Management

The underlying condition causing the syndrome should be identified and treated. For example, carotid artery dissection may require stenting. Recovery is rare if the syndrome follows a sympathectomy.

Apical lung tumours (Pancoast's tumour) are rarely operable and may be palliated by radiotherapy and chemotherapy. Surgery can be considered to correct the ptosis.

The prognosis depends on how the underlying cause responds to treatment.

ECTROPION

Ectropion is abnormal eversion of the lower eyelid. The common causes are weak musculature associated with old age, facial trauma and burns.

Investigation
Diagnostic clinical indicators

Patients complain of tears running down their face (epiphoria).

There may be a history of facial trauma or burns. A facial nerve palsy may be present.

The lower lid sags away from the sclera, which is very often inflamed and red. There may be corneal ulceration or corneal keratinization.

The diagnosis is based solely on the clinical signs.

The **differential diagnoses** include cancers of the eyelid (e.g. basal cell carcinoma, squamous cell carcinoma), icthyosis, Bell's palsy and floppy eyelid syndrome.

Management

Lubricating drops and local anaesthetics can give symptomatic relief.

Surgical correction is achieved by full-thickness resection of part of the eyelid combined with tightening of the orbicularis occuli muscle.

ENTROPION

Entropion is inversion of the eyelid, usually a consequence of scarring from trachoma or persistent screwing up of the eyelids and rubbing in older people.

Investigation

Diagnostic clinical indicators

There may be a history of eye irritation and discomfort caused by the lashes rubbing against the conjunctiva and cornea. The eyelids appear inverted. Corneal abrasions and scars may be apparent.

The diagnosis is based solely on the clinical signs. The **differential diagnoses** include distichiasis and trichiasis.

Management

Strapping the lower eyelid into a normal position is a temporizing measure.

Surgical treatment involves shortening the tarsal plate and excising a portion of the orbicularis oculi muscle to cause scarring and weakness of the muscle and prevent inversion. There is a risk of late recurrence.

EXOPHTHALMOS

Exophthalmos, or proptosis, is forward protrusion of the eye from its normal position in the orbit. Any swelling or a tumour within the orbital space can push the eyeball forwards.

Investigation

Diagnostic clinical indicators

The physical signs are described in detail in *Symptoms and Signs*.

The abnormality is usually noticed by the patient, their relatives or friends. Pain, loss of visual fields or loss of visual acuity may develop. Diplopia is common especially if there is an eccentric swelling within the orbit. There may be a history of head and neck trauma. Thyrotoxicosis is an important cause of exopthalmos. The patient should be questioned on about the symptoms associated with hyperthyroidism (see Chapter 13).

The conjunctiva may be oedematous and wrinkled (chemosis). Corneal ulcers may be present. The globe may be pulsatile, suggesting the presence of an arteriovenous malformation. Auscultation may reveal a bruit indicative of **carotid cavernous fistula**. Signs of thyrotoxicosis may be apparent. Orbital cellulitis may cause a cavernous sinus thrombosis.

Local infection causes pain, periorbital swelling and erythema before the orbit becomes immobile and blindness develops.

Eye tests

Visual acuity, visual fields and eye movements should be tested.

Blood studies

Patients with suspected orbital cellulitis should have a **full blood count** and measurement of **inflammatory markers**.

Thyroid function tests should be carried out.

Imaging

A **CT or MRI scan** should be carried out if orbital or periorbital tumours are suspected. **CT angiography** of the head should display carotid cavernous fistula or a cavernous sinus thrombosis.

Management

Orbital cellulitis requires urgent **broad-spectrum antibiotic** treatment and carries a good prognosis if diagnosed and treated promptly. Pus should be urgently drained to avoid blindness if there is evidence of compression of the optic nerve.

Patients with thyrotoxicosis require treatment of the underlying condition (see Chapter 13).

A **lateral tarsorrhaphy** (suture of the eyelids to each other) can protect the cornea from abrasions and ulcers. Part of the orbit can be removed to reduce the orbital pressure.

A cavernous sinus thrombosis requires urgent treatment with **antibiotics**, but despite treatment carries a poor prognosis with a mortality rate of 30 per cent and a serious complications rate (e.g. blindness, ophthalmoplegia) in a further 30 per cent of cases.

A carotid cavernous fistula can be treated with **embolization**.

XANTHALASMA

Xanthalasma are intradermal creamy/yellow plaques usually in the medial aspect of the upper and lower eyelids. In up to half of patients they are associated with elevated plasma lipid levels.

Investigation

Diagnostic clinical indicators

The diagnosis is made on the clinical appearance. Patients often present because they are worried about their appearance: they are soft, yellow plaques.

The **differential diagnoses** include rodent ulcers, deposits secondary to sarcoidosis and necrobiosis lipoidica.

Blood tests

Plasma lipid levels, high-density lipoprotein (HDL) cholesterol and low-density lipoprotein (LDL) cholesterol should be measured

Management

These small slightly raised yellow patches are usually inconsequential and should be left alone.

They can be removed by surgical excision or using a carbon dioxide and argon laser but the recurrence rate is up to 30 per cent.

Statins should be prescribed if the blood lipids and cholesterol are elevated.

MICROGNATHISM

In this abnormality the lower third of the face is undersized compared with the rest of the face and skull giving the patient a 'bird face' type appearance.

Table 4.12
The causes of micrognathism

Pierre Robin syndrome
Treacher Collins syndrome
Foetal alcohol syndrome
Di George's syndrome
Trisomy 13
Trisomy 18
Cri du chat syndrome

The causes of micrognathism are listed in Table 4.12.

Investigation

Dental and skull X-rays confirm malgrowth of the bones. Appropriate **chromosome and genetic testing** for associated syndromes should be carried out.

Management

The lower jaw can be advanced and reshaped by osteotomies. This is done in conjunction with an orthodontist to ensure that a good dental occlusion is restored.

LUMPS ON THE HEAD

There are many conditions that cause localized swellings on the head, such as:

- lipomata
- sebaceous cysts
- dermoid cysts
- osteomata
- neurofibromata
- vascular malformations
- squamous cell carcinomas.

The treatment of the majority is by simple surgical excision.

CRANIOSYNOSTOSIS

This is a deformity of the skull as a consequence of premature fusion of the sutures between individual bones. The most common is premature fusion of

Table 4.13
The causes of craniosynostosis

Primary

Defects in the fibroblast growth factor receptors

Defective osteoclastic activity

Secondary

Hypercalcaemia

Vitamin D deficiency

Hyperthyroidism

Hypophosphataemia

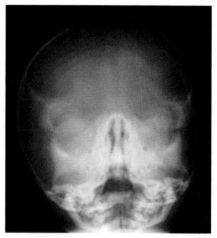

FIGURE 4.7 AP Skull X-ray showing the absence of suture lines in a baby with craniosynostosis

the sagittal suture causing an elongated head with a keel-shaped vault (scaphocephaly).

The causes of craniosynostosis are listed in Table 4.13.

Premature fusion of the coronal suture (brachycephaly) causes the skull to enlarge laterally and upwards.

There may be co-existing congenital abnormalities such as Crouzon's syndrome and Apert's syndrome. The head appears deformed and the patient may complain of headaches and loss of vision.

Signs of raised intracranial pressure, visual field defects and cranial nerve deficits may be present.

Investigation

Imaging

A **plain skull X-ray** will demonstrate the fused sutures and the shape of the skull (Fig 4.7). A **CT scan** is useful for demonstrating intracranial pathology and to plan surgery.

Management

This condition must be recognized early in order to prevent neurological damage and allow normal development of the brain. Cosmetic results are also poor if the diagnosis is delayed.

Surgical correction may only require the excision of a single suture. In more complex cases facial osteotomies and orbital reconstructions are indicated. A multidisciplinary approach between neurosurgeons and plastic surgeons is desirable.

The prognosis for craniosynostosis is better for those with single suture involvement and no associated intracranial abnormalities.

ENCEPHALOCELE

This neural tube defect causes an embryological defect in the skull, usually the occiput, which allows herniation of the meninges and brain tissue. The extent of neurological damage is dependent on the amount and location of protruding brain matter. Visual and motor deficits are common, as are developmental problems.

The **differential diagnoses** include a cystic hygroma, branchial cleft cysts or a meningocele.

Investigation

Ultrasound scanning of the foetus may provide a prenatal diagnosis.

An **MRI scan** of the head delineates brain tissue and spinal cord abnormalities in the newborn.

Angiography may be required to assess the intracranial vasculature prior to carrying out surgical repair of the defect.

Management

One-third of infants with this condition are stillborn. There is a high rate of mental retardation among those that survive. The decision to close a significant defect or to not intervene can be difficult and poses ethical dilemmas. The defect should be closed within 48 hours of birth once a decision has been taken that this is the correct option.

HYDROCEPHALUS

Hydrocephalus is caused by an obstruction to drainage or failure to absorb cerebrospinal fluid. The causes of hydrocephalus are listed in Table 4.14.

Investigation

Diagnostic clinical indicators

Signs of hydrocephalus in the infant include an enlarged head, sunken and turned down eyes ('setting-sun' appearance) and bulging fontanelles. Adults may complain of symptoms of raised intracranial pressure: headaches, papilloedema and ataxia. They will eventually become comatose.

Imaging

The size of the ventricles in infants with a patent fontanelle can be measured using **ultrasound**.

A **CT scan** of the brain demonstrates hydrocephalus and identifies the underlying cause. **MRI** scanning is better at diagnosing pathology of the spine such as syringomyelia and Arnold–Chiari malformation.

Management

Early diagnosis is important to avoid permanent brain damage.

Table 4.14
The causes of hydrocephalus

Infants

Congenital aqueduct stenosis

Congenital posterior fossa malformations, e.g. Arnold-Chiari malformation

Myelomeningocele

Meningitis

Intraventricular haemorrhage

Adults

Subarachnoid haemorrhage

Meningitis

Neoplasm deforming the third ventricle, e.g. astrocytoma

Neoplasm of fourth ventricle, e.g. ependymoma

Brain metastases causing obstruction

Intracranial pressure is usually reduced by placing a shunt that drains cerebrospinal fluid from the lateral ventricle into either the right atrium or, more commonly, the peritoneum. These **ventriculo-peritoneal** or **ventriculo-atrial shunts** are tubes that are inserted into the brain through a burr hole, and tunnelled subcutaneously into the appropriate cavity. There is a relatively high incidence of shunt complications, including shunt infection, shunt obstruction, shunt migration/disconnection and intracerebral haemorrhage.

Hydrocephalus may be fatal if left untreated and, even with treatment, cognitive and physical impairment are common, depending on the success of shunting and the associated cerebral anomalies.

BAT EARS

This term describes prominent jutting out ears. True bat ears are a congenital deformity. The trait is passed on as an autosomal dominant entity. The **differential diagnosis** is mainly from the cup-shaped ears associated with Down's syndrome.

No investigations are necessary.

Management

Bat ears can be **corrected surgically** if their appearance causes the patient distress (often because of teasing at school). Operations should be carried out after the age of 7 when the development of the ear cartilage is complete.

An incision is made behind the ear to expose the cartilage. The cartilage is then scored with a scalpel to allow it to fold back, the skin incision closed and a firm head bandage applied for 10 days.

CAULIFLOWER EARS

Repeated trauma to the ear can cause multiple subperichondral haematomata which resolve very slowly and often incompletely.

Aside from the deformity that the haematoma causes, there is an associated risk of necrosis of the cartilage of the ear and infection.

The patient complains of swelling and deformity of the ear. Contact sports such as rugby, boxing and wrestling can cause cauliflower ears.

No investigations are necessary.

Management

A large fresh haematoma should be drained promptly through a surgical incision followed by a firm compression bandage to prevent re-accumulation of fluid. **Antibiotic prophylaxis** is advocated by some to prevent infection.

Protective headgear worn during contact sports can help prevent this condition.

KELOID EAR LOBES

Keloid scar tissue can develop following a cut to the ear or ear piercing. After the latter it appears as a firm nodule behind the earlobe and can be pedunculated. It is more common in black-skinned people and oriental people.

Inclusion dermoid cysts are sometimes confused with keloid scars of the ear.

Management

Custom-made **mechanical compression** devices have been used with some success to treat earlobe keloids.

Multiple injections of **triamcilonone acetonide** (a corticosteroid) into the keloid can cause shrinkage but the recurrence rate after 5 years can be as high as 50 per cent.

Surgical excision of the keloid with triamcilonone injection into the surrounding tissues, or **radiotherapy** to the site of excision has been shown to lower the recurrence rate. Malignant transformation several years after radiotherapy has been reported.

ACCESSORY AURICLES

Accessory auricles are extra pieces of cartilage that are usually found in front of the tragus of the ear. They are present from birth and are symptomless. The history distinguishes them from an enlarged pre-auricular lymph gland or a parotid tumour.

Surgical excision can be performed for cosmetic reasons.

RHINOPHYMA

This condition is caused by excessive growth of the sebaceous glands of the nose. It has no relation to excessive alcohol intake. It is more common in men and usually appears after the fifth decade.

Management

The excessive tissue can be shaved down to the base of the sebaceous glands with a Humby knife, curette, scalpel or laser.

The raw area can be left open or covered with a non-adherent dressing until it eventually re-epithelializes.

CLEFT LIP/CLEFT PALATE

The failure of the maxillary, mandibular and frontonasal processes to fuse properly results in cleft lips and cleft palates.

The condition is thought to arise from a combination of genetic and environmental factors (Table 4.15). Mutations in the gene coding for transforming growth factor (TGF) are thought to play a role.

Most deformities are recognized at birth. This can cause disfigurement, airway obstruction and problems with speech. The infant may not be able to suckle.

Otitis media, secondary to problems with the eustation tubes, is common.

Special investigations are rarely required.

Management

Feeding the infant can be a major problem. Prosthodontists and orthodontists can construct aids for feeding.

Surgical reconstruction of the lip should be carried out by the age of 3 months. The base of the nose is repaired, the alar cartilage is repositioned, the orbicularis muscle is reconstructed and finally the skin defect is closed.

Table 4.15
The environmental risk factors for cleft lip/palate

Folic acid deficiency
Phenytoin
Retinoids
Alcohol
Steroids

Surgical correction of the cleft palate should be carried out by the time the child is 1 year old to allow the development of normal speech. A speech therapist should be involved early.

Problems that may need to be addressed later in life include dental deformities, collapse of the dental arch, and further restorative surgery to improve the cosmetic appearance of the face.

BODY HABITUS/DEFORMITY

MARFAN'S SYNDROME

Marfan's syndrome has an autosomal dominant inheritance. It is caused by a defect in the fibrillin-1 gene, which results in the production of defective microfibrils that make up connective tissue components such as elastin and the suspensory ligament of the ocular lens.

Investigation
Diagnostic clinical indicators

Patients are tall, slim with a high arched palate, long arms and long fingers. Presentations include chest pain (aortic dissection or rupture), breathlessness (spontaneous pneumothorax), diastolic cardiac murmurs (aortic regurgitation) and loss of vision (lens dislocation). Shock and abdominal pain may indicate a ruptured abdominal aortic aneurysm.

The **differential diagnoses** include:

- Ehlers–Danlos syndrome
- Kleinfelter's syndrome
- hyperpituitarism
- acromegaly.

Genetic screening

Genetic screening for mutations in the fibrillin-1 gene should be obtained.

Imaging

Chest radiography may reveal a widened mediastinum if the aorta is dilated, a pneumothroax or heart failure in the breathless patient.

A **CT or MRI** scan of the aorta is used to diagnose aortic dissection and dilatation of the aorta and the aortic root.

An **electrocardiogram** may demonstrate arrythmias and conduction abnormalities. **Cardiac echocardiography** (transthoracic or transoesophageal) is useful to assess aortic and mitral valve regurgitation and to measure the aortic root.

Ophthalmoscopy

An examination of the anterior chamber of the eyes may confirm displacement or partial dislocation of the lens.

Management

Patients should be discouraged from taking part in contact sports.

Beta-adrenergic receptor antagonists (e.g. labetalol, atenolol) and angiotensin-converting enzyme (ACE) inhibitors are used to **lower the blood pressure** and reduce the rate of aortic expansion and protect against aortic dissection.

The patient may require cardiac surgery to replace a dilated aortic root and regurgitant aortic valve. The mitral valve can also become incompetent. Both the thoracic and the abdominal portions of the aorta are prone to aneurysmal degeneration and may need to be repaired (see Chapter 11). An aortic dissection may require emergency treatment by open repair or an endovascular stent graft.

A dislocated lens may have to be removed and replaced with a plastic prosthesis.

Patients should be **counselled** about the risk of their offspring inheriting Marfan's syndrome. Improved means of detecting cardiovascular complications and the prophylactic use of beta-blockers have improved the prognosis associated with this condition. The average patient now survives to 70 years of age.

ACHONDROPLASIA

This condition is passed on to siblings as an autosomal dominant trait and there may be a history of dwarfism in the family. It is caused by a mutation in the gene coding for fibroblast growth factor receptor-3 (FGFR3), which is transmitted as an autosomal dominant trait. Eighty per cent of cases are, however, caused by spontaneous mutations.

Differential diagnoses include:

- rickets
- renal dwarfism
- cretinism
- dwarfism.

Investigation

Diagnostic clinical indicators

Achondroplasia is one of the causes of dwarfism where the patient is of short stature with a large head, prominent forehead and flattened bridge of the nose. The hands and fingers are stunted, the legs bowed and the patient has a waddling gait.

Genetic screening

DNA analysis shows a mutation in the gene coding for FGFR3. Pre-natal screening for the FGFR3 mutation is now possible.

Imaging

Plain **X-rays** of the skeleton demonstrate square-shaped long bones, radiolucency of the proximal femur and a shrunken skull base.

MRI or CT scanning of the brain and base of skull may show evidence of spinal cord/brainstem compression, cervical instability or hydrocephalus.

Management

The patient's height and weight should be monitored closely. Dietary advice should be given in order to avoid obesity. **Growth hormone** is now accepted as a treatment for short stature achondroplasia.

Obstructive sleep apnoea can be a problem and may require adenotonsillectomy, weight loss or even continuous positive airways pressure or tracheostomy.

Spinal cord compression and compression at the craniocervical region may require surgical decompression.

Frequent otitis media is a sequelae of achondroplasia and should be treated vigorously.

The patient and their family may require **counselling** to cope with the social stigma associated with the physical appearance of achondroplasia. In up to 5 per cent of cases newborns do not survive longer than 1 year. In less severe cases, patients should expect a normal lifespan with normal cognitive development.

NEURAL TUBE DEFECTS

Defects of the neural tube, the embryonic structure that gives rise to the brain and spinal cord, are also associated with abnormal development of the vertebral canal – known as **spina bifida**.

A **meningocele** is a protrusion of the meninges through a defect in the spinal canal.

When both the meninges and spinal cord protrude it is called a **meningomyelocele**.

The least severe defect is referred to as **spina bifida occulta**, where there is no visible abnormality and is often an incidental finding on an X-ray showing a defect in the vertebral arch of the lumbosacral region. The defect may be covered by a tuft of hair or skin dimple. The predisposing causes are shown in Table 4.16.

Investigation

Diagnostic clinical indicators

Neural tube defects usually present as a soft translucent mass in the midline of the lower back or skull. There may be lower limb motor and sensory loss and bladder and bowel dysfunction.

The **differential diagnoses** of neural tube defects include:

- syringomyelia
- neonatal meningitis
- spinal epidural abscess
- spinal cord infarction.

Blood tests

Prenatal diagnosis is established by detecting a high **maternal serum alpha-fetoprotein** level.

Table 4.16
Factors associated with neural tube defects

Advanced maternal age

Zinc deficiency

Folate deficiency

Maternal diabetes

High maternal alcohol intake

Drugs, e.g. sodium valproate

Genetic abnormalities, e.g. trisomy 13 and trisomy 21

Imaging

Plain X-rays can be used to assess vertebral abnormalities and the presence of a scoliosis. **MRI scanning** of the brain and spinal cord will show any abnormalities of nervous tissue and the extent of spinal cord and nerve root involvement.

CT scanning is preferred for diagnosing hydrocephalus.

Management

Some children with neural tube defects die at birth. Many of those who survive are left with considerable problems that require management by a multidisciplinary team consisting of surgeons, therapists, psychologists and social workers. *Neonates with an open neural tube defect require prompt closure of the defect by a neurosurgical team.*

Many patients have an associated hydrocephalus, which will require a ventriculo-peritoneal shunt (see above).

Bladder dysfunction is common and needs to be assessed by a urologist.

Flexion contractures of the knees and dislocations of the hips prevents mobility, and many patients are wheelchair bound by the time they reach their late teens.

Prognosis The prognosis depends on the severity of abnormality. Up to 15 per cent of children with a meningomyelocele die by the age of 10 years, and mental retardation is present in up to 15 per cent.

CHEST WALL DEFORMITIES

These are discussed in Chapter 14.

5

The skin and subcutaneous tissues

Pari-Naz Mohanna and David Ross

LESIONS IN THE SKIN

BENIGN PAPILLOMA (SKIN TAG)

This is a simple pedunculated overgrowth of the skin that can occur anywhere. It has no potential for malignant change. No investigations are required.

Management

- **Reassurance**
- **Surgical excision** – if symptomatic, e.g. catches on clothes.

SEBORRHOEIC KERATOSIS (SEBORRHOEIC WART, SENILE WART, BASAL CELL PAPILLOMA)

Seborrhoeic keratosis is the most common benign tumour in the skin of older individuals. There is a keratotic proliferation of epidermal cells. Some cases are inherited through an autosomal dominant mode of inheritance.

Investigation

Clinical diagnostic indicators

Seborrhoeic keratoses have a variety of clinical appearances. They rarely protrude more than 3 mm, but catch on clothing and sometimes itch. They are usually grey but may become deep brown, when they may be mistaken for a melanoma. They occur more frequently in sunlight-exposed areas.

The sudden appearance of multiple pruritic seborrhoeic keratoses (Leser–Trélat sign) has been associated with the development of adenocarcinoma of the gastrointestinal tract, lymphoma and acute leukaemia.

No special investigations are needed. **Excisional biopsy** may be required if the diagnosis is in doubt.

Differential diagnosis

- Basal cell carcinoma
- Squamous cell carcinoma
- Melanoma
- Bowen's disease
- Sebaceous naevus
- Melanocytic naevus

Management

Reassurance that the lesion is benign is usually sufficient. Some patients ask that they be removed for cosmetic reasons and itching.

A variety of techniques may be employed to treat seborrhoeic keratoses:

- topical trichloroacetic acid
- cryotherapy
- electrodesiccation ± curettage
- curettage alone
- shave biopsy
- surgical excision.

With cryotherapy, liquid nitrogen is used to lower the temperature of the skin and produce cell death. Keratinocytes die when exposed to approximately −40 to −50°C, while other structures in the skin (e.g. collagen, blood vessels and nerves) are more resistant to the lethal effects of cold.

Recurrence is rare but new lesions often develop in adjacent skin.

BACTERIAL INFECTIONS

IMPETIGO

Impetigo is a highly contagious Gram-positive bacterial infection of the superficial layers of the epidermis. Impetigo is caused by *Staphylococcus aureus* and group A beta-haemolytic streptococci (GABHS), also known as *Streptococcus pyogenes*.

Investigation
Clinical diagnostic indicators
There are two clinical forms of the disease – bullous impetigo and non-bullous impetigo.

The pustules are discrete and in a few days dry into yellow scabs, which eventually fall off. They may occur anywhere, but are most often seen around the mouth and on the face and hands.

Impetigo is usually diagnosed clinically.

Bacteriology
The exudate from underneath the crust should be sent for culture and sensitivity especially if post-streptococcal glomerulonephritis is present.

Methicillin-resistant *Staphylococcus aureus* (MRSA) must be excluded if an outbreak of impetigo has occurred.

Management
Oral antibiotics are the mainstay of therapy. The chosen agent must provide coverage against both *Streptococcus aureus* and *Streptococcus pyogenes*. For empiric antibiotic therapy, a **cephalosporin**, **semisynthetic penicillin**, or **beta-lactam/beta-lactamase** inhibitor is recommended.

Topical antibiotics can be applied to affected areas twice or thrice daily for 7–10 days in patients with small or few lesions.

Good **hygiene** with antibacterial washes, such as **chlorhexidine**, may prevent the spread of impetigo and prevent recurrences.

Consult a nephrologist if signs and symptoms of acute glomerulonephritis develop.

Prognosis Resolution of lesions usually occurs after 7–10 days of treatment. If lesions have not resolved within 7–10 days of antibiotic therapy, cultures should be performed to look for resistant organisms.

Lesions do not leave scars if not scratched.

FURUNCULOSIS

Furuncles and boils are caused by infection entering hair follicles. The causative organism is usually *S. aureus*. When the lesion contains only pus it is called a furuncle; when it contains a solid core it is called a boil. Although most patients with furuncles and boils are otherwise healthy, these lesions are sometimes related to immune deficiency, anaemia, diabetes or iron deficiency.

Investigation
Clinical diagnostic indicators
The diagnosis is usually made clinically when a painful cutaneous lump is red and fluctuant. The central area may become white, yellow or black.

Blood tests
A **full blood count** and **blood glucose** may be done to exclude conditions that predispose to furunculosis.

Bacteriology
A microbiology swab should be sent for culture and sensitivity.

Management
General measures include:

- weight loss advice
- improvement of diabetic control
- improvement of hygiene and use of antiseptic cleaners.

Specific measures:

- An oral **antibiotic** (usually flucloxacillin) may sometimes be needed for several weeks.
- Surgical **incision and drainage** is required if the area involved is large.

ERYSIPELAS/CELLULITIS

Erysipelas is a superficial bacterial infection in the skin that characteristically extends into the cutaneous lymphatics. This disease was known in the Middle Ages, when it was referred to as 'St Anthony's Fire', named after an Egyptian healer who was known for successfully treating the infection. Historically, it occurred on the face and was caused by *S. pyogenes*. However, a shift in the distribution and aetiology of the disease has occurred, with most erysipelas infections now occurring on the legs and with *non-group A streptococci* sometimes being the aetiological agents.

Investigation

Clinical diagnostic indicators

The infected skin is red, tender and oedematous. The oedema makes the advancing edge raised and palpable, a feature that provides a way of assessing progression or regression. There will usually be pyrexia.

Predisposing factors include a pre-existing oedema such as lymphoedema, diabetes, alcohol abuse, HIV infection, nephrotic syndrome, other immunocompromising conditions and a vagrant lifestyle.

Bacteriology

Routine blood and tissue cultures are not cost-effective because they have an extremely low yield and results have a minimal impact on management. Cultures are perhaps best reserved for very immunosuppressed hosts in whom an atypical aetiological agent might be more likely.

Management

Elevate and rest the affected limb to reduce local swelling, inflammation and pain.

- **Antibiotic therapy** is the mainstay of treatment, with **penicillin** as the first-line of therapy. **Oral antibiotics** are sufficient in most cases. **Intravenous antibiotics** are recommended in severe cases and in infants, elderly patients and the immunocompromised.
- **Patient education** is important with recurrent erysipelas – focused on local antisepsis and general wound care.
- **Surgical excision** may be necessary only in severe infections with skin necrosis or gangrene.

HIDRADENITIS SUPPURATIVA

Hidradenitis suppurativa (HS) is an infection of the apocrine sweat glands. Its exact aetiology remains obscure but all the following have been proposed: occlusion and bacterial infection, genetics, host defence defects, diabetes, hormonal imbalance, cigarette smoking, chemical and mechanical irritants.

Investigation

Clinical diagnostic indicators

The condition most commonly affects the axillae and the groin. The site and chronic recurring nature of the condition make it debilitating. It presents with **tender swellings** (often multiple) which coalesce and discharge pus. The **differential diagnosis** is furunculosis.

Bacteriology

A microbiology swab may be sent for **culture** in severe infections. Almost every micro-organism may be isolated. Among the most frequently found species are *S. aureus* and coagulase-negative staphylococci, anaerobic streptococci (e.g. microaerophilic *Streptococcus milleri*) and *Bacteroides* species.

Management

Medical management

Non-surgical procedures are important both before and after surgery. If the disease is diagnosed and treated early, secondary systemic complications can be prevented and the extent of surgery can be limited.

Medical management includes:

- **improvement of hygiene**, use of antiseptic cleaners and antiperspirant agents
- **weight loss** in obese patients
- wearing **loose-fitting clothing**.

Surgical management

Surgery is the definitive treatment, especially in patients with chronic HS.

Radical surgical excision reduces the likelihood of recurrence. The excision margins must be well beyond the apocrine glands, both horizontally and radially. To define the apocrine gland-bearing area, the **iodine starch test** is used. Where the sweat makes contact with the iodine starch little black spots appear.

Following resection it may be possible to close the skin directly, but more often closure requires a skin graft (Fig 5.1) or reconstruction with local, regional or free cutaneous and myocutaneous flaps.

Limited surgical intervention, consisting of deroofing abscesses and sinus tracts, with vigorous

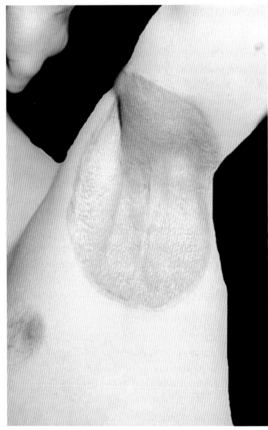

FIGURE 5.1   Split skin graft to the left axilla following excision of hidradenitis suppurativa

curettage of their base, and healing by secondary intention can be valuable in some cases.

Surgical excision using the **carbon dioxide laser** and healing by secondary intention can be used particularly in severe perianal hiradenitis. Healing usually occurs in 4–8 weeks.

Results The recurrence rate in patients treated with radical surgery varies considerably but has been reported to be as high as 50 per cent in the sub-mammary region.

ANTHRAX

Anthrax is caused by exposure to the spores of the bacterium *Bacillus anthracis*, which are primarily found in association with grazing animals, their skin, hides, fur and bones.

The bacteria can lie in a dormant phase as spores and can exist in the environment for decades. Under the right conditions, the dormant spores can germinate and multiply. Most cases are mild but anthrax can be lethal.

Investigation
Clinical diagnostic indicators
There are three clinical manifestations:

- **Cutaneous anthrax**: the skin lesion begins as a papule, which then becomes a serous or haemorrhagic vesicle, which bursts and becomes a black slough.
- **Gastrointestional anthrax**: associated with severe vomiting and diarrhoea.
- **Pulmonary anthrax**: presents with the sudden onset of dyspnoea and chest pain.

Bacteriology
A fluid sample or microbiology **swab** should be taken from the cutaneous lesion. **A sputum sample** should be taken if there is clinical evidence of inhalation anthrax. **Blood cultures** should be taken if there is clinical evidence of systemic infection.

Imaging
A **chest X-ray** or **CT scan** is required if inhalational anthrax is suspected.

Management
Antibiotics are the first line of therapy. Many are effective including **doxycycline**, **penicillin**, **amoxicillin** and **ciprofloxacin**. In severe infections intravenous antibiotics should be given.

Patients exposed to anthrax may be given **prophylactic antibiotics** for up to 60 days.

SYPHILIS

Syphilis is a chronic systemic venereal disease with multiple clinical presentations (i.e. the great imitator). It is caused by *Treponema pallidum*, a microaerophilic spirochaete. It is characterized by episodes of active disease (primary, secondary, tertiary stages) interrupted by periods of latency.

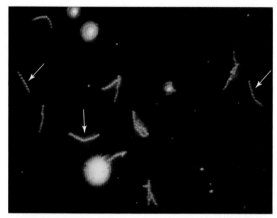

FIGURE 5.2 Immunofluorescence staining of fixed smears from moist cutaneous lesions demonstrating the presence of spirochetes in syphilis

Syphilis is transmitted in three ways, either from intimate contact with infectious lesions (most common) or blood transfusions (blood collected during early syphilis), or transmitted transplacentally from an infected mother to her foetus. Although syphilis is uncommon in the United Kingdom its incidence has slightly increased in recent years.

Investigation
Clinical diagnostic indicators
The many forms of clinical presentation are described in *Symptoms and Signs*.

Blood tests
- The rapid plasma reagin (RPR) test
- The Venereal Disease Research Laboratory (VDRL) test
- The fluorescent treponemal antibody absorption (FTA-ABS)
- The T-pallidum hemagglutination (TPHA) test.

Smears from lesions
Dark-field microscopy and **immunofluorescence staining** of fixed smears from moist cutaneous lesions should be examined for the presence of spirochetes (Fig 5.2).

Imaging
The investigation of extracutaneous syphilis will require **X-rays, ECG, angiography, lumbar puncture** and **biopsies.**

Management
Penicillin remains the mainstay of treatment and the standard by which other modes of therapy are judged. Skin testing and desensitization are recommended for patients with an allergy to penicillin.

LEPROSY

Leprosy is a chronic granulomatous disease principally affecting the skin and peripheral nervous system, caused by *Mycobacterium leprae*. Although much improved in the last 25 years, knowledge of its pathogenesis, course, treatment and prevention continues to evolve. Affected patients need to be managed by a multidisciplinary team, including an ophthalmologist, a plastic surgeon, an orthopaedic surgeon, an otolaryngologist, a neurosurgeon, a neurologist, a physiotherapist and an occupational therapist.

Investigation
Clinical diagnostic indicators
The classical symptoms and signs are described in *Symptoms and Signs.*

Serology
Serology and polymerase chain reaction (PCR) testing can be diagnostic but may fail to detect early or mild forms. Reverse transcriptase PCR (RT-PCR) is more sensitive in detecting bacilli.

Lepromin testing
Lepromin testing indicates host resistance to *M. leprae*. Although the results do not confirm the diagnosis, they are useful in determining the type of leprosy.

Although laboratory studies may help in making a definitive diagnosis, these tests are usually unavailable in remote areas and in some developing countries.

Imaging
X-rays may be useful to detect and monitor leprosy-induced bone changes.

Tissue biopsy
A skin biopsy is examined for the presence of acid-fast bacilli (Fig 5.3) and the characteristic morphological feature of an inflamed nerve.

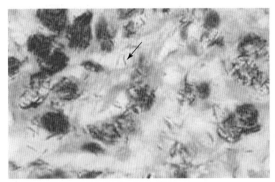

FIGURE 5.3 Red acid-fast bacilli on Ziehl–Nielsen staining of a skin biopsy from a patient with leprosy

Management

Medical care

- **Pharmacotherapy** needs to be started early to stop the infection, reduce morbidity, prevent complications and eradicate the disease. The agent most commonly used is **Dapsone** as well as **rifampin, ofloxacin** and **minocycline**. The length of treatment ranges from 6 months to 2 years. Patients are considered non-infectious within 1–2 weeks of treatment.
- **Physical, social and psychological rehabilitation**

Surgical care

Emergency surgery may be needed to decompress inflamed nerves and incise and drain abscesses. **Elective surgery** is often needed to correct lagophthalmos, reconstructive nasal collapse, release of contractures and improve function and appearance.

NON-GENITAL VIRAL WARTS

Warts are benign proliferations of the skin and mucosa caused by the human papilloma virus (HPV). Currently, more than 100 types of HPV have been identified. Certain HPV types tend to occur at particular anatomic sites; however, warts of any HPV type may occur at any site. A small subset of HPV types is associated with the development of malignancies. This is most commonly is seen in patients with genital warts and in immunocompromised patients.

Investigation

Clinical diagnostic indicators

The primary clinical manifestations of HPV infection include common warts, genital warts, flat warts and deep palmoplantar warts (myrmecia).

The diagnosis is suggested by finding elevated pale papilliferous growths covered with greyish epithelium.

Immunohistochemistry

Immunohistochemical detection of HPV may confirm the presence of virus in a lesion, but it has a low sensitivity.

Virus identification

Viral DNA identification is more sensitive and specific.

Management

The treatment of warts can be difficult, with frequent failures and recurrences. Many warts resolve spontaneously within a few years.

Medical care

Multiple modalities are available for the treatment of warts, but none is uniformly effective. Start with the least painful, least expensive and least time-consuming methods and reserve the more expensive and invasive procedures for refractory extensive warts.

Benign neglect is recommended in many cases as sixty-five per cent of warts regress spontaneously within 2 years.

Treatment of **topical agents** is recommended for patients with extensive, spreading or symptomatic warts or warts that have been present for more than 2 years.

Salicylic acid is a first-line therapy that is available without a prescription. Cure rates of 70–80 per cent are reported.

Other topical agents only to be applied by trained personnel include **cantharidin** and **trichloroacetic acid**.

Intralesional injections of **immunotherapeutic and chemotherapeutic agents** can be used for warts that are persistent and refractory to topical agents.

Systemic agents such as cimetidine, retinoids and intravenous cidofovir may help.

Surgical care

Cryosurgery with liquid nitrogen (−196°C) is the most effective method.

Paring the wart, in addition to two freeze–thaw cycles, is a valuable adjunct to cryosurgery for plantar warts.

Laser therapy is reserved for large or refractory warts. Carbon dioxide lasers are the most effective, although there can be residual scarring.

Surgical excision carries the risks of scarring and recurrence.

FUNGAL INFECTIONS

CANDIDIOSIS (MONILIASIS)

Candidiosis is an infection caused by the yeast *Candida albicans* or other candida species. Candida is a normal component of the body's flora, being present in the skin, vagina and throughout the gastrointestinal tract (mouth through anus). Superficial infections of the skin and mucous membranes are the most common types and present clinically as candidiosis of the buccal mucosa and tongue, intertrigo, diaper dermatitis, perianal dermatitis, balanitis and paronychia.

Candidiosis has increased in prevalence in recent years, mirroring an increase in immunocompromised patients. Other predisposing factors include tissue trauma, endocrine disease such as diabetes, nutritional deficiency and prolonged use of antibiotics.

Investigation

Clinical diagnostic indicators

The candida grows into typical yellow-white plaques on the surface of the infected epithelium.

Microscopy

Microscopic examination and culture of skin scrapings is diagnostic (Fig 5.4).

Management

Treat any predisposing factors. Simple **skin care** measures including exposure and drying of affected area. **Topical antifungal agents** including miconazole nitrate or clotrimazole. **Oral therapy** including nystatin, clotrimazole, itraconazole, ketoconazole and fluconazole.

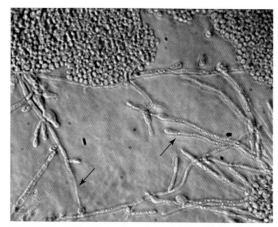

FIGURE 5.4 Light microscopy demonstrating the yeast of *Candida albicans*. Some cells have assumed a small, round form, whereas others are long, filamentous hyphale. The ability to shift forms is thought to be crucial for invasion of – and survival within – the different tissues that *Candida* infects

TINEA PEDIS (ATHLETE'S FOOT)

Tinea pedis is a dermatophyte infection of the soles of the feet and the interdigital spaces, most commonly caused by *Trichophyton rubrum*. Wars, with the accompanying mass movements of troops and refugees, the general increase in available means of travel and the rise in the use of occlusive footwear have all combined to make *T. rubrum* the world's most prevalent dermatophyte.

Investigation

Clinical diagnostic indicators

The presence of soggy white skin in the interdigital clefts and a distinctive smell are diagnostic.

Skin scrapings

The diagnosis can be confirmed from skin scrapings sent for potassium hydroxide (KOH) staining and culture.

Management

Simple **skin care measures** include exposure and drying of the affected area.

- **Topical antifungals** – clotrimazole, econazole and ketoconazole
- **Oral antifungals** – fluconazole and itraconazole.

BENIGN PIGMENTED NAEVI

Benign pigmented naevi can be subdivided into those containing naevus cells and those containing melanocytes. Naevus cell naevi are either congenital or acquired. Melanocytic naevi originate in either the epidermis or the dermis.

CONGENITAL NAEVUS CELL NAEVI

Giant hairy naevi

They are brown/black and hairy and have to be >20 cm in diameter in the adult or cover >5 per cent of the body surface area.

The lifetime risk of malignant change is in the region of 2–4 per cent, although figures of up to 40 per cent have been reported. Melanomata arising within GHN (Fig 5.5) have a worse prognosis than other melanomata. Lesions overlying the sacrum may be associated with a meningocele or spina bifida.

Management

The best method of treatment is controversial. Some advocate **close surveillance** with excision of any abnormal areas. Others prefer **prophylactic removal** by

- excision ± reconstruction with skin grafts, local flaps with or without tissue expansion (Fig 5.6).
- dermabrasion
- curettage
- laser ablation.

Acquired naevus cell naevi

These lesions are rare in infancy with their incidence steadily increasing during childhood, sharply during adolescence, more slowly in early adulthood and plateaus in middle age.

Investigation

Clinical diagnostic indicators

They are subdivided into the following groups with the following clinical features.

- **Junctional naevi** are composed of nests of naevus cells clustered around the epidermal–dermal

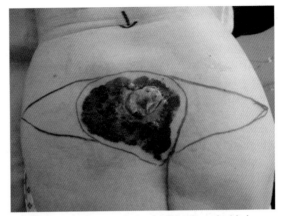

FIGURE 5.5   Malignant melanoma arising in a giant hairy naevus in an 82-year-old woman

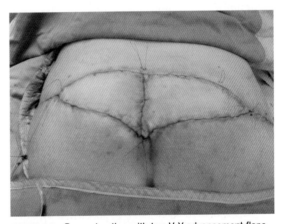

FIGURE 5.6   Reconstruction with two V-Y advancement flaps.

junction. They present as flat, smooth and irregularly pigmented lesions, usually in childhood or adolescence.

- **Compound naevi** consist of nests of naevus cells clustered at the epidermal–dermal junction extending into the dermis. They present as a round well-circumscribed slightly raised lesion, usually in adolescence.
- **Intradermal naevi** are composed of nests of naevus cells clustered within the dermis. They are dome shaped lesions which may be non-pigmented or hairy and present in adults.

Management

None is associated with malignant transformation; therefore, their management is conservative unless excision is requested for aesthetic reasons.

Special naevus cell naevi

Spitz naevi (juvenile melanoma)

These lesions are benign melanocytic tumours with cellular atypia. They predominately present in childhood as reddish-brown nodules, commonly on the face and legs. Management is by **excision** with a narrow margin.

Dysplastic naevi

These lesions characteristically occur in sun-exposed areas and have

- an irregular outline
- patchy pigmentation
- a diameter >5 mm.

'Atypical naevus syndrome' is defined as >100 dysplastic naevi present in one patient. They have a 5–10 per cent risk of malignant change.

Management

- Atypical naevus syndrome: excision of representative lesions to confirm diagnosis and watch.
- Dysplastic naevi: excision to confirm diagnosis.

Halo naevi

They are relatively common in older children and teenagers. They are caused by destruction of the naevus by the immune system. The naevus is surrounded by a depigmented area of skin. Management is **expectant** – they tend to regress leaving a small scar.

Epidermal melanocytic naevi

Ephelis/freckle

Freckles are macular pigmented lesions arising as a result of increased melanin production by the melanocytes. They contain a normal number of melanocytes. They can disappear in the absence of sunlight.

Lentigo

These lesions contain an increased number of melanocytes and persist in the absence of sunlight.

Café au lait macule

These are pale-brown patches. Five or more such lesions measuring >1.5 cm in diameter are required to support the diagnosis of neurofibromatosis.

Dermal melanocytic naevi

These lesions are characterized by the presence of melanocytes within the dermis.

Blue naevus

These arise as a result of the arrested migration of melanocytes bound for the dermal–epidermal junction. The presence of macrophages distinguishes them from the Mongolian blue spot. They present as nodular blue-black lesions on the extremities, buttocks and face. Malignant transformation is rare. No treatment is required other than for cosmesis.

Mongolian blue spot

These are common in Asians and Afro-Caribbeans, but rare in Caucasians. They are present in 90 per cent of Mongolian infants. They form a characteristic blue-grey pigmentation over the sacrum. The pigmentation increases after birth and regresses in childhood. No treatment is required.

Naevus of Ota

The condition is uncommon in Caucasians but prevalent among Japanese people. The pigmentation arises from intradermal melanocytes. This lesion is characterized by blue-brown pigmentation of the sclera and the adjacent periorbital skin in the distribution of the ophthalmic and maxillary divisions of the fifth cranial nerve. No treatment is required.

Naevus of Ito

Like the naevus of Ota, this condition is also uncommon in Caucasians but prevalent among Japanese. The pigmentation arises from intradermal melanocytes. This lesion is characterized by blue-grey discoloration in the shoulder region. No treatment is required.

LUMPS IN THE SKIN

KELOID AND HYPERTROPHIC SCARS

Keloid scars result from an overgrowth of dense fibrous scar tissue that extends beyond the borders of the original wound into normal tissue. They do not usually regress spontaneously, and tend to recur after excision. Keloid scars continue to enlarge for 6–12 months after the initial injury.

In contrast, **hypertrophic scars** (HTSs) are characterized by an overgrowth of dense fibrous scar tissue that is confined to the borders of the original wound and does not extend into normal tissue. HTSs only enlarge for 2–3 months after the initial injury and may undergo spontaneous resolution. If excised they do not recur if the causative factors such as infection and excessive tension on the wound are eliminated.

Investigation

Diagnosis is usually based on clinical findings. Rarely, a biopsy may be needed to confirm the diagnosis.

Management

Medical care

No single therapeutic modality is best for all keloids. The location, size and depth of the lesion; the age of the patient; and the past response to treatment determine the type of therapy used. Prevention is key.

Prevention

- Avoid performing non-essential cosmetic surgery in patients known to form keloids.
- Close all surgical wounds with minimal tension.
- Do not place incisions across joint creases.
- Avoid making mid-chest incisions, and ensure that incisions follow the skin creases whenever possible.

Medical treatments

Occlusive dressings, including silicone gel sheets and non-silicone occlusive sheets. (The effect results from a combination of occlusion and hydration.)

Compression therapy such as pressure earrings or pressure garments that produce a thinning effect on the skin.

Intralesional corticosteroid injections reduce excessive scarring by reducing collagen synthesis, altering glucosaminoglycan synthesis, and reducing production of inflammatory mediators and fibroblast proliferation during wound healing. The most commonly used corticosteroid is **triamcinolone acetonide** (TAC) in concentrations of 10–40 mg/mL at 4- to 6-week intervals. The complications of repeated corticosteroid injections include atrophy, telangiectasia formation and pigmentary alteration.

Recent innovations include intralesional interferon, 5-FU, doxorubicin, bleomycin, verapamil, retinoic acid, imiquimod 5 per cent cream, tacrolimus, tamoxifen, botulinum toxin and TGF-β3.

Radiation therapy

The use of radiotherapy to treat keloids remains controversial. Although many studies have demonstrated efficacy and decreased recurrence rates, the safety of radiotherapy has been questioned. It is usually given within 24 hours of keloid excision.

Surgical management

Cryotherapy affects the microvasculature and causes cell damage via intracellular crystals, leading to tissue anoxia.

Excision minimizes chances of recurrence by placing the wound in the relaxed skin tension lines, careful tissue handling and closure with minimal tension.

Decreased recurrence rates have been reported with excision when combined with other postoperative modalities, such as **radiotherapy** or **intralesional corticosteroid therapy**.

Laser therapy using carbon dioxide, argon and Nd:Yag lasers have been used but all are associated with a high recurrence rate.

SEBACEOUS CYSTS (EPIDERMOID/PILAR CYSTS)

Sebaceous cysts are smooth fluctuant lumps that are attached to the skin and have a punctum. These features differentiate them from a lipoma and other benign skin tumours.

Investigation

The diagnosis is usually based on the clinical findings.

Management

- **Reassurance** and benign neglect.
- **Excision**, ensuring that the entire sac is removed intact to reduce the chances of recurrence.
- **Incision and drainage** if infected. The wound should be packed and allowed to heal by secondary intention. At a later date the cyst wall can be excised.

DERMOID CYST

A dermoid cyst is a cystic teratoma that contains developmentally mature skin. Depending on its location it can also contain hair follicles, sweat glands, clumps of hair, sebum, blood, fat, bone, nails, teeth, eyes, cartilage and thyroid tissue.

Dermoid cysts may be **congenital**, arising *in utero* as a result of entrapment of the epidermis during fusion of the facial planes; or **acquired**, usually secondary to a penetrating injury implanting epithelium subcutaneously, often in the digits. Most commonly they arise in the head and neck region but can also be intracranial, intraspinal, perispinal and intra-abdominal.

Congenital dermoids are classified according to their location. Their distinction is crucial as it dictates their management.

- **Angular dermoids** are situated lateral to the orbit.
- **Central dermoids** occur anywhere in the midline between the forehead and the nasal tip. They may have intracranial extensions.

Investigation

CT and **magnetic resonance imaging** (MRI) are only indicated in central dermoids to establish if there is an intracranial extension (Fig 5.7).

Management

Surgical excision is the treatment of choice but the techniques used vary according to the locality of the cyst:

- acquired dermoids – simple excision
- angular dermoids – open or endoscopic excision

- central dermoids – excision is more complex and may require the involvement of craniofacial and or neurosurgeons to address any intracranial extension.

ACQUIRED IMPLANTATION DERMOID CYST

These cysts usually arise secondary to a sharp injury breaching the skin and forcibly implanting a piece of skin into the subcutaneous tissue. There may be a scar overlying the fluctuant swelling.

Investigation

The history and examination findings are usually sufficient for diagnosis.

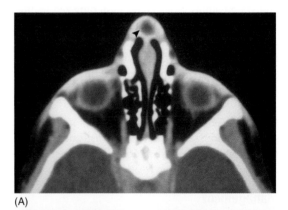

(A)

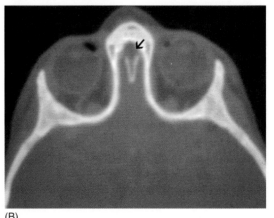

(B)

FIGURE 5.7 (A) Computed tomography (CT) scan demonstrates the nasal dermoid (arrow head). (B) CT scan demonstrates intracranial extension (arrow)

Imaging

X-ray or MRI: implantation dermoid cysts of the digits may require radiological imaging to identify any underlying bony erosion and to exclude a differential diagnosis of a giant cell tumour.

Management

Surgical excision of the cyst.

PYOGENIC GRANULOMA

Pyogenic granuloma is a relatively common benign vascular lesion of skin or mucosa whose exact cause is unknown.

Investigation

Clinical diagnostic indicators

Pyogenic granulomas usually appear in children and young adults as a solitary glistening red papule or nodule that is prone to bleed and ulcerate. They most often occur on the head, neck, extremities and upper trunk, and may be associated with trauma and typically grow rapidly over a period of a few weeks.

Tissue biopsy

A number of malignant tumours may mimic pyogenic granuloma, so if there is diagnostic uncertainty, histopathological confirmation of the diagnosis is essential before advising treatment.

Management

Excision of the lesion is indicated to alleviate any bleeding, discomfort, cosmetic distress, and diagnostic uncertainty. This may be achieved by shaving, punch biopsy, scalpel or laser and is curative if the lesion is completely removed.

FAT NECROSIS

Fat necrosis arises when the vascularity to the fat is compromised, usually by repetitive trauma, e.g. subcutaneous injections. Common sites include the buttocks and breast.

Investigation

Clinical diagnostic indicators

Two clinical features – its hardness and tethering to its overlying skin – make it mimic a neoplastic lesion, particularly in the breast. Therefore, the following may be useful to exclude a malignant lesion:

- tissue biopsy
- fine needle aspiration biopsy.

Imaging

US, MRI and **CT** are rarely required.

Management

- **Reassurance** and regular observation.
- **Surgical excision** ± reconstruction.

DERMATOFIBROMA/HISTIOCYTOMA

Dermatofibroma is a common cutaneous nodule that occurs most often in the lower legs of women after minor trauma, such as an insect bite. A number of well-described, histological subtypes have been reported. The diagnosis is usually based on the clinical features.

Removal of the tumour is not necessary unless diagnostic uncertainty exists or there are particularly troubling symptoms.

NEUROFIBROMA

Neurofibromas are benign tumours that contain a mixture of neural (ectodermal) and fibrous (mesodermal) elements. They are often multiple and may become plexiform, usually in association with the V cranial nerve. Neurofibromatosis is characterized by multiple neurofibromas, café au lait spots, Lisch nodules, axillary freckles and acoustic neuroma.

The diagnosis is usually based on the clinical findings of rubbery subcutaneous fusiform lumps which are sometimes pedunculated and pale in colour.

Management

- **Reassurance** and benign observation.
- **Surgical resection** is indicated if the patient has symptoms but can be challenging, as neurofibromas often surround important nerves.

KERATOACANTHOMA

Keratoacanthomas (KAs) are relatively rare. They originate in the pilosebaceous glands.

Investigation

Clinical diagnostic indicators

Clinically and pathologically they resemble squamous cell carcinoma (SCC). In fact, some authorities maintain that they are well-differentiated SCCs rather than a distinct clinical entity. KAs are characterized by rapid growth over a few weeks to months, followed by spontaneous resolution over 4–6 months, in most cases, and leave a deep scar.

Tissue biopsy

Although often performed, biopsies are rarely helpful, as KAs are very difficult to distinguish from SCCs histologically.

Management

Observe and wait for spontaneous resolution with weekly follow-up for the measurement of the lesion and photography. This approach is not very popular as it accepts healing with residual, puckered scarring.

Surgical excision must include adequate margins (3–5 mm) and histopathological evaluation to exclude invasive SCCs.

Mohs micrographic surgery can be used to treat large or recurrent keratoacanthomas located in specific anatomical areas with cosmetic or functional considerations. It involves tangential excision with a narrow margin followed by complete examination of the surgical margin using frozen sections. If the margins are not complete, further excisions are perfomed and examined until clearance is obtained.

Radiotherapy is also an option as KAs are radiosensitive and respond well to low doses of radiation. Radiation therapy may be useful in selected patients with large tumours in whom resection will result in cosmetic deformity.

TUMOURS OF THE SKIN AND ITS APPENDAGES

SEBACEOUS HYPERPLASIA

Sebaceous hyperplasia is a common, benign condition of sebaceous glands in adults of middle and later age. Lesions can be single or multiple and can be confused with basal cell carcinomata. When the skin of the nose is involved the condition is called **rhinophyma**.

Management

Sebaceous hyperplasia is completely benign and does not require treatment; however, lesions can be cosmetically disfiguring and sometimes bothersome when irritated.

A biopsy may be necessary to exclude a basal cell carcinoma.

Treatment options include photodynamic therapy, cauterization, electrodessication, topical chemical treatments or laser treatment.

SEBACEOUS ADENOMA

This is a rare benign tumour usually occurring on the scalp of elderly people, comprising incompletely differentiated sebaceous cells. It can be excised if symptomatic.

SEBACEOUS NAEVI (SEBACEOUS NAEVUS OF JADASSOHN)

This warty naevus is usually present at birth but tends to enlarge and become prominent at puberty, when the sebaceous glands enlarge. There is a 20–30 per cent chance of malignant transformation into a basal cell carcinoma or less commonly a mixed skin appendiceal tumour (see later).

Management

In view of the high chance of malignant transformation they should be **excised**.

SEBACEOUS CARCINOMA

This is a rare skin cancer that may arise many years following radiotherapy, usually involving the scalp and face.

Management
Surgical excision.

SWEAT GLAND TUMOURS

These solitary subcutaneous lumps include eccrine poromas, cylindromas and syringomas. All are benign sweat gland tumours that can be treated by **surgical excision**.

TUMOURS OF THE HAIR FOLLICLES

These solitary nodules are of variable colour. They include trichoepithelioma, trichofolliculoma, tricholemmoma and pilomatrixoma (calcifying epithelioma of Malherbe). All can be treated by **surgical excision**.

SOLAR/ACTINIC KERATOSIS

This is an ultraviolet light-induced premalignant keratosis of the skin.

Investigation

There are thickened yellow or brown plaques of variable diameter involving the sun-exposed areas of the face and dorsum of the hand.

Tissue biopsy

Punch, incision or excision biopsy is indicated to confirm the diagnosis. The lesion is characterized by dysplasia and architectural disorder of the epidermis.

Management
Medical

Educate the patient to limit sun exposure. Patients should be cautioned to avoid sun exposure between 10:00 am and 3:00 pm and always wear adequate sunscreens and protective clothing daily.

Topical agents are 5-fluorouracil (5-FU) (Fig 5.8) and 5 per cent imiquimod cream.

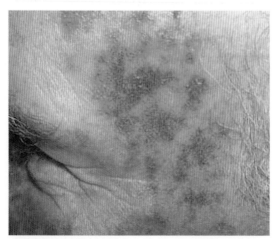

FIGURE 5.8 Normal reaction of an area of actinic keratosis treated with 5-fluorouracil

Photodynamic therapy (PDT) with topical delta-aminolevulinic acid utilises a light-sensitizing compound that preferentially accumulates in actinic keratosis cells, where it can be activated by the appropriate wavelength of light, causing cell death.

Surgical

Cryosurgery is the use of a cryogen (usually liquid nitrogen) to lower the temperature of the skin and produce cell death. Keratinocytes die when exposed to approximately −40 to −50°C, whereas other structures in the skin, such as collagen, blood vessels and nerves, are more resistant to the lethal effects of cold.

Curettage, shave excision and conventional excision all provide a sample for histological evaluation.

HUTCHINSON'S LENTIGO (LENTIGO MALIGNA)

Sir John Hutchinson first described lentigo maligna in 1890; the disease continues to be called Hutchinson melanotic freckle on occasion. The Hutchinson melanotic freckle was originally thought to be infectious because of its slow yet progressive growth.

Investigation
Clinical diagnostic indicators

This premalignant lesion commonly arises in the head and neck. It is believed to be a pre-invasive lesion induced by long-term cumulative ultraviolet injury. It presents as a large pigmented patch which may be nodular and variegated and slowly enlarges with time.

Tissue biopsy

An incision or **excision biopsy** is essential.

Management

- **Surgical excision** with a 0.5-cm margin.
- **Close and regular observation** are necessary if the lesion is too large to simply excise and close directly or the patient is unwilling to undergo surgery.
- If any changes occur then a biopsy is required.

BOWEN'S DISEASE

Bowen's disease is a squamous cell carcinoma (SCC) *in situ* with the potential to progress to become an invasive SCC. It is associated with chronic sun exposure and exposure to arsenic.

Investigation

Clinical diagnostic indicators

The patches of flat, pink, papular patches caused by this condition are often misdiagnosed as eczema.

Tissue biopsy

An incisional or excisional biopsy is essential.

Management

Medical care

- **Topical therapy** with 5-FU.
- **Photodynamic therapy** (PDT) has shown promise in the treatment of superficial carcinomata.

Surgical care

Simple excision with conventional margins Although lesions are typically well demarcated, the actual extent of the disease may extend well beyond the clinical margins. For this reason, the excision should be made at least 4 mm outside the clinical margin.

Mohs micrographic surgery This is an excellent method for treating larger areas, recurrent Bowen's or specific anatomical areas with cosmetic or functional considerations.

Curettage and electrodesiccation, cryotherapy and carbon dioxide laser ablation Compared with simple excision and Mohs surgery, these methods are less likely to remove tumours that are present in the adnexal structures.

BASAL CELL CARCINOMA (BASAL CELL EPITHELIOMA, BALALOM, RODENT ULCER, TRICHOBLASTIC CARCINOMA)

Basal cell carcinoma is a malignant tumour of cells derived from the basal layer of the epidermis, pluripotential cells in the epithelium and hair follicles. It is the commonest skin tumour in Caucasians with 95 per cent occurring between 40 and 80 years and 85 per cent in the head and neck region. Only 200 cases of metastatic BCCs have been reported worldwide. The ratio of basal to squamous cell carainoma is 3:1.

Investigation

Clinical diagnostic indicators

Characteristically it presents in sun-exposed areas as an ulcerated skin nodule with a rolled pearly edge and fine blood vessels. However it may have many clinical appearances and these are shown in *Symptoms and Signs*.

Basal cell carcinoma is associated with:

- chronic sun exposure
- exposure to chemicals such as arsenic
- immunosuppression
- sebaceous naevus
- Gorlin's syndrome, an autosomal dominant condition with many characterizing features, one being multiple basal cell carcinomas.

Differential diagnosis

- Squamous cell carcinoma
- Malignant melanoma
- Bowen disease
- Sebaceous hyperplasia
- Naevus
- Seborrheic keratosis.

Tissue biopsy

A **punch, incisional or excisional biopsy** is required to confirm the diagnosis and to identify the histological subtype (Table 5.1).

Table 5.1
Histological types of basal cell carcinoma

Localized
Nodular
Nodulocystic
Micronodular
Pigmented

Superficial/multifocal

Infiltrative
Morpheaform (sclerosing/fibrosing)

Management

Basal cell carcinoma must be managed by a multi-disciplinary team.

Medical care

Topical therapy with 5-FU is effective for superficial lesions only.

Cryotherapy is an effective treatment for non-aggressive cases, with cure rates near 90 per cent Its success is dependent on the experience of the operator.

Photodynamic therapy is good for pre-cancerous lesions and superficial basal cell carcinomas (Gorlin's).

Radiotherapy is useful for patients who cannot easily tolerate surgery, such as elderly or debilitated individuals and for lesions in cosmetically sensitive areas. Its cure rates approach 90 per cent. Unfortunately, tumours recurring in previously radiated sites tend to be more aggressive.

Surgical care

The goal of surgical treatment is to destroy or remove the tumour so that no malignant tissue is allowed to proliferate further. Factors to consider when choosing therapy include the histological subtype, the location and size of tumours, the age of the patient and the patient's ability to tolerate surgery. Recurrent tumours are generally more aggressive than primary ones. Tumours that are aggressive and those occurring near vital or cosmetically sensitive structures are best treated with methods that allow for an examination of the tissue margins.

Simple excision biopsy This should include 2- to 5-mm margins (7 mm for morphoeic), but even so 5 per cent of lesions will be incompletely excised and 30–50 per cent of these will recur (Fig 5.9).

Mohs micrographic surgery This method gives cure rates of 98–99 per cent for primary cancers and 94–96 per cent for recurrent basal cell carcinomas. The indications for its use are:

- tumours located in high-risk sites (periorbital, periauricular, and perineal)
- tumours with poorly delineated clinical borders
- tumours arising from scar tissue
- tumours that are larger than 2 cm or have aggressive malignant features
- morpheaform or sclerosing basal cell carcinoma
- recurrent basal cell carcinomas.

Curettage and electrodessication with diathermy of the base should only be used for non-aggressive tumours in low-risk sites. The specimen cannot be examined for margin control.

Follow-up

Well-circumscribed completely excised basal cell carcinomas in low-risk sites can be discharged from follow-up with advice regarding sun protection and self-examination.

Poorly circumscribed, incompletely excised, recurrent tumours in high-risk areas require 3–6 months' follow-up.

SQUAMOUS CELL CARCINOMA

Squamous cell carcinoma is a malignant tumour arising in the cells of the stratum spinosum layer of the epidermis. It frequently arises on the sun-exposed skin of middle-aged and elderly individuals as well as in immunosuppressed people and patients exposed to ionizing radiation. Tumours can be preceded by a keratin horn, Bowen's disease and leukoplakia as well as arising in chronic wounds, in which case they are termed Marjolin's ulcer.

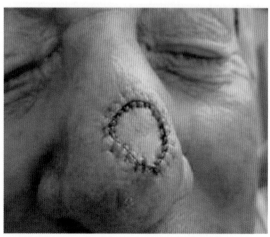

FIGURE 5.9 Excision of basal cell carcinoma from nose and full thickness skin graft

Tumours are staged according to American Joint Committee on Cancer guidelines, which use the TNM classification system.

Investigation

Clinical diagnostic indicators

The clinical appearance is highly variable, but usually the tumour presents as an ulcerated lesion with hard, raised everted edges (see *Symptoms and Signs*).

Differential diagnosis

▦ Keratoacanthoma,
▦ Basal cell carcinoma
▦ Bowen's disease
▦ Cutaneous horn
▦ Actinic keratosis.

Tissue biopsy

A **punch, incisional or excisional biopsy** is required to confirm the diagnosis, variants and prognostic indicators.

Tumours are characterized by dysplastic epidermal keratinocytes, extending down through the basement membrane into the dermis, and the presence of keratin pearls. Differentiation may be well, moderate or poor.

Bad prognostic indicators include increased depth of invasion, vascular invasion, perineural invasion and lymphocytic infiltration.

Imaging

Ultrasound or CT scan is required for patients with clinically palpable regional lymphadenopathy. **Ultrasound-guided fine needle aspiration cytology** of the lymph node or an excision node biopsy is required to confirm the diagnosis. The incision for an open biopsy must not compromise the incision which might be required for a subsequent block dissection.

Management

Tumours should be treated within a multidisciplinary team.

▦ **Surgical excision** with margins of at least 0.5–1 cm, if possible, followed if necessary by reconstruction with a graft.
▦ **Moh's micrographic surgery**

▦ **Lymphadenectomy** in patients with proven nodal disease
▦ **Radiotherapy**: primary or adjuvant radiotherapy after excision or lymphadenectomy.

Follow-up

Patients who develop one squamous cell carcinoma have a 40 per cent risk of developing additional tumours within the next 2 years. As this risk increases as more time elapses, patients should be evaluated every 3–6 months to assess for local and regional recurrence as well as new disease.

MALIGNANT MELANOMA

Malignant melanoma is a tumour that develops as a result of the malignant transformation of melanocytes. These cells are derived from the neural crest. Melanomata usually occur in the skin but can arise in other locations to which neural crest cells migrate, such as the gastrointestinal tract, brain or retina. Although malignant melanoma only constitutes 5–10 per cent of all skin cancers it causes 80 per cent of all skin cancer deaths. Its incidence varies from <1 per 100 000 in China to 45 per 100 000 in Australia and is rising by almost 6 per cent per year. Melanoma predominantly affects adults, with a peak incidence in the fourth decade, and has no sex prevalence. A patient's risk of developing a second primary melanoma after diagnosis of the first one is 3–5 per cent.

Investigation of the primary lesion

Clinical diagnostic indicators

The frequency of the various clinical varieties of melanoma is given in Table 5.2.

Table 5.2
Frequency of clinical varieties of melanoma

Superficial spreading: 60 per cent

Nodular: 30 per cent

Lentigo maligna: 7 per cent

Acral lentiginous: <2 per cent

Amelanotic melanoma: <1 per cent

Desmoplasic melanoma: <1 per cent

Classically, the 'ABCD' mnemonic is used to describe the clinical features that suggest malignant change in a pigmented lesion:

A = Asymmetry of the mole
B = Border irregularity of the mole
C = Colour change or variability
D = Diameter increasing especially to >6 mm
E = Extra features; pruritis, ulceration and bleeding.

Risk factors

- History of a changing mole
- Atypical naevus syndrome
- Personal history of melanoma
- Family history of melanoma
- Congenital giant hairy naevus
- Blue eyes, fair and/or red hair, pale complexion
- Regular tanning bed use before age 30
- Multiple naevi
- Immunosuppression: transplant patients, haematological malignancies
- Non-melanoma skin cancer
- Sun sensitivity (tendency to sunburn).

Differential diagnosis

- Seborrheic keratosis
- Traumatized or irritated naevus
- Pigmented basal cell carcinoma
- Lentigo
- Blue naevus
- Angiokeratoma
- Traumatic haematoma
- Dermatofibroma
- Pigmented actinic keratosis.

Tissue biopsy

Excisional biopsy with a 2-mm margin and cuff of fat. You must have a low threshold to perform a biopsy if a lesion is suspicious.

Histological report is crucial for treatment planning and assessment of prognosis.

Incisional or punch biopsies are rarely indicated except in very large lesions, e.g. suspicion of malignant change within a congenital giant hairy naevus or for a possible subungual melanoma.

A shave biopsy or curettage should never be performed as it renders subsequent Breslow and Clark staging inaccurate.

Table 5.3
The Breslow thickness

Breslow thickness is the distance between the granular layer of the epidermis and the deepest part of the melanoma measured in millimetres. The Breslow thickness is used as part of the TNM classification and is directly related to survival:

- thickness of 0.75 mm or less
- thickness of 0.75–1.5 mm
- thickness of 1.5–4 mm
- thickness greater than 4 mm.

Table 5.4
The Clark level

Clark's level is based on the depth of tumour invasion:

- level I: involves only epidermis (*in situ* melanoma); no invasion
- level II: invades papillary dermis but not papillary-reticular dermal interface
- level III: invades and expands papillary dermis up to the interface with, but not into, reticular dermis
- level IV: invades reticular dermis but not into subcutaneous tissue
- level V: invades into subcutaneous tissue.

Histological classification

Melanomata may be classified according to their clinical and histological characteristics, their Breslow thickness (Table 5.3), their Clark level (Table 5.4) and their TNM staging (Table 5.5).

Imaging

CT scan may be used to assess any palpable lymph nodes. **Ultrasound- or CT-guided fine needle aspiration cytology** of the lymph node is usually diagnostic. If clinical suspicion remains despite a negative cytology, an **open excision biopsy** is required.

Staging

The following staging investigations are required as the presence of palpable lymph glands suggests the possibility of more distant spread.

Table 5.5
TNM staging

The TNM (tumour, node, metastasis) system is used for clinical staging. (American Joint Committee on Cancer (AJCC) staging system)

- ■ T = tumour
  - ☐ Tis: *in situ* melanoma
  - ☐ T1: depth <0.75 mm
  - ☐ T2: depth 0.75–1.5 mm
  - ☐ T3: depth 1.5–4 mm
  - ☐ T4: depth >4 mm
- ■ N = regional lymph nodes
  - ☐ N0: no regional lymph node metastasis
  - ☐ N1: node <3 cm or <3 in-transit metastases
  - ☐ N2: node >3 cm or >3 in-transit metastases
- ■ M = distant metastasis
  - ☐ M0: no distant metastasis
  - ☐ M1: Distant metastasis

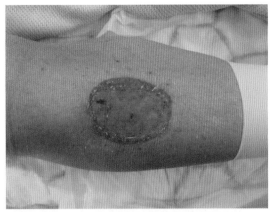

FIGURE 5.10   Split skin graft to right lower leg following a 2-cm wide excision of a malignant melanoma

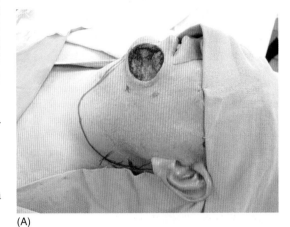

(A)

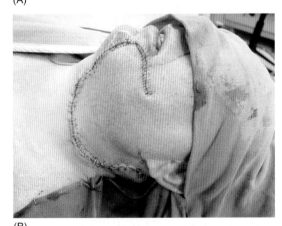

(B)

FIGURE 5.11   (A) Wide excision of melanoma left chin and (B) reverse cheek rotation flap

Chest X-ray, **liver function tests** and an **ultrasound, CT** or **MRI** of the abdomen and pelvis.

Management

Malignant melanomata must be treated within a multidisciplinary team.

Widely excise the primary lesion. Once the diagnosis of melanoma has been confirmed histologically the patient should undergo a wider excision down to the fascia. Numerous studies have been carried out and the following excision margins are presently recommended:

- ▥ melanoma *in situ* **5–10 mm** excision margin
- ▥ Breslow thickness <1 mm: **1 cm** excision margin
- ▥ Breslow thickness 1–2 mm: **1–2 cm** excision margin
- ▥ Breslow thickness >2 mm: **2 cm** excision margin.

Reconstruction of the defect may be performed using either a skin graft (Fig 5.10) or a flap (Fig 5.11).

Lymphadenectomy. If the regional lymph nodes are involved a lymphadenectomy must be performed.

No survival benefit has yet been shown from **elective lymph node dissection** (ELND) and so this procedure should not be performed outside of a clinical trial.

Similarly, although no studies have demonstrated a survival benefit from **sentinel lymph node biopsy**

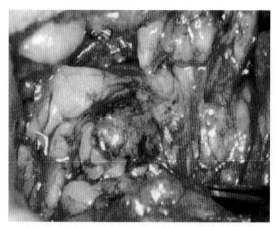

FIGURE 5.12   Blue lymphatic channel and lymph node

(SLNB) it is used as a staging tool and the UK National Guidelines recommend that all patients with melanoma greater than 1 mm thick should be offered a SLNB at the time of wide local excision.

The technique aims to identify and remove and study the first draining lymph node within a regional lymphatic basin when no clinically positive nodes are present. Double labelling is used with pre-operative lymphoscintigraphy and peri-operative vital blue dye injection into the melanoma site. The sentinel node is identified with the gamma probe and sent for histological assessment. If the SLNB is positive the patient is offered a completion lymphadenectomy (block dissection).

Adjuvant therapies The following therapies have been tried over the years, usually for advanced disease and with variable, usually little, long-term success:

- isolated limb perfusion for extremity melanomas
- high-dose interferon α-2b
- biological agents
- vaccines
- radiotherapy may provide symptomatic relief for metastases to bone, brain, or viscera
- surgical resection of isolated metastases may be performed for palliation.

Prognosis These factors adversely affect prognosis:

- sex and age: males have a worse prognosis; elderly people have a worse prognosis
- site: lesions on the trunk, scalp, mucosa and perineum have a worse prognosis
- ulcerated lesions have a worse prognosis

- acral lentiginous melanomata have a worse prognosis
- Breslow thickness and Clark's level
- lymphocytic infiltration.

The survival rate at 10 years

- for tumours <0.75 mm thick is 98 per cent
- for tumours 0.75–1.5 mm thick is 91 per cent
- for tumours >3 mm thick is 55 per cent.

Follow-up care

Close follow-up care is essential to detect new primary lesions, recurrence or metastases. History and physical examination are the cornerstones plus further testing (e.g. chest radiography, blood chemistry) if suggestive findings are encountered. Most practitioners observe patients every 3–6 months initially and then yearly. Some physicians advocate observing patients with thicker tumours more frequently than patients with thinner lesions. Follow-up care with a dermatologist is strongly recommended.

Repeatedly educate patients on sun protection, self-examination for detection of new or recurrent lesions and for recognition of the signs and symptoms of metastatic disease.

MYCOSIS FUNGOIDES

The term mycosis fungoides (MF) was first used by Alibert, a French dermatologist, in 1806, when he described a severe disorder in which large necrotic tumours resembling mushrooms presented on a patient's skin. Mycosis fungoides is the most common type of cutaneous T-cell lymphoma and usually presents as a patch of thickened red skin.

The principal investigation should be a **tissue biopsy**.

Once the diagnosis is confirmed histologically the patient should be referred for cytotoxic chemotherapy as for other lymphomas.

KAPOSI'S SARCOMA

This is a cutaneous sarcoma that is often associated with HIV and AIDS. It presents as crops of painless red-purple nodules which often develop on the lower limbs.

Once the diagnosis is confirmed by biopsy the patient should be managed by a multidisciplinary team to treat the underlying cause and the cutaneous sarcomas.

VASCULAR MALFORMATIONS

Vascular malformations (VMs) are inborn errors of vascular morphogenesis which are present at birth, permanent and progressive. They may either be **low-flow** capillary, lymphatic or venous; or **high-flow** arterial and arteriovenous.

Most lesions are mixed. The predominant vessel is used to describe the le sion.

They occur anywhere on the head and neck but are most common in the lips, tongue, cheeks and muscle. When bone is involved there is resulting bone hypertrophy.

VMs grow in proportion with the child as well as with puberty, infection and trauma.

HAEMANGIOMATA

Haemangiomata are the most common vascular tumours of childhood. They are benign neoplasms of vasoformative tissue that may involve any part of the body but most commonly the head and neck region. They are usually absent at birth but have a characteristic clinical course, marked by early proliferation followed by spontaneous involution. The enlargement of these lesions during the proliferative phase in the neonatal period or early infancy is caused by a rapidly dividing endothelial cell proliferation. Following the involutional phase, 90 per cent of patients, by age of 9 years, are left with a fibrofatty remnant.

Occasionally, haemangiomata may impinge on vital structures, ulcerate, bleed or cause high-output cardiac failure or significant structural abnormalities. Rarely, they may be associated with one or more congenital anomalies.

Investigation

The diagnosis is made by finding a localized abnormality with features of veins, arteries or lymphatics.

Management

Reassurance and observation by the parents. Parents need to be supported and educated regarding the natural history.

Active treatment is indicated if the haemangioma impinges on vital structures, ulcerates, bleeds, causes high-output cardiac failure or significant structural abnormalities. These cases should be managed by a multidisciplinary team.

Medical treatment includes:

- systemic steroids
- interferon-α-2a
- vincristine
- antiplatelet agents.

Invasive therapy includes:

- intralesional steroid
- intralesional OK-432
- intralesional sclerosant
- laser treatment
- surgical debulking – particularly when obstructing vision, hearing, airway or feeding
- selective embolization.

LOW-FLOW VMS

Venous and mixed VMs

Clinical diagnostic indicators

- They grow slowly and do not expand beyond the local region.
- They may be associated with pain, bleeding and facial asymmetry.
- They are easily compressible and swell when dependent.
- They may contain phleboliths (seen on X-ray).

Management

This is indicated if bleeding or causing obstruction:

- **Sclerotherapy** with 95 per cent ethanol, or detergent or bleomycin
- **Surgical excision**.

Lymphatic VMs

There are two main types:

- lymphangiomas, which are microcystic, e.g. lymphangioma circumscriptum
- cystic hygromas, which are macrocystic.

Clinical diagnostic indicators

The diagnosis is based on the clinical features of a soft fluctuant translucent swelling. They tend to expand and contract depending on the movement of lymphatic fluid and can suddenly increase in size as a result.

Patients can present with macrocheilia, macroglossia and macrodontia, which may cause airway obstruction.

Management

Management is largely supportive.

- **Intralesional OK-432** can cause sclerosis or regression.
- **Surgery** is reserved for cases in which there is airway compromise. Lymphatic malformations recur if they are not fully excised. Surgery is often complicated by poor wound healing.
- **Nd:Yag laser.**

Capillary VM/Port wine stain

These are progressive ectatic dilatations of mature superficial dermal vessels occurring as a result of developmental weakness of the vessel wall.

Sturge–Weber syndrome is when they arise in the distribution of the ophthalmic and maxillary regions of the trigeminal nerve.

Management

Obliteration with the pulsed dye laser.

HIGH-FLOW VM

Arteriovenous malformations (AVM)

These are high-flow lesions that are interconnections between the venous and arterial systems and most commonly arise intracranially.

Clinical diagnostic indicators

They usually present at birth but only become clinically apparent in infancy or childhood. Trauma or puberty can trigger their expansion. They are characterized by a pulsation, a palpable thrill, and an audible bruit.

The high-flow shunt can cause heart failure.

Blood tests

Full blood count and **clotting screen**.

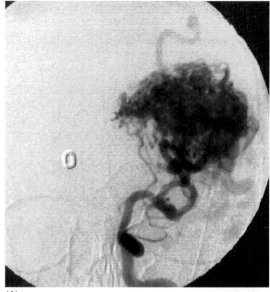

(A)

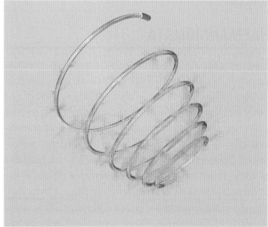

(B)

FIGURE 5.13 (A) Arteriogram demonstrating an arteriovenous malformation (AVM). (B) Coil used for preoperative embolization into the nidus of the malformation

Imaging

MRI angiography and **arteriography** are used to determine involved vessels.

Management

- Correct any clotting abnormality.
- **Preoperative embolization** (Fig 5.13) into the nidus of the malformation followed by **surgical resection** within 24–72 hours. The limits of the resection are guided by preoperative MRI and

angiography and during operation by Doppler flow detection, frozen section and the pattern of the bleeding at the wound edges.

- **Reconstruction** of the defect may be required.

SPIDER NAEVI

A spider naevus consists of a solitary dilated skin arteriole feeding a number of small branches that leave it in a radial manner. They are common, benign, acquired lesions present in 10–15 per cent of healthy adults and young children. Numerous prominent spider naevi are observed in patients with significant hepatic disease.

Investigation

Clinical diagnostic indicators

Diagnosis is made clinically by compression of the central vessel, which produces blanching and temporarily obliterates it. When released, the threadlike vessels quickly refill with blood from the central arteriole.

Blood tests

Patients with extensive lesions need to be investigated for underlying liver disease.

Management

Medical treatment

Reassurance and advice as the lesions are harmless and usually resolve spontaneously.

Surgical treatment

Laser therapy or electrodesiccation. With the latter, the spider is compressed to empty it of blood and the central arteriole is then gently electrodesiccated. Once this is destroyed, the radiating capillaries empty. Incompletely destroyed lesions may recur.

CAMPBELL DE MORGAN SPOT

This is a bright red clearly defined macule caused by a collection of dilated capillaries. They are usually found on the neck, chest, abdomen, back or arms and are seen more commonly with increasing age.

The diagnosis is made from their characteristic appearance and the fact that they do not blanch on pressure, unlike the spider naevus.

Management

Treatment is recommended only for irritation or haemorrhage or in instances in which the lesions are deemed by the patient to be cosmetically undesirable.

These lesions can be obliterated by **cryotherapy**, **pulsed dye laser**, **electrodesiccation** or **shave excision**.

HYPERHIDROSIS

Hyperhidrosis is a condition characterized by sweating in excess of that required for normal thermoregulation. It usually begins in childhood or adolescence. It may occur on any site but those most commonly affected are the palms, soles and axillae. It may be idiopathic or secondary to other diseases, metabolic disorders, febrile illnesses or medication use.

Investigation

The excess sweating is obvious but a search should be made for a cause especially if the sweating is generalized. This may require:

- **thyroid function tests**, which may reveal underlying hyperthyroidism or thyrotoxicosis
- **blood glucose levels**, which may reveal diabetes mellitus or hypoglycaemia
- **urinary catecholamines**, which may reveal a possible phaeochromocytoma.

Management

Medical care

Topical agents include topical anticholinergics, boric acid, 2–5 per cent tannic acid solutions, resorcinol, potassium permanganate. Drysol (20 per cent aluminium chloride hexahydrate in absolute anhydrous ethyl alcohol) is usually the most effective topical agent.

Systemic agents used to treat hyperhidrosis include anticholinergic medications. The use of anticholinergics may be unappealing because their adverse effect profile includes mydriasis, blurry vision, dry mouth and eyes, difficulty with micturition and constipation.

Iontophoresis consists of passing a direct current across the skin. Numerous agents have been used to induce hypohidrosis, including tap water and anticholinergics; however, treatment with anticholinergic iontophoresis is more effective than tap water iontophoresis.

Botulinum toxin injections are effective because of their anticholinergic effects at the neuromuscular junction and in the postganglionic sympathetic cholinergic nerves in the sweat glands (Fig 5.14). The effect can last between 6 and 12 months.

Surgery

Local excision. When the area of excess sweating is localized, surgical excision of the affected area (identified with iodine starch testing) to remove the appropriate sweat glands will eliminate the sweating. This technique is particularly useful for axillary hyperhidrosis.

Sympathectomy. The activity of the sweat glands is controlled by the sympathetic nerves. Open or endoscopic surgical sympathectomy is a particularly effective method of stopping hyperhidrosis of the hands and feet, but cervical sympathectomy carries a small risk of the patient developing Horner's syndrome.

Subcutaneous liposuction is another means of removing the eccrine sweat glands responsible for axillary hyperhidrosis. Compared with classic surgical excision, this modality results in less disruption to the overlying skin, resulting in smaller surgical scars and a diminished area of hair loss.

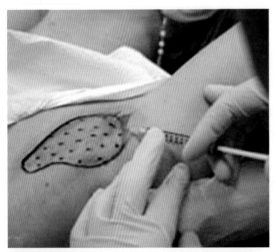

FIGURE 5.14 The area of hyperhidrosis to be treated with botulinum toxin is marked and the injections are given

SUBCUTANEOUS INFECTIONS

SUBCUTANEOUS ABSCESS

Subcutaneous abscesses are very common.

Investigation

The physical signs are usually pathognomonic – a painful, hot, red and swollen area.

Blood and urine tests
Full blood count and blood glucose
Urine dipstick for glucose

Imaging
Ultrasound is a valuable diagnostic tool when the clinical presentation is not clear. It will differentiate between cellulitis and an abscess.

Management

Surgical incision and drainage should be performed when the abscess is fluctuant. A microbiology swab should be sent for microscopy, culture and sensitivity.

The cavity is drained and, if deep, packed to keep it open to allow healing from below upwards. The pack needs to be changed daily until the wound has healed by secondary intention.

Intravenous or oral antibiotics may be required.

SINUSES AND FISTULAE

SINUS

A sinus is a tract lined by granulation tissue connecting a cavity to an epithelial surface. The reasons for delayed or non-healing are listed in *Symptoms and Signs*.

Investigation

A **microbiology swab** taken from the wall of the sinus and any discharge should be sent for microscopy, culture and sensitivity.

Sinogram, using **MRI or CT** $\pm$ contrast, delineates the complexity and anatomy of the sinus tract to exclude tuberculosis or actinomycosis.

Management

Any underlying conditions such as diabetes should be treated. **Surgical drainage** of deep infection and excision of the sinus tract removes epithelium and foreign bodies allowing healing by secondary intention. Resultant wounds can be closed by local flaps.

FISTULA

A fistula is a pathological connection between two epithelial surfaces.

Investigation

Bacteriology

A microbiology swab taken from the wall of the fistula and any discharge should be sent for microscopy, culture and sensitivity to exclude tuberculosis.

    Fistulogram (Fig 5.15), using **MRI or CT** ± contrast, delineates the complexity and anatomy of the fistula tract.

Management

Treatment is dependent on the site and underlying cause of the fistula.

    Treatment is dependent on the site and underlying cause of the fistula.

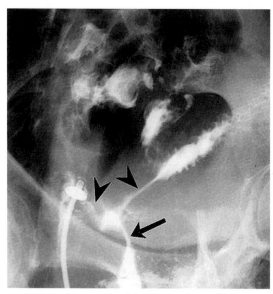

FIGURE 5.15 A conventional fistulogram demonstrating an enterocutaneous fistula (arrowheads) and a second cutaneous fistula (arrow) communicating with the contrast injection site

- Diabetes, malnutrition and infection should be treated.
- Treat the underlying disease process.
- Divert any potential cause of persistence eg. the faecal stream.
- Excise or lay open the fistula tract.
- Closure of dead space with flaps.

LUMPS BENEATH THE SKIN

LIPOMA

Lipomata are benign tumours composed of mature fat cells. They are the most common benign mesenchymal tumour.

Investigation

Clinical diagnostic indicators

They are usually solitary and found in the subcutaneous tissues and, less commonly, in internal organs. Typically, they develop as discrete rubbery masses in the subcutaneous tissues of the trunk and proximal extremity. Multiple painful lipomas are the hallmark of Dercum's disease.

Differential diagnosis

- Sebaceous cyst
- Neurofibroma
- Dermoid cyst
- Tumour of skin appendages
- Soft tissue sarcoma.

Imaging

Although this is invariably a clinical diagnosis, **CT scanning** may be useful for distinguishing between lipomas and liposarcomas and their relation to adjacent structures.

Management

Careful preoperative assessment is required to determine whether the lipoma is supra-, intra- or submuscular as this will determine whether the procedure should be performed under local or general anaesthesia. They may be removed by two methods:

- **Surgical enucleation**
- **Liposuction:** this is very effective and results in a smaller incision.

GANGLION CYST

Ganglions commonly occur around the hand and wrist joints, in patients of any age. They are smooth, spherical and usually firm. They fluctuate, transilluminate and are attached to either the ligament or the joint capsule.

Investigation
Imaging

Plain X-rays can be obtained to evaluate any potential underlying bone or joint abnormality but are rarely necessary. **MRI** is only useful in cases with an atypical presentation or when a synovioma is suspected.

Management

Pain and cosmesis are indicators for treatment. When a ganglion is in proximity to the radial artery, care must be taken to avoid damaging this structure as well as the palmar cutaneous branch of the median nerve.

Aspiration and steroid injection or traumatic disruption. Recurrence rates after non-operative ganglion treatment are high (30–60 per cent).

Surgical excision should be performed under regional or general anaesthesia with an arm tourniquet. The whole ganglion should be removed together with a modest portion of the capsule or ligament to which it is attached.

Total ganglionectomy results in an 85–95 per cent cure rate.

THE NAILS

PARONYCHIA

Acute paronychia is an acute inflammation of the nail fold. It is frequently caused by minor trauma, such as a splinter in the distal edge of the nail or excessive nail biting.

Investigation
Clinical diagnostic indicators

The infectious process begins in the lateral perionychium and is followed by the development of erythema, intense inflammation, swelling, pain and local tenderness. Vesicles and blisters may also form. Chronic paronychia commonly occurs in hands that are repeatedly exposed to water.

Bacteriology

Swab the discharge for microbiological culture and sensitivity.

Imaging

A **plain X-ray** is useful in chronic paronychia to exclude underlying osteomyelitis.

Management

- **Appropriate antibiotic therapy**.
- **Incision and drainage** if there is no response to antibiotic therapy. An incision should be made parallel to the nail fold directly over the abscess. The wound is packed and allowed to heal by secondary intention.
- In recalcitrant disease the diseased nail fold together with the proximal nail plate is excised and healing occurs by secondary intention.

INGROWING TOENAIL (ONYCHOCRYPTOSIS)

Predisposing factors include congenital malalignment of the digit, hyperhidrosis, diabetes, increased pressure from external sources (e.g. trauma), poorly fitted shoes, poor posture and gait, incorrectly trimmed nails or naturally short nails. In onychocryptosis, the primary direction of nail growth is lateral instead of forward. The laterally curved edge of the nail plate penetrates the lateral nail fold resulting in inflammation and pain. Infection and abscess formation develop if left untreated.

Investigation

Plain X-ray to exclude underlying osteomyelitis in chronic cases.

Management
Medical care

The foot should be washed regularly with soap and water and kept dry during the rest of the day. After washing the corner of the nail digging into the skin, the skin should be lifted and a small piece of cotton or gauze should be placed between the nail and the skin to keep it elevated. High heels or tight-fitting shoes should not be worn.

Antibiotics are prescribed if there is a superimposed infection.

Surgical treatment

Surgical removal of the nail and drainage of the abscess is followed by **obliteration of the nail bed** by the application of phenol to stop the nail regrowth. **Zadek's procedure** involves removal of a wedge of the entire nail and its bed. It has a 10 per cent chance of recurrence.

PERIUNGAL AND SUBUNGAL WARTS

These develop in the paronychial region of the nail unit and are caused by the human papillomavirus. They may cause squamous atypia and can be painful.

Investigation

They have to be differentiated from ingrowing toenails and paronychia.

Management

Treatment is difficult and recurrence is common. **Cryosurgery** with liquid nitrogen is the most commonly used treatment.

SUBUNGUAL EXOSTOSIS

Subungual exostoses are painful outgrowths of healthy bone or remnants of calcified cartilage that frequently occur on the great toe in young people. Trauma has been implicated as the inciting cause.

Investigation

Clinical diagnostic indicators

The exostosis begins as a small elevation on the dorsal surface of the terminal phalanx but with time it may appear as an outgrowth under the distal nail edge, or it may even completely destroy the nail plate. Patients present with pain, which may be accompanied by an abnormal gait because

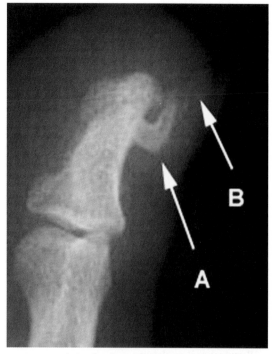

FIGURE 5.16   Lateral radiograph of the right thumb showing a trabeculated bony growth (A) with an expanded distal area layered by radiolucent cartilage (B)

of difficulty walking and a deformed nail. The differential diagnosis is an ingrowing toenail or a paronychia.

Imaging

On **plain X-ray,** the diagnostic appearances are a trabeculated bony growth with an expanded distal area layered by radiolucent cartilage (Fig 5.16).

Management

The exostosis can be approached and **excised** either through a fish mouth incision leaving the nail plate in place or, after partial nail avulsion, through a longitudinal incision in the nail bed.

ONYCHOMYCOSIS

Onychomycosis (OM) refers to a fungal infection that affects the nails. It may involve any component of the nail unit, including the nail matrix, the nail bed or the nail plate.

Investigation

Clinical diagnostic indicators

It can present with pain, discomfort and disfigurement and may produce serious physical, psychosocial and occupational limitations that have a significant impact on quality of life.

Microbiology

Microscopy and culture should be obtained of either clippings of the nail plate or a sample taken from the proximal nail where the concentration of hyphae is greatest.

Management

A combination of oral, topical and surgical therapy can increase efficacy.

- **Topical antifungals** are beneficial only for mild cases involving the very distal nail plate.
- **Oral antifungals** (itraconazole and terbinafine) are useful for severe and recalcitrant cases.
- **Surgical nail avulsion.**

ONYCHOGRYPHOSIS

Onychogryphosis (thickened toenail) is caused by damage to the germinal matrix, which can be acute, such as dropping a heavy object on to the toe, or chronic trauma over the years. It is occasionally mistaken for a fungal infection of the nail and mistreated with antifungal therapy. This diagnosis must be excluded with the appropriate tests (see above).

Management

- **Cutting and filing** the nail to reduce its thickness.
- **Nail ablation**, ensuring that the entire germinal matrix is either surgically removed or chemically destroyed with phenol.

BURNS

About 250 000 people are burnt each year in the United Kingdom. Of these, almost 112 000 attend an emergency department, and about 210 die of their injuries. At least 250 000 others attend their general practitioner for treatment of their injury.

EMERGENCY EXAMINATION AND TREATMENT OF BURNS

In a patient with multiple injuries, the most obvious injury may be their burn, but careful assessment and treatment of other injuries is vital before burn management.

All patients with facial burns or suspected of having an inhalational injury should be assessed by an anaesthetist before being transferred to a specialist unit.

Rapid assessment and treatment can be life saving.

The essential points needed from the history are summarized in Table 5.6.

FIRST AID
Stop the burning process

The person should be removed from the burning source without endangering the rescuers.

Flame burns	Extinguish flames safely Remove hot charred clothes.
Scald burns	Remove fluid soaked clothing.
Electrical burns	Turn off the electric power before administering first aid. Remove all jewellery.

Cool the burn wound

Cool with lukewarm running water ideally at 15°C for 20 minutes. This period should be increased for those with chemical burns. Cooling the surface reduces the inflammatory reaction and stops the progression of burn depth as well as acting as an analgesic.

Remember children are at significant risk of hypothermia; therefore, raise the ambient room temperature to 30°C and keep the rest of the child well wrapped.

Dressings

Cover the burn with a **clean sheet or cling film**. These are simple to use and allow wound inspection so that definitive assessment can be performed. Sterile burn cooling gels are also available.

Do not use tight dressings as this can constrict the limbs and compromise circulation.

Elevate the burnt area to reduce swelling.

Table 5.6
Essential points to determine in the history of a burn

Timing of injury and duration of exposure	
Mechanism of injury	Enclosed space (consider inhalational injury)
	Blast or explosion
	Electrocution
	Jump or fall
	Road traffic accident
Scald	Assess temperature and nature of fluid (recently boiled, milk etc.)
Electrical injury	High or low voltage
Duration of time in contact	
Chemical injury	Type of chemical
Duration of contact	
Any first aid given	
Evidence of non-accidental injury (NAI)	
Pre-morbid state	
Medications/allergies	

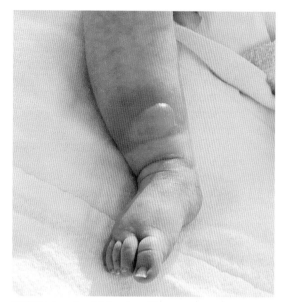

FIGURE 5.17   Small intact burn blisters

MANAGEMENT OF MINOR BURNS

Cleaning

Burn debris should be removed with mild soap and water, sterile saline or a topical antiseptic solution before dressings are applied.

The dead skin of open blisters should be removed, and large or friable blisters should also be 'deroofed' (the outer layer removed). Small blisters may be left intact (Fig 5.17).

Antibiotics are not routinely prescribed in minor burns.

The tetanus status of the patient should be checked.

Dressings

In the simple, clean, partial thickness burn, dressings such as paraffin gauze (for example, Jelonet), chlorhexidine impregnated gauze (Bactigras) or similar dressings such as soft silicone (Mepitel) can be used with an overlying gauze pad.

Hydrocolloid dressings are particularly good for use on hands and other small areas of superficial or partial thickness burns, although they leave a 'skim' of exudate that needs to be removed to allow appropriate assessment of the wound.

In bigger burns, several layers of dressing are usually required to absorb exudate and to prevent shear or friction of the skin.

MANAGEMENT OF MAJOR BURNS

Primary survey

Immediate life-threatening conditions are identified and emergency management begun.

Remember the ABC of emergency management (Table 5.7).

- **A** – Airway maintenance with cervical spine control
  - ☐ Clear the airway of foreign material and open the airway with chin lift/jaw thrust.
  - ☐ Ensure inline immobilization of the cervical spine, avoiding hyperflexion or extension of the neck.

□ Singed nasal and facial hair, swollen lips and tongue and carbonaceous sputum imply an inhalational injury unless proven otherwise. Urgent assessment is required by an anaesthetist.

B – Breathing and ventilation

□ Expose the chest ensuring that expansion is adequate and equal.

□ Provide supplemental 100% oxygen through a humidified non-rebreathing mask.

□ Remember carbon monoxide poisoning can give a cherry pink, non-breathing patient.

□ Beware a respiratory rate >20/minute.

□ Beware, circumferential chest burns may need an escharotomy.

C – Circulation with haemorrhage control

□ Check the pulse.

□ Capillary refill – normal return is 2 seconds, longer indicates hypovolaemia, or indicates need for escharotomy on that limb.

□ Intavenous access with 2 large bore cannulas and send blood for full blood count, urea and creatinine, clotting and blood group.

D – Disability: neurological status

□ Establish level of consciousness:

A alert

V response to vocal stimuli

P response to painful stimuli

U unresponsive

□ Examine the papillary response to light, which should be brisk and equal.

E – Exposure with environmental control

□ Remove all clothing and jewellery and keep the patient warm.

F – Fluid resuscitation

□ Insert two large-bore, peripheral intravenous catheters, preferably though unburned tissue.

□ Take blood for full blood count, urea and electrolytes, coagulation studies, amylase and carboxyhaemoglobin.

Fluid resuscitation is indicated after a serious burn, i.e.

- 10 per cent of total body surface area in children
- 15 per cent of total body surface area in adults.

Table 5.7
The primary survey of a burnt patient

A Airway maintenance and cervical spine control

B Breathing and ventilation

C Circulation with haemorrhage control

D Disability – neurological status

E Exposure and environmental control

F Fluid resuscitation

The size of the burnt area is estimated by using Wallace's rule of nines (Fig 5.18), a Lund and Browder Chart or by using the palmar surface of the patient's hand, which approximates 1 per cent body surface area.

The British Burn Association recommends the use of the Parkland formula (Table 5.8) to calculate the fluid requirement, but all these aids are only guidelines. The patient's circulation must be closely monitored and fluid replacement adjusted accordingly and guided by the patient's response to resuscitation.

Monitor the adequacy of resuscitation from:

- the urine output (urinary catheter): 0.5–1.0 mL/kg hourly in adults and 1.0–1.5 mL/kg in children
- pulse and blood pressure
- central line, arterial line
- respiratory rate
- pulse oximetry
- an ECG
- venous blood tests at 4 to 6 hours intervals
- arterial blood gases.

If haemorrhage occurs from other injuries, replace with blood.

X-ray the cervical spine (lateral) chest and pelvis. **Pain relief** with morphine should be given only intravenously slowly and cautiously in small incremental doses until the pain is controlled.

SECONDARY SURVEY

This is a comprehensive head to toe examination that commences after life-threatening conditions have been excluded or treated (see Chapter 6).

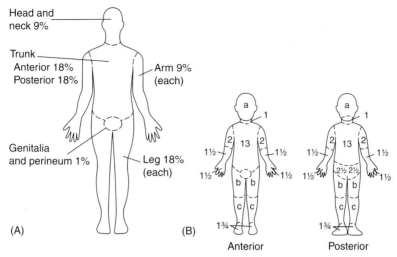

	Head and neck 9%
Trunk	Anterior 18% / Posterior 18%
Arm 9% (each)	
Genitalia and perineum 1%	Leg 18% (each)

Relative percentage of body surface area (%BSA) affected by growth

Body Part	Age				
	0 yr	1 yr	5 yr	10 yr	15 yr
a = 1/2 of head	9 1/2	8 1/2	6 1/2	5 1/2	4 1/2
b = 1/2 of 1 thigh	2 3/4	3 1/4	4	4 1/4	4 1/2
c = 1/2 of 1 lower leg	2 1/2	2 1/4	2 3/4	3	3 1/4

FIGURE 5.18   Wallace's rule of nines and the Lund and Browder chart (the relative proportions of body area differ in children)

Table 5.8
The Parkland formula

Total fluid requirement in the first 24 hours following a burn is

3–4 mL/kg of Hartmann solution for each percentage of total body surface area (TBSA)

Half is given in the first 8 hours from the time of the burn

Half is given in the next 16 hours

Children receive maintenance fluid in addition, at an hourly rate of:

    4 mL/kg for the first 10 kg of body weight
    2 mL/kg for the second 10 kg of body weight
    1 mL/kg for extra weight

End point
Urine output of 0.5–1.0 mL/kg/h in adults
Urine output of 1.0–1.5 mL/kg/h in children

History Use the mnemonic AMPLE:

    Allergies
    Medications
    Past medical history
    Last meal
    Events: environment related to injury and information about the mechanism of injury.

Examination The patient should be thoroughly examined from head to toe and any additional radiological investigations carried out where indicated.

The burnt areas need to be further assessed and the depth of the burns documented on a chart. Accurate assessment of burn depth is vital as it differentiates between burns that will heal spontaneously and those that require surgical intervention (Table 5.9, Figs 5.19 and 5.20). Circumferential burns will require escharotomy.

INDICATIONS FOR REFERRAL TO A BURNS UNIT

The burn injuries requiring referral to a Burns Unit are shown in Table 5.10.

Table 5.9
Assessment of burn depth

Depth	Colour	Blisters	Capillary refill	Sensation	Healing
Epidermal	Red	No	Present	Present	Yes
Superficial dermal	Pale pink	Small	Present	Painful	Yes
Mid-dermal	Dark pink	Present	Sluggish	±	Usually
Deep dermal	Blotchy red	±	Absent	Absent	No
Full thickness	White	No	Absent	Absent	No

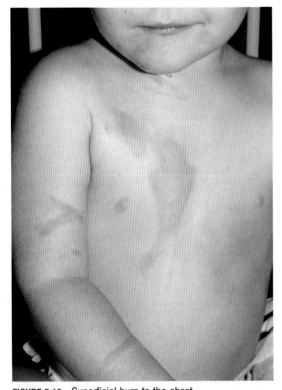

FIGURE 5.19   Superficial burn to the chest

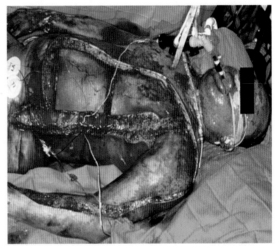

FIGURE 5.20   Circumferential full thickness burns requiring escharotomies

INTENSIVE CARE MANAGEMENT

The goal in the management of an acute burn is to limit the extent of the systemic insult. Intensive care management aims to prevent organ failure in high-risk patients. The burn may be the 'tip of the iceberg', and the following sequlae must be anticipated and treated.

Inhalational injury

This can result in mucosal burns, mucosal inflammation, bronchorrhoea, bronchospasm ciliary paralysis, reduced surfactant, obstruction by debris and systemic inflammatory response. The **management** is:

- intubation and ventilation
- adequate oxygenation
- aggressive airway toilet
- substantial increase in fluid resuscitation.

Heart failure

This can result from circulating myocardial depressant factors and myocardial oedema. **Inotropic drugs** should not be used in management until adequate fluid resuscitation has been ensured.

Table 5.10
Conditions that require referral to a specialist burns centre

Associated airway injury

Partial thickness burns >5 per cent of total burn surface area (TBSA) in a child

Partial thickness burns >10 per cent of TBSA in an adult

Full thickness burns >1 per cent TBSA

Burns of special areas: face, hands, feet, genitalia, perineum and major joints

Electrical burns

Chemical burns

Circumferential burns

Burns at the extremes of age

Burn injury in patients with pre-existing medical disorders

Any burn with associated trauma

Non-accidental injury

Renal failure

This can arise early on as a result of delayed or inadequate fluid resuscitation or from substantial muscle breakdown or haemolysis. Delayed renal failure is usually a consequence of sepsis and is associated with other organ failure. The first signs are a reduced urine output despite adequate fluid resuscitation, followed by rising serum creatinine and urea. Management is with **haemodialysis**.

Cerebral failure

This can arise as a result of hypoxia, head injury or cerebral oedema from excessive fluid resuscitation.

Nutrition

This is an essential part of intensive care management as burn injuries are associated with a hypermetabolic response that can persist for a many months. Close attention to nutritional needs is critical to prevent protein breakdown, decreased wound healing, immune suppression and an increase in infective complication. **Management**:

- Reduce heat loss – environmental conditioning
- Excision and closure of burn wound
- Early enteral feeding – prevents stress ulcers and maintains the intestinal flora. Use a nasojejunal tube to bypass gastric stasis.

Infection

This is responsible for up to 75 per cent mortality in burns after the initial resuscitation. Prevention, recognition and treatment present considerable challenges. Infection can occur at any site but pulmonary infection is the most common.

Diagnosis can be challenging as extensive colonization of wounds makes interpretation of surface cultures difficult.

Signs of wound infection include:
- change in wound appearance (discoloration of surrounding skin, offensive smell)
- delayed healing
- graft failure
- deepening of burn depth.

Preventive measures should include:
- regular cleaning of wounds
- regular change of dressings
- surgical excision and closure
- topical antimicrobials; flamazine.

Treatment:
- systemic antibiotics
- excision of necrotic and infective tissue and cover

MANAGEMENT OF THE BURN WOUND

Epidermal and superficial dermal burns
- Healing occurs within two weeks.
- Clean and dress on alternate days with a non-adherent primary dressing (e.g. Jelonet, Mepitel) and an absorbent secondary dressing such as gauze or gamgee.
- Antimicrobial agents are added where infection is likely (perineum and feet), heavy colonization is evident or invasive infection is suspected.
- Any burn not healed within 2 weeks should be referred for assessment.

Deep dermal burns
- These are unlikely to heal within 3 weeks.
- There is a high incidence of hypertrophic scarring, so they should be excised to a viable depth and skin grafted within 5–10 days.

Full-thickness burns
- These have no regeneration elements left.
- Unless they are very small so that healing can occur from the edges, they will take weeks to heal and undergo severe contraction.
- They should be excised, and skin grafted.

Timing of surgery

Ideally all wounds should have epithelial cover within 3 weeks to minimize scarring. **Early excision** of the burn is essential as it terminates the physiological response leading to multiple organ failure as well as reducing the likelihood of infection. Ideally this should be performed and the wounds grafted within 5 days of injury.

- **Tangential excision** is a slower process with increased blood loss but results in tissue preservation, thereby improving function and cosmesis.
- **Fascial excision** is a faster technique with less blood loss, but more tissue is removed resulting in poorer function and cosmesis.

Wound coverage following excision

After burn excision, wound coverage is required either to achieve healing or to act as a temporary dressing and reduce loss of exudate and development of infection, while the donor sites regenerate and can then be re-harvested.

Split skin graft (autograft)

- **Sheet grafts** provide a superior cosmetic and functional result.
- **Meshed grafts** allow expansion of the graft, contouring to the excision defect and drainage of exudate from the wound bed, thereby improving the 'take'. However, the cosmetic result is inferior as the mesh pattern is permanent.

Skin substitutes

Biological substitutes are acellular or cellular:

- acellular: allograft (glycerol preserved), alloderm and xenograft (porcine)
- cellular: allograft (cryopreserved), cultured keratinocytes, transcyte and dermagraft.

Non-biological substitutes are Integra (dermal substitute) and biobrane.

Essentials of burn reconstruction

- Requires a strong patient–surgeon relationship and psychological support.
- Clarify expectations and explain priorities.
- Note all available donor sites.
- Start with a 'winner', an easy and quick operation.
- Complete as many surgeries as possible in preschool years.
- Offer multiple simultaneous procedures.
- Reassure and support patient and family.

Timing of reconstruction

Urgent procedures
- Exposure of vital structures (such as eyelid releases).
- Entrapment or compression of neurovasculare bundles.
- Fourth-degree contractures.
- Severe microstomia.

Essential procedures
- Reconstruction of function (such as a limited range of motion).
- Progressive deformities.

Desirable procedures
- Reconstruction of passive areas.
- Aesthetics.

Techniques for reconstruction

- Excision and primary closure.
- Z-plasty.
- Skin graft

- Dermal templates and skin grafts.
- Local, regional free flaps.
- Tissue expansion.

REHABILITATION AFTER BURN TREATMENT

- Rehabilitation starts from the time of injury. Consistent and often repetitive education is a vital part of patient care.
- Pain control is essential in order to allow rehabilitation.
- Respiratory rehabilitation involves chest physiotherapy to remove secretions, normalizing breathing mechanics and preventing complications.
- Movement and function should be passive and active with the assistance of physiotherapy and occupational therapy.
- Oedema must be managed using compression, movement, elevation and lymphatic massage.
- Scar management involves massage, silicone gel sheets, elastomer moulds, compression garments, sun protection, ultrasound and intralesional steroids.
- The psychological needs of the burn patient differ at each stage and require the involvement of social workers, vocational counsellors and psychologists.
- Outpatient follow-up should be regular and comprehensive.

ELECTRICAL BURNS

Electrical injuries are divided into three groups: low voltage, high voltage and lightning strike.

Low voltage

The energy imparted from 240 V usually gives a deep burn in the form of a small entry and exit wound (Fig 5.21). Such burns are commonly seen on the hands. If alternating current crosses the myocardium, arrhythmias may arise. If the electrocardiogram is normal and there is no history of loss of consciousness, admission to hospital for cardiac monitoring is not required.

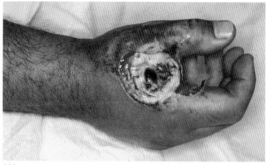

(A)

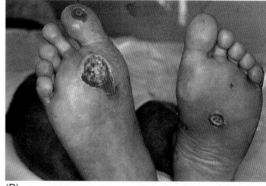

(B)

FIGURE 5.21   Entrance and exit wounds from a low voltage electrical injury

High voltage

High voltage burns occur as a result of injury from 1000 V or more. These are catastrophic injuries that cause extensive tissue damage and often rhabdomyolysis and subsequent renal failure.

Lightning

These injuries result from an ultra-high tension, high amperage, short duration electrical discharge of direct current. The pattern of injury is variable. A direct strike is when the discharge is through the victim and this has a high mortality. More commonly, a side flash (Fig 5.22) occurs when lighting strikes an object of high resistance such as a tree and the current is then deflected through a victim on its way to the ground.

Important points to remember when dealing with electric burns are summarized in Table 5.11.

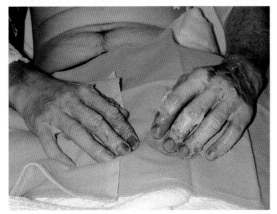

FIGURE 5.22   Flash burns to both hands

CHEMICAL BURNS

Acid burns

Acid causes coagulative necrosis and denatures proteins. Acid burns are usually painful.

Hydrofluoric acid penetrates tissues deeply and can cause fatal systemic toxicity even in small burns.

They should be treated immediately with copious lavage and topical calcium gluconate gel. Systemic calcium may be required as hydrofluoric acid sequesters calcium with the burn.

Alkali burns

Common household alkalis such as bleaches, cleaning agents and cement cause a liquefactive

Table 5.11
Important points to remember when managing electrical burns

Avoid injury to those rendering assistance

Treat cardiac and respiratory arrest

Assess and manage associated trauma

Continuous cardiac monitoring for 24 hours for significant injuries

Patterns of injury are specific to high voltage, low voltage and lightning strikes

Standard burns resuscitation formulae may be inadequate

Haemoglobinuria is common in high-voltage injury and requires maintenance of urine output 75–100 mL/hour until urine clears

High-voltage injury involving limbs may require fasciotomy

All electrical burns should be referred to a Burns Unit

necrosis. They have the potential to penetrate tissues deeper than most acids. Progressive injury dehydrates the cells and denatures the collagen and protein. Often the onset of pain is delayed, thus postponing first aid and allowing more tissue damage.

6

Major trauma

Kevin G. Burnand

The common causes of civilian trauma are road traffic, household, work place (especially the construction industry) and sports accidents plus civilian violence. All vary greatly in incidence in different parts of the world. Military and police force injuries mainly occur as a consequence of war and civil unrest and are usually caused by missiles, gunshot, shrapnel, glass and burns (the management of burns is covered in Chapter 5).

Most injuries are first seen at the site where they occur and then later, often by a different group of doctors, in a hospital Accident and Emergency Department (A&E).

The management of major trauma can therefore be divided into three stages – at the site of injury, immediately after hospital admission and following a secondary survey. Quite often this involves repeating and adding to the investigations and sometimes changing management. The overall process can be summarized as:

- First stage: first aid (pre-hospital)
- Second stage: immediate urgent assessment and resuscitation on arrival at hospital
- Third stage: a more detailed assessment – the 'secondary survey' – and the definitive treatment of specific injuries.

Running parallel and associated with this pathway is **triage** – *priority selection*: first, at the place of injury (especially when many patients are injured at once); second, in the A&E (where priority must be given to the resuscitation of the most severely injured); and third for treatment, especially when facilities are limited and priority must be given to patients who require urgent intervention to save their lives.

INVESTIGATION AND MANAGEMENT AT THE SITE OF THE ACCIDENT/INJURY: FIRST AID

The objective behind developing the skills of ambulance crew paramedics and emergency response trauma teams, based at trauma centres, has been to reduce early deaths from injury by providing rapid help and resuscitation at or close to the point of injury. The hope was that 'immediate' resuscitation in the first '*golden hour*' would reduce the mortality of serious injury.

The value of sending super specialized teams to administer complex rather than basic skilled treatment at the site of an injury/accident has, however, never been proven in either a civilian or military context; consequently, opinion has gradually moved away from prolonged complex attempts to fully stabilize the injured patient, often by relatively inexperienced staff, before transporting them to hospital to the now favoured '**scoop and run**' approach, in which rapid resuscitation – CABC (**c**ontrol of immediate life-threatening events, the **a**irway, **b**reathing and the **c**irculation) – is followed by rapid transfer to the nearest emergency department or base hospital. Prolonged assessment and resuscitation at the site of the accident/injury, '**stay and play**', has now largely been abandoned.

Assess the cause and extent of the injury/accident

It has to be recognized that initial estimates of the number of casualties are often inaccurate because of confused communications and the shock experienced at the scene of the disaster by many of those involved, including the eye witnesses. It should also be remembered that it may take some time to reach and extricate those trapped by collapsed buildings or tunnels.

In any major catastrophe, some are killed outright and many have relatively minor injuries, leaving a small group of patients in whom early appropriate intervention can save life and sometimes achieve a satisfactory outcome with no permanent sequelae.

In civilian life (mainly road traffic injuries), an eye witness assessment of the speed of travel of the vehicles involved and the mechanisms of injury (e.g. behind the wheel of a car, thrown clear, wearing seat belts) can provide a useful indication of the type of injury sustained. Equally, it is helpful if the height of any fall can be relayed to the trauma centre (a soft landing area can result in a favourable outcome).

Inform the recipient emergency services

After a major injury alert, the emergency services will ask the major trauma centres (often more than one if a large number of injuries are expected) to activate their 'major disaster plan' and inform them how many injuries to expect. When a small number of casualties is expected, one or more trauma teams should be assembled.

CLINICAL ASSESSMENT AND TREATMENT AT THE SITE OF INJURY

The first task at the site of the accident is to stabilize the injured as rapidly as possible to enable and ensure their safe transport to hospital. To stay alive a patient must be able to breathe, for which they must have a patent airway, functioning respiratory muscles and a circulation.

The presence of these vital attributes – an open airway, breathing and an adequate circulation – must be assessed immediately. First-aiders use the mnemonic **ABC** to remind them of this first task.

It is usual to assess the **airway** and **breathing** first *but the order of assessment will depend upon the clinical problem.*

There is no point in breathing if there is no blood in the blood vessels to oxygenate, **so catastrophic, exsanguinating bleeding must be dealt with first**.

Similarly, there is no point in being able to breathe if the patient is engulfed in a poisonous gas such as carbon monoxide, so a **C** has been added before the **ABC** to remind the first-aider that any catastrophic life-threatening situation has to be dealt with first. The old first-aid books summarized this with the statement that the first-aider's first task was to '*remove the cause from the patient or, if this was not possible, the patient from the cause*'.

It is normally possible to deal with CAB and C at the same time if the patient is being attended to by a team.

Begin with a rapid CABC assessment.

C. Catastrophic circumstances

Deal with these first.

Exsanguinating bleeding should be stopped whenever possible by **direct digital pressure** or in military casualties the application of a **tourniquet** applied by a buddy.

The value of local pressure in preventing arterial haemorrhage has been recognized by the first-aid manuals for many years.

Most of the studies of the use of tourniquets in *war injuries* made before the 1950s showed their use to be associated with a high rate of subsequent amputation because of the time taken between tourniquet application and the patient's arrival at a base hospital. The realization in the 1950s that early arterial reconstruction could save threatened limbs provided the distal tissues were alive led to the exaggerated view that the use of tourniquets should be abandoned because the irreversible distal tissue ischaemia they caused made arterial reconstruction worthless.

The current rapid transfer of casualties to base hospitals by helicopters (often in less than an hour unless there are other extenuating circumstances) has led to the realization that tourniquets can save lives but that it is important that the tourniquet should only overcome diastolic arterial pressure and not occlude all the veins, so permitting some arterial inflow and tissue perfusion. With these provisos, tourniquets can be used to prevent exsanguination during the transfer of patients with major limb haemorrhage.

Careful **recording of the time of application** is important. The **maximum period of application should be kept below 6 hours** to avoid an inevitable amputation.

Occasionally, haemostasis may be obtained by the application of haemostatic forceps or a suture.

A. Airway

The airway should be assessed and secured first, provided there are no catastrophic circumstances.

Although the importance of damage to the spinal cord by moving an unstable cervical spine while attempting to clear the airway has been emphasized by the advanced trauma life support training system (ATLS), it is now recognized that clearance of the airway with rapid re-establishment of breathing is the overriding priority. Nevertheless, every effort should be made to stabilize the cervical spine while this is being achieved (see below).

The airway and breathing can be assumed to be satisfactory if the patient can speak, but extreme agitation may indicate the onset of hypoxia, which can lead to rapid unconsciousness and death if not correctly managed.

Unconscious patients should have their airway cleared of any obstructing agent (e.g. false teeth, blood and debris) by inserting a finger or a sucker under direct vision. Vomit and blood runs to the back of the throat and can only be removed with a sucker.

The chin and jaw should then be lifted to prevent the tongue from falling back and occluding the airway.

A **Guedel airway** should be inserted if this is available (Fig 6.1). A *nasopharyngeal airway* may be extremely valuable if there is massive oral trauma with fractures of the jaw and severe bleeding into the mouth.

An **endotracheal tube** is required if breathing is not restored or the patient remains deeply unconscious with an absent gag reflex.

Alternatives include the insertion of a **laryngeal mask**, a needle **cricothyroidostomy** or a **tracheostomy**, all of which can be life-saving in certain circumstances.

B. Breathing

Once an open airway has been established, breathing can be taken over by a **bag valve mask** or by direct connection to the tube. An inflation bag giving oxygen at 10–12 L per minute can be used to control ventilation until a **mechanical ventilator** becomes available.

The cervical spine must be immobilized while airway access is obtained and ventilation commenced by **manual support of the neck** in the early stages or by the application of **a cervical collar** (Fig 6.2).

Once the patient has been intubated, the cervical spine protection must be continued. Flexion and extension of the neck should be avoided. Patients should be transferred lying on a rigid board with their neck in a neutral position.

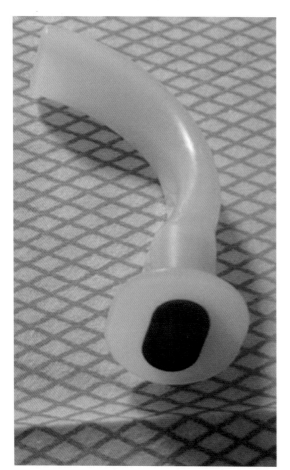

FIGURE 6.1 Guedel airway

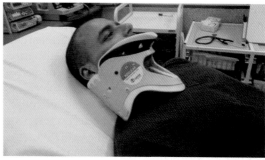

FIGURE 6.2 Neck collar

The emphasis on spinal cord protection has been very important in focusing the attention of first-aiders to the prevention of iatrogenic secondary spinal cord injury during resuscitation and assessment, but it is also now recognized that slavishly following neck protection policies at the expense of preventing other major causes of mortality such as overt bleeding has probably cost lives. The **B** of breathing and the **C** of circulation should take precedence in patients with limb injuries and no evidence of head or neck injuries.

C. Circulation

Almost all patients who have a major injury will be in 'hypovolaemic shock' as evidenced by the presence of tachycardia, hypotension, pale and clammy extremities. The treatment of shock requires restoration of the circulation. Two intravenous cannulae should be inserted, one in each antecubital fossa. Bone marrow infusion can be used as an alternative route for filling the circulation if a peripheral vein cannot be cannulated. This requires a specially adapted cannula. Another alternative is to cut down over, expose and insert a catheter directly into the long saphenous vein at the ankle.

A total of 500 mL of normal saline or Hartmann's or Ringer's lactate should be rapidly infused.

Further aliquots of fluid, in the form of colloid, should be infused until the pulse can be palpated at the wrist and the blood pressure is recordable with a sphygmomanometer. Fluid infusion should be slowed when the systolic blood pressure reaches 100 mmHg.

There are two schools of thought on the subsequent management of fluid replacement in patients presenting with hypovolaemic shock. It was originally thought that fluid administration should continue to maintain the blood pressure at a satisfactory level, i.e. a systolic pressure greater than 100 mmHg. The rationale was that this would enable the patient to better overcome a rapid decompensation from further bleeding and reduce the risk of developing some of the complications of prolonged hypotension such as acute tubular necrosis and acute respiratory distress syndrome (ARDS).

The other school of thought, perhaps influenced by the management of leaking abdominal aortic aneurysms, holds that permissible, controlled hypotension, i.e. a systolic blood pressure between 70 and 85 mmHg, reduces the risk of promoting further bleeding by encouraging the natural homeostatic mechanisms induced by hypotension. This approach reduces the risk of entering the vicious circle of raising the blood pressure, restarting bleeding and having to give further transfusions. It may also avoid the marked reduction of mesenteric and renal perfusion, which is the normal homeostatic response to hypovolaemic shock.

Keeping the infusion of crystalloids to a minimum also reduces the complications of interstitial fluid overload – heart failure, pulmonary oedema, peripheral oedema and paralytic ileus – and prevents the dilution of clotting factors, which may ultimately lead to more bleeding problems.

Animal experiments suggest that the rapid restoration of blood volume results in a lower mortality, but it is difficult to translate the results of such studies to injured human beings. It seems probable that both approaches may be beneficial in different clinical circumstances, e.g. fit young individuals probably benefit from an early and complete restoration of their blood volume, whereas elderly patients do better if their blood volume is restored slowly.

Fractured limbs should be stabilized by inflatable splints which, with traction and reduction, may provide considerable pain relief and improve the limb's circulation.

Analgesia and prophylactic antibiotics should be given if available, especially if the wounds are extensive and heavily contaminated.

TRANSPORT TO HOSPITAL

Before transfer, wounds should be covered (especially chest wounds). Pressure dressings or digital pressure may be appropriate.

The most common mode of transfer in the United Kingdom is the ambulance, which has usually been summoned by an eye witness with a mobile phone. Satellite locating devices now allow a rapid response to a recognized position.

Helicopter air ambulances have become popular in many parts of the world where long distances are involved or roads are congested with traffic. Helicopters are expensive and their value for money in major cities with many hospitals is arguable. They have their own inherent difficulties, which include inadequate landing sites and poor access to the patient during transfer.

INVESTIGATION AND MANAGEMENT AT THE ACCIDENT & EMERGENCY DEPARTMENT (MAJOR TRAUMA CENTRE)

The recipient A&E or major trauma centre should have been informed by ambulance control or by the paramedic ambulance team of the number of seriously injured patients it can expect to receive to enable it to activate its major disaster plan or, for smaller numbers of casualties, assemble a trauma team in the resuscitation area.

The hospital telephone exchange has the responsibility of contacting and requesting all the key personnel to assemble at the A&E. The key contacts are shown in Table 6.1.

Each trauma team should be under the control of an A&E consultant or a consultant general surgeon and should include an anaesthetist capable of intubating difficult airways, an orthopaedic surgeon and at least one senior A&E nurse. A junior doctor should record the progress of the resuscitation and ensure that all the injuries and the clinical course of the patient are carefully recorded. All members of the team must be clearly identified by an appropriate tabard (a labelled overall or tunic).

A senior doctor (either the on-call A&E consultant or the on-call general surgeon) should take overall control of the incident and be clearly identifiable. He/she should have the ability to contact the operating theatres, the blood bank, intensive care and the wards in order to arrange the transfer of major casualties out of A&E as soon as they have been assessed and resuscitated. The doctor in overall charge should undertake the initial triage of the patients into one of the following categories:

- P1 – life threatening
- P2 – urgent
- P3 – minor
- P4 – dead.

This triage is based on information given by the paramedics, together with the quick ABC assessment

Table 6.1
Personnel to be contacted following a major disaster

The accident and emergency (A&E) consultant on call

The other A&E consultants

The general surgeon on call

The other general surgeons

The orthopaedic consultant on call

The other orthopaedic consultants

The consultant anaesthetists on call

The other consultant anaesthetists

All junior doctors on call

The intensive care consultants on call

The other intensive care consultants

The nurse in charge of theatres

The blood transfusion consultants + consultants in charge of other laboratories

The consultant radiologists and senior radiographers

The hospital bed manager

The hospital manager on call

The communications department

The specialist services
- plastic
- vascular
- otolaryngology
- ophthalmology
- cardiothoracic

The portering services

The mortuary

made at the site of the accident (described above) and ensures that appropriate priority is given to the patients who require the most urgent treatment.

In each of the assembled trauma teams, the team leader must coordinate and ensure that the appropriate resuscitation is carried out. The junior members of the team should concentrate on ensuring an adequate airway and ventilation and obtaining access to the circulation. The more senior members of the team should monitor the circulation and oxygenation of the patient and carry out a rapid secondary survey before determining the additional investigations required (usually plain X-rays, computed tomography (CT) scans and ultrasounds).

It is important to avoid overwhelming the resuscitation area with well-meaning volunteer doctors who are keen to provide help.

It is also helpful if some surgeons go directly to the operating theatres to help staff prepare for the amputations, laparotomies, fracture fixations and thoracotomies that may be required.

Initial resuscitation

This follows the same system described above for the scene of the accident, taking note of the valuable information about the extent and cause of the injuries provided by the transporting team.

THE RAPID IN-HOSPITAL PRIMARY SURVEY

This should be repeated by the doctor in charge of the triage to confirm initial reports and ensure that nothing has altered or been missed in the initial survey. The primary survey is again considered as CABC but C2, D and E are now added.

C is for catastrophic haemorrhage This must be controlled at once.

A is for airway Consideration is given to the cervical spine, which should be immobilized in a collar or by sand bags if there is any hint of a neck injury. Blood, vomitus, teeth, etc., should be cleared from the mouth if this hasn't already been done by the paramedics. Endotracheal intubation of the airway is carried out for deep coma – a Glasgow Coma Scale less than 8 (described later). Surgical approaches can be considered if endotracheal intubation is impossible.

B is for breathing This is assessed once a clear airway has been secured. If the patient is breathing spontaneously, has a good colour and is talking no further action needs to be taken.

Ventilation is indicated if the breathing is laboured or ineffective or if the oxygen saturation is low poor while the patient is being given oxygen. Physical examination of the chest helped by a chest

X-ray or a CT scan should concentrate on detecting the following common chest injuries:

- sucking wounds
- a pneumothorax or pneumothorax tension
- haemothorax
- flail segment
- cardiac tamponade
- ventilatory failure.

A sucking wound should be occluded. A chest drain may need to be inserted.

A **pneumothorax** should be treated by the insertion of a chest drain through the second anterior intercostal space or, alternatively, urgent insertion through the fifth intercostal space in the mid-axillary line if it is a tension pneumothorax. A simple hollow needle or other hollow device may be used as an alternative to deflate a life-threatening tension pneumothorax.

A **suspected haemothorax** should be treated, initially, by inserting a chest drain through the tenth posterior intercostal space *(air rises, fluid falls!)*.

A **flail segment** is treated by positive pressure ventilation.

Cardiac tamponade is one of the most difficult clinical diagnoses to make but should be suspected if there are congested neck veins, muffled heart sounds and occasionally the presence of pulsus paradoxus. It should be treated by needle aspiration of the pericardial sac using ultrasound guidance.

C is for circulation The injured patients will often have had intravenous catheters inserted before they reach hospital but, if this has not occurred, two large-bore needles or catheters should be inserted into the antecubital veins of both arms. A long saphenous vein cut-down or bone marrow infusion can be life-saving if these approaches fail.

Central venous and **arterial pressure** catheters may be inserted to aid monitoring.

Blood should be sent for blood grouping and if a transfusion is likely to be needed, cross-matching.

All known wounds should be inspected for overt bleeding. It may be helpful to let down any tourniquet, temporarily, to assess the amount and source of the bleeding it is controlling. All other major bleeding is likely to be *covert* rather than *overt* and usually comes from injuries in the chest and abdomen, and pelvic or limb fractures.

Warm crystalloid or colloid should be administered while blood is awaited and their effect monitored by measuring the pulse rate and blood pressure. **Overloading with crystalloid is not helpful. Blood and blood products should be given as soon as possible, especially if there is evidence of continuing haemorrhage. Some colloid is permissible but more than 1 L is undesirable.**

A **urethral catheter** should be passed provided there is no evidence of a urethral or bladder injury, when a **suprapubic catheter** is preferred. Urine output is a reliable indication of rehydration and renal function.

C2, the additional C This is now a multislice urgent CT scan in the A&E (if available). Its value has now been firmly established. The alternative is a limited **ultrasound scan**.

Plain radiographs should be taken of the skull, neck, chest, abdomen, pelvis and limbs.

Continued hypotension is an indication for surgical exploration of the bleeding site as demonstrated by the CT findings, unless the bleeding is thought to be from pelvic or long bone fractures when external fixation and pelvic immobilization may be preferable.

Cardiac massage should be performed if the heart stops despite fluid administration. Cardiac tamponade must be reconsidered. Pericardiocentesis can be life-saving.

D is for disability Primarily disability can be caused by any associated brain injury. A quick simple mnemonic coding is AVPU:

A = alert
V = responding to verbal stimuli
P = responding to painful stimuli
U = unresponsive.

This can be used to provide a rapid assessment of cerebral function until, as soon as possible, a full Glasgow Coma Scale has been calculated (see later).

E is for exposure All clothing should be removed or cut off to ensure that the whole body can be examined during the secondary survey, but it is important to ensure that the patient does not become hypothermic at this stage during the examination.

THE SECONDARY SURVEY

Once the patient has been stabilized and the major systems briefly assessed, a secondary survey is carefully carried out to ensure that important injuries have not been missed during the early drama and haste of the resuscitation. It is important to monitor the patient carefully while this is taking place, as instability or deterioration may require urgent remedial action. The pulse, blood pressure, ECG, respiration, oxygen saturation, Glasgow score and urine output should be monitored continuously. An arterial and a CVP catheter provide valuable information on the state of the circulation.

The history A more detailed history should be taken from the patient, if conscious, focusing on their recollection of the accident. Any obvious symptoms of pain, loss of function or loss of consciousness should be recorded. Any known past medical history, drug allergies and sensitivities should be documented.

The examination Passive neck movements should be avoided during the secondary examination of a patient with a suspected neck injury until a rapid CT scan has been performed. The important advantage of a rapid CT scan is the exclusion of major spinal injury. Until this has been done, the patient should be '**log-rolled**' by several staff to inspect their back for wounds and burns and to carry out a rectal examination to assess sphincter tone.

The rest of the secondary survey can be performed with the patient prone, starting at the top of the head and finishing at the toes.

Head and neck

The scalp should be inspected and palpated for wounds, swellings and depressions. A deeply depressed area, especially if there is an overlying scalp wound, suggests there may be a **depressed** or **compound fracture of the skull**.

Battle's sign and **racoon eyes** suggest the presence of a fracture of the base of the skull (see *Symptoms and Signs*).

The ears and the nose should be inspected for **cerebrospinal fluid (CSF) leakage**, which, if found, should be tested for glucose with a dipstick. Facial asymmetry and bruising should be assessed and all bony promontories felt. The outline of the nose should be felt and any tenderness assessed.

The pupils and eye movements should be inspected. The presence of **diplopia** on upward gaze suggests there may be a **blow-out fracture of the orbital floor**.

Anaesthesia over the cheek with **bruising** and **enophthalmos** suggests the presence of a **fractured zygoma**.

The cornea and conjuctiva of both eyes should be inspected and the visual acuity checked with a Snellen's chart.

All the cranial nerves should be examined.

The mouth should be opened and the stability of the upper jaw checked by putting a finger and thumb inside the mouth and pulling it backwards and forwards. This demonstrates a **Le Fort's fracture of the maxilla**.

The neck should be carefully palpated and active neck movements assessed. Spasm prevents active neck movements if there is a major cervical spine injury. All wounds in the neck should be carefully assessed to indicate the possibility of damage to major vessels, the airway or, rarely, the gullet.

Chest (upper torso)

The presence of respiratory distress should have been detected in the primary survey, but it is worthwhile rechecking that the chest movement is equal and full and that there is no evidence of any **stridor**.

The trachea must be palpated to see if it is central. The chest wall should be carefully inspected for bruising, asymmetry and possible penetrating lacerations.

Look for the presence of a **flail segment**, a condition in which an area of chest wall is sucked inwards as the chest expands during inspiration (Fig 6.3).

The apex beat should be felt to ensure that it is not displaced (e.g. by a tension pneumothorax).

The neck veins should also be examined or the CVP checked, as a marked rise in venous pressure together with the presence of pulsus paradoxus and muffled or inaudible heart sounds is one of the main signs of **cardiac tamponade**.

The chest wall should be carefully palpated to detect **tenderness** (rib fractures), **unusual movement** (flail chest) and the presence of **crepitus** (indicating a pneumothorax or damage to the

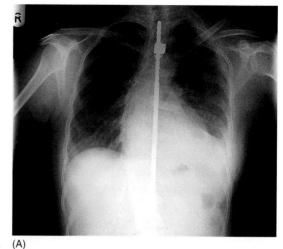

(A)

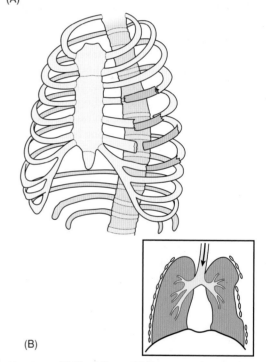

(B)

FIGURE 6.3 (A) Chest X-ray of flail segment; the left clavicle is fractured, and a spinal fixator is in place. (B) flail segment

oesophagus). The lungs should be percussed to check for dullness (a haemothorax or ruptured diaphragm) or excessive resonance (a pneumothorax). Air entry at the bases and vocal resonance completes the examination.

An **erect chest X-ray** or **CT scan** of the chest should be obtained if any abnormality is suspected. An **echocardiogram** is useful for confirming the presence of tamponade and indicating the need for pericardiocentesis.

Abdomen and pelvis (lower torso)

The abdomen must be inspected, palpated, percussed and auscultated. Any wounds are documented, especially if they could have breached the abdominal cavity. There may be signs of visible bruising (seat belt) or distension. Local tenderness in a conscious patient can be helpful, especially if there is tenderness on percussion. The bladder area should be percussed (if a catheter has not been passed), to detect any bladder distention. The presence of normal bowel sounds is encouraging but these may disappear in the face of continuing intra-abdominal haemorrhage or spreading peritonitis from a traumatized bowel or pancreas.

The genitalia must be checked and the external urethral meatus inspected for the presence of blood. Bruising of the perineum or lower abdomen, especially if associated with urethral bleeding, suggests a fracture of the pelvis with **urethral** or **bladder damage**. In these circumstances a **suprapubic** rather than a urethral **catheter** may be a better means of draining a full bladder.

Pelvic instability should be checked for by 'springing' the pelvis in both the anteroposterior and lateral directions. If a fracture is suspected, **plain X-rays** or **CT scans** are indicated.

The rectum and buttocks, which should have been examined when the patient was rolled into the prone position, should be checked again.

Displaced sacral fractures can be felt on rectal examination.

There is debate over the value in the assessment of abdominal injuries in an unconscious patient of rapid **ultrasound, paracentesis** and **CT scanning**. All can be helpful. Although CT scanning is probably the most useful, it will not pick up early bowel injury or mesenteric tears until there is free fluid and/or gas within the abdominal cavity.

The limbs

The upper and lower limbs must be carefully examined for lacerations, swelling, bruising, deformity and, in the conscious patient, loss of power. All the pulses in the limbs must be palpated and recorded and, in a conscious patient, the motor and cutaneous nerves tested.

The reflexes and the Babinski reflex should be tested on unconscious patients.

Plain radiographs and **duplex scanning** of the vessels should be carried out if a vascular injury is suspected (see below).

Disposal

After completing the secondary survey the patient may require further imaging or may need to be transferred to the intensive care or high dependency unit, the ward or the operating theatre.

A further rapid assessment of the patient should be carried out before they are transferred.

All patients with major injuries should be admitted for at least 24 hours, as a number of patients develop late symptoms and problems.

It is important that the admitting teams repeat the secondary survey to avoid missing injuries that may have been overlooked in the resuscitation room. The whole process should be repeated the next day to ensure that other injuries have not been missed.

Further investigations and management should be guided by the progress and further assessment of the injured patient.

HEAD INJURIES

OVERALL MANAGEMENT OF HEAD INJURIES

All patients who are thought to have multiple injuries should have a brain scan, any neck injuries excluded by a careful secondary survey, and be monitored with the Glasgow Coma Scale (Table 6.2).

CT brain scanning should be carried out on all patients who have been unconscious (knocked out) and those who cannot remember their injury.

CT scans should also be obtained if a patient's level of consciousness deteriorates, if the pupils dilate or if neurological signs develop (e.g. reduction in power, loss of speech, upgoing plantar responses).

A brain CT scan should also be obtained in all deeply unconscious patients.

Patients who are fully responsive with a Glasgow score of 15 can be discharged home with a responsible person who can bring them back to hospital should they develop new symptoms (e.g. vomiting or drowsiness).

Table 6.2
Glasgow coma scale

Eyes open	Spontaneously	4
	To verbal command	3
	To pain	2
	No response	1
Best motor response		
to verbal command	Obeys verbal command	6
to painful stimulus	Localizes pain	5
	Flexion withdrawal (decorticate rigidity)	4
	Abnormal flexion	3
	Extension (decerebrate rigidity)	2
	No response	1
Best verbal response	Orientated and converses	5
	Disorientated and converses	4
	Inappropriate words	3
	Incomprehensible sounds	2
	No response	1
	Maximum score **is 15 (min 3)**	

Patients with a Glasgow score of less than 13 should have a CT scan but can be discharged if it is normal and they have no associated injuries.

Patients with a history of head injury, a period of unconsciousness or retrograde amnesia used to be admitted to hospital for 24 hours observation after skull X-rays had been taken. **New guidelines have suggested that an early CT scan may reduce the need for hospital admission in many patients.** This may produce a modest cost saving without a deterioration in care.

Any patient with abnormalities on CT scanning (e.g. a skull fracture or cerebral injury), those with a persisting abnormality on the Glasgow Coma Scale or where there is a question of alcohol or drug intoxication should be admitted to hospital. Other reasons for admission include CSF leakage, persistent

vomiting and severe headache and the possibility of a non-accidental injury.

Patients with severe localized head injuries should be resuscitated and transferred to a neurosurgical unit. Those found to have a **cerebral haematoma** on CT scanning should also be transferred.

Patients who do not require transfer to a neurosurgical unit but require further observation as well as those with multiple injuries should be admitted to an Intensive Care Unit where they can be sedated, ventilated (if necessary), their pupils assessed and intracranial pressure monitored.

Intracranial pressure

The signs of a raised intracranial pressure (called compression in the first-aid books) are:

- a reduction in the level of consciousness
- respiratory depression
- a fall in the pulse rate
- a fall in blood pressure.

The '**cerebral perfusion pressure**', which is the intracerebral pressure subtracted from the blood pressure, should, ideally, be maintained between 60 and 80 mmHg. A further CT scan should be obtained if it rises unexpectedly.

Cerebral oedema is the usual cause of a raised pressure if a haematoma has been excluded.

The pressure may be lowered by continued **hyperventilation, head elevation, manitol** in repeated aliquots (0.2 g/kg) and **intravenous steroids. Hypothermia** and **barbiturates** can also be tried as cerebral protecting agents and **a single large dose of manitol** (0.5 g/kg) can be used if coning is felt to be imminent.

MANAGEMENT OF COMMON HEAD INJURIES

PRIMARY BRAIN INJURIES

When the head hits a solid surface at high speed, the frontal and temporal regions of the brain hit the inside of the skull. Rotational and **contre-coup** injuries may also occur. The brain injuries caused by a direct blow to the head include neuronal damage, brain lacerations, haemorrhage and oedema.

These injuries can be reduced or prevented by wearing suitable protection (e.g. a helmet) during high-risk activities such as motor cycling.

These injuries are often very difficult to treat and have a poor outcome.

SECONDARY BRAIN INJURIES

Secondary injuries occur as a consequence of hypoxia, ischaemia, poor cerebral blood flow in a very hypotensive patient and compression by cerebral haematomata or depressed skull fractures. This damage is potentially avoidable by careful management including intubation and ventilation. A third of these patients have major injuries in other systems.

SCALP INJURIES

Scalp injuries include swelling, bruising, lacerations or complex wounds with areas of skin loss. All scalp injuries must be taken seriously as they can be complicated by the presence of an associated skull fracture which may be linear, stellate or depressed (see below). They should, therefore, be carefully debrided before being primarily closed by sutures under local anaesthesia. Any suspicion that there could be an associated skull fracture should lead to this being excluded by CT scanning. Skin flaps can be used to close areas of skin loss. Skin grafts and free flaps are rarely required.

SCALP HAEMATOMATA

These usually occur as a consequence of birth canal trauma or an external injury. They usually resolve spontaneously.

COMPOUND OPEN FRACTURES OF THE SKULL

These occur when there is a scalp laceration or a skull fracture and the dura is also torn. There is a considerable risk of infection, especially meningitis. The risk of infection can be reduced by the early removal of damaged tissue on the edge of the scalp wound and closure of the dura mater and the skin if possible.

Compound fractures also occur when a base of skull fracture breaches a potentially infected space such as the nose, pharynx, sinuses or middle ear.

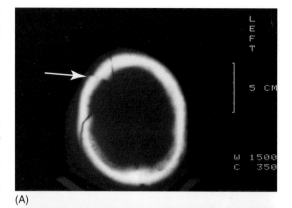

(A)

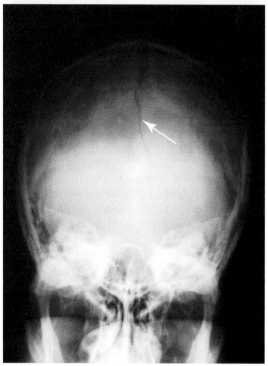

(B)

FIGURE 6.4   Two examples of fractured skull. (A) CT scan and (B) plain X-ray

Panda eyes, Battle's sign and CSF rhinorrhoea or otorrhea all indicate this diagnosis. Cranial nerve injuries are also often present. CT scanning using bone windows confirms the diagnosis (Fig 6.4).

Treatment is to give **antibiotics** while the risk persists (e.g. while there is CSF leakage) and for a few days after the risk has passed. Patients with CSF rhinorrhoea should be advised not to blow their nose to avoid forcing air and bacteria inside the skull.

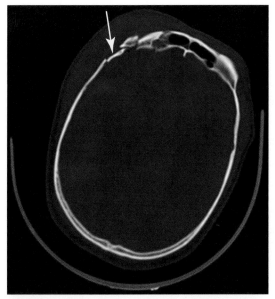

FIGURE 6.5   CT of a depressed fracture of skull

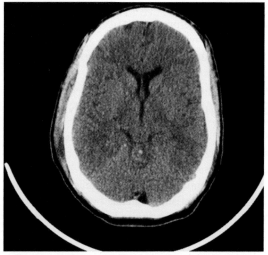

FIGURE 6.6   CT of diffuse axonal injury of brain with cerebral oedema, compressing the ventricles and removing the contrast of grey and white matter

DEPRESSED FRACTURES OF THE SKULL

A depressed skull fracture is usually caused by a localized direct blow. The overlying scalp is usually lacerated or forms a boggy swelling over the fracture. A stellate fracture may coexist. The depression can occasionally be felt but should be visible on a **plain X-ray** of the skull or a **CT scan** with bone windows (Fig 6.5).

Severely depressed bone fragments can cause secondary brain injury. They should be elevated through a separate burr hole. Many patients do not like the appearance of a depressed fracture even though it is symptomless and request that it be elevated for aesthetic reasons.

Any scalp wounds overlying a fracture should be sutured to cover the fracture.

CONCUSSION

Concussion is defined as a brief loss of consciousness that fully recovers within 24 hours. It is often associated with amnesia. Its importance lies in its possible association with skull fracture and extradural haemorrhage. Skull X-rays or CT scans are often required to exclude such possibilities and help decide whether the patient should be admitted to hospital for observation or sent home.

DIFFUSE AXONAL INJURY

This may follow moderate or severe head trauma and is often visible on high-quality CT scans (Fig 6.6). It can result in memory disturbances, headaches, loss of consciousness, anxiety, depression and even personality changes. The treatment is expectant. **Steroids** and **mannitol** may be given in the initial stages if cerebral oedema is suspected.

CEREBRAL LACERATION, HAEMORRHAGE, HAEMATOMA, CONTUSION AND NEURONAL INJURIES

All these forms of brain damage may be associated with skull fractures or penetrating injuries.

- CT scans should demonstrate the extent of the problem.
- Direct cerebral pressure monitoring can be helpful.
- Most patients present in coma and require hyperventilation, steroids and manitol.
- Failure to respond to conservative measures can be taken as an indication to explore the brain, but the results are usually poor and at best leave a severely brain damaged patient.

CEREBRAL HYPOXIA, ISCHAEMIA AND CEREBRAL OEDEMA

These problems may result from strangulation but are more commonly associated with multiple trauma, poor ventilation and prolonged hypovolaemic shock. Prevention is by early adequate correction of the blood volume and adequate restoration of oxygenation. The onset of cerebral oedema can be monitored by the application of a cerebral pressure sensor.

Large doses of **manitol** and **steroids** can reduce cerebral oedema, as can deliberate hyperventilation to reduce carbon dioxide levels.

INTRACRANIAL HAEMATOMA

An intracranial haematoma results from an intracranial haemorrhage. It may cause a rise in intracranial pressure and cause a reduction in the level of consciousness, respiratory depression, a fall in the pulse rate and a fall in blood pressure.

Haematomata may develop in the extradural, subarachnoid or subdural spaces or within the substance of the brain, an intracerebral haematoma.

EXTRADURAL HAEMATOMA

Extradural haematomata complicate about 10 percent of all severe head injuries. They are caused by a tear of the middle meningeal artery or one of its branches and are often associated with a temporoparietal linear fracture. As the thin temporal bone fractures it tears the middle meningeal artery, which then rapidly bleeds into the extradural space.

Investigation
Clinical diagnostic indicators

The injury is often not severe but followed by increasing headache, vomiting and drowsiness. Consciousness may be lost after a so-called 'lucid interval'. The diagnosis should be made before coma develops.

Lateralizing signs develop with **ipsilateral pupil dilatation** preceding the development of a **contralateral hemiparesis**.

If the condition is left untreated, **fixed dilated pupils** and **coma** eventually presage **respiratory arrest**.

An extradural haematoma must be excluded in any patient presenting with coma.

Imaging

A **plain skull X-ray** may show a linear fracture in the temporoparietal region. If it does, it should lead to admission and a careful neurological assessment. Any injured patient who has unexpectedly lost consciousness should be similarly assessed.

A **CT scan of the brain** should be obtained in any patient whose level of consciousness is deteriorating especially if there are any localizing neurological signs.

Brain CT scanning should also be carried out on patients who are admitted unconscious. An extradural haemorrhage is seen as a dense mass between the dura and the bone (Fig 6.7). Cerebral pressure monitoring is rarely useful or practicable.

Management
Surgical decompression

Once the diagnosis has been confirmed by a CT scan, the haematoma should be evacuated as quickly as possible through a **burr hole** placed directly over it.

If the patient deteriorates rapidly before a CT scan is available, burr holes should be made on the side of the fracture or on the side of the pupil dilatation This is now rarely required as time can usually be bought by giving **mannitol** 0.5 g/kg of bodyweight and hyperventilating the patient while transferring them to a scanner.

After the haematoma has been evacuated the burr hole often has to be extended to become a **craniotomy** to expose the bleeding point and secure the bleeding vessel.

Prognosis

The mortality following an extradural haematoma is about 5–10 per cent because many cases are complicated by other injuries.

ACUTE SUBDURAL/SUBARACHNOID HAEMATOMA

These haematomata commonly complicate high-speed road injuries and are more common than extradural haematomata. They are also more

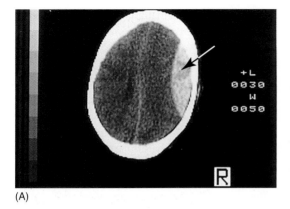

(A)

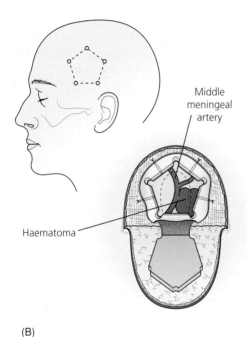

(B)

FIGURE 6.7   (A) CT Scan of an extradural haemorrhage, seen as a white area on the right. (B) Craniotomy to drain an extradural haemorrhage and ligate the middle meningeal artery

frequent (30 per cent of all severe head injuries) and carry a worse prognosis because of the associated injuries – usually major damage to the cerebral hemisphere with bleeding from torn veins on the damaged surface of the brain. The large subdural/subarachnoid space allows the blood to spread out over a wide area.

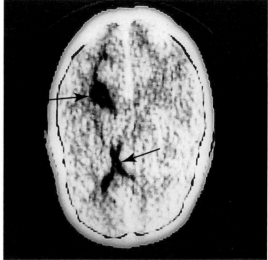

FIGURE 6.8   CT scan of a subdural haematoma that is compressing the lateral ventricles (arrows) and causing a midline shift

Investigation

Clinical diagnostic indicators

These patients are often unconscious on arrival in the A&E and there are often associated injuries. Monitoring may show a deterioration in their Glasgow score with the development of localizing signs, although these may be present *ab initio*.

Imaging

CT scans are extremely helpful in making the diagnosis (Fig 6.8).

Management

The aims of treatment are to evacuate the haematoma, control the bleeding and prevent brain swelling. This is achieved through burr holes and flaps (see Fig. 6.7).

Prognosis Early evacuation may reduce the morbidity and mortality. Thirty per cent of patients treated by drainage make only a moderate recovery and 30 per cent usually die.

CHRONIC SUBDURAL HAEMATOMA

These haematomata are far more common in elderly people and often follow minor trauma. The cerebral atrophy of old age increases the mobility of the brain within the skull and consequently increases the chance of the veins on the surface of the atrophied brain tearing. They are common in epileptic and alcoholic patients and in patients on anticoagulants.

Investigation

Clinical diagnostic indicators

Patients often develop symptoms days or weeks after an injury that may have been forgotten. **Headache, loss of intellect, fluctuations in consciousness and eventually localizing signs (hemiparesis)** are the common modes of presentation.

Imaging

A **CT scan** will confirm the diagnosis.

Management

Surgical decompression

The haematoma should be evacuated through a burr hole or craniotomy.

Prognosis Ninety per cent recover.

INTRACEREBRAL HAEMORRHAGE

These patients are usually unconscious when they arrive at the A&E with a Glasgow score of 3.

There is an overlap between the symptoms and signs of intracerebral haemorrhage, primary brain injury and acute subdural/subarachnoid haematoma. The diagnosis can be resolved by a **CT scan** (Fig 6.9).

The management, when possible, should be expectant with **ventilation, cerebral pressure monitoring, mannitol and steroids**.

Evidence of an expanding haematoma on serial CT scans is an indication for an attempt at surgical evacuation, but the results are extremely poor.

Prognosis The mortality rate exceeds 50 per cent.

GENERAL COMPLICATIONS OF HEAD INJURIES

Meningitis can follow compound skull vault and basal skull fractures. Treatment is with antibiotics, which should also be given prophylactically in this type of injury to prevent infection developing.

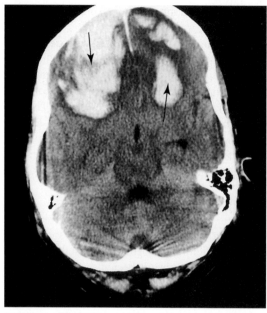

FIGURE 6.9   CT of intracranial haemorrhage seen as dense white masses within the swollen and featureless brain matter

Post-traumatic epilepsy often follows brain contusion, an intracranial haematoma or a depressed fracture. The overall risk is 5 per cent. Prophylaxis with anticonvulsants remains controversial as their value has not been proven, but they should be given if a fit occurs.

A **carotid cavernous sinus fistula** may develop if a fracture of the floor of the middle cranial fossa tears the carotid artery as it enters the cavernous sinus. It presents with unilateral proptosis and hyperaemia and oedema of the conjunctiva of the affected eye. The patient may hear the buzz of the fistula and a machinery murmur can be auscultated over the globe. The proptosis is pulsatile.

Its complications include blindness, diplopia and catastrophic nasal haemorrhage. Treatment is by occlusion of the fistula with balloons, coils or glue through a catheter passed up the carotid artery. This carries a risk of cerebral embolization and stroke.

Anosmia (loss of sense of smell) is common after basal fractures of the anterior cranial fossa and is untreatable.

Headache, irritability and lack of attention are common after all serious head injuries but tend to improve with time.

A patient's **personality** can change after a severe head injury.

Post-traumatic stress disorder with depression and anxiety is often diagnosed but difficult to prove.

Neurodisability occurs in many patients with severe brain injuries and requires prolonged treatment in Physiotherapy and Occupational Therapy Departments, preferably dedicated to head-injured patients. Many may require long-term care at home or need to be looked after permanently in facilities for the chronically disabled.

THE CERVICAL SPINE

The importance of not exacerbating a spinal cord injury by failing to recognize an unstable cervical spine fracture has already been discussed at length.

Conscious patients without neck symptoms have never been found to have an unstable cervical spine or have subsequently progressed to develop neurological deterioration. It is, therefore, unnecessary to go to great lengths to maintain spinal cord protection in a conscious patient who has not had a head injury and does not complain of neck pain.

The neck should be examined for deformity or bruising and the patient asked to move the neck in all directions. There is no need for further investigations if all neck movements are full and pain-free and there are no neurological signs in the limbs.

Difficulties arise in the unconscious patient, especially if they are intubated and ventilated. In these circumstances the management options include:

- Treat the cervical spine as if it is unstable until the patient regains full consciousness.
- Obtain plain X-rays of the cervical spine (lateral, anteroposterior and open-mouth views) and then decide how to proceed.
- Obtain an MRI or CT scan of the cervical spine.
- Carry out dynamic flexion and extension cervical spine X-rays using an image intensifier. This procedure must be terminated if subluxation occurs.

The spine should be considered unstable if both the anterior and posterior columns have been disrupted.

A stiff collar is effective unless there is overt bleeding from a wound in the neck. Displaced unstable injuries are treated by halo traction until surgical stabilization can be undertaken (see Chapter 10).

MAXILLOFACIAL INJURIES

The common causes of maxillofacial injuries are

- fights
- road traffic injuries
- sports injuries
- falls
- industrial injuries
- wars
- insurgencies.

Maxillofacial trauma is often associated with airway problems, haemorrhage, neck and head injuries, and fractures of the mandible, maxilla, zygoma, nasal bones and orbit.

Investigation

Clinical diagnostic routines

When examining the **skull, eye and orbit:**

- inspect and palpate the cranium
- palpate the orbital margins
- test visual acuity
- examine the eyelids
- note the pupil size
- inspect the corneae and anterior chamber
- test the red reflex
- check for diplopia and eye movements
- test for infra-orbital nerve paraesthesia.

When examining the **nose** check for:

- lacerations
- contusions
- epistaxis
- CSF rhinorrhoea
- deformity, e.g. deviated nasal septum.

When examining the **Zygoma** (cheek) check for:

- pain and tenderness
- a 'step' deformity
- flattening of face
- trismus
- hypo-aesthesia of the infra-orbital nerve
- diplopia.

When examining the **maxilla** check for:

- mid-face asymmetry, deformity or swelling
- missing teeth
- dental malocclusion

- jaw opening
- panda or racoon eyes
- epistaxis
- CSF rhinorrhoea
- mobility of the fractured segment.

When examining the **mandible** check for:

- laceration over the point of the chin
- pain (pre-auricular tenderness)
- swelling
- reduced jaw opening
- malocclusion
- trismus
- deformity
- missing teeth.

Table 6.3 is a quick checklist that covers the majority of the above clinical investigations.

Imaging

Occipital plain radiographs are useful for diagnosing maxillary, zygomatic and orbital fractures. Orbital floor injuries are associated with the hanging drop sign (Fig 6.10).

Nasal X-rays, **plain X-rays** and **orthopantomographs** are required for fractures of the nose and mandible.

Posteroanterior plain X-rays of the mandible may be needed to reveal condylar fractures.

CT scans can be helpful when looking for the complex displacements associated with mid-face fractures. They can also show up herniation of the orbital contents.

Angiography may be used to diagnose and manage major bleeding by therapeutic embolization of the external carotid artery or its branches.

Table 6.3
A quick checklist for maxillofacial injuries

Check the contour of the facial bones for pain, tenderness and deformity

Examine the eyes to test their movement

Check the bite

Look for missing teeth in the mouth

Check jaw opening

Test all the cranial nerves

Management

Conscious patients can usually protect their **airway** by sitting up and leaning forwards. Unconscious patients must have any debris cleared from their mouths by using MacGill forceps, fingers and a suction catheter.

Oropharyngeal and nasopharyngeal airways may need to be inserted if the soft palate and tongue are displaced backwards by a posteriorly displaced Le Fort fracture or a mandibular fracture. The displacement may have to be manually disimpacted before an endotracheal tube can be passed.

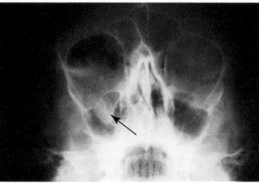

(A)

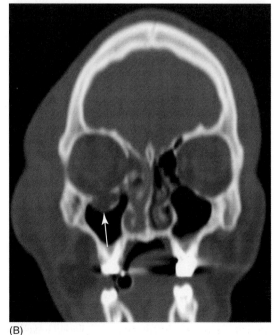

(B)

FIGURE 6.10 Fracture of orbit with 'hanging drop' sign (blowout fracture). (A) Plain X-ray. (B) CT scan

Massive haemorrhage, though rare, may require posterior nasal packing, an emergency cricothyroidostomy or tracheostomy. Once the airway has been secured, the source of haemorrhage can be confirmed by catheter angiography and stopped by therapeutic embolization.

Fractures

Most fractures are now treated by open exploration, reduction and fixation with microplates. Surgery should be carried out as soon as possible (Fig 6.11).

Most of the incisions needed for access to fractures of the maxilla and mandible can be made in the mouth. The orbit can be reached through the conjunctiva and fractures of the upper maxilla and zygoma can be dealt with through incisions made above the hairline.

Orbital (blowout) fractures The herniated orbital contents must be replaced and the floor of the orbit restored with a plastic sheet or bone graft (Fig 6.10).

Nasal fractures These are usually treated by closed reduction and external plaster splinting (Fig 6.11).

Zygomatic fractures Undisplaced fractures do not require treatment.

Displaced fractures These can be treated by closed temporal reduction or, in complex or comminuted fractures, by open reduction and fixation with microplates (Fig 6.11).

Undisplaced maxillary fractures These can be treated with analgesia and a soft diet. Displaced fractures require open reduction and internal fixation with microplates. Closed reduction and external fixation is sometimes still used (Fig 6.11).

Mandibular fractures Fractures of the condylar head are usually treated conservatively with analgesia and a soft diet. The mandible can be immobilized with mandibulomaxillary wires if there is evidence of malocclusion.

Open reduction and internal fixation is required if the condyle is dislocated and associated with malocclusion (Fig 6.11). When the bony condyles are fractured and displaced or the maxilla is also fractured and displaced, open reduction is again necessary.

Undisplaced fractures of the angle or body of the mandible are treated conservatively if there is no mobility or malocclusion but, if these are present, open reduction and fixation by microplates is indicated.

Complications of maxillofacial injuries

The complications include:

- **Airway obstruction** at the time of injury or by an acutely deviated nasal septum.
- **Malreduction** causing facial deformity, e.g. untreated nasal or zygomatic fractures are common. Untreated blowout fractures can cause persistent **diplopia** and **ophthalmoplegia**.
- **Dental malocclusion** can follow inadequate treatment of maxillary and mandibular fractures.
- **Growth retardation** and **deformity** can follow condylar fractures of the mandible in children and the condyle may fuse with the temporal bone, making it impossible to open the jaw.
- **Haemorrhage,** which can be life-threatening.
- **Infection** (osteomyelitis is rare).
- **Trismus** is also rare.
- **Delayed union and non-union** are rare but **nerve damage** may persist.
- **Tooth injury:** teeth, can be pushed back and reimplanted. If a broken tooth is found, a chest X-ray should be considered as it might have been inhaled.

NECK INJURIES

The neck is divided into three zones (Fig 6.12). Zone 1 is between the thoracic outlet and the cricoid cartilage. Zone II is between the cricoid and the angle of the mandible. Zone III is above the angle of the mandible and below the base of the skull. Injuries in zones I and II are not easily accessible.

All deep neck wounds used to be explored but this approach has been challenged in recent years with improved imaging and endoscopy.

Angiography and interventional radiology may be useful in both the diagnosis and management of injuries in zones I and II, particularly injuries of the vessels.

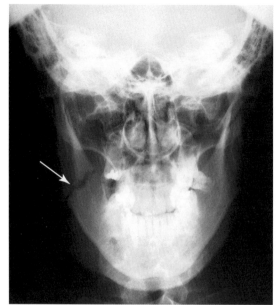

(A)

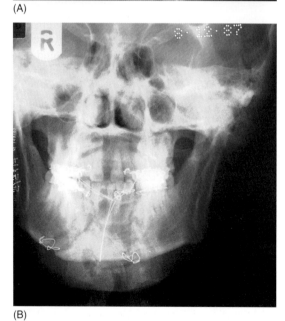

(B)

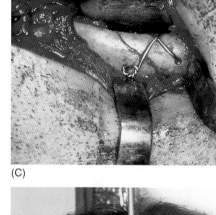

(C)

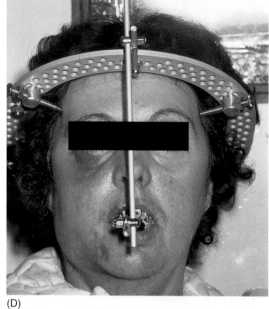

(D)

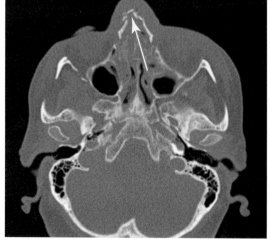

(E)

FIGURE 6.11   (A) Fractured mandible (arrow). (B) Wiring of a fractured mandible. (C) Wiring across a fractured mandible. (D) Stabilization of a maxillary fracture using a Haloframe with external fixation. (E) Nasal fracture

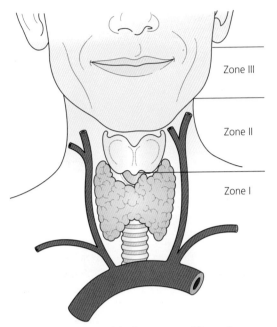

FIGURE 6.12   Drawing of the three zones of the neck

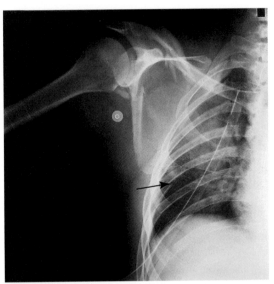

FIGURE 6.13   X-ray of fractured ribs

Duplex scanning and CT angiography may also provide useful preliminary information about blunt or penetrating vascular injuries, which can be treated by stenting, embolization or surgical exploration and repair.

Endoscopy of the airways and gullet may also provide useful information.

TORSO TRAUMA

The chest and abdomen are often injured simultaneously in patients with major trauma and are the main sites of concealed haemorrhage. For simplicity, it is easier to consider both separately but it must be remembered that the pleura extends above the clavicle and that the lower chest and upper abdomen overlap. A ruptured spleen and liver damage are often associated with fractured ribs. Bullets and knives often traverse both cavities.

CHEST WALL AND LUNG INJURIES

These can be subdivided into penetrating, blast and blunt injuries. The majority of penetrating injuries are caused by knives but bullet wounds are now increasing in all parts of the world. In conflicts,

high-velocity bullets and shrapnel are the major causes of penetrating chest wounds, although the widespread use of Kevlar jackets has reduced their incidence in military personnel.

Blunt chest trauma is more often associated with road traffic accidents and crushing injuries. The use of seat belts and air bags has reduced the incidence of these injuries, although seat belts, while saving life, can themselves cause fractures of the ribs and/ or sternum (Fig 6.13).

Occasionally, patients *in extremis* with severe hypotension and a presumed chest injury can have an emergency thoracotomy through a 'clam shell' incision before a diagnosis is made. At the very least, this allows a tamponade to be released, a cardiac puncture to be closed, cardiac massage to be carried out and a clamp put on the aorta or the hilum of the lung, although few patients survive these heroic manoeuvres.

FRACTURES OF THE RIBS

Fractures of the ribs are usually caused by a compressing blunt injury but can be caused by a direct blow.

A fractured rib may cause a **pneumothorax** (Fig 6.14) if a sharp spicule of bone at its end punctures the pleura and the lung, or cause a **haemothorax** if a chest wall vessel (intercostal or

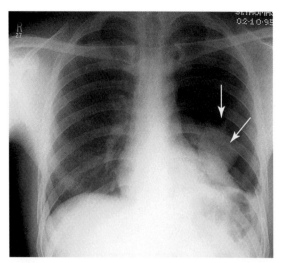

FIGURE 6.14   X-ray of pneumothorax collapsed lung (arrows)

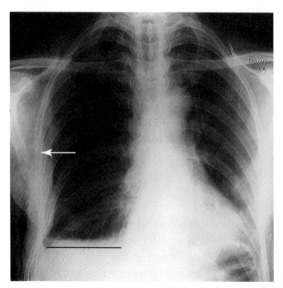

FIGURE 6.15   X-ray of haemothorax (above black line) fractured rib arrowed

internal mammary) is torn or a lung vessel pierced (Fig 6.15).

An underlying **lung contusion** must always be suspected.

When a number of adjacent ribs are fractured in two places, the segment between the breaks is sucked in during inspiration and pushed outwards during expiration. This is called a '**flail segment**'. The loss of chest wall rigidity can cause severe respiratory distress (Fig 6.3).

Investigation

Clinical diagnostic indicators

Fractured ribs are suspected from the history of injury and pain in the chest wall on inspiration. Local tenderness on palpation and 'rib springing' supports the diagnosis. Seat belt marks or local bruising are also suggestive.

Blood tests

Blood gas levels should be measured if the patient is showing air hunger.

Imaging

An erect chest X-ray should be taken, with additional rib views if there are areas of local tenderness, to confirm the diagnosis. It is important to carry out the chest X-ray with the patient in the erect position, if possible, to detect a small pneumothorax at the apex and, more importantly, a moderate or even large haemothorax at the base of the chest cavity, which can be missed if the patient is lying down.

A CT scan should be ordered if a lung injury is suspected, especially if the oxygen saturation is reduced or blood gasses show evidence of a ventilation perfusion mismatch (a low pO_2 and a normal or reduced pCO_2).

Management

Pain relief

Patients with fractured ribs require analgesia. Oral or intramuscular analgesics may be supplemented by local infiltration around the origins of the intercostal nerves, just below the fractures, with a long-acting local anaesthetic agent such as **marcaine 0.5 per cent.**

Suspect other injuries

Those suspected of having an associated lung injury, a flail segment, a haemothorax or a pneumothorax should be admitted to hospital because they may require further treatment (see below). Blood gas monitoring, repeated chest radiographs and physiotherapy with appropriate analgesia should be instituted. Supplemental oxygen should be given by a mask.

Patients with uncomplicated rib fractures can be sent home, but remember that lower rib fractures on the left and right can cause splenic and liver injuries which are best diagnosed by CT scanning.

The pain may take several weeks to settle, even in uncomplicated rib fractures, and may persist even longer.

FLAIL SEGMENT

Investigation

Once this has been diagnosed from the clinical signs (see above), **chest** and **rib X-rays** should be taken to confirm the presence of double rib fractures. A **CT scan** should be obtained if the oxygen saturation is impaired to exclude an underlying lung injury.

Management

In the past, many patients were treated by endotracheal intubation and positive pressure ventilation until the fractured ribs began to unite, but it is now recognized that this is often overtreatment. In many cases conservative management with pain relief (see above), supplemental oxygen, physiotherapy and careful monitoring is sufficient, but intubation and ventilation may become indicated if the patient shows signs of increasing respiratory distress and respiratory failure (reduced oxygen saturation). **Early rib fixation with interosseus wires** may be considered as an alternative treatment should prolonged ventilation not be available, especially in young fit patients with a large flail segment.

Prognosis The prognosis is usually good but a severe associated lung injury can lead to ARDS, which has a 20 per cent mortality. The prognosis of rib fractures depends upon the associated intrathoracic injuries.

PNEUMOTHORAX

A pneumothorax may be **open** or **closed, simple** or **tension**.

Investigation

Clinical diagnostic indicators

Patients with a simple large closed pneumothorax present with difficulty in breathing and the physical signs of a collapsed lung – no or reduced air entry and hyper-resonance to percussion. Small pneumothoraces may cause no physical signs and are diagnosed on chest X-ray.

Open pneumothoraces are caused by penetrating injuries and may present with a **sucking wound**, which can cause a **tension pneumothorax**. A tension pneumothorax causes respiratory distress,

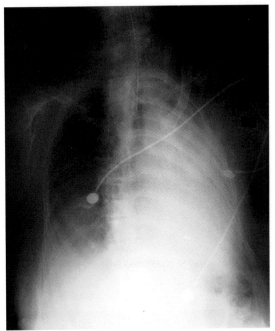

FIGURE 6.16   Tension pneumothorax on right side: Mediastinum and heart have shifted to the left

mediastinal shift, reduced cardiac output and reduced air entry into the contralateral lung.

A **chest X-ray** should be taken to confirm the diagnosis (Fig 6.16), but patients in extremis require urgent decompression based on the clinical signs alone.

Management

Small pneumothoraces with no signs of impaired oxygenation (normal blood gas saturations) can be treated by observation plus **analgesia** for any associated rib fracture, physiotherapy and blood gas saturation monitoring.

Oxygen should be administered by a mask.

A **thoracostomy tube** should be inserted if there are signs of respiratory distress.

The tube is removed when air stops bubbling through the tube's underwater seal drain (Fig 6.17) and a chest X-ray shows the lung to be fully expanded.

Sucking wounds must be covered with an occlusive dressing to prevent further air entering the pleural cavity.

Tension pneumothoraces must be treated urgently by the immediate insertion of a tube to relieve the tension. In an emergency situation, outside of hospital, any hollow tube will suffice, preferably one whose open end can be held under water to prevent the re-entry of air.

A few patients will develop a **continuous air leak**, which suggests there is major bronchial damage (a **bronchopleural fistula**) or the tube has been incorrectly placed in the lung. Applying suction to the underwater seal drain may close the leak, but some patients require open or endoscopic closure of the fistula by direct suture.

A **tracheal injury**, a very rare event, may require direct surgical repair, preferably after endotracheal intubation.

HAEMOTHORAX

Investigation

Clinical diagnostic indicators

In contrast to a pneumothorax, which is hyper-resonant to percussion, a haemothorax is dull. Both are associated with a reduced air entry to the lung with reduced breath sounds. A large haemothorax may cause dyspnoea and be associated with the signs of hypovolaemic shock.

Blood tests

The haemoglobin and the blood gas saturations should be measured.

Imaging

An **erect chest X-ray** will confirm the diagnosis (Fig 6.15).

Management

Intravenous catheters should be inserted. Four units of blood should be cross-matched and supplemental oxygen given by mask.

A **thoracostomy tube** should be inserted through the tenth intercostal space posteriorly and connected to an underwater seal drain (Fig 6.17). In most patients, the chest drain removes the blood and as the lung expands, the bleeding stops.

In some patients, however, a large volume of blood drains out (more than 1 or 2 L) and the blood loss continues. Various formulae have been devised to indicate when to perform a **thoracotomy**, e.g. an initial drainage of more than 1.5 L or more than

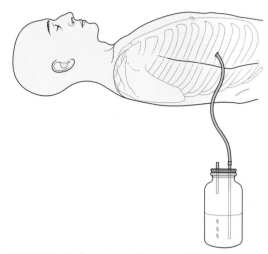

FIGURE 6.17   Underwater seal drainage of pleura

200 mL/hour for 3–4 hours; but, in reality, it soon becomes apparent when the blood replacement is failing to keep up with the blood loss and surgery to stop the bleeding becomes essential.

The bleeding may be coming from the chest wall (intercostal or internal mammary arteries) or one of the lung vessels. Rarely, the lung has been avulsed causing catastrophic haemorrhage. Many such patients never reach hospital alive. Emergency thoracotomy with pneumonectomy can occasionally be life-saving.

Prognosis Most patients with a straightforward haemothorax recover completely, but a failure to remove all the clotted blood can leave a layer of clotted blood restricting respiration. In these circumstances the layer of fibrin around the lung may have to be removed by an operation called **decortication**.

Very rarely, the thoracotomy tube can be the route for the entry of infection. It may also damage the lung during insertion.

LUNG CONTUSION (DIRECT INJURY)

It is now recognized that this is an important cause of major morbidity in many patients with chest injuries. A **plain chest X-ray** in patients with poor oxygen saturations may show severe consolidation of the underlying lung (Fig 6.18). These patients can rapidly develop ARDS, which carries

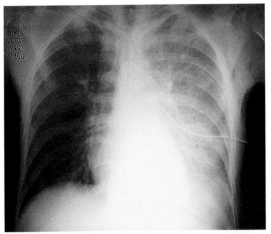

FIGURE 6.18 Chest X-ray of underlying contusion of left lung: penetration is much poorer on this lung field compared with the normal right lung

a considerable mortality (20 per cent). Oxygen supplementation, analgesia and physiotherapy may help, but some patients require endotracheal intubation and prolonged ventilation. A tracheostomy will need to be inserted if ventilation is required for more than a week.

CARDIAC INJURIES

The heart may be **contused** by blunt trauma, often associated with sternal fractures, or **punctured** by a penetrating sharp injury. In the latter type of injury the blood collecting within the pericardium may compromise cardiac function by compressing the heart within the inelastic pericardial sac. This is know as cardiac **tamponade**.

CARDIAC CONTUSION

This is suspected when the blood pressure is low in the absence of hypovolaemia.

Investigations

An **ECG** showing evidence of ST elevation and inverted T waves is highly suggestive of the diagnosis, which can be confirmed by finding an **elevated troponin level** within 24 hours.

Echocardiography may show an inadequate cardiac output without evidence of tamponade.

Management

Conservative treatment is indicated in the absence of tamponade unless the valves have been damaged, when urgent surgical repair must be considered.

Inotropes (adrenaline, dobutamine and noradrenaline) may be required and **anti-arrhythmics** used to treat any abnormal rhythms that develop. Most patient recover completely.

PENETRATING CARDIAC INJURIES AND TAMPONADE

A sharp injury in an appropriate site makes a cardiac laceration and the associated risk of tamponade a possibility.

Investigations

Clinical diagnostic indicators

Tamponade should be suspected if there are signs of poor cardiac output in the presence of raised neck veins. The heart sounds are muffled and the radial pulse is weak. Pulsus paradoxus may be present but is not essential for the diagnosis.

Imaging

A **chest X-ray** will show a globular cardiac shadow (Fig 6.19A). **Echocardiography** may show blood in the pericardial sac (Fig 6.19B).

Management

Blood in the pericardial sac can be aspirated under imaging control through a needle inserted below the xiphisternum with ultrasound guidance.

Immediate reaccumulation of blood is an indication for surgical exploration and the suture of any cardiac lacerations. Most cardiac lacerations can be closed with simple sutures but care must be taken to avoid damage to a coronary artery.

RUPTURED THORACIC AORTA

This is the commonest cause of death in those who have suffered a massive deceleration injury (e.g. an aeroplane crash) and can be present in patients who survive deceleration injuries in road traffic accidents.

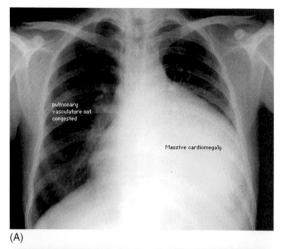

pulmonary
vasculature not
congested

Massive cardiomegaly

(A)

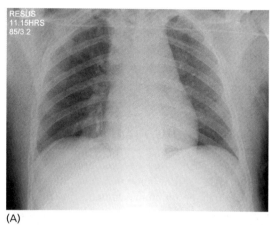

(A)

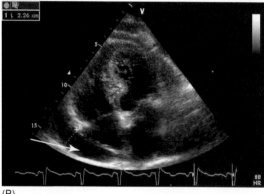

(B)

FIGURE 6.19   Haemopericardium. (A) Chest X-ray showing globular heart; (B) echocardiogram of blood in pericardium (arrowed)

The descending thoracic aorta is fixed by fascia to the posterior chest wall just below the level of the left subclavian artery, whereas the heart and ascending aorta are mobile. Massive deceleration can cause a tear at the junction of the aorta's fixed and mobile parts.

Provided the adventitia remains intact the patient will not immediately die of blood loss and may arrive in the A&E with few, if any, physical signs; but this diagnosis should be suspected in any patient who has suffered a head-on deceleration injury.

Investigation

A **chest X-ray** may show a **widening of the mediastinum** (Fig 6.20A). The diagnosis can be confirmed by a **CT scan with contrast enhancement** (Fig 6.20B).

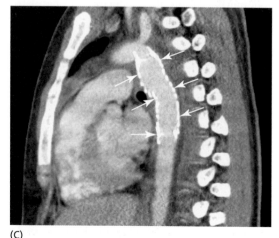

(B)

(C)

FIGURE 6.20   (A) Chest X-ray showing a wide mediastinum; (B) CT showing thoracic aortic disruption haematoma (arrowed); (C) stent graft

Management

This injury is now treated by **endovascular stent grafting** (see Chapter 11, Fig 6.20C), which has been shown to have reduced the morbidity and mortality in follow-up studies extending for more than 5 years. This has replaced open surgical repair.

RUPTURE OF THE DIAPHRAGM

This is usually caused by a compression injury of the chest and/or abdomen and followed by herniation of the abdominal contents into the chest. Knives may also cut through the diaphragm but almost never cause it to split extensively.

Investigation

Clinical diagnostic indicators

Patients may complain of shortness of breath and have poor air entry over the left lung base with a dull percussion note.

Imaging

Plain chest X-rays and **CT scans** can confirm the diagnosis (Fig 6.21).

The **differential diagnosis** is from a long-standing eventration of the diaphragm and, rarely, a haemothorax or pneumothorax.

Management

The diaphragm should be repaired through an abdominal incision after reducing any herniated contents back into the abdomen.

OESOPHAGEAL INJURY

Oesophageal injuries in the chest are extremely rare, but the oesophagus can be damaged in the neck by stab wounds or bullets.

Investigation

Clinical diagnostic indicators

The presence of **surgical emphysema** in the neck suggests the diagnosis.

A **chest X-ray** or **CT scan** (see Fig 6.22) will confirm the diagnosis if it shows air in the mediastinum.

Contrast radiography and **oesophagoscopy** can be useful to determine the site of the damage.

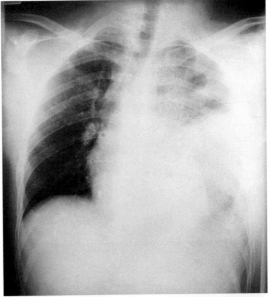

(A)

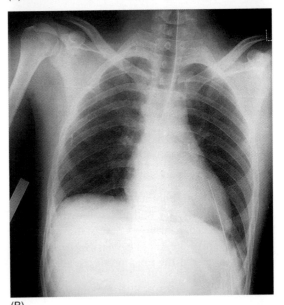

(B)

FIGURE 6.21   (A, B) Rupture of the diaphragm before and after treatment

Management

Surgical repair is used to close any tears provided they are found early. Late presentations can be treated by **drainage**, defunctioning by a **cervical oesophagostomy** and **stenting** across the damaged segment (see Chapter 14).

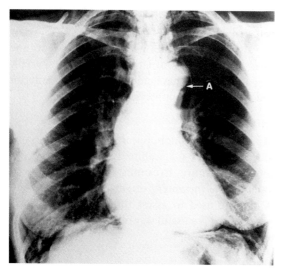

FIGURE 6.22 Surgical emphysema/air in the mediastinum; air can be seen tracking along muscle fibres between pleura and mediastinum (A)

ABDOMINAL INJURIES

BLUNT INJURIES

The usual causes of blunt abdominal injuries are road traffic accidents, but sporting injuries and interpersonal blunt violence can also damage the abdominal organs. Seat belts can cause damage to the small bowel, colon and mesentery. Fractures of the lower ribs on the left are associated with splenic damage and fractures on the right with liver injuries. Both of these organs can be burst by external compression, which can give rise to major intra-abdominal bleeding.

Intra-abdominal blunt injuries should be suspected in any patient who has sustained a severe injury and is showing signs of hypovolaemic shock but no overt signs of bleeding in the chest or from other injuries. A fractured pelvis or femur can bleed a considerable amount (see page 158), but persistent hypotension after adequate resuscitation is always suggestive of bleeding into the abdomen.

PENETRATING INJURIES

Penetrating injuries of the abdomen are common. Most people survive knife wounds unless they are multiple or damage the abdominal aorta, inferior vena cava, liver or spleen.

Bullet wounds, especially from high-velocity weapons and shrapnel, can cause very severe injuries. The injuries associated with low-velocity weapons depend on the course of the bullet. This can be roughly estimated from the entry and exit wound, if present. The course of any bullet can vary considerably if it hits bone. The entry wound gives a rough idea of the organs likely to have been hit first.

High-velocity bullets cause much damage around their trajectory.

The resulting **cavitation** sucks clothing and other contaminants into the wound track, making wide excision of damaged tissue essential.

The increasing use of Kevlar protection by Western armed forces has reduced the incidence, morbidity and mortality of high-velocity wounds of the torso.

Investigation

Clinical diagnostic indicators

Provided the patient is conscious, clinical examination and repeated re-examination of the abdomen is helpful if blunt trauma is suspected. Genital, vaginal and rectal examinations should be performed to exclude perineal trauma. The pulse and blood pressure should be monitored but **there is no evidence that repeated measurement of abdominal girth is of any value**. Abdominal assessment is very difficult in the unconscious patient, as the local signs of peritonitis cannot be detected.

Blood tests

A baseline full blood count should be taken and blood sent for cross-matching (4 units) if an abdominal injury is suspected.

External wound exploration

This is a very inaccurate technique for assessing abdominal wounds (false-positive rate 90 per cent) and it should only be carried out in the operating theatre before surgery.

Imaging

Plain X-rays should be taken of the chest, abdomen and pelvis in anyone suspected of having an abdominal injury. The bullet entry wounds should be marked and the bullet may be seen (Fig 6.23).

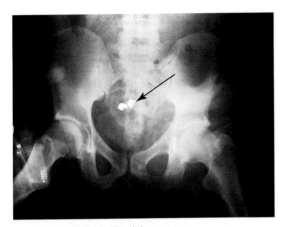

FIGURE 6.23   Bullet in the abdomen

The **FAST technique** (focused **a**bdominal **s**onography for **t**rauma) attempts to detect blood in the abdomen, not to assess injuries to individual organs. The right upper quadrant, left upper quadrant and pelvis are scanned by ultrasound. The technique has a specificity of 95 per cent and a sensitivity of 85 per cent. It can guide the management of unstable patients (e.g. laparotomy) or precede further evaluation in stable patients (CT scan). It is easy to repeat.

Contrast-enhanced **ultrafast 68-slice CT scanning** has revolutionized the assessment of the stable patient with suspected abdominal trauma. The head, back and chest can be imaged at the same time. CT is good for assessing damage to individual organs and the retroperitoneal tissues, including the pancreas and major vessels. It can be used to detect small quantities of air as well as assessing the amount of blood present in the abdominal cavity.

MRI is not helpful. **Arteriography** may be considered if therapeutic embolization or stenting is being considered.

Diagnostic peritoneal lavage

Peritoneal lavage has been a very popular method for assessing the likelihood of the presence of an intra-abdominal injury in unconscious patients but has been largely superseded by ultrasound and CT scanning.

If the lavage fluid contains more than 100 000 red cells/mm or more than 500 white cells/mm, it has a 90 per cent sensitivity and 97 per cent accuracy for detecting abdominal bleeding.

Bile, blood and vegetable matter can also be detected.

False positives and negatives can occur and there is a small risk of iatrogenic injury, especially in patients who have adhesions to the anterior abdominal wall from previous surgery.

Laparoscopy

Laparoscopy does not appear to add value to peritoneal lavage or CT scanning in diagnosing blunt abdominal injury. It cannot assess the retroperitoneum, the mesentery or small bowel accurately. It may be used to assess thoracoabdominal stab wounds and is a useful way of confirming a rupture of the diaphragm.

Management

As a general rule, all gunshot wounds of the abdomen, pelvis, perineum and lower chest should be explored after appropriate resuscitation and the investigations described above.

Diagnostic laparotomy is the ultimate investigation and the first step in management, but with increasingly accurate methods of investigation many more patients with abdominal injuries are now being treated conservatively.

SPECIFIC INTRA-ABDOMINAL INJURIES

SPLENIC INJURY

This is the commonest abdominal injury. A **CT scan** is helpful in determining the severity of the splenic injury.

Most splenic injuries used to be treated by splenectomy until the late risk of overwhelming post-splenectomy infection (OPSI) was recognized. This severe and potentially lethal complication is greatest in children. As a consequence, many children and fit young adults are considered for non-operative management of splenic trauma if they are not severely shocked, i.e. have a systolic blood pressure greater than 90 mmHg, and require only minimal resuscitation (less than 1 unit of blood).

Elderly patients, however, tend to do badly with non-operative management and should be treated surgically the moment they show signs of becoming haemodynamically unstable.

Occasionally, the spleen can be repaired. Fragmented spleens can be sliced up and placed within an omental pocket in an attempt to reduce the risk of OPSI, but in these circumstances splenectomy is usually unavoidable.

LIVER INJURY

Many liver injuries are treated non-operatively after **CT scan** assessment (Fig 6.24). Laparoscopic haemostasis, selective angio-embolization and image-guided drainage of haematomata may extend conservative management and avoid open surgery.

ERCP and biliary drainage can be used to control biliary leaks.

Unstable patients require laparotomy through a Mercedes-Benz upper abdominal incision when packing, debridement, haemostasis and even liver resection may be needed, depending on the findings and the experience of the surgeon.

The 'second look laparotomy' for removal of packs at 48 hours should be carried out by an experienced hepatobiliary surgeon.

PANCREATICO-DUODENAL INJURY

These rare injuries (the organs are well protected) have a high morbidity and mortality and are difficult to manage. Injuries of the pancreas and duodenum rarely occur in isolation. Both can be seen preoperatively on **CT scans**.

Evidence of leakage of duodenal or pancreatic secretions is an indication for surgical exploration.

At operation, Kocher's manoeuvre is employed to mobilize and examine the duodenum. The pancreas

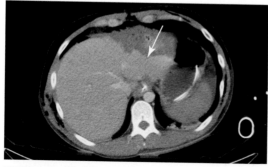

FIGURE 6.24   CT of liver injury (arrow)

is explored through the greater sac. Bile staining in the retroperitoneal tissues or a large haematoma in the pancreas supports the diagnosis.

Duodenal and pancreas injuries can be repaired and drained, but a distal fistula may develop if the pancreatic duct has been damaged.

Distal pancreatectomy, a **Whipple's procedure** and **exclusion** using pyloric division and a Roux loop can all be utilized to deal with a damaged pancreas, depending on the findings and the state of the patient. All carry a considerable mortality and morbidity.

BOWEL INJURY

Abdominal compression can split the bowel wall directly, by increasing the intraluminal pressure or by shearing the fixed and mobile portions of the gut apart (e.g. at the duodenojejunal flexure, ileocaecal junction or sigmoid colon).

Rapid deceleration can tear the mesentery and so cause bleeding and bowel ischaemia.

The whole intestine must be assessed at a **laparotomy** for abdominal trauma. Almost all bowel injuries are treated by laparotomy and **primary repair** or **resection and primary anastomosis**.

Colonic injuries may need exteriorization or defunctioning, especially if they involve the upper rectum.

KIDNEY INJURY

Most renal injuries can be managed non-operatively. They usually present with loin pain and/or haematuria. A mass is rarely present. A CT scan is an accurate way of making the diagnosis. Open surgery usually results in nephrectomy.

Local embolization of a bleeding cortical vessel is effective for iatrogenic bleeding after biopsy.

PELVIC INJURIES

Pelvic fractures are associated with massive blood loss and have a considerable mortality. The bleeding is reduced by the application of an **external fixator**. The bleeding can sometimes be controlled by **arterial embolization**.

VASCULAR INJURIES

These are usually the result of penetrating trauma, but bullets passing close to arteries can cause contusions and internal damage. Venous bleeding can be massive if major veins are torn.

Investigation

Clinical diagnostic indicators

The main indicators of an intra-abdominal vascular injury are hypovolaemic shock and acute abdominal pain.

Imaging

The **Doppler pressures** in the lower limbs are usually reduced by damage to the iliac arteries.

Duplex scans of the abdominal vessels may reveal the site of an arterial occlusion or disruption.

CT angiography or **catheter arteriography** can be used to define the exact site and extent of the arterial damage if the patient is stable.

Management

Major bleeding requires surgical exploration and vascular repair.

Stent grafts can sometimes be used to occlude partially damaged vessels, but most other vascular injuries should be approached directly, controlled and repaired.

Shunts can be used to maintain perfusion while other injuries are assessed and treated, but blood flow should be restored as soon as possible, if necessary by the insertion of a **vein graft** taken from an undamaged limb.

Vessels, especially veins, can be ligated if the patient is unstable or the organ the vessel supplies cannot be salvaged.

THE ABDOMINAL COMPARTMENT SYNDROME

This condition can be caused by a large retroperitoneal haematoma or continuing intra-abdominal bleeding. It can be confirmed by finding a bladder pressure above 30 mmHg.

The raised intra-abdominal pressure can cause renal, respiratory and cardiovascular problems which may lead to multi-organ failure and, if left untreated, death. The onset of oliguria or anuria or respiratory distress indicates the development of ARDS.

The management is to **open the abdomen** to relieve the pressure and to close it with a plastic sheet, which allows the wound edges to bulge. The abdomen is resutured when the pressure has declined.

GENERAL MANAGEMENT ISSUES

POST-INJURY CRITICAL CARE

Patients must be continuously monitored and reassessed to detect injuries missed in the initial survey.

The three most important complications that may follow all major injuries that must be detected and treated are **sepsis, electrolyte imbalance** and **multi-organ failure. Acidosis** must be corrected with bicarbonate, **hypothermia** reversed and **coagulopathy** treated with clotting factors.

Ventilation needs to be continuously reassessed and adjusted, especially when the patient is intubated.

The circulation must be adequately filled with crystalloid, colloid, fresh frozen plasma, blood and platelets. Inotropic drugs can be used to boost a faltering circulation.

Haemofiltration can be used to remove excess fluid, treat hyperkalaemia and remove waste products until the kidneys are functioning normally.

Prophylaxis must be given against deep vein thrombosis with low molecular weight heparin. Some patients may benefit from the placement of a temporary inferior vena cava filter.

Patients with brainstem death should be considered for organ donation.

REHABILITATION

Many patients with severe head and spinal injuries require prolonged rehabilitation and many end up with permanent disabilities. Rehabilitation services should aim to restore maximum function and provide facilities to those who are permanently disabled, giving them the chance to obtain the best quality of life. Physiotherapy, occupational therapy, psychotherapy and social services all play a part in rehabilitation, which, if possible, should be managed by a specialist centre.

SCORING SYSTEMS

These have been developed primarily as an audit tool for testing the value of physical signs and investigations as predictors of outcome. The anatomical damage and the physiological responses of the body to the injury are combined to give a *trauma injury severity score*. The aim of management is not to lose any predicted survivors, and do everything possible to have survivors among those predicted to do badly.

7

Fractures, joint injuries and diseases of bones

Steven A. Corbett

FRACTURES

A fracture is a structural discontinuity of bone. It is important to recognize that the injury is rarely just to the bone itself but almost always involves the soft tissue. Fractures in normal or diseased bone are caused by direct and indirect trauma and repetitive stress.

Trauma

A fracture may be caused by *direct* force, where the fracture occurs at the point of impact, or an *indirect* force, where the fracture occurs away from the site of the applied force.

An indirect force can be **rotational**, e.g. a twisting injury of the ankle causing a lower leg fracture; **compressive**, e.g. a vertebral crush fracture; on **distractive**, e.g. an avulsion fracture.

Stress

Fractures can be caused by low levels of stress below the normal yield strength of the bone. Stress fractures commonly occur in the lower extremity, i.e. in the tibia, tarsal and metatarsal bones. They are common in athletes, and white women with advancing age, especially those with underlying metabolic bone disease (known as 'fragility fractures').

Pathological bone

Fractures can be caused by low-energy injuries in bone which has been weakened by a pre-existing abnormality such as

- **metabolic conditions** (osteoporosis, Paget's disease, renal osteodystrophy)
- **bone tumours** (benign and malignant, primary, secondary or metastatic)
- **infections** (osteomyelitis tubercolosis).

Classifications of bone injury

Fractures may be classified into complete or incomplete, closed or open.

Incomplete fractures occur where the bone is incompletely divided, often leaving part of the periosteum intact. In a greenstick fracture in a child, the bone bends, such that one cortex buckles while the other remains intact.

Complete fractures may be subclassified on the appearance of the fracture into *transverse, oblique/spiral, comminuted* (when there is more than one fragment) and *crush* (where the fracture is impacted) (Fig 7.1).

Closed fractures can be classified according to bone damage (see above) and the accompanying soft tissue injuries as categorized by Tscherne.

Grade 0   Negligible soft tissue injury.
Grade I   Superficial abrasion or contusion of the soft tissues overlying the fracture.
Grade II   Significant contusion of the muscle with contaminated skin abrasions or both; the bone injury is usually severe.
Grade III   Significant injury to the soft tissues associated with degloving, crushing, compartment syndrome or vascular injury.

Open fractures have an injury that allows communication between the fracture and the outside environment and can be classified according to the method of Gustilo (see p. 153).

Site

Fractures can occur in any part of a bone – in the diaphysis (shaft), metaphysis (the part of the diaphysis next to the growth plate) or epiphysis (secondary ossification centre beside the growth plate).

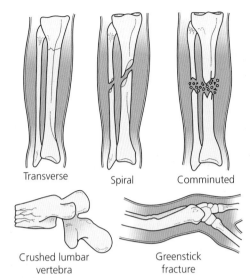

Transverse   Spiral   Comminuted

Crushed lumbar   Greenstick
vertebra   fracture

FIGURE 7.1   Diagram of types of bone damage

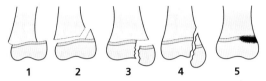

1   2   3   4   5

FIGURE 7.2   Diagram of Salter–Harris classification of children's fractures

Blood tests

Routine blood investigations are seldom required for most fractures. The preoperative blood tests required will depend on the patient's age and co-morbidities.

In the presence of major trauma, especially long bone and pelvic fractures, a **full blood count** and **urea and electrolyte measurement** should be obtained. **Blood grouping or immediate cross-matching** may be required depending on the severity of the injuries (see Chapter 6).

Imaging

X-rays of the fracture are mandatory. In order to assess all the necessary information, the X-rays must be taken in a minimum of two views, usually in anteroposterior and lateral directions, and include the joint above and below the injury. This is to assess whether there are other associated fractures or joint dislocation.

The important features to note (see also Appendices, Revision panel 3) are

■ the site of the fracture, which may involve the middle, proximal or distal thirds of the bone
■ the shape of the fracture, i.e. transverse, oblique, spiral, comminuted or segmental
■ the displacement of the fracture which represents the translation of the fracture, and may be described as
  □ the percentage of one bone displacement relative to the other;
  □ the alignment or angulation of the fracture in respect of the tilt of the bones relative to each other;
  □ the rotation of the fracture which may be recognized by comparing the cortical width on one side of the fracture with the other.

Epiphyseal fractures which occur around the physis of a growing bone can cause deformity in later life, as a bone bridge may grow across the fracture site and prevent growth on one side of the bone. Epiphyseal injuries have been classified by Salter and Harris (Fig 7.2) as

Type 1:   A fracture through the growth plate separating the epiphysis from the metaphysis (6 per cent incidence).
Type 2:   A fracture through the growth plate with division of the epiphysis and metaphysis except for a flake of metaphyseal bone (75 per cent).
Type 3:   Separation of part of the epiphysis and its growth plate from the rest of the epiphysis (8 per cent).
Type 4:   A fracture line crossing the physis with bone involvement on both sides of the physis (10 per cent).
Type 5:   A fracture where there is compression of the growth plate (1 per cent).

Investigation

Clinical diagnostic indicators

The symptoms and signs of a fractured bone include pain, tenderness, swelling, deformity, loss of function and mobility, abnormal movement and crepitus.

In children, the presence of physeal growth plates can make interpretation of X-rays difficult.

Knowledge of the dates of ossification within a bone is often necessary.

Contrast radiography involves injecting radio opaque dye into cavities during X-ray examination in order to outline structures and increase the sensitivity and specificity of the examination. This is most commonly used for fractures involving the hip and shoulder joints, especially when the bones are not ossified and hence difficult to visualize on plain X-rays.

CT scanning is able to reveal soft parts not seen on a standard X-ray. Multiple images are taken and compiled into a series of cross-sectional pictures. These image 'slices' can be reconstructed to provide three-dimensional images. By focusing on the site of interest the difficulties of interpreting the overlapping injuries seen on an X-ray are avoided. CT is a useful way of delineating fracture patterns and can have an important role when determining whether a patient needs operative intervention. They can also help planning the intervention.

Magnetic resonance imaging uses external magnets to cause realignment of protons of hydrogen nuclei. These then resonate and emit signals which can be detected. This allows a 3D image to be constructed. Pictures may be obtained from any angle. Tissues which contain abundant hydrogen, e.g. fat and cancellous bone marrow, produce a high-intensity signal giving bright images. The image of tissues with little hydrogen, e.g. cortical bone, ligaments and tendons, usually appear black. Cartilage and muscle produce an intermediate signal which is a grey colour.

T1 images are weighted towards fat so that fat appears bright and cortical bone dark.

T2 images are weighted towards water so that fluid, haemorrhage, soft tissue tumours and cerebrospinal fluid (CSF) that appear dark on T1 studies are bright on T2. T1 images are best for demonstrating anatomical structure and T2 images are most useful for contrasting normal and abnormal tissue.

The advantage of the MRI scan is that it can take pictures from almost every angle, whereas CT scans can only take horizontal pictures, unless reconstruction is undertaken. The patient is not exposed to ionizing radiation involved in an MRI scan.

MRI is contraindicated in patients with pacemakers, cerebral or aneurysmal clips, shrapnel or metal work in certain anatomical locations.

MRI scanning can be used to demonstrate fresh haemorrhage, infection or evaluate occult fractures, e.g. in the elderly hip.

Ultrasonography can be used to image muscle and soft tissue. The advantage of the ultrasound scan is that it is a dynamic rather than a static technique and has no reported significant side-effects. It is commonly used to assess soft tissue injuries, especially tendon tears in the shoulder rotator cuff tendons, which may occur in combination with a fracture.

Dexa scanning is a non-invasive and quantitative method of measuring bone mineral density (BMD) and bone mineral content (BMC). It is a quick and easy tool for detecting bone loss and for assessing the changes in mineralization associated with fracture repair. It is most frequently used to detect osteoporosis in patients suspected of having changes within the bone predisposing them to fragility fractures, or to detect osteoporosis in those with a fracture without a previously identified risk.

Radioisotope scans may be used to outline fractures sustained in an abnormal bone, and to illicit stress fractures not seen on plain X-ray. Metabolically active bone constituents are labelled or tagged with different isotopes and are administered by intravenous injection. Common radioisotopes are technetium-99m, gallium-67 and indium-111. Their activity is measured by a gamma camera accessed twice – immediately after injection during the blood phase and a few hours later. The first image indicates hyperaemia/vascularity and shows how quickly the radioisotope reaches the lesion. The second image detects new bone formation and activity.

Occasionally single photon emission computerized tomography (SPECT) can be performed to give 3D information about a lesion.

GENERAL MANAGEMENT OF FRACTURES
Resuscitation

The management of any fracture begins with the resuscitation of the patient following the ATLS (Advanced Trauma Life Support System) guidelines (see Chapter 6). Once the overall condition of the patient is stabilized, the management of the fracture can begin.

The treatment of any fracture should follow Apley's principles. These are

- **reduce** (the fracture)
- **hold and stabilize** (the fracture)
- **mobilize and exercise** (as healing progresses).

Non-operative management should ensure that the fracture is in a good position so that once it has healed the patient has a good functional outcome.

Not all fractures need to be reduced. Some displacement or angulation may be acceptable provided it does not compromise the eventual functional outcome.

Fractures that are displaced, angulated or impacted require disimpaction and manipulation to correct any malalignment and angulation and restore apposition of the bones.

It should be recognized that absolute anatomical reduction is not always necessary.

Methods of reduction

Reduction can be achieved by gravity, manipulation with anaesthetic provision, traction or surgical intervention, involving open reduction of the injury.

- **Gravity** is used, particularly for treatment of upper limb fractures, e.g. placing the patient with a humeral neck fracture in a collar and cuff sling.
- **Manipulation of fractures** can be performed under local, regional or general anaesthesia. The former are most often used in the treatment of distal radial fractures, which may be disimpacted, and the displacement and angulation corrected under intrahaematoma anaesthesia or a regional block (Bier's block).
- **Mechanical traction** is now less frequently applied but can be used in the treatment of cervical, supracondylar humeral and long bone fractures The traction overcomes muscular spasm and allows disimpaction.

If a fracture cannot be reduced by closed methods an **open surgical procedure** will be required. The interposition of soft tissue between the fracture ends, and muscle pull on the fracture sustaining residual displacement are reasons why closed reductions fail.

If an open approach is employed, the fracture is invariably stabilized with a mechanical form of fixation.

Methods of maintaining stability

Once the fracture is reduced, it needs to be held in the position achieved by the manipulation.

When non-operative intervention is selected, fractures are held by splintage or the application of a cast or brace.

Casts of **plaster of Paris** are still used, but lighter products incorporating **fibreglass** are often better tolerated by patients.

Functional bracing allows movement of a joint, either above or below the fracture, thereby preventing undue stiffness. (Fig 7.3). The brace may be fashioned with a hinge using plaster of Paris or fibreglass. Specially manufactured braces are also available. In some instances, the joint above a fracture can be left free while a plaster still provides support, e.g. a Sarmiento brace for a tibial fracture allows movement of the knee joint, although the plaster itself extends to the anterior aspect of the knee allowing weight-bearing.

Traction was traditionally the mainstay in fracture management to maintain reduction (Fig 7.4). In recent times, its reduced usage has led to a loss of expertise in its application. In many cases, it has been superseded by operative techniques and a better understanding of the factors that influence fracture healing. Nevertheless, it still can provide an important treatment option.

Traction can be applied to the skin or through a bone.

Skin traction requires the application of an adhesive strapping to a limb with traction cords connecting to the mode of traction, e.g. weights.

Skeletal traction usually requires the placement of a Steinmann or Denholm pin through a bone, which is generally either the tibial tuberosity or the calcaneum, to which the traction is fixed.

Traction can either be balanced or fixed.

Balanced traction is achieved on a limb by applying a force in one direction, either with skin

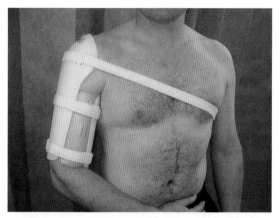

FIGURE 7.3   Humeral functional brace

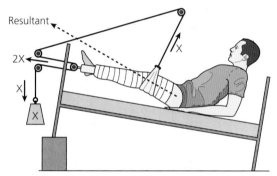

FIGURE 7.4   Diagram of Hamilton–Russell balanced traction

traction or skeletal traction, which is counteracted by the patient's body weight, usually by raising the end of the bed. Pulleys can be used to ensure the correct line of pull.

Fixed traction uses the same principle, but the lower limb is placed in a Thomas splint so the traction, which is applied to the distal part of the limb and connected to the end of the splint, is counteracted by the proximal ring of the splint pressing against the pelvis.

Surgical interventions

Surgical intervention may be required to reduce the fracture to a satisfactory position and hold the fracture in an acceptable position by external or internal fixation and intramedullary or extramedullary techniques.

External fixation includes the use of frames and external fixators (Fig 7.5). The basic principle is to place screws in the bone, each side of the fracture, and hold them in place with an external frame (a fixator). The screws may be inserted into the injured bone which has sustained the fracture or in other bones on either side of the fractured bone. In the latter case, ligamentotaxis (tension in the soft tissues) may be employed to reduce the injury, e.g. distal radial fractures. Fixators may be uni-axial, bi-axial or circular. In the last case, wires rather than screws are utilized and a frame is constructed resembling Meccano (the Ilizarov frame).

External fixation is most commonly used when there is an associated severe soft tissue, nerve or blood vessel injury. It can also be used for severely comminuted or unstable fractures where internal fixation may not be possible. The advantage of external fixation is that it allows access to the soft tissues, allowing interventions such as skin or soft tissue grafting.

Internal fixation requires either extramedullary or intramedullary devices.

Extramedullary fixation includes the use of pins, plates, screws and wires (Fig 7.6). The objective of this type of fixation aims to achieve anatomical reduction of the fracture fragments and hold them in position. This is especially important for the fractures close to joints where fixation is necessary to fulfil the local biomechanical demands. Effort should be made to preserve the bone fragments and the soft tissue by means of an 'atraumatic' surgical technique. This should be followed by early active pain-free mobilization of the muscles and joints adjacent to the fracture to prevent the development of pain and stiffness.

Internal fixation is indicated

- when long-lasting immobilization of the soft tissues, especially around joints, may result in pain and stiffness;
- when a fracture involves a load-bearing articular surface. Precise reconstruction of these surfaces is important, as any incongruity of the articulating surfaces will give rise to areas of high stress and the risk of developing post-traumatic arthritis;
- when recovery of function of long bones is dependent on early exact and stable reconstruction, as well as immediate mobilization to prevent permanent impairment, e.g. supracondylar femur and forearm fractures.

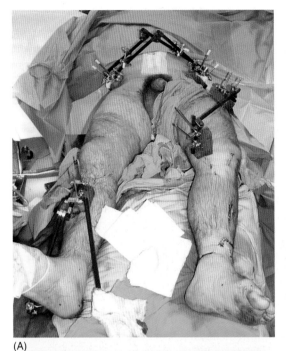

(A)

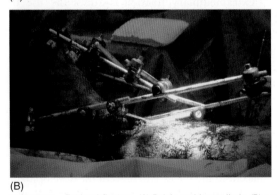

(B)

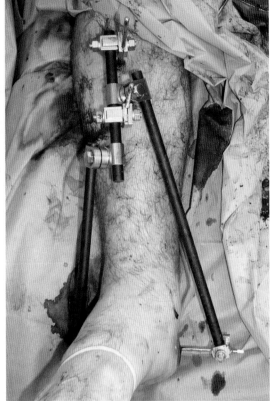

(C)

FIGURE 7.5   External fixators. (A) Pelvic and lower limb; (B) open tibia; (C) tibia

Most bones heal by endochondral ossification and callus formation, rigid internal fixation allows the fracture to heal primarily without a callus phase.

In **Intramedullary fixation** a nail is inserted into the intramedullary cavity (Fig 7.7). The nail may either be solid or flexible. Solid nails are secured with locking screws at each end. This confers stability in both axial alignment and rotation. The bone may have to be reamed before insertion. Solid nails are generally used for long bone fractures, particularly of the humerus, femur and tibia. Flexible nails are sometimes used in childhood fractures. Inflatable nails are also available.

A fracture sometimes cannot be reduced or held in an acceptable position. It is then necessary to **replace the bone**, e.g. patients with neck of femur or humeral head fractures may have to have a hemiarthroplasty (replacement of the femoral or humeral head) or a total joint replacement (Fig 7.8).

MANAGEMENT OF OPEN FRACTURES

An open or compound fracture is an orthopaedic emergency (Fig 7.9). Patients should be operated on within 6–8 hours of the injury because of the risk of

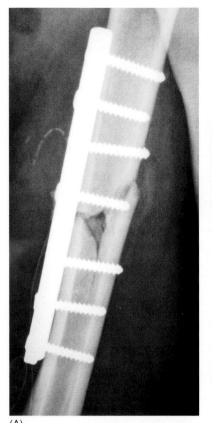 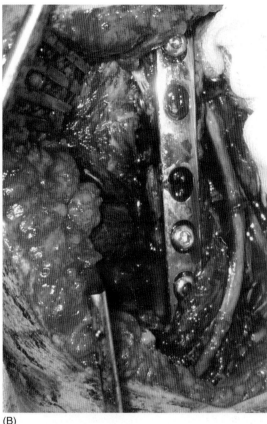

(A)   (B)

FIGURE 7.6   Extramedullary fixation. (A) Humeral plate X-ray; (B) Intraoperative photo of humeral plate and radial nerve

wound contamination becoming wound infection. There is also often the additional presence, in an open fracture, of significant soft tissue and neurovascular injury.

On arrival in the Accident and Emergency Department, it is important that once the patient has been assessed in respect of any life-threatening conditions and a full ATLS assessment made, attention is directed to the fracture.

The fracture will have been temporarily splinted and any wound covered at the scene of the incident (see Chapter 6).

Within the Accident and Emergency Department:

▪ The patient should be given appropriate intravenous antibiotics to guard against possible infection. Intravenous flucloxacillin and amoxicillin or cefuroxime are currently the antibiotics of choice as the most commonly infecting organism is a staphylococcus.

▪ The patient's tetanus immunization status should be ascertained. Some wounds are known to be tetanus-prone, e.g. those that are more than 6 hours old and deeper than 1 cm, those that are the result of a projectile injury and may contain devitalized tissue and gross contamination, and crush, burn or frostbite injuries.

▪ Those patients with an unknown tetanus status or those who have not had recent immunization should be given tetanus and diphtheria toxoids and tetanus immunoglobulin.

▪ Patients who are fully immunized should be given tetanus toxoid, particularly if they have not received a booster dose within the previous 5 years.

▪ The neurovascular status of the limb should be ascertained and recorded.

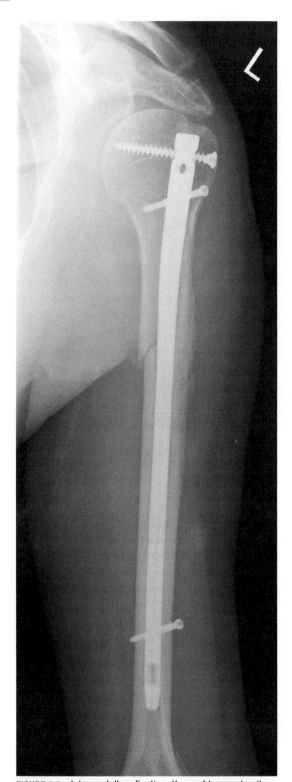

FIGURE 7.7   Intramedullary fixation. X-ray of humeral nail

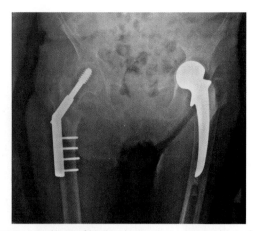

FIGURE 7.8   X-ray of hip hemiarthroplasty showing internal fixation for bilateral hip fractures

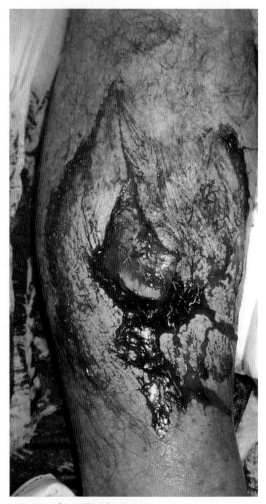

FIGURE 7.9   Open tibial fracture

- Appropriate splintage should be applied before transfer to the operating room even if this is only a temporary measure.
- The patient should be given appropriate analgesia.
- A betadine-soaked dressing should be applied over the wound and should not be removed once an accurate description of the wound has been recorded in the notes. If possible, this should be supplemented with a photograph.

The **Gustilo classification** of open wounds (see below) can be used to record and assess the degree of soft tissue damage. There is a tendency for the Gustilo classification category to 'increase' with time as the patient receives treatment.

Type I   Open fractures with a small, <1 cm, clean wound with minimal injury to the musculature and no significant stripping of the periosteum from the bone. The bone injury is simple with minimal comminution.

Type II   Open fractures with 1–10 cm wounds but no significant soft tissue damage or avulsion. The fracture contains moderate comminution.

Type III   Open fractures with larger wounds and associated extensive injury to the muscle, periosteum and bone which is often associated with significant contamination of the wound. The fracture may be segmental. Such injuries can be subdivided into:

  IIIa   Extensive contamination or injury to the underlying soft tissues but adequate viable soft tissue is present to cover the bone and neurovascular structures without muscle transfer.

  IIIb   Extensive injury to the soft tissues requiring a rotational or free muscle transfer to achieve coverage of the bone and neurovascular structures. These usually have massive contamination.

  IIIc   Open fractures with associated vascular injuries that require arterial repair.

The category of Gustilo injury generally reflects the velocity of the trauma sustained by the patient:

Type I	low energy
Type II	moderate energy
Type III	high-energy fractures.

On transfer to the operating room, the management should follow the same principles and routine applied in the Emergency Department.

The patient should be given further **antibiotic cover** suitable for the organisms which may ultimately lead to infection. Flucloxacillin and penicillin can be used in combination or a second-generation cephalosporin, such as cefuroxime. If the wound is heavily contaminated, metronidazole may be added to prevent infection by Gram-negative and anaerobic organisms. The intravenous antibiotics should be continued for 2–3 days.

Once the patient has been anaesthetized, attention can be directed towards the wound, the fracture and any other associated injuries.

The dressings are removed before the skin is prepared and draped. The wound should be irrigated with normal saline. A minimum of 6 L of fluid is usually needed, depending on the size of the wound. A pulsed lavage pressure irrigation system may be advantageous.

All foreign material and dead tissue must be removed until the wound edges are clean, and healthy viable underlying tissue is visible. The area of injured soft tissues is often much larger than the size of the wound suggests. Careful assessment and the excision of unhealthy tissue may involve extending the wound in the knowledge that subsequent closure may not be possible. It is however far better to have a zone of clean healthy tissue around the fracture.

At the time of the injury, the skin may have been pealed back over the bone and soft tissue for a considerable distance. This is called a *degloving injury* and is most commonly seen inassociation with lower limb fractures. Because of the disruption from its underlying attachments, the degloved skin will not survive and, hence, will need to be excised.

The viability of soft tissues and muscle can be assessed from their

Colour
Consistency
Contraction
Circulation

remembered as the **four Cs.**

The most valuable indicator of viability is bleeding during excision. If it has a dark colour, mushy consistency, fails to contact when pinched with forceps and is not bleeding from a cut surface, the muscle is not viable and should be excised. If muscle is found to be non-viable, then a **fasciotomy** should be considered. This involves incising the whole length of the skin and fascia covering the muscles, parallel to the muscle fibres, in order to decompress the fascial compartment. Failure to do so may result in increasing pressure within the compartment leading to a compartment syndrome (see later).

Arterial injuries need to be addressed immediately.

Severed nerves are best left and repaired at a later stage, unless the patient is going to undergo primary closure of the wounds.

The management of devascularized bone fragments is controversial. Large, free, contaminated or devascularized fragments of cortical bone may be replaced, in order to add to the mechanical integrity of internal fixation or, in grade III open fractures, removed to reduce the risk of infection.

Primary closure of the wound can be performed after the removal of all the dead tissue and washout provided there is negligible skin loss, the wound is clean and its edges come together without tension. Primary closure is often possible in Type I and Type II injuries.

If there has been considerable contamination, tension when attempting to close the wound, or there are Type III injuries, the wound should be left open, packed with gauze soaked in Betadine and reassessed 48 hours later when **a delayed primary closure** can be undertaken, provided the wound can be closed without tension and there is no evidence of infection.

In cases of gross contamination, **antibiotic-loaded chains** can be applied to the wound to deliver a high level of local antibiotics to the fracture site. In some instances, a vacuum-assisted closure device (Vac pump) can be used to help reduce and close the wound. This consists of a polyurethane sponge with transparent self-adhesive sheets which are applied over the wound and connected to a vacuum pump set to negative pressure. The vacuum draws fluid from the zone of injury and promotes wound healing.

If wound closure still cannot be undertaken, a **delayed secondary closure** should be considered. Plastic surgical techniques such as split skin grafts, whole thickness skin grafts, local rotational skin and combination flaps and free flaps are used depending on the vascularity of the underlying surface and the absence of infection.

In a well-vascularized area, split skin grafts taken from a healthy area can be applied directly to the defect. They usually take well but the cosmetic result is often poor.

An area with a poor blood supply, especially when there is extensive skin loss overlying a fracture, may be covered with a local fasciocutaneous or musculocutaneous flap or occasionally a free flap in which the flap's blood vessels are anastomosed by microsurgery to vessels in the affected area.

All these full thickness grafts are less reliable and leave a significant scar at the donor site, but when successful produce a grafted area of good quality.

The fracture itself should be managed according to established practice. Stabilization is imperative, particularly after performing the above measures to preserve the integrity of the soft tissues. If the fracture is not stabilized further soft tissue damage may occur, which increases the risk of developing infection.

Long bone fractures of the upper and lower limbs are usually stabilized by an intramedullary nailing technique, although plate fixation can also be used.

In high-energy trauma, with Gustilo classification Type IIIb/c injuries, more specialized stabilization is often required, using circular frames (Ilizarov) to allow access to the zone of soft tissue injury for subsequent plastic surgical procedures.

COMPLICATIONS OF FRACTURES

The complications of a fracture may be classified according to the time of its occurrence and its site, i.e. immediate/early/late and local or general.

The local complications relate to the bone, soft tissues, neurovascular structures and any adjacent joint.

The general complications include

- blood loss
- deep vein thrombosis
- pulmonary thromboembolism
- fat embolism
- acute respiratory distress syndrome.

The immediate complications of fractures are:

- bleeding (haemorrhage)
- vascular injury
- nerve injury
- visceral injury.

Bleeding

Although a fracture may be associated with an injury to a major blood vessel, the local soft tissue trauma and, indeed, bleeding from the bone itself can lead to significant blood loss. Hypovolaemic shock can arise.

The degree of blood loss varies with the bones involved:

- Major pelvic fractures may cause a 3L blood loss
- Femoral and humeral fractures a 1–3L blood loss
- Tibia and forearm fractures a 0.5–1.5L blood loss.

A pelvic fracture may cause the loss of 50 per cent of the circulating blood volume without any obvious evidence of impending circulatory disaster.

The significance of such fractures must never be underestimated, especially if there are other injuries.

The state of the circulation should be assessed frequently and appropriate volume replacement given in the form of crystalloid or colloid fluids and blood (see Chapter 6).

It is crucial to anticipate these requirements and be 'proactive' rather than 'reactive'.

Vascular injuries

Arteries and veins may be damaged by sharp or blunt trauma (see Chapter 6 and 11). An artery may be cut, torn, contused, compressed or simply go into spasm, in association with a fracture. This may result in haemorrhage, thrombosis or both. Arterial bleeding is generally pulsatile and can be torrential. Venous bleeding tends to well up from the wound. Both may be contained and concealed within a cavity or a fascial compartment.

The arteries most often injured in association with specific fractures are:

- the axillary artery in proximal humeral fractures
- the brachial artery in supracondylar fractures of the humerus in children
- the popliteal artery in fractures and dislocations of the knee

- the femoral artery in a supracondylar fracture of the femur
- the internal iliac and superior gluteal arteries in association with pelvic fractures.

In pelvic fractures the haemorrhage is often from injured veins and retroperitoneal blood vessels.

An artery may appear normal externally, but following a blunt injury may contain an intimal tear or flap which restricts blood flow causing intravascular thrombus formation leading to distal embolism or total vascular occlusion.

Arterial injuries are suspected on clinical examination and are confirmed by measuring doppler pressures.

The classic features of a vascular injury in a limb are pallor, coldness, a weak or absent pulse and paraesthesia or numbness (see Chapter 11). A duplex examination may confirm the injury and a CT angiography gives more precise information. Treatment is dependent on the nature of the vascular injury. If an angiography shows the vessels are intact with no intimal tear, then the injury may be treated expectantly.

When an artery is cut or torn, it can either be repaired primarily with sutures or a vein patch or replaced with a vein graft. Thrombosed vessels can be cleared by a balloon catheter.

When an arterial repair is performed the fracture must be stabilized simultaneously to prevent further injury to the blood vessel.

Nerve injuries

The effects of a nerve injury are seen in the anatomical distribution of the nerve, and may include Sensory, Motor, Autonomic, Reflex and Trophic changes (SMART).

The axons, their containing sheaths and the myelin may be injured in three ways.

Neuropraxia This is considered to be a bruising of the nerve with transient loss of function and early recovery. It is the least severe injury because the continuity of the nerve is preserved. It is characterized by a conduction block. Wallerian degeneration of the myelin sheath does not occur and there is no axonal loss. Recovery is usually evident within 3–6 weeks.

Axonotmesis This is disruption in the axons and surrounding endoneural sheath but with the perineurium and epinuerium, however, remaining intact. Wallerian degeneration occurs, with Schwann cells ingesting the fragmented myelin to restore the endoneural tubes and allow the advancement of the regenerating axons. Recovery is good but may take weeks to months.

Neurotmesis This is complete division of the nerve leaving no neural continuity. No recovery is seen unless the nerve is repaired.

The fractures/joint injuries most often associated with nerve injuries are:

- humeral fractures: the radial nerve
- humeral supracondylar fractures in children: the ulna nerve, median nerve are radial nerve
- medial condyle fractures of the elbow: the ulna nerve
- tibial plateau fractures: the common peroneal nerve
- shoulder dislocation: the axillary nerve
- hip dislocation: the sciatic nerve
- knee dislocation: the common peroneal nerve.

Investigation

All patients with a fracture should have a detailed clinical examination of the neurological status of the limb at the time of admission. Should the status change, particularly during or after an intervention such as a manipulation or the application of a cast or splint, early exploration of the nerve may be required.

If after an observation period of 3–6 weeks no recovery is observed, **nerve conduction** (NCS) and **electromyography** (EMG) studies should be performed.

The velocity of nerve conduction should be measured between two points above and below the site of the injury. If the nerve is compressed or damaged the conduction velocity in both motor and sensory nerves may be slowed. It will be absent if the nerve has been divided.

An EMG requires an electrode to be inserted into muscle to record motor unit activity. Denervation and reinervation potentials can be detected at rest, dependent on the severity and any recovery if there has been a nerve injury.

Management

The management of a nerve injury depends on the nature of the underlying injury. Unless there is clear evidence that a nerve has been transected (neurotmesis) a period of observation is indicated. During this time it may be appropriate, if there is significant motor functional loss, to provide joint support with a splint.

If NCS/EMG studies show no evidence of recovery the nerve should be explored.

A nerve that is known to be divided, should be repaired primarily or secondarily as part of management of the fracture.

EARLY COMPLICATIONS OF FRACTURES

- Local infection
- Septicaemia
- Gas gangrene
- Deep vein thrombosis/pulmonary embolism
- Fat embolism
- Adult respiratory distress syndrome
- Compartment syndromes
- Blisters/pressure sores

Infection

It is rare that a closed fracture will progress to infection unless there is secondary haematogenous seeding of the fracture haematoma from pre-existing infection at another site in the body. Infection in open fractures can lead to septicaemia and multi-organ failure.

Tetanus is a potentially lethal neuroparalytic disease caused by an exotoxin of *Clostridium tetani*.

Gas gangrene is a bacterial infection which produces gas within the tissues and constitutes a medical emergency (Fig 7.10). It is caused by an exotoxin-producing Clostridium species, most often *Clostridium perfringens*, which survives in low-oxygen anaerobic conditions. It can also be caused by *group A streptococcus*. It causes local muscle necrosis, gas production and sepsis leading to toxaemia and shock. The toxins damage tissues, blood cells and blood vessels. The area of infection becomes inflamed, very painful and tender. The

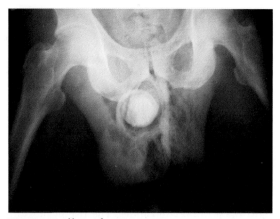

FIGURE 7.10   X-ray of gas gangrene

air in the swollen tissue gives it a crackly popping texture – subcutaneous emphysema. There may be associated blisters filled with a brown-red, foul-smelling fluid. If left untreated, the patient develops shock with hypotension, kidney failure, coma and death if left untreated.

Investigation must be initiated on clinical suspicion. Local tissue culture and a Gram stain of the affected tissue may show Gram-positive rods (clostridia). Blood culture may grow the bacteria.

A plain **X-ray or MRI scan** may show gas in the tissue.

Management

Supportive intervention as well as the appropriate intravenous **antibiotics and analgesia** for pain are essential. All dead tissue must be excised. Hyperbaric oxygen has been used with varying degrees of success as an aid to treatment. The patient needs to be nursed in intensive care when respiratory, renal and cardiac junctions can be assisted.

Fat embolism

Fat embolism is the embolism of both the pulmonary and systemic microvasculature with lipid globules and fibrin platelet thrombi. Fractures cause the blood triglyceride concentration to rise and allow the release of lipid globules from the damaged bone marrow into the circulation. The increased triglycerides reduce the uptake of oxygen by haemoglobin, increase blood viscosity, reduce microcirculatory blood flow, promote

platelet aggregation and activates the coagulation pathways. Fat emboli can affect the function of the organs in the following ways:

- lungs: ventilation perfusion mismatch causes hypoperfusion, hypoxia, tissue ischaemia and infarction
- brain: oedema causes confusion and convulsion
- heart: increased risk of arrhythmia
- kidneys: tubular damage and renal failure with lipid globules appearing in the urine
- skin: petechial haemorrhages.

This widespread damage can lead to multi-organ failure.

The patient becomes hypoxic with confusion, often aggressive behaviour and subsequently drowsiness and loss of consciousness. The respiratory rate increases, the pulse may be irregular and petechiae may be seen, particularly on the chest wall or within the conjunctivae.

Arterial blood gasses will show a low arterial oxygen content. Fat globules may be present in the urine, the platelet count is often low, and a chest X-ray may show patchy consolidation.

Treatment is with oxygen and assisted ventilation. The role of corticosteroids and heparin is controversial but may be used to treat the pathology.

Adult respiratory distress syndrome

Adult respiratory distress syndrome (ARDS) occurs secondary to the pulmonary oedema that may follow trauma, shock or infection. It is characterized by inflammation of the lung parenchyma causing impaired gas exchange and concomitant systemic release of inflammatory mediators that cause inflammation, hypoxaemia and frequently multiple organ failure.

Patients present with tachypnoea, dypsnoea and hypoxia. If multi-organ failure occurs, further symptoms relevant to the affected organs become apparent.

Investigation involves routine **blood** investigation, arterial **blood gases** and a **chest X-ray**.

Treatment is supportive. Patients often require mechanical ventilation with positive end-expiratory pressure (PEEP). The role of steroids and nitric oxide remains controversial.

Deep vein thrombosis and pulmonary embolism

Deep vein thrombosis (DVT) occurs in 30–50 per cent of patients with lower limb fractures, The risk of a pulmonary embolus in fractures, such as pelvic fractures, can be as high as 10 per cent, with fatal embolism occurring in 1 per cent (see Chapters 2 and 11). The injury is the main risk factor but this is amplified if the patient is immobilized and has other problems which increase the risk, such as obesity, carcinoma, a family or past history of DVT or a coagulation abnormality.

Investigation

Clinical diagnostic indicators

Although a DVT may present with calf tenderness and limb swelling it should be recognized that it is often symptomless.

Pulmonary embolism (PE) may present with chest pain, tachycardia, tachypnoea, haemoptysis, hypoxia, confusion, pyrexia, an arrhythmia or sudden collapse and death.

Blood tests

The investigation of DVT should include **D-dimer** and **blood gas** measurements.

Imaging

Venography and duplex Doppler **ultrasound scans** will confirm the presence of thrombus in the peripheral veins. An **MRI** can also be considered.

Ventilation/perfusion (V/Q) or **spiral CT scan** will reveal the size and effect of the emboli.

Management

The optimum management of DVT/PE is prevention rather than cure. This can be achieved by physical means with elastic stockings and intermittent leg compression pumps (see Chapter 2) or by administering prophylactic subcutaneous low molecular weight heparin, which has now largely superseded the use of unfractionated heparin (see Chapters 2, 6 and 11).

When a patient has a demonstrable DVT, treatment should be started with a loading dose of heparin followed by a maintenance dose.

Anticoagulation should be maintained for 3–6 months with warfarin.

Thrombolysis, **thrombectomy** and a **vena cava filter** are all considered in Chapter 11.

Compartment syndromes

A compartment syndrome is a serious complication, often associated with high-energy fractures of the forearm bones and tibia.

It results from a change in the pressure–volume relationship within a tight fascial compartment, most often in the extremities. The rise in pressure may be secondary to bleeding, oedema, inflammation or infection.

As the pressure within a compartment rises venous drainage is impaired and ultimately arterial inflow is restricted. The vascular insufficiency causes cell death and necrosis of both muscles and nerves which in itself causes further oedema and swelling, thereby exacerbating the problem.

A compartment syndrome can lead to the loss of a limb if left untreated. If the limb survives, the dead muscle which cannot regenerate becomes fibrotic and contracts, leading to permanent discomfort and disability, e.g. Volkmann's ischaemic contracture.

Investigation

Clinical diagnostic indicators

The classical signs and symptoms of a compartment syndrome are remembered as the five Ps (see Chapter 11):

Pain
Paraesthesia
Pallor
Paralysis
Pulselessness.

The main indication of a compartment syndrome is pain disproportionate to the apparent injury and increasing analgesic requirements, The development of paraesthesia and the absence of pulses are late signs, but beware, the presence of a distal pulse does not exclude a compartment syndrome. Passive stretching of the toes and fingers moved by the muscles in the affected compartment is painful.

Caution It should be remembered that the symptoms of a compartment syndrome may develop after a patient's limb has been placed in a plaster cast or splint if the limb swells and/or the cast has been applied too tightly. In these circumstances any constricting bandages or splints must be released immediately. If there is no improvement within 1–2 hours of releasing the dressings, a decision to decompress must be made on clinical grounds or compartment pressure measurements.

The most commonly affected compartments are:

lower leg	4 groups: superficial and deep posterior, anterior and lateral
forearm	3 groups: volar, dorsal and mobile wad
hand	10 groups: dorsal interossei (4), palmar interossei (3), adductor pollicis, thenar and hyperthenar compartments
foot	9 groups: intrinsic, medial, central and lateral.

Compartment syndrome can also occur in the thigh and buttock and elsewhere.

Further investigation often has to be based on a high index of suspicion of the condition.

Compartment pressure monitoring

The compartment pressure can be measured with specially designed needles. If the compartment pressure is >30 mmHg or if the diastolic blood pressure minus the measured compartment pressure is <30 mmHg, urgent treatment is required. Necrosis of muscle may begin when the interstitial pressure is as low as 30 mmHg.

Management

Fasciotomies open the fascial enclosures and reduce the compartment pressures and include division of the skin. **The fasciotomies must be complete**. A limited partial approach is not acceptable and they should include, not only the compartment under most pressure, but all relevant compartments adjacent to the region of injury.

The wounds are left open and a second procedure is undertaken approximately 46–48 hours later to assess the viability of the muscle and decide if further excision is necessary.

Delayed primary closure is undertaken when all the tissues in the compartment are viable. This may involve several visits to the operating room. The wounds may be closed gradually using vascular slings in a bootlace type approach tightened over a period of days to approximate the wound edges.

Sometimes it is not possible to close the wounds and split skin grafts may be required. Although this management may lead to cosmetic deformity, it is essential if the survival and normal function of the limb are to be ensured.

Fracture blisters, pressure sores, plaster sores

Blisters and sores that develop following a fracture may be caused by either the patient's immobility or the nature of the fracture immobilization. The injury itself may also cause blistering, especially if there is considerable swelling – 'fracture blisters' (Fig 7.11).

Such complications can be prevented by elevating the limb, encouraging movement and ensuring that dressings or casts are well padded and not too tight. Pressure mattresses should be available if required.

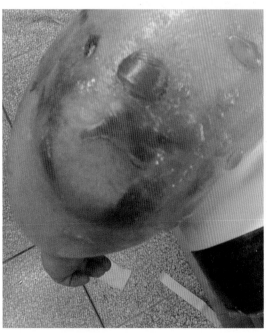

FIGURE 7.11   Fracture blisters

Pressure sores are graded as:

Stage I: superficial damage indicated by non blanchable redness

Stage II: damage to the epidermis extending into, but no deeper than, the dermis

Stage III: damage to the full thickness of the skin which may extend into the subcutaneous tissue layer.

Stage IV: damage extending into muscle, tendon or even bone.

Management

▥ Management includes removal of dead tissue with topical agents, excision or surgical. **Infection control** using antiseptics and antimicrobials and the application of Vacpump dressings to reduce the zone of injury and encourage granulation tissue.

▥ **Nutritional support** with review by a dietician (polytrauma patients are often protein and nutrient deficient which can impair healing).

▥ Plastic surgical grafting often fails.

LATE COMPLICATIONS OF FRACTURES

▥ Malunion
▥ Delayed union
▥ Non-union
▥ Heterotopic ossification (myositis ossificans)
▥ Avascular necrosis
▥ Joint instability and osteoarthritis
▥ Volkmann's ischaemic contracture
▥ Complex regional pain syndrome.

Malunion

If a fracture is not reduced satisfactorily and held in an appropriate position it may heal in an abnormal position. This is termed a malunion and, as a consequence, the broken bone may be shortened, maligned, angulated or rotated. Malunion may cause visible deformity and also compromise function.

Malunion is investigated and confirmed by **X-ray**, often supplemented by a **CT scan**.

Management

The malunion may have to be accepted; but if there is a significant functional deficit or deformity, the bone may have to be refractured and fixed in a more appropriate position.

Alternatively, corrective osteotomies can be undertaken, away from the original fracture site, to restore the limb to a satisfactory shape and alignment.

Delayed union

Delayed union occurs when a bone does not heal within the expected timeframe. The normal timeframe of healing varies between different bones and is

▥ upper limb humeral fractures: 6–12 weeks
▥ forearm fractures: 6–8 weeks
▥ wrist fractures: 6–8 weeks
▥ femoral fractures: 12–24 weeks
▥ tibial fractures: 12–24 weeks
▥ ankle fractures: 6–8 weeks

Delayed union can be caused by local and systemic factors and by the patient and the surgeon.

Local factors that may cause delayed union include:

▥ Disturbance of the local blood supply. The blood supply to a bone is usually though a main nutrient artery, which divides into ascending and descending medullary arteries with branches radiating out to the cortex. The periosteum also provides a separate circulation which may be compromised if, with the soft tissues, it is stripped from the bone during the trauma.

▥ Excessive movement at the fracture site if the splinting is inadequate.

▥ Inadequate movement because of over rigid fixation.

▥ Infection. Although fractures can heal even in the presence of infection, the healing process is often delayed.

▥ Soft tissue interposition between the bone ends.

▥ Separation of the bone ends caused by excessive traction or when internal fixation has been misapplied and holds the fracture apart.

Patient factors that contribute to delayed union include:

▥ smoking
▥ malnutrition
▥ metabolic bone disease.

The type of bone is important. Cancellous (spongy) bone heals more quickly than cortical (compact) bone.

The patient's age is also important. The union of childhood fractures is rapid but the speed of healing decreases as the skeleton matures.

The surgeon may contribute to delayed healing by inadequate fixation, excessive periosteal stripping or failing to formulate the most appropriate initial management.

Investigation

Plain X-rays of delayed healing show a visible fracture line and little evidence of callus formation. A **CT scan** may provide additional information.

Simple blood investigations may be appropriate if malnutrition or metabolic bone disease are suspected.

N.B. It is important to distinguish between simply a slow union, passing through the normal clinical and radiological stages of healing but which will ultimately unite, and those fractures where delayed union will progress to a non-union.

Management

Any obvious cause must be addressed and an attempt to promote healing made. The method of immobilization should be reviewed and altered as necessary.

Patients should be encouraged to stop smoking and excessive activity may need to be reduced; alternatively activity may need to be encouraged, e.g. partial weight-bearing on a lower limb fracture may stimulate fracture healing.

Low-intensity ultrasound delivered to the skin overlying the fracture has been shown to have potential benefit in the treatment of some delayed unions.

Non-union

In some instances a delayed union progresses to non-union. This is generally considered to have occurred when there is absence of radiological union with clinically detectable painful movement at the fracture site 6 months after injury (Fig 7.12).

Two types of non-union are recognized.

- With **hypertrophic non-union** the bone ends are sclerotic and flared (giving the bone ends

the appearance of an 'elephant's foot') with a clear fracture line still visible. The gap is filled with fibrous tissue not bone.

- With atrophic non-union the bone ends become narrow, rounded and sclerotic and there is no suggestion of new bone formation.

The causes of non-union are the same as those that cause delayed union.

Non-union is investigated by performing **plain X-rays and CT scans**. Contributing factors should be investigated as for delayed union.

Management

The treatment of non-union depends on its type.

If an hypertrophic un-united fracture can be fixed with absolute rigidity by mechanical means, the fibrous and cartilaginous tissue between the bone ends may mineralize and be converted to bone. The fixation may be internal or external.

Healing may be enhanced with ultrasound or the local application of bone morphogenic protein or artificial bone grafts.

Atrophic non-union is more difficult to treat. The fracture must be held rigid (usually by internal fixation) after the fibrous tissue between the bone ends has been excised, the bones decorticated back to healthy bone and bone grafts, either auto- or allograft, are placed around the fracture.

Avascular necrosis

Following a fracture, the blood supply to the bone may be permanently disrupted and the bone becomes ischaemic and necrotic. A progressive cycle then ensues of bone collapse with areas of revascularization, but ultimately the bone collapses and secondary arthritis develops.

Avascular necrosis (AVN) most often occurs in

- the head of the femur following fractures of the neck of the femur
- the head of the humerus following fractures of the proximal humerus
- the scaphoid following fractures of its waist or proximal pole
- the lunate following injury or dislocation
- the talus following a fracture of its neck.

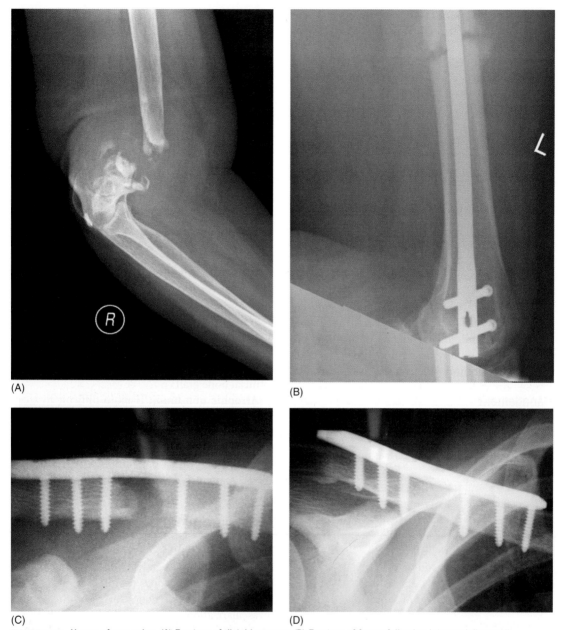

(A)

(B)

(C)

(D)

FIGURE 7.12   X-rays of non-union. (A) Fracture of distal humerus; (B) Fracture of femur following intramedullary nail treatment; (C) Fracture of clavicle treated by plating and grafting; (D) Healed fracture of clavicle after treatment.

The diagnosis is made with **plain X-rays**, but the initial X-ray images may be normal and only show the diagnostic changes, i.e. subchondral osteolytic areas, a crescent sign caused by collapse of the subchondral bone, and osteoarthritis, in the later stages of the disease.

Magnetic resonance imaging scans and **bone scans** are more useful especially in the early stages of avascular necrosis (Fig 7.13).

Treatment options include core decompression of the bone or grafting in an attempt to stop the process, or at a later stage an osteotomy or an arthroplasty.

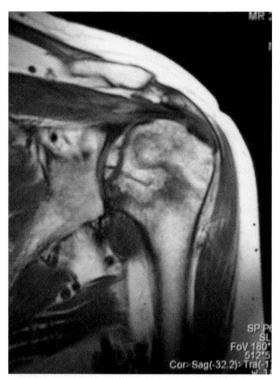

FIGURE 7.13   Magnetic resonance image of avascular necrosis humeral head

Heterotopic ossification (myositis ossificans)

This is ossification in the muscle surrounding a fracture. A calcific mass develops within the tissue leading to restriction of movement. Ultimately a joint may become encased within the calcific mass. Initially the mass is painful but the pain usually resolves leaving stiffness and restricted movement.

Plain X-rays will confirm the diagnosis and show progressive calcification within the soft tissues (Fig 7.14). This is best evaluated with **serial CT scans**.

A bone scan may also be performed to assess the osteogenic activity within the tissues.

Established cases can be treated by **excision of the heterotopic bone**. **Indomethacin** and **radiotherapy** have both been shown to reduce the risk of recurrence.

Volkmann's ischaemic contracture

This condition is caused by the ischaemia that occurs in a compartment syndrome or following

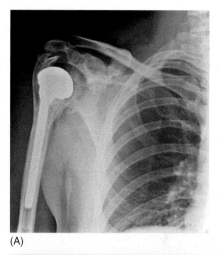

(A)

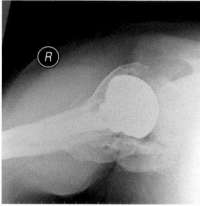

(B)

FIGURE 7.14   (A, B) X-rays of myositis ossificans following hemiarthroplasty for fracture

an arterial injury. Dead muscles become fibrotic and contract. Contractures cause deformity and stiffness which compromise function.

The hand and forearm are most commonly affected, but the leg and foot can also be involved. In a severe case, for example where there is clawing of the hand and fingers (claw hand), **tendon releases, tendon transfers** and **nerve grafts** may help.

Joint instability and osteoarthritis

Fractures around a joint may lead to joint instability if there is bone loss, malunion, soft tissue, ligament and tendon injury. Damage to an articular cartilage surface may predispose to osteoarthritis in later life.

Great attention must be paid to fractures that involve joints to ensure that they are reduced satisfactorily, leaving no **steps** in the articular surface. Not only does the direct injury increase the risk of later osteoarthritis, but if there is incongruity of the joint, local sheer forces cause further cartilage destruction.

Complex regional pain syndrome

Complex regional pain syndrome (CRPS) is a chronic condition characterized by severe pain, swelling and changes in the skin. Two varieties are recognized, dependent on the presence or absence of an obvious nerve injury.

- Type 1 occurs in the absence of a nerve injury and is also known as **Sudek's atrophy**, **algodystrophy** or **reflex sympathetic dystrophy (RSD)**.
- Type 2 occurs in the presence of a nerve injury and is also termed **causalgia**. The syndrome can occur after fractures or trauma.

Patients present with severe pain, swelling and stiffness usually of the hand (glass hand). There is a change in colour of the skin and an increased sweat response. The nails become cracked and brittle.

There is no specific test for the condition. **X-rays** may show osteoporosis.

Treatment is multidisciplinary and involves advice from a pain specialist and a physiotherapist. Medication including **gabapentin, anti-inflammatory** and **antidepressant drugs** are generally used. Neurostimulation with spinal cord stimulators can also be used. Sympathectomy is a last resort.

PATHOLOGICAL FRACTURES

Pathological fractures occur in bone which is abnormal or diseased. They may follow direct trauma in weakened bone or can be caused by repetitive microtrauma. This may, therefore, be inevitable or may occur because of an underlying problem. The degree of trauma is usually less than that expected to cause such a fracture. These fractures may be caused by congenital or acquired conditions.

Congenital causes of pathological fractures include the following:

- **Osteogenesis imperfecta** in which there is autosomal dominant or recessive gene causing transmission of a collagen disorder leading to bone fragility. It may be associated with short stature, scoliosis, tooth defect (dentinogenesis imperfecta), hearing defects, ligamentous laxity and blue sclerae.
- **Metabolic bone disorders**, e.g. osteoporosis, osteomalacia, Paget's disease.

Acquired causes include:

- **Infection**, i.e. acute and chronic osteomyelitis.
- **Primary neoplasms**, e.g. simple bone tumours and cysts; primary bone tumours include osteogenic sarcoma, chondrosarcoma, fibrosarcoma and Ewing's tumour.
- **Secondary malignant bone tumours** including metastatic deposits, most frequently from primary growths in the lung, bronchus, breast, prostate and kidney, most commonly affecting the humeral shaft, the femoral shaft, the pelvis and the spine.

The presentation of these fractures can be age dependent. Under the age of 20 years, the most common causes of pathological fractures are benign bone tumours and cysts. Over the age of 40 years the most common causes are metabolic bone disease, myeloma, secondary carcinoma and Paget's disease.

An **X-ray** is the main method of diagnosis (Fig 7.15). **Bone scans, MRI or positron emission tomography (PET) scans** are often used. Sometimes the diagnosis is not made until a **tissue biopsy** is examined.

Other investigations, usually used to seek the cause and should include a full blood count, erythrocyte sedimentation rate (ESR), serum calcium phosphate, alkaline phosphatase, acid phosphatase (prostate), serum electrophoresis, urinalysis for Bence Jones proteins (myeloma), an X-ray skeletal survey including the skull, chest and pelvis, bone marrow biopsy and bone biopsy.

Pathological fractures are treated in the same way as other fractures. If there is generalized bone disease, the fracture will heal with appropriate treatment. Internal fixation is the usual method.

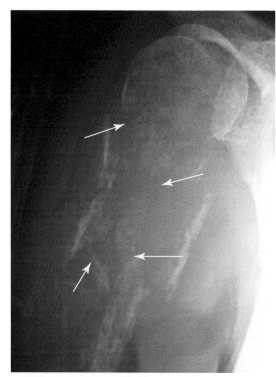

FIGURE 7.15 Pathological fracture secondary to tumour

Benign cysts which cause a fracture may heal with immobilization. Once a cyst has caused a fracture it will often 'heal' spontaneously, e.g. aneurysmal bone cysts. The injection of steroids or sclerosants may be used to encourage the cyst to heal.

Primary bone tumours need definitive treatment, which may include a resection and prosthetic replacement.

The treatment of **metastatic tumours** depends on the patient's life expectancy. It may include internal fixation with an intramedullary nail, excision and prosthetic replacement or radiotherapy. Prophylactic surgery may be performed before a fracture occurs if a susceptible bone lesion has been identified.

JOINT INJURIES

These consist of

- **dislocation**; joint disruption with complete discontinuity
- **subluxation**; joint disruption with partial discontinuity
- **fracture associated with a dislocation.**

Associated with these joint injuries may be

- **soft tissue damage**; ligaments, tendons and intra-articular structures
- **joint surface damage**: including chondral defects which may ultimately lead to osteoarthritis and
- **adjacent neurovascular structure damage**, followed by
- **chronic instability of the joint**
- **recurrent dislocation**
- **aseptic necrosis.**

The principles of management are similar to those of a fracture, in that the joint needs to be

- reduced: usually with analgesia, sedation and/or general anaesthesia
- held in position
- mobilized.

The problems caused by the dislocation of a joint include

- pain
- immobility
- abnormal mobility
- deformity
- loss of function.

The joints commonly affected are the shoulder, acromioclavicular, elbow, finger, hip and knee joints.

Dislocation of the glenohumeral (shoulder) joint

Dislocation of the glenohumeral joint is very common. In 98 per cent of cases the humeral head dislocates anteriorly, but it can also dislocate posteriorly or, rarely, inferiorly (luxatio erecta). The cause is usually trauma but it can occur secondary to generalized joint hyperlaxity, or abnormal muscle patterning conditions.

A dislocation may occur in a unidirectional or multidirectional manner. Anterior dislocation usually occurs when the shoulder is abducted and externally rotated, such as when an opponent is running past an individual while playing rugby.

The typical traumatic injury pathology profile is a tear of the anterior inferior labrum – the Bankart injury – with a corresponding defect on the posterolateral aspect of the humeral head – the Hill–Sachs lesion.

Investigation

Clinical diagnostic indicators

Clinical examination should include assessment of the neurovascular structures, particularly the axillary nerve, which should be documented. Brachial plexus injuries, especially involving the posterior cord, although rare, can also occur.

Imaging

Plain X-rays should be taken in two planes, AP and lateral scapular or axillary views are essential (Fig 7.16). (*Any joint dislocation requires X-rays to be taken in more than a single plane.*)

Although an anterior dislocation is normally obvious, a posterior dislocation can be easily missed on a single view. **MRI scans** demonstrate soft tissue damage associated with the dislocation.

Management

Treatment is by **reduction** using a variety of methods.

Kocher's method: Traction is applied to the arm. The arm is then gently externally rotated to reduce spasm. The elbow is then gently adducted across the chest and once reduction is achieved the arm is internally rotated.

Gravity: The patient is laid prone on a table with the affected arm hanging over its side. The weight of the arm and the relaxed position gently pull the head of the humerus back into place. A small weight can be attached to the arm to provide additional traction.

Hippocratic method: The surgeon's stockinged heel is placed against the chest to provide counter traction that is applied to the arm to pull the humeral head back into position.

Once reduced, the arm is placed into a sling for a period of 1–3 weeks before mobilization and strengthening with **physiotherapy** is commenced.

The neurovascular status should be checked once reduction has been achieved.

Surgery: In the younger patient or in recurrent dislocation, operative stabilization of the joint may be undertaken.

An arthroscopic approach is usually used to repair and fix the Bankart labral injury back to its correct position on the glenoid.

Open surgery is still used especially if a bone block is required on the glenoid neck – the coracoid transfer of Bristow–Latarjet.

Tightening of the subscapularis muscle to limit external rotation – the Putti–Platt operation – is now largely of historical interest.

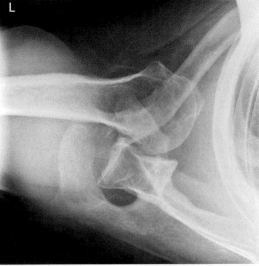

(A)

(B)

FIGURE 7.16   (A–B) X-rays of glenohumeral joint dislocation

Dislocation of the acromioclavicular joint

Injury to the acromioclavicular joint is usually caused by a fall on to the outer aspect of the shoulder. A spectrum of injuries occur dependent on the number of ligaments that are torn.

Investigation

Clinical diagnostic indicators

If only the acromioclavicular ligaments are injured, then the joint is only partially dislocated. If the coracoclavicular ligaments are torn a significant displacement of the joint will occur which will be clinically evident. On rare occasions, the clavicle may be displaced posteriorly or inferiorly.

Imaging

Plain X-rays will reveal the extent of the disruption (Fig 7.17).

Management

If there is still residual congruency of the joint, then a **non-operative** course is generally followed – rest, immobilization, followed by physiotherapy as the pain and tenderness subsides.

If the clavicle is displaced from the joint by more than 100 per cent of its width, surgical intervention is usually the treatment of choice. If there is suspicion that the X-ray underestimates the instability of the joint, then the patient is asked to hold a weight in the hand, to reveal the potential unrecognized instability.

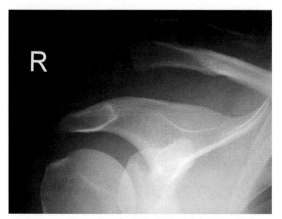

FIGURE 7.17 X-ray of acromioclavicular joint dislocation

Surgical options include both arthroscopic and open approaches. The most common procedures are:

- transfer of coracoacromial ligament or utilization of an artificial ligament to replace the coracoclavicular ligament
- reduction and internal fixation of the joint using a clavicular hook plate or Bosworth screw.

Dislocation of the elbow joint

This is relatively common in both children and adults, following a fall on to the outstretched hand. There may be associated fractures, particularly of the coronoid, radial head and the olecranon. Associated injury to the ulnar nerve, median nerve or brachial artery is uncommon but must be assessed.

Plain X-rays should be taken in two planes prior to any attempt at reduction.

The dislocation is reduced by applying **traction**. The arm is then placed into a backslab with more than 90 degrees of flexion and the arm supported in a sling.

In the absence of an associated fracture, mobilization is commenced at 2 weeks after the injury. If a fracture has been sustained, then a longer period of immobilization may be required.

Dislocation of the wrist joint

Dislocation of the carpal bones is relatively uncommon. It is usually caused by a fall on to the outstretched hand. The dislocation may occur in the proximal row of the carpal bones while the distal row remains aligned. Alternatively, the distal row of the carpus dislocates, sometimes in association with partial proximal row dislocation dorsally.

Plain X-rays are required to assess the injury (Fig 7.18).

The dislocation is then reduced under **traction** and the result checked with further radiographs.

The palm is then placed in **a plaster of Paris cast** followed by further X-ray assessment for a period of approximately 4 weeks.

In many cases the carpal bones need to be stabilized with the **insertion of K-wires** which are subsequently removed.

Median nerve palsy can occur if in spite of continuing discomfort the reduction is delayed.

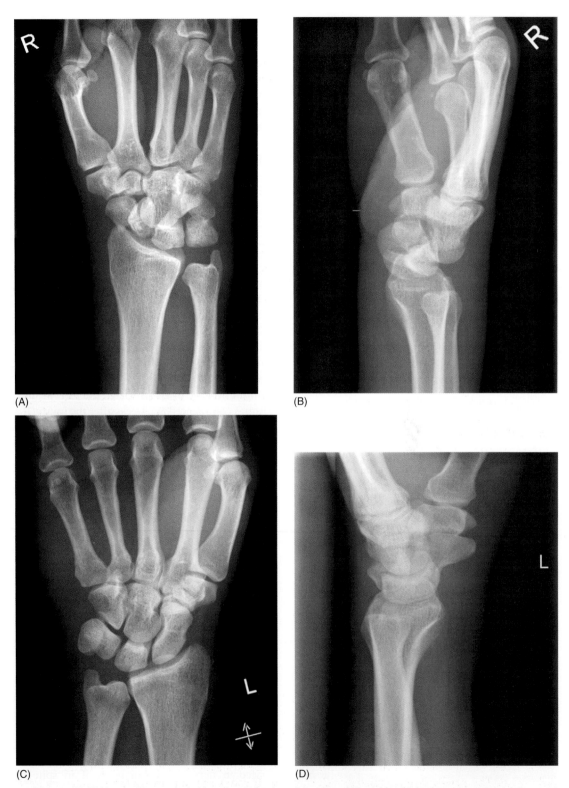

FIGURE 7.18   (A–D) X-rays of trans-scaphoid perilunate fracture dislocation of the right wrist (and normal comparison)

Dislocation of the hip joint

Traumatic dislocation of the hip usually occurs posteriorly. This often occurs when a force is transmitted through the knee to a flexed hip, such as a dashboard impact during a road traffic accident. It can also occur following a fall. Associated injuries include acetabular fracture or fracture of the femoral head/shaft. In 10 per cent of cases, avascular necrosis occurs from a disturbance of the capsular blood supply of the femoral head.

Investigation

Clinical diagnostic indicators

Clinically, the hip is flexed and shortened with internal rotation. Approximately 10 per cent of dislocations are associated with a sciatic nerve palsy.

Imaging

Plain X-rays should be taken in two planes: AP and lateral. If there is an associated fracture, pelvic inlet and outlet views should also be obtained.

A **CT scan** may also be performed to ensure that no associated fractures have been missed.

Management

The dislocation should be **reduced** by traction and manipulation as soon as possible, as this lowers the incidence of complications. General anaesthesia is often required.

Following reduction, the leg is placed in traction during a **period of bed rest**. Further plain X-rays should be taken to confirm the reduction and a **CT scan** performed to ensure that no associated fractures have been missed and that no bone fragments are retained within the joint.

If significant fractures are recognized, **open reduction and internal fixation** may be required.

Dislocations of the knee joint

Patella dislocation This can be caused by a direct blow at the side of the knee or a sudden muscular contraction. It may be associated with underlying hyperlaxity. The patella usually dislocates laterally.

Plain X-rays should be taken to confirm the dislocation. The patella is manipulated back into place and the knee joint immobilized in plaster or

a brace for approximately 6 weeks. Physiotherapy is then instituted.

Knee joint dislocation This is a relatively uncommon injury. The joint usually dislocates anteriorly but it can dislocate posteriorly, medially or laterally. Some of the knee joint ligaments – the medial collateral, lateral collateral, anterior and posterior cruciate ligaments – are inevitably injured and there may be soft tissue injuries to the menisci.

Chondral injury and/or fracture may also be present. Neurovascular structures are at risk, particularly the common peroneal nerve and the popliteal artery.

Investigation

The integrity of the popliteal nerve and its branches and the popliteal artery must be clinically assessed and recorded.

Plain X-rays must be taken to confirm the dislocation. **MRI scans** may be performed to assess the severity of the associated soft tissue injuries.

Management

The dislocation is **reduced** by traction and manipulation followed by either a period of immobilization or an immediate or delayed direct surgical repair of the damaged structures, including the ligaments within the joint.

Ankle joint dislocation

This rarely occurs without an associated fracture. If there is no fracture there is likely to be an associated rupture of the medial and/or lateral ligaments.

Investigation is by **plain X-ray** and **MRI scan**.

Surgical repair of the ligamentous structures followed by a period of immobilization is required.

PRIMARY TUMOURS OF BONE

Malignant tumours of bone are rare and their management is highly specialised. Therefore a detailed description of their investigation and management would be out of place in this introductory student's textbook. Nevertheless the basic principles can be summarised as:

▨ Be suspicious of their possible presence
▨ If your suspicions are confirmed, refer urgently to a specialist multidisciplinary centre.

Investigation

Clinical Diagnostic Indicators

Most tumours present with musculoskeletal pain, which is dull, deep-seated and progressive. Any non-mechanical unexplained skeletal pain, especially at night, unrelieved by rest or anti-inflammatory medication should arouse suspicion. Unexplained deep swelling, especially in an adolescent, must be thoroughly investigated.

Further symptoms and signs of bone tumours are well described in our companion volume.

Blood test and urine analysis

A full blood count with differential, biochemistry including calcium and phosphate measurement, and an ESR is requested. An ESR >100 mm, the presence of Bence-Jones protein and monoclonal gammopathy, are highly suggestive of multiple myeloma – a common primary malignancy of bone.

Imaging

Plain X-rays of the painful bone may show a space occupying lesion.

Ultrasound is more valuable for soft tissue lesions.

An **isotope bone scan** may detect isolated lesions or multiple metastases.

These tests should be sufficient to confirm your clinical suspicions and justify referral to a specialist centre. However if possible, they should be supplemented with an **MRI and CT scan** to delineate the extent of the tumour and its relationship with the surrounding tissues.

A tissue biopsy is best performed in the specialist referral centre, as inappropriate sampling can lead to tumour spread and also potentially compromise surgical planes of resection.

Management

Once the diagnosis has been confirmed, treatment will vary according to the lesion's degree of malignancy and spread.

Simple cysts and aneurysmal bone cysts may undergo **curettage, bone grafting or injection**.

Such measures combined with **radio frequency or laser ablation** may be used to treat an osteoid osteoma.

In general terms, confined low grade lesions can be treated with **wide excision with a good margin of healthy surrounding tissue**. In higher grade tumours, more **radical excision** is necessary, often followed by **bone graft** and **prosthetic replacement**.

Amputation can be a last resort and is not indicated until the absence of metastatic spread is confirmed.

Chemotherapy may be required before and after surgery.

Radiotherapy is suitable for some sensitive tumours such as Ewing's sarcoma.

Table 7.1
Major primary bone tumours

	Benign	Malignant
Tumours of bone	Osteoid osteoma Osteoblastoma	Osteosarcoma
Tumours of cartilage	Osteochondroma Chondroma Chondroblastoma	Chondrosarcoma
Tumours of haemopoiesis	Myeloma Lymphoma	
Others	Simple bone cyst Aneurysmal bone cyst Giant cell tumour Fibroma	Ewing's tumour Fibrosarcoma

8

The bones, joints and soft tissues of the upper limb

Steven A. Corbett

Most of the clinical problems that arise in the upper limb are caused by diseases in and around the limb's many joints.

The problems that affect all joints are:

- pain
- stiffness
- fixity
- laxity
- loss of stability
- deformity.

The diseases that cause these problems affect all joints to varying degrees. This chapter describes the investigation and management of the mechanical disturbances and diseases of the shoulder, elbow and hand that give rise to the common problems listed above.

It is important to understand the anatomy of each joint in order to appreciate how mechanical disturbances can cause a clinical problem.

The investigation and management of the problems that arise from vascular disease in the upper limb are described in Chapter 11.

THE SHOULDER

Anatomy

The shoulder comprises a series of complex bones and joints linked by ligaments, tendons and muscle to the breast bone (sternum), neck, cervical spine and chest (thorax). Shoulder pain is a common problem and may arise from any of these structures or less commonly be referred from the neck, the heart or the abdomen.

The **rotator cuff** comprises the supraspinatus, infraspinatus, teres minor and subscapularis tendons, which insert into the greater and lesser tuberosities of the humerus. This forms a musculotendinous cover to the front, top and back of the head of the humerus

overlying the shoulder joint's capsule. Its functions include elevating the arm (supraspinatus) rotating the humeral head externally (infraspinatus and teres minor) and rotating the humeral head internally (subscapularis). The rotator cuff also plays an important role in holding the humeral head stable in the glenoid fossa of the scapula when the arm is moved.

The long head of biceps, which arises from the superior labrum of the glenoid fossa and traverses the shoulder joint, is often considered to be part of the rotator cuff. The short head of biceps arises from the coracoid process and is outside the joint.

The **subacromial bursa** is the largest bursa within the shoulder and lies between the cuff's tendons and the coracoacromial arch. The coracoacromial arch is formed by the acromion, the coracoid, the coracoacromial ligament and the acromion processes. This bursa allows the rotator cuff to glide during movement.

CAUSES OF SHOULDER PAIN

ROTATOR CUFF CAUSES OF SHOULDER PAIN

- The impingement syndrome (often also called supraspinatus tendonitis or subacromial bursitis)
- Rotator cuff tears, which may be partial or complete.
- Calcific tendonitis, which may be acute or chronic.

THE IMPINGEMENT SYNDROME

Investigation

Clinical diagnostic indicators

The impingement syndrome is **pain in the subacromial space when the humerus is elevated or internally rotated**. This is classically described as **the painful arc between 60 degrees and 120 degrees**,

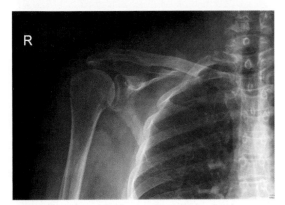

FIGURE 8.1   X-ray of impingement syndrome showing sclerosis of undersurface of acromion (sourcil sign)

when the arm is abducted. The range may however, vary and pain is sometimes experienced in a higher range. The impingement can occur between the rotator cuff, the subacromial bursa, the anterior third of the acromion, the coracoacromial ligament and the acromioclavicular joint.

Patients present with pain at 90 degrees elevation and also when internally rotating the shoulder in this position. Impingement tests may be performed in which local anaesthetic is injected into the subacromial space. This is deemed positive if the impingement sign disappears.

Imaging

Plain X-rays may show narrowing of the acromiohumeral distance together with sclerosis on the under-surface of the acromion (sourcil sign) (Fig 8.1). Changes in the bone around the greater tuberosity may also be seen (enthesiopathy).

Ultrasound scanning may demonstrate evidence of inflammation and of structural changes within the tendons and the subacromial bursa. Impingement can also be demonstrated. The scan can be used as a dynamic test to show the impingement as the patient moves their arm.

An **MRI scan** will also demonstrate the pathology, but only gives a static image.

Management

Non-operative treatment Approximately 65 per cent of patients can expect significant relief of symptoms with non-operative treatment.

Physiotherapy and a short course of **anti-inflammatory medication** are the first-line management.

Injection of local anaesthetic and cortisone into the subacromial space is performed if this fails. This may be done under ultrasound guidance to improve accuracy. The number of injections should be limited. Patients should not be subjected to numerous injections as other potentially successful treatment options are available.

Subacromial decompression can be performed if the patient fails to improve with non-operative measures, either as an arthroscopic or now less commonly as an open procedure. The under-surface of the anterolateral acromion is cleared and smoothed, the coracoacromial ligament is released and the subacromial bursa excised.

Patient satisfaction rates are reported to be 98 per cent following this procedure.

ROTATOR CUFF TEARS

Tears of the rotator cuff may occur in any of the tendons but the supraspinatus is most frequently affected. The tear can be partial or complete and can be caused by trauma or, more commonly, following degenerative age-related change within the tendon.

Investigation
Clinical diagnostic indicators

The patient may be symtomless, or have pain or weakness, which may manifest in an inability to raise the arm. Muscle wasting may develop if the condition becomes chronic (Fig 8.2).

Imaging

X-rays may show a reduction of the space between the acromion and the humerus together with the features of impingement (see above)

An **ultrasound scan** can demonstrate partial and complete tears, the number of tendons involved and the degree of retraction of the tendons. The radiologist may comment on the volume (bulk) of the supplying muscles if the tears are longstanding.

An **MRI scan** shows similar features and can also assess the degree of fatty change within the musculature which suggests chronicity.

Arthroscopy will reveal the tear.

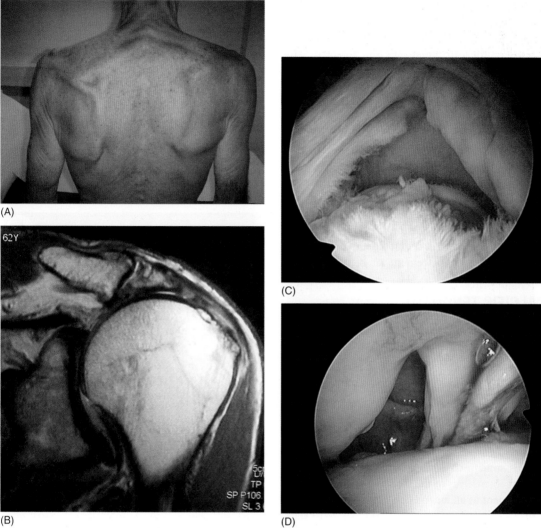

(A)

(B)

(C)

(D)

FIGURE 8.2   Rotator cuff injury. (A) Associated muscle wasting; (B) MRI of the tear; (C, D) two arthroscopic photographs of a tear

Management

Conservative treatment

Non-operative treatment is often the initial management, particularly for partial tears and for complete tears in patients over the age of 65 years.

Physiotherapy and a short course of **anti-inflammatory medication** are instituted.

Corticosteroid injection into the **subacromial space** may also be tried, but repeat injections should be limited to avoid further weakening of the rotator cuff structures.

Surgical repair

The following questions must be considered before surgical intervention:

- Is the patient symptomatic, i.e. do they have night pain, pain with overhead activity or loss of activities of daily living?
- What is the age of the patient?
- What was the activity level of the patient before the tear?
- Has the tendon tear caused retraction, muscle atrophy and fat deposition in the muscle?

Surgical repair is the treatment of choice in symptomatic patients less than 65 years old with complete tears. The edges of a partial tear may be excised or the tear completed and repaired. This can be achieved either by an arthroscopic or by an open surgical technique and is generally combined with a subacromial decompression. The results from surgery are very good, particularly in this age group.

In the older age group, the edges of the tear can be excised arthroscopically and a subacromial decompression performed.

Muscle transfer procedures using latissimus dorsi may be tried if a rotator cuff tear is massive and irreparable.

If there is associated glenohumeral joint arthritis (cuff tear arthropathy) a shoulder **hemiarthroplasty** or **shoulder joint replacement** can be performed.

CALCIFIC TENDINITIS

Investigation

Clinical diagnostic indicators

Patients with acute calcific tendonitis present with a sudden onset of **severe pain** with a **restricted range of movement** in the shoulder caused by the deposition of calcium hydroxyapatite within the supraspinatus tendon. The pain, which is caused by swelling and pressure within the tendon, is sometimes so intense that the patient will present themselves to the Accident and Emergency Department as an emergency. The symptoms however, usually improve over a period of 7–10 days, with the shoulder returning to normal within a 6-week period.

In chronic calcific tendonitis, the patient will present with signs and symptoms more consistent with impingement.

Imaging

A **plain X-ray** will show an area of calcium, usually just above the greater tuberosity and beneath the acromion (Fig 8.3). In the acute phase this is marked, but, with time, it disappears.

An **ultrasound scan** can also be used to assess the rotator cuff and sometimes shows evidence of residual calcium deposits not seen on a plain X-ray.

MRI scanning is less useful in this condition.

If these investigations show no evidence of ectopic calcium, blood investigations, including measuring inflammatory markers, should be considered as the differential diagnosis of acute calcific tendonitis includes septic arthritis of the glenohumeral joint.

Management

In the early phase, the arm should be rested with a short course of **anti-inflammatory medication**.

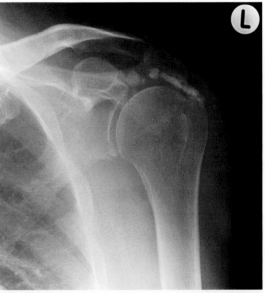

(A)

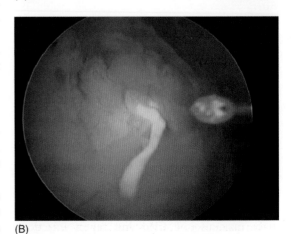

(B)

FIGURE 8.3 (A) X-ray of calcific tendonitis; (B) a calcific deposit

Subacromial injection of corticosteroid and local anaesthetic into the subacromial space can relieve pain, provided the diagnosis has been confirmed.

Needling of the deposit and barbotage of the calcium may also be performed. This is best achieved under ultrasound guidance. An arthroscopic excision of the calcific lesion combined with an arthroscopic subacromial decompression can be performed if the symptoms become chronic.

ADHESIVE CAPSULITIS (FROZEN SHOULDER)

In this condition, the shoulder joint capsule becomes contracted, thickened and inflamed, secondary to an ill-defined condition, which may have similar features to Dupuytren's disease.

Investigation

Clinical diagnostic indicators

Characteristically, there are three clinical phases as the process progresses:

- **freezing**: characterized by severe pain especially at night, with a restricted range of movement. Active and passive arm elevation is restricted to below shoulder height, and there is a marked loss of external rotation (often 0 degrees)
- **frozen**: when the pain improves but the shoulder remains stiff
- **thawing or resolution**: when the patient regains movement.

Blood tests

Blood investigations should be performed to exclude **diabetes mellitus and thyroid disease** as there is an association between adhesive capsulitis and these conditions. Auto antibodies should be measured to exclude an inflammatory arthritis or other rheumatological conditions, including polymyalgia rheumatica.

Imaging

Plain X-rays may show bone osteopenia secondary to disuse.

Ultrasound and MRI scans may show contracture of the joint capsule with obliteration of the axillary fold.

Arthroscopy demonstrates the adhesions (Fig 8.4).

Management

In the first (inflammatory, freezing) phase, the key component of treatment is **pain relief**.

Anti-inflammatory medication can be given combined with **intra-articular injections of corticosteroid** into the glenohumeral joint – best achieved under radiological guidance.

Alternatively, an injection may be given into the subacromial space, although this may be less successful. Physiotherapy at this stage is best avoided.

Operative intervention is often contraindicated in the first phase as it is likely to leave the patient with significant postoperative pain, which will reduce their ability in the second and third stages to mobilize the shoulder.

In the second (frozen) phase, when the pain is less severe yet the shoulder remains stiff, a physiotherapy **exercise programme** should be undertaken. There is, however, some evidence that this does not speed recovery. Injection of corticosteroid during this phase is not necessary, as it does not affect residual positional pain. The newer technique of injecting a volume of solution to distend the joint (**hydrodilatation**), is sometimes employed.

Manipulation under anaesthesia may be performed to break the capsular adhesions, but care must be taken not to fracture the humerus.

Alternatively, an arthroscopic release of the glenohumeral joint capsule combined with division of the rotator interval (between subscapularis and

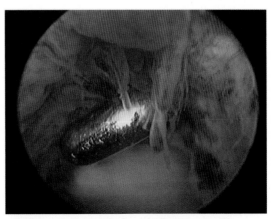

FIGURE 8.4 Arthroscopic view of adhesive capsulitis

supraspinatus tendons), may dramatically improve the range of movement.

In the third (thawing) phase, physiotherapy may have a role, but other forms of treatment are rarely required, as the condition continues to resolve.

BICEPS TENDONITIS

The long head of biceps is often considered to be part of the rotator cuff and can be involved in an impingement syndrome. It can also be associated with isolated inflammation, tenderness and fraying of the tendon over the bicipital groove (Fig 8.5).

Investigation

Clinical diagnostic indicators

Clinical investigation should include Speed's test, which assesses the pain caused by elbow flexion, and Yergason's test, which assesses the pain caused by flexion and supination of the elbow.

Imaging

Plain X-rays may show evidence of associated rotator cuff pathology which is similar to that of the impingement syndrome. An ultrasound scan can be used to assess inflammation and swelling, particularly in the bicipital groove.

Management

Initially, non-operative treatment consists of rest and the use of anti-inflammatory medication. Physiotherapy is then commenced.

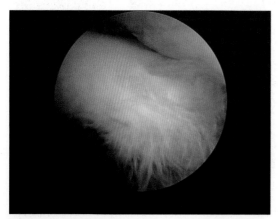

FIGURE 8.5   Biceps tendon fraying

An ultrasound-guided injection of steroids around the biceps tendon can be employed if symptoms persist.

An arthroscopic subacromial decompression is performed if the symptoms fail to resolve. This may be combined with a biceps tenodesis, in which the proximal biceps tendon is implanted into the humerus, excising the intra-articular portion.

Alternatively, in elderly patients, a biceps tenotomy can be performed, in which the long head of biceps is simply cut.

Occasionally, a patient presents with a rupture of the long head of biceps, often preceded by chronic symptoms of bicipital tendonitis commonly found in association with other rotator cuff pathology. The patient will present with a lump in the arm, often referred to as 'Popeye's sign' (see *Symptoms and Signs*).

Operative repair of the tendon should only be considered in the younger patient.

OSTEOARTHRITIS OF THE GLENOHUMERAL JOINT

Investigation

Osteoarthritis in the glenohumeral joint causes pain and progressive restriction of shoulder movement, particularly abduction and forward elevation.

Imaging

Plain X-rays show the standard features of arthritis – loss of joint space, sclerosis, osteophyte formation, osteopenia and subchondral cysts (Fig 8.6A).

An ultrasound scan is used to assess the status of the rotator cuff and any associated rotator cuff tears.

A CT scan and arthroscopy may be needed prior to a shoulder replacement to assess the degree of any bone loss, especially within the glenoid, and the orientation of the humeral head with the glenoid (Fig 8.6B).

Management

Physiotherapy and anti-inflammatory medication is helpful. Exercises may improve mobility. Modification of activity may also help reduce pain.

Surgery can be performed if the patient's symptoms are severe. The humeral head may be resurfaced or a hemiarthroplasty performed (Fig 8.6C). On occasion, a total shoulder replacement may be required (Fig 8.6D).

Arthroscopy and a washout of the joint can give symptomatic relief but does not alter the underlying arthritic process.

OSTEOARTHRITIS OF THE ACROMIOCLAVICULAR JOINT

Osteoarthritis of the acromioclavicular joint is common and, indeed, X-ray changes are often seen in many patients over the age of 40 even though they may be symptomless.

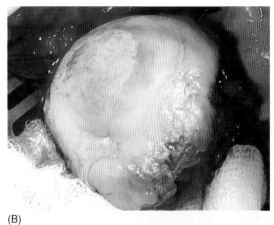

(B)

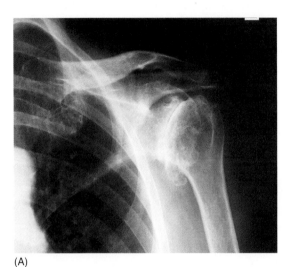

(A)

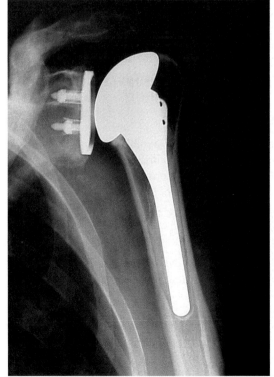

(D)

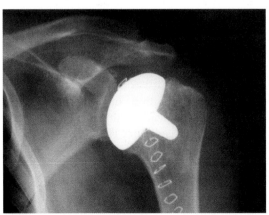

(C)

FIGURE 8.6 Osteoarthritic degeneration of the shoulder. (A) Plain X-ray showing loss of jointspace, osteophytes and severe sclerosis of the bones; (B) a clinical photograph of a degenerate humeral head; (C) shoulder resurfacing and hemiarthroplasty; (D) total shoulder replacement

Investigation

Clinical diagnostic indicators

The patient presents with pain when using the arm overhead (particularly on cross-arm activity), tenderness and swelling.

Imaging

X-rays show the typical features of osteoarthritis.

Management

The treatment is **rest** and the use of **anti-inflammatory medication**. Occasionally, **corticosteroid injection** is performed.

    Operative intervention with an arthroscopic or open **acromioclavicular joint excision**, which involves resection of the lateral end of the clavicle, can be undertaken if conservative measures fail.

    Reconstructive surgery If the acromioclavicular joint is unstable, often secondary to trauma with rupture of the coracoclavicular ligaments, it can be stabilized by transferring other ligaments such as the coraco-acromial ligament or by inserting an artificial woven ligament, or by screw fixation of the clavicle to the coracoid.

RHEUMATOID ARTHRITIS OF THE SHOULDER JOINT

Rheumatoid arthritis can affect both the glenohumeral joint and acromioclavicular joint. The synovitis causes rupture of the rotator cuff with secondary cartilaginous change which can lead to superior migration of the head of the humerus and the development of a rotator cuff arthropathy.

Investigation

Imaging

The **X-ray** features of a rheumatoid arthritic disease will be present, including narrowing of the acromiohumeral distance.

    In chronic cases the acromion may remodel around the humeral head forming a secondary joint (acetabularization) (Fig 8.7).

    An **ultrasound** or **MRI scan** will show the features of arthritic change together with the status of the rotator cuff by delineating the tendons involved, the extent of any tears and the degree of their retraction.

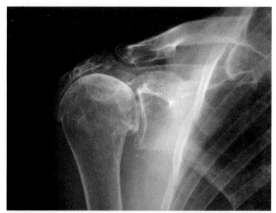

FIGURE 8.7   Rotator cuff arthritis and acetabularization

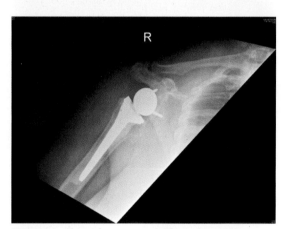

FIGURE 8.8   X-ray of reverse-geometry replacement

Management

Medical treatment includes disease-modifying drugs (steroids, gold, anti-TNFX) and anti-inflammatory medication with physiotherapy and allied therapies.

    Surgical intervention includes arthroscopic clearing of the synovium and washout of the joint to try to alleviate symptoms. This is often combined with a subacromial decompression.

    A **hemiarthroplasty** can relieve pain if the above measures fail but may not improve function if the rotator cuff tendons are affected. Under these circumstances a **reverse-geometry shoulder replacement** in the elderly patient can provide both symptomatic relief and restore function (Fig 8.8). This involves replacing the glenoid with a 'ball' and converting the head of the humerus to a socket (reversing the joint) so that the deltoid muscle can take over the role of the rotator cuff.

SHOULDER INSTABILITY

The glenohumeral joint is remarkable for its great range of movement. It has virtually no intrinsic bony stability and, therefore, the stability is provided by static and dynamic restraints.

The static stabilizers consist of the glenoid labrum and the capsular ligaments, while the dynamic stabilization is provided by the muscles, principally those of the rotator cuff.

In addition, there is a negative intra-articular pressure within the joint. If there is a disturbance of this balance the shoulder becomes unstable and may dislocate or subluxate.

There are three major causes of instability:

▧ trauma
▧ hyperlaxity
▧ muscle patterning disorders.

A combination of these factors may be present.

The direction of the instability may be anterior, posterior or multidirectional and episodes may be acute, chronic or recurrent.

Anterior instability is the most common and frequently arises after an anterior dislocation of the head of the humerus causing a tear of the anterior labrum (as described by Bankart), together with an injury to the posterior superior humeral head (as described by Hill–Sachs) (Fig 8.9).

Investigation

Clinical diagnostic indicators

The patient may present with pain and reduced range of movement in the shoulder, secondary to apprehension and loss of confidence. There may also be a history of recurrent dislocation.

Imaging

Plain X-rays demonstrate an injury to the posterosuperior humeral head (the Hill–Sachs lesion), i.e. a depression in its surface where it engages with the anterior aspect of the glenoid. This is often best seen on an **axillary view**.

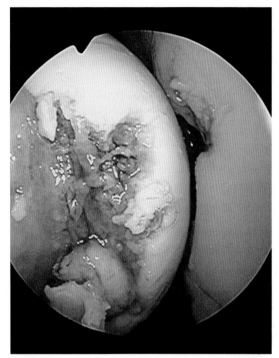

FIGURE 8.9 Arthroscopic photograph of a Hill–Sachs lesion: injury to the posterior superior humeral head

A bone injury of the anterior inferior quadrant of the glenoid may be visible, related to the labral injury described by Bankart, known as a 'bone Bankart'.

A **CT scan** should be performed if there is concern regarding the extent of bone loss.

An **MRI scan** can be used to assess the extent of labral injury and the degree of displacement of the labrum from the glenoid.

An examination under anaesthesia (**EUA**) and a diagnostic **glenohumeral joint arthroscopy** may help if the above investigations are inconclusive.

Management

When a patient under the age of 20 years dislocates their glenohumeral joint for the first time, they have at least a 60 per cent chance of a further dislocation in the next 2 years, which is independent of physiotherapy provision. Surgical intervention should therefore be considered for such patients.

In patients over the age of 40 years, who undergo a primary dislocation, the chance of recurrence is considered to be <10 per cent. In these patients, early surgery is contraindicated. These patients often benefit from **physiotherapy** designed to improve **scapulothoracic muscle stabilization, coordination and strengthening**.

It should be recognized, however, that in this age group the risk of an associated rotator cuff injury increases with advancing years.

The indications for surgical stabilization are:

- primary dislocation in the younger age group, especially for those with significant recreational and sporting demands
- recurrent dislocation
- patients with apprehension and lack of confidence promoted by the instability.

Operative intervention may be undertaken as either an arthroscopic or open procedure. There are two main types of operative intervention:

- **repair of the capsulolabral tear** (Bankart lesion)
- **open bone transport procedures** (Laterjet/ Bristow) where bone is transported from the coracoid to fill the glenoid bone defect and reinforce the anterior inferior joint capsule.

Following surgery the arm is generally immobilized for a period of 2 weeks to allow the capsulolabral complex to heal before physiotherapy is commenced.

Posterior instability can occur following a previous posterior dislocation. This is far less common than anterior instability. Diagnosis is confirmed by X-ray and MRI scan investigation. Operative intervention may include arthroscopic labral repair and open surgical techniques.

CAUSES OF ELBOW PAIN

The elbow is a synovial hinge joint between the distal end of the humerus and the proximal ends of the radius and ulna. Elbow pain is a common complaint and can arise from any of the bones, tendons, muscles and ligaments that support the joint.

Less commonly pain can be referred to the elbow from the neck, the shoulder or distal structures.

LATERAL EPICONDYLITIS (TENNIS ELBOW)

Tennis elbow is caused by repeated small interstitial tears, followed by neovascularization and inflammation in the common origin of the extensor tendons on the lateral epicondyle.

Investigation
Clinical diagnostic indicators

The patient presents with **pain on the lateral aspect** of the elbow, often aggravated by lifting objects, shaking hands and exercise, particularly when wielding a tennis racket.

There is tenderness and occasionally swelling over the lateral epicondyle. There may be a loss of elbow extension. The patient has a positive finger extension test – pain when the extensor tendons are loaded.

Imaging

A **plain X-ray** may show sclerosis of the lateral epicondyle in the region of the insertion of the common extensor tendons. A calcific focus may be seen.

An **ultrasound scan** may show disruption of the tendon insertions with interstitial tears or neovascularization.

Management

Rest followed by physiotherapy with stretching and strengthening of the extensor tendons should be the initial treatment. **Anti-inflammatory medication** may also be prescribed.

Injection of a corticosteroid may prove beneficial initially but, in the long term, seldom conveys any advantage over physiotherapy alone.

The **injection of autologous blood** at the site of the pain and tenderness has been described.

Success of non-operative treatment is approximately 85–90 per cent.

Surgical intervention can be undertaken if the symptoms are not relieved by the above management. **The extensor tendon origin is released from the lateral epicondyle of the humerus** and any damaged tissue and bone is also removed. The success rate of such surgery is approximately 80–85 per cent.

MEDIAL EPICONDYLITIS (GOLFER'S ELBOW)

This condition is similar to tennis elbow, except that it affects the **common flexor tendon origin**, which inserts to the medial epicondyle of the humerus. The same pathological processes arise. Pain is reproduced on activity or by passive extension of the wrist.

Neither tennis nor golfer's elbow are confined to sportsmen. Both can affect any one of the general population.

Investigation and treatments are the same as those for tennis elbow.

OLECRANON BURSITIS

Investigation

Clinical diagnostic indicators

Olecranon bursitis presents with a large **swelling** over the posterior aspect of the elbow (Fig 8.10). It is usually caused by the accumulation of inflammatory fluid in the olecranon bursa in response to repeated minor trauma. The swelling may be hot, but pain varies. It may be associated with infection, gout or rheumatoid arthritis.

Blood tests

Routine blood investigations may be required to detect the presence of underlying causative conditions and exclude potential infection.

Imaging

A **plain X-ray** may confirm the diagnosis of an underlying arthritis.

Management

Treatment is with **anti-inflammatory medication and rest** to generally allow the bursitis to settle.

Aspiration and **injection** of the bursa with a **corticosteroid** can be considered if rest and oral medication fail to produce any improvement; but the patient should be told that injection carries the risk of introducing infection, which can lead to skin breakdown and the development of a sinus. This complication which can represent a significantly greater problem for the patient than an uncomplicated bursa.

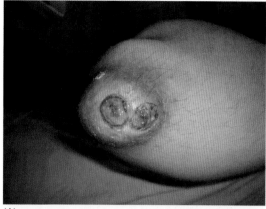

(A)

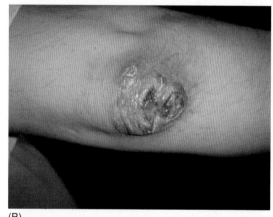

(B)

FIGURE 8.10   (A, B) Ulcerated olecranon bursitis

Aspiration alone often fails because the fluid reaccumulates.

The whole bursa can be **excised** if the swelling is a cosmetic and physical inconvenience.

An infected bursa should be treated with rest and an appropriate antibiotic. If this fails to resolve the situation, the bursa can be drained and excised, but this may leave a problem with wound closure.

LOOSE BODIES

Loose bodies can occur in the elbow joint and present with pain and mechanical locking. Depending on their site within the joint they may limit extension, flexion, supination and pronation.

Investigation

A **plain X-ray** may demonstrate their presence.

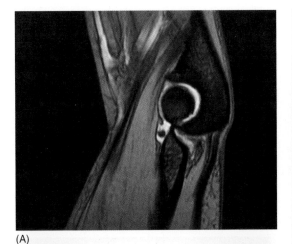

(A)

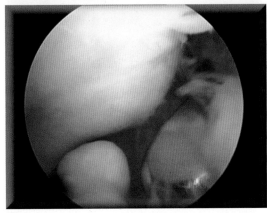

(B)

FIGURE 8.11   (A) MRI of a loose body in the elbow. (B) An arthroscopic view of an elbow loose body

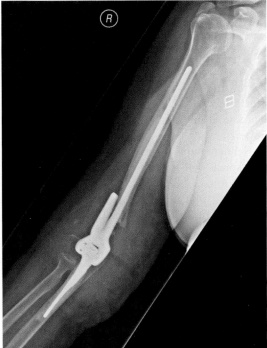

FIGURE 8.12   X-ray of a total elbow replacement

A **CT scan** and **arthroscopy** will further delineate their presence and show any associated degenerative changes (Fig 8.11).

Management

Loose bodies may be removed from the elbow joint through an arthroscope.

OSTEOARTHRITIS OF THE ELBOW JOINT

Osteoarthritis can occur at the elbow joint. It is uncommon as a primary disorder, more likely to occur as a sequel to a previous injury. It causes pain and limitation of movement.

Investigation

Plain X-rays show a loss of joint space, subchondral sclerosis and osteophytes. Loose bodies may be evident. Other forms of radiological investigation seldom provide further useful information.

Management

The symptoms are first treated with **anti-inflammatory medication** and an alteration of daily activity.

Associated loose bodies may be removed through an arthroscope. **Arthoscopic or open removal of osteophytes** can sometimes improve the joint's range of movement.

In severe cases, **elbow replacement** can be undertaken with **resurfacing replacements** and **hinged implants** (Fig 8.12). The results of replacement surgery are not as good as hip and shoulder replacement, as there is a greater risk of the prosthesis becoming loose.

RHEUMATOID ARTHRITIS OF THE ELBOW JOINT

Rheumatoid arthritis commonly affects both the elbow and the superior radioulnar joint. In addition to swelling, pain and tenderness, the elbow becomes unstable because of the soft tissue involvement. All movements may become limited.

Management

During an attack of acute synovitis, the **elbow should be rested** and the patient given **anti-inflammatory drugs**.

Disease-modifying drugs have significantly reduced the incidence of rheumatoid disease.

For the chronically painful elbow, with failed non-operative measures, open or **arthroscopic excision of the radial head** and **synovectomy** may improve symptoms.

If this fails, a **total elbow replacement** may be performed (Fig 8.12).

DISTAL BICEPS TENDON RUPTURE

Investigation

Clinical diagnostic indicators

The distal biceps may separate from its insertion into the radial tuberosity or rupture within the substance of the tendon and causing a painful swollen elbow. This usually occurs following a traumatic incident when the elbow is flexed against resistance. A gap can often be felt in the tendon.

Imaging

The diagnosis may be confirmed by an **ultrasound or MRI scan**.

Management

The pain and swelling usually settle but, in the longer term, the biceps will ultimately atroph and patients experience a loss of approximately 50 per cent supination and 30 per cent flexion. They consequently have difficulty performing tasks involving these movements, e.g. using a screwdriver.

Operative repair of the distal biceps can be performed using either a single- or two-incision approach. The tendon is repaired either by inserting anchors into the radial tuberosity or by tunnelling it within the bone.

If presentation is delayed, the biceps may be joined to another muscle, e.g. the brachialis, or a tendon graft can be inserted.

PAIN IN THE FOREARM (NERVE ENTRAPMENT)

ULNAR NERVE COMPRESSION

The site where the ulnar nerve passes behind the elbow through the cubital tunnel is a common site of compression.

Investigation

Clinical diagnostic indicators

The patient will present with **pain extending down to the hand** with a variety of clinically detectable sensory, motor, reflex, autonomic and trophic changes in its region of innervation.

Imaging

Plain X-rays should be used to detect any osteophyte formation in the region of the cubital tunnel or nearby degenerative joint disease.

Function studies

EMG studies, which assess the conduction velocity within the nerve, can be used to confirm the diagnosis.

Management

Treatment includes **extension splinting at night** and the avoidance of repetitive elbow movement.

Non-steroidal anti-inflammatory medication should be given.

If these measures fail to resolve the problem, **ulnar nerve decompression** and/or **transposition of the nerve** to the anterior aspect of the elbow will relieve the symptoms, but nerve function does not always recover completely.

RADIAL NERVE COMPRESSION

The radial nerve may be compressed at different points along its course resulting in **pain and paraesthesia** in the distribution of its sensory branch and weakness of the forearm and wrist extensor muscles.

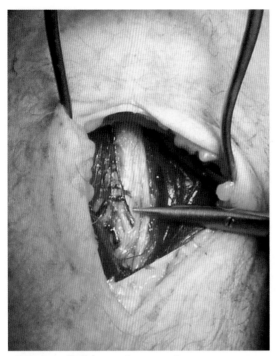

FIGURE 8.13   Radial nerve decompression

In the radial tunnel, compression can be caused by fibrous bands, recurrent radial vessels, a tendinous origin of the extensor carpi radialis brevis, and thickening along the distal margin of the supinator.

Investigation

Clinical diagnostic indicators

The pain is generally centred over the anterolateral proximal forearm in the region of the neck of the radius. Maximum tenderness is usually found four finger breadths distal to the lateral epicondyle.

Active finger extension, especially of the middle finger, is painful.

Imaging

Plain X-ray and other radiological imaging seldom reveal a significant abnormality.

Function studies

EMG studies are often normal.

Management

Treatment is **operative decompression** of the nerve.

PAIN IN THE HAND AND WRIST

CARPAL TUNNEL SYNDROME

This is the most common nerve compression syndrome. It is caused by compression of the median nerve as it passes through the carpal tunnel – the tunnel formed by the carpal bones and the flexor retinaculum. In addition to the median nerve, the tendons to the finger flexors (flexor digitorum superficialis, flexor digitorum profundus and flexor pollicus longus) pass through the carpal tunnel.

There is very little space within the tunnel and any change in the volume of adjacent structures causes pressure on the median nerve which affects its function.

Investigation

Clinical diagnostic indicators

Compression of the nerve results in **pain, altered sensation** and eventually, **muscle denervation**. Pain that develops during the night is a diagnostic feature.

Clinical examination may reveal neurological abnormalities. Sensory symptoms can often be reproduced by percussing the median nerve (Tinel's sign) or by compressing the carpal tunnel with the wrist flexed for 1–2 minutes (Phalen's test).

Function studies

The clinical diagnosis may be confirmed by **nerve conduction/EMG studies**.

Blood tests

Blood investigations may be needed to elicit or exclude a precipitating cause such as rheumatoid arthritis, diabetes, myxoedema and pregnancy.

Management

Non-operative treatment includes the provision of a **splint** to prevent movement, **particularly at night**. An **injection of steroid** can be effective in the short term. Any associated underlying condition should be treated.

The **carpal tunnel can be decompressed** using an open or arthroscopic technique under local, regional or general anaesthesia by **dividing the flexor retinaculum**, which in effect 'deroofs' the tunnel. It is a very effective operation.

TENOSYNOVITIS AND TENOVAGINITIS

Tenosynovitis of the extensor tendons can be caused by overuse or repetitive minor trauma. It most commonly affects the first dorsal compartment (abductor pollicis longus and extensor pollicis brevis) and the second dorsal compartment (extensor carpi radialis, longus and brevis). These tendons pass beneath a tight fibrous bridge just proximal to the styloid process of the radius. The tendon swells and becomes painful.

Investigation

Clinical diagnostic indicators

The patient develops a **firm tender swelling** on the radial aspect of the wrist which is often considered to be a bony outgrowth.

Pain can be demonstrated when the thumb is opposed the wrist is forced into ulnar deviation – **a positive Finkelstein's test**.

Imaging

An **X-ray** may show a calcific deposit but is generally normal.

An **ultrasound or MRI scan** will confirm the inflammation and the swelling of the tendon but is rarely indicated, as this is generally a clinical diagnosis.

Management

Conservative treatment comprises **rest, splintage and anti-inflammatory medication**. Subsequently hand therapy may be useful.

For chronic symptoms, the **injection of a corticosteroid** into the tendon sheath can be undertaken. If this fails, then **operative release** of the tendon sheath under local anaesthesia can be performed.

Extensor tenosynovitis can also occur in other extensor tendons about the wrist, e.g. De Quervain's tenosynovitis. Non-operative measures are usually successful.

OSTEOARTHRITIS OF THE WRIST

Osteoarthritis of the wrist is uncommon as a primary disease but may occur secondary to previous injury.

Plain X-rays show narrowing of the radiocarpal joint, sclerosis, cyst formation and osteophytes (Fig 8.14).

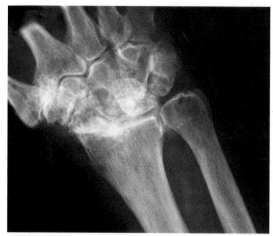

FIGURE 8.14   X-ray of osteoarthritis of the wrist. Loss of joint space and bone sclerosis

Treatment comprises **rest and splintage**. If symptoms progress an **arthrodesis** of the wrist can be performed.

SCAPHOID NON-UNION

The scaphoid bone has a high incidence of non-union following fracture, particularly if the initial diagnosis is missed.

Investigation

Clinical diagnostic indicators

The patient will have had troublesome **wrist pain** following a fracture of the scaphoid or following an injury when a fracture was not detected. The pain is caused by the un-united fracture and secondary changes in the radiocarpal joint and between the scaphoid and the neighbouring small bones of the hands.

Imaging

Plain X-rays will confirm non-union and show secondary changes consistent with avascular necrosis and bone degeneration.

CT and MRI scans can be used to delineate avascular necrosis.

Management

Operative fixation of the non-union is made with a special screw (Herbert's screw) which has a differential pitch and thereby compresses the fracture.

A **bone graft** may also be used and may be vascularized. This can be taken from the iliac crest or the radial styloid.

If secondary changes are present, partial or complete **arthrodesis** is indicated.

KIENBOCK'S DISEASE

Kienbock's disease is **osteochondrosis of the carpal lunate bone**. Avascular necrosis of the bone leads to its fragmentation and collapse.

Investigation
Clinical diagnostic indicators

The patient complains of **aching and stiffness** with tenderness localized to the centre of the dorsum of the wrist.

Imaging

Plain X-rays usually show an intact lunate but, depending on the stage of disease, subsequent X-rays may show sclerosis followed by collapse and fragmentation and, ultimately, superimposed arthritic change.

An **MRI scan** will show a lack of blood flow to the bone and attempted revascularization.

Management

Treatment depends on the stage of the disease. In some cases, where there is an abnormally large difference in length between the radius and ulna, which potentially could cause pressure on the lunate contributing to the avascularity, a radial shortening may be performed.

Revascularization techniques involving a bone graft taken from elsewhere in the body can be undertaken.

As the disease progresses, **removal of the lunate together with the proximal row of carpal bones** (lunate, scaphoid and triquetrum) may be required.

Partial or total wrist **arthrodesis** are also options.

CARPOMETACARPAL OSTEOARTHRITIS

The carpometacarpal joint is the hand joint most commonly affected by osteoarthritis. Its incidence is greater in women. A third of women over the age of 40 have X-ray changes.

Investigation
Clinical diagnostic indicators

The **pain** it causes is centred over the carpometacarpal joint at the base of the thumb approximately 1 cm distal to the radial styloid process.

Imaging

Plain X-rays show joint space narrowing, subchondral sclerosis, osteophyte formation and cystic change. There may be radial and dorsal subluxation of the joint (Fig 8.15).

Management

Splintage, hand therapy and non-steroidal anti-inflammatory agents can be used in the initial management. If this fails to control symptoms, then **corticosteroid injection into the joint** can be undertaken.

If symptoms continue to progress, then **excision of the trapezium** and **ligament reconstruction** and **tendon interposition** may help.

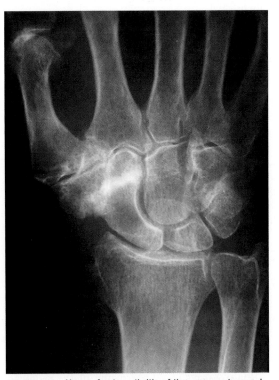

FIGURE 8.15   X-ray of osteoarthritis of the carpometacarpal joint

Carpometacarpal joint fusion is another option.

Prosthetic replacement has been described but there is an incidence of instability and dislocation of the prosthesis. Other alternatives include **excision arthroplasty, interposition arthroplasty** and **silastic replacement arthroplasty**.

INTERPHALANGEAL JOINT OSTEOARTHRITIS

Generalized osteoarthritis of the interphalangeal joints is very common. It mostly affects the distal interphalangeal joints, causing **pain and swelling** spreading to involve all the fingers of the hands. Osteophytic **lumps** develop at the margins of the joints, at the distal interphalangeal joints (**Heberden's nodes**), and, less frequently, the proximal interphalangeal joints (**Bouchard's nodes**).

Plain X-rays show the typical features of osteoarthritis.

Treatment is dependent on the patient's symptoms. The pain often subsides such that no operative treatment is necessary. Occasionally, fusion of the joint is performed.

RHEUMATOID ARTHRITIS OF THE WRIST

The wrist is commonly affected by rheumatoid arthritis as the radiocarpal and distal radioulnar joints have a large amount of synovium.

Investigation

Clinical diagnostic indicators

As the radioulnar joint and the extensor tendons become involved in the disease process they become **painful, swollen and tender**. The tendons which cross the joint may erode and rupture (Vaughn–Jack syndrome), more commonly on the ulnar side of the wrist. The extensor pollicis longus can be eroded and rupture as it rubs against Lister's tubercle at the lower end of the radius.

Imaging

X-rays show periarticular osteoporosis, destructive **osteolysis** and arthritis of the distal radioulnar joint. Ultimately, volar and ulnar carpal subluxation occurs with radial deviation of the wrist and ulnar deviation of the fingers.

Management

Non-operative management with **splintage, anti-inflammatory drugs and disease-modifying medication** can be effective.

Persistent synovitis and progressive bony change may require **synovectomy, repair of ruptured tendons, excision of the distal ulna, arthroplasty or arthrodesis**.

Tendon transfers may also be undertaken.

RHEUMATOID ARTHRITIS OF THE HAND

Rheumatoid arthritis affects the hand more frequently than elsewhere in the body leading to **pain, deformity and disability**. In the initial phases there is synovitis of the metacarpal–phalangeal joint and tendon sheaths. As the disease progresses the small joints are destroyed and tendon erosions lead to instability and progressive fixed deformity.

Investigation

X-rays initially show **periarticular osteoporosis** leading to **periarticular erosion** and **joint space narrowing**. Ultimately, deviation of the fingers and subluxation of the metacarpal–phalangeal joints develops, the changes that underlie the **swan neck** and **boutonnière deformities**.

Management

Initial treatment is non-operative with **resting splints, hand therapy and drugs** but although this may relieve the symptoms it does not control the local disease.

Injection of corticosteroids may reduce synovial inflammation.

Surgical intervention includes repair of ruptured tendons, transfer of tendons, joint replacement, synovectomy, arthroplasty and arthrodesis.

DUPUYTREN'S DISEASE/CONTRACTURE

Dupuytren's disease is a thickening of the palmar fascia that causes **contracture of the fingers**.

Investigation
Clinical diagnostic indicators

Dupuytren's disease is often bilateral, and most common in men aged 40–60 years. It is associated with:

- a positive family history
- alcoholism
- epilepsy secondary to medication eg phenytoin
- diabetes
- human immunodeficiency virus (HIV).

The diagnosis is made on the history and physical signs. No specific investigation is warranted other than those needed to elicit the presence of associated co-morbidities.

Management

Injection of **corticosteroid** has been used to soften the nodules.

If the patient is unable to place their hand flat on a table, a test implying a fixed flexion contracture, surgical treatment is worthwhile although many elderly people are content to live with quite a severe deformity.

Surgical treatments include **local, regional and total palmar fasciectomy. Fasciotomies** may also be performed.

After surgery the hand is splinted and followed by hand therapy to maintain the operative correction.

An improvement of any accompanying fixed flexion of the metacarpal-phalangeal joints is more likely than a reduction of any flexion deformity involving the interphalangeal joints.

TRIGGER FINGER/TRIGGER THUMB

Thickening of the flexor profundus longus tendon to a finger or the flexor pollicis longus to the thumb can result in the tendon becoming trapped in its tendon sheath. This results in the digit becoming stuck in a flexed position. Extension is only possible passively.

No specific investigation is required if the triggering can be demonstrated and there is the expected palpable swelling on the volar aspect of the hand overlying the heads of the metacarpals.

Management

Rest may allow the swelling to resolve and the condition improve. Corticosteroid injection can also be used.

Incision of the flexor tendon sheath to allow free passage of the tendon along its sheath is most effective. This condition can occur in children, usually under the age of 2. It resolves spontaneously without the need for any specific treatment.

GANGLION

A ganglion is a swelling that frequently occurs around the wrist following cystic degeneration in the fibrous tissue of the joint capsule or tendon sheath.

No specific investigation is required.

Management

A ganglion may disappear spontaneously. If it persists it can be **excised**.

Aspiration and/or corticosteroid injection of the ganglion is associated with a high rate of recurrence. Even following surgical excision, 10 per cent recur.

PEARL GANGLIA

Pearl ganglia occur in the hand and fingers. They are small, hard swellings, usually in the mid-line of the flexor tendon sheaths. When compressed during a grip they can be acutely painful.

No specific investigation is required.

Management

They often rupture and disappear spontaneously or can be aspirated. If they remain troublesome they can be **excised**.

INFECTION IN THE HAND

Infections can develop in the hand, the nail folds (paronychia), the pulp spaces (whitlow), the tendon sheaths, the web spaces, the deep fascial spaces and the joints; i.e. the infection is usually compartmentalized.

Investigation
Blood tests

Inflammatory/infective markers should be measured.

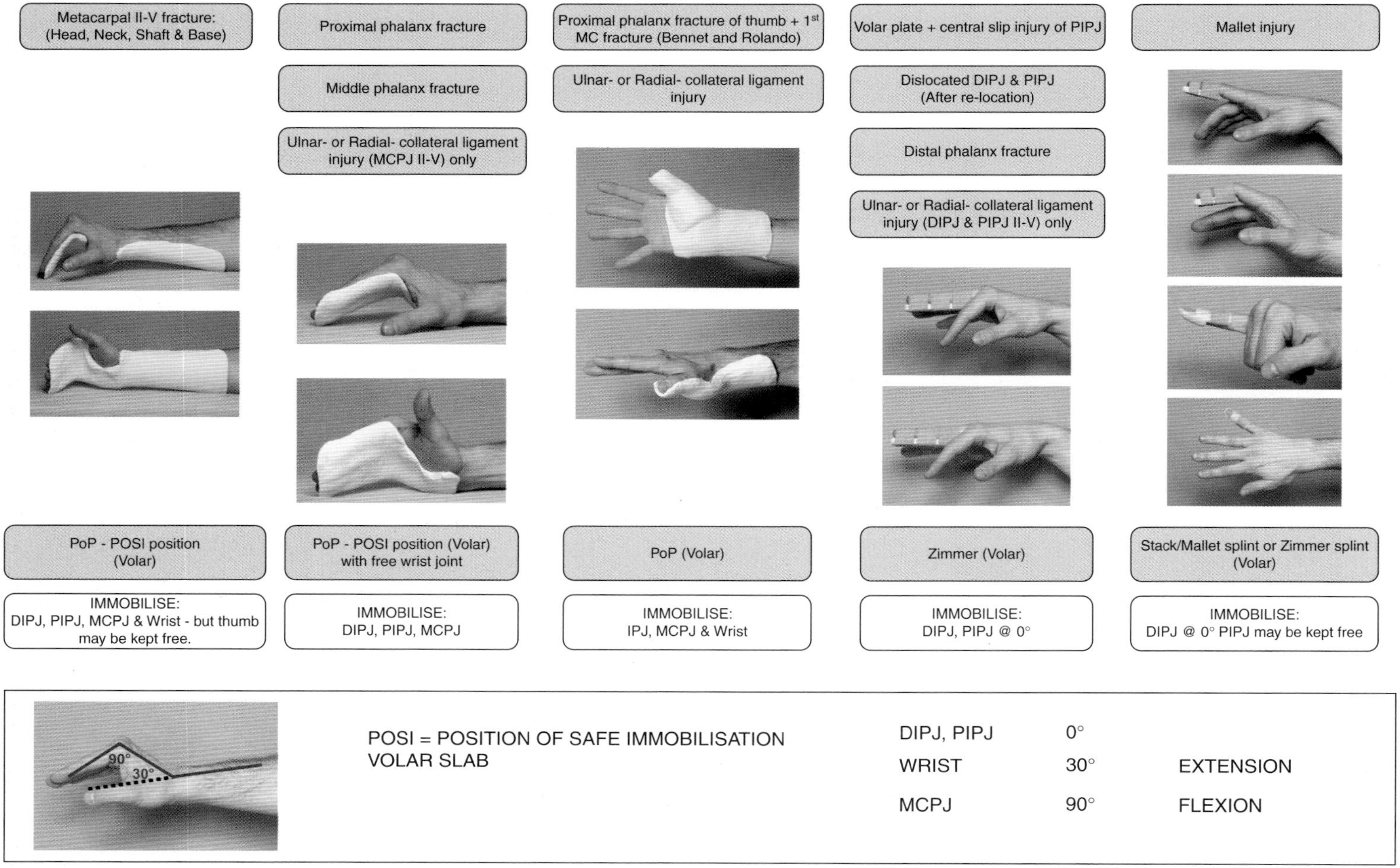

FIGURE 8.16 Guidelines for initial splinting of hand injuries in A&E

Bacteriological tests

Samples of pus, if available, should be sent for culture to identify the infecting organism and its antibiotic sensitivities.

Management

The infecting organism is most commonly a staphylococcus. **Appropriate antibiotics** should be given, which, depending on the severity of the infection, may need to be given intravenously.

The hand should be elevated and **rested in a sling**.

If an **abscess** develops it should be **incised and drained**. The hand should then be splinted in a neutral position of function to avoid a contracture.

The position for safe immobilization of the wrist and hand is slight extension of the wrist, flexion of the metacarpal-phalangeal joints, and extension of the interphalangeal joint with the thumb in abduction (Fig 8.16).

9

The bones, joints and soft tissues of the lower limb

Sam Singh and Diane L. Back

THE HIP

The hip joint is a ball and socket joint formed between the head of the femur and the three bones that comprise the acetabulum, the ilium, ischium and pubis. It is surrounded by a tough membranous capsule lined by synovium and contains the synovial fluid that lubricates the joint.

This very stable configuration allows flexion, extension, abduction, adduction, internal and external rotation. The numerous muscles and tendons between the pelvic bones and the greater and lesser trochanters of the femur assist in movements of the hip.

The main problems caused by diseases of the hip are **pain** and **restriction of movement**.

Pain in the hip joint is classically felt in the groin, but may also be referred down to the knee. It may arise from either the soft tissues or the joint itself.

Restriction of movement as well as activity-related symptoms, night pain and stiffness in the morning are common, especially in the degenerate hip. The patient may walk with a limp, use a walking stick and complain of functional inabilities, such as being unable to put on their socks and shoes.

Do not forget that pain felt in the hip may be a referred pain from the lower lumbar spine and sacro-iliac joints because of their shared nerve supply from the L2, 3 and 4 nerve roots.

SOFT TISSUE CAUSES OF HIP PAIN

Many of the muscles that insert around the hip are associated with bursae, which may become inflamed and painful. The following are the three most common causes of soft tissue pain around the hip. Their investigation and treatment are similar.

TROCHANTERIC BURSITIS

The gluteus medius, gluteus minimus and tensor fascia lata muscles attach to the greater trochanter and assist in abduction, a few degrees of internal rotation and hip flexion.

There are two bursae between these muscles which may become inflamed.

Clinical diagnostic indicators

Patients with trochanteric bursitis are often athletes or older overweight women. They present with pain over the greater trochanter when they lie down and worsening pain on walking and climbing stairs. The pain can be reproduced on examination by deep palpation and by resisted abduction.

ADDUCTOR TENDONITIS

The adductor muscles, pectineus, adductor magnus, adductor longus and adductor brevis arise from the inferior pubic ramus and insert sequentially along the medial aspect of the femoral shaft.

Clinical diagnostic indicators

Adductor tendonitis is most common in athletes, particularly horse riders. It causes pain in the groin and along the medial aspect of the thigh which can be reproduced by resisted adduction of the hip.

ILIOPSOAS TENDONITIS

The iliopsoas originates in two parts: the iliacus from the ilium of the pelvis and the psoas from the first to fifth lumbar vertebrae. The two muscles merge to form a large tendon which inserts into the lesser trochanter.

The pain of iliopsoas tendonitis is experienced over the lesser trochanter, where there may be palpable tenderness, although the overlying structures may mask this sign. The pain is exacerbated by flexion of the hip, as iliopsoas is the primary flexor of the hip.

Investigation

All of the above soft tissue causes of pain can be investigated in the same way.

Imaging

Plain X-ray in chronic cases may show calcification of the bursae (Fig 9.1).

Ultrasound scanning may demonstrate a thickened and inflamed bursa.

Management

A combination of **rest, massage and simple analgesia** should be advised as first-line treatment, combined as the acute symptoms settle with gentle mobilization and stretching exercises.

If conservative treatment fails, an **injection** with local anaesthetic and cortisone, preferably under ultrasound guidance, will usually help.

Rarely, a **surgical exploration** and excision of the bursae or division of the iliopsoas tendon may be required.

SNAPPING HIP

Although this is generally not a painful condition, it causes the patient anxiety.

A clunking or a snapping sensation may occur as the iliotibial band passes over the greater trochanter,

particularly when the patient flexes the hip and extends the knee, in a standing position.

No specific investigation or treatment is required, other than **reassurance**.

BONY CAUSES OF HIP PAIN

The bony causes of hip pain differ with the age of the patient.

In the child, the recognized causes of hip pain are **developmental dysplasia of the hip** (0–4 years), **Legg–Calve–Perthes disease** (4–9 years) and **slipped upper femoral epiphysis** (SUFE) (9–14 years). Other pathologies such as infection and trauma may occur but both are rare.

In the older population, hip pain is usually related to the development of **osteoarthritis**, which may be primary – caused by wear and tear of the articular cartilage – or secondary – caused by another disease process altering the bony anatomy of the joint.

DEVELOPMENTAL DYSPLASIA OF THE HIP

Developmental dysplasia of the hip (DDH) was previously known as 'congenital dislocation of the hip' and represents abnormal development or dislocation of the hip caused by capsular laxity or mechanical factors. It affects 1.5 per 1000 live births and it is recognized to be more common in females (85 per cent), breech presentation at birth and a positive family history. The left hip is most commonly affected (67 per cent).

Investigation

Early diagnosis is crucial to prevent the development of irreversible changes which will lead to pain and deformity.

Clinical diagnostic indicators

All children should be clinically screened at a routine postnatal examination.

The clinical examination involves **Ortolani's test** (elevation and abduction of the femur relocates a dislocated hip) and **Barlow's test** (adduction and depression of the femur dislocates a dislocatable hip) (Fig 9.2).

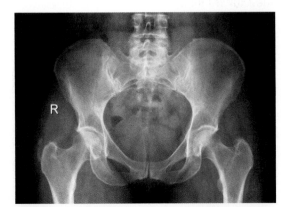

FIGURE 9.1   Calcification of a hip bursa

Imaging

Plain X-rays are generally not helpful at this stage, as the femoral head has not ossified.

Clinical examination may be supplemented by an **ultrasound assessment**.

Management

Treatment should be designed to achieve and maintain a concentric reduction of the joint, and varies with age.

When Developmental Dysplasia of the hip is diagnosed *at birth* then the child may be placed into a **Pavlik harness** or a splintage device, which holds the hips in an abducted and flexed position, taking care to avoid 'excessive' positions which may cause avascular necrosis. This is generally worn for 12 weeks. It can be removed when a stable reduction is confirmed radiographically.

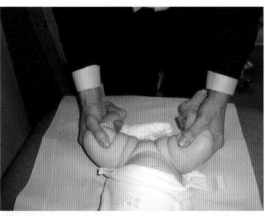

(A)

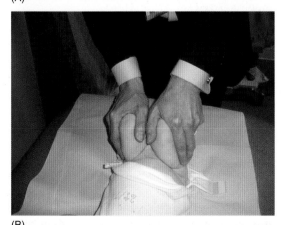

(B)

FIGURE 9.2   Ortolani's and Barlow's test

If Developmental Dysplasia of the Hip is diagnosed *after 2–3 months*, bracing or more commonly **plaster immobilization** of the hip is employed.

If, *after 9–12 months*, the dislocation is irreducible to closed techniques, an **open reduction** may be necessary followed by **immobilization in a hip spica**.

In children where the hip joint is not satisfactorily reduced, further surgery may be necessary to obtain coverage of the femoral head within the acetabulum. **Osteotomies** of both the pelvis and the femur may be used to achieve this.

LEGG–CALVE–PERTHES DISEASE

This is non-inflammatory **osteochondritis of the proximal femoral epiphysis** caused by a vascular disturbance. The femoral head undergoes osteonecrosis, becomes softer and deformed and then remodels.

Investigation

Clinical diagnostic indicators

Legg–Calve–Perthes disease usually occurs in males aged 4–9 years. There may be a family history. It is bilateral in 10–15 per cent of patients. It can cause pain in the groin, hip and knee and cause a limp. Clinical examination reveals decreased abduction and internal rotation of the hip joint.

Imaging

A **plain X-ray** will usually show a flattened femoral head. A crescent sign may be present, a lucent area in the subchondral bone (Fig 9.3). As the disease progresses, the femoral head fragments and the bony anatomy becomes more distorted.

Management

The aim of treatment is to contain the femoral head within the acetabulum and so prevent

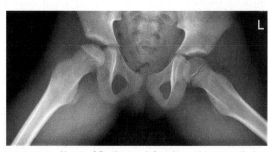

FIGURE 9.3   X-ray of Perthes – deformity and 'crescent' sign

gross bony anatomical distortion. This can be achieved by:

- avoidance of weight-bearing, and non-steroidal analgesia for the young patient with early changes
- braces or splints in older patients with more advanced disease.

Surgery involving osteotomies about the hip joint can be considered if the above methods fail.

SLIPPED UPPER FEMORAL EPIPHYSIS

Slipped upper femoral epiphysis (SUFE) is essentially a fracture in the growth plate of the upper femoral epiphysis, which causes the femoral epiphysis to slip. Although the femoral head remains in the acetabulum, the neck of the femur displaces anteriorly and externally rotates. This can occur acutely, as a result of trauma, but more commonly develops slowly.

Investigation

Clinical diagnostic indicators

Slipped femoral epiphysis is most common in 10- to 14-year-old obese males with a positive family history. Thirty per cent of cases are bilateral.

The **pain** it causes is felt in the groin and often referred to the knee. The patient prefers to hold the leg in an externally rotated position.

There may be an associated hormone imbalance, such as hypothyroidism.

Imaging

Anteroposterior (AP) and 'frog-leg' X-rays of the pelvis to assess the degree of any slippage is the principal investigation.

An **MRI scan** may show subtle features of the impending problem in early cases.

It is important to assess the symptomless hip.

Management

Surgical treatment, varied according to the degree of displacement, is essential.

If there is only slight or moderate displacement, the **epiphysis should be pinned** *in situ* **using cannulated screws**, without attempting a reduction.

An **osteotomy** to correct the deformity may be needed at a later date if there is gross displacement. **Continued surveillance** is essential as the epiphysis may become avascular if the blood supply does not recover adequately.

It is not uncommon for these patients to develop secondary osteoarthritis later in life and require a hip replacement.

IRRITABLE HIP: TRANSIENT SYNOVITIS

The aetiology of this condition is unknown; however, it is the most common cause of painful hips in childhood. It may follow a recent viral infection, particularly of the upper respiratory tract. It is usually self-limiting and improves over a 3–4 day period. The diagnosis is reached by excluding other pathologies such as sepsis and hence routine blood investigations and plain X-rays should be performed.

An **ultrasound scan** and possible **aspiration of the joint** for microbiology investigation may assist in the diagnosis.

Treatment is symptomatic with bed rest, or a period of non-weight-bearing on crutches, and anti-inflammatory medication. If there is any doubt about the presence of sepsis in the hip, antibiotics should be given until the results of the haematological and microbiological investigations on the joint fluid are received.

OSTEOARTHRITIS OF THE HIP

Osteoarthritis of the hip is one of the commonest conditions causing pain in the joints. The exact aetiology is not known, but we do know that the following factors predispose to development of secondary osteoarthritis:

- developmental dysplasia of the hip
- abnormal biomechanics
- fracture
- Legg–Calve–Perthes disease
- SUFE
- DDH.

Investigation

Clinical diagnostic indicators

Pain and the effects of restriction of movement are the common symptoms and signs.

Imaging

Plain X-rays of the pelvis and the affected hip are the essential investigations (Fig 9.4) supplemented with **CT** or **MRI scans** depending on the underlying aetiology. The diagnostic radiographic findings

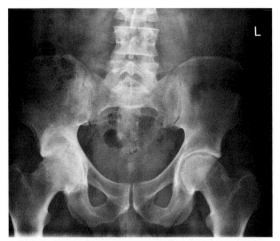

FIGURE 9.4 X-ray of osteoarthritic hip

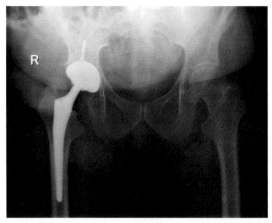

FIGURE 9.5 X-ray of hip prostheses

include **loss of joint space, subchondral sclerosis, cyst formation and osteophyte formation**.

Management

Conservative treatment consists of initial symptom modifying activities, **simple analgesics** and **walking aids**, e.g. a walking stick.

If there is a leg length discrepancy, a **shoe raise** may be employed to help balance the pelvis and relieve strains across the pelvis and lower back.

Surgical intervention is often required as the disease progresses.

The most common procedures are **total hip arthroplasty** and **resurfacing operations**, in which both the acetabulum and the femoral head are replaced (Fig 9.5).

Most implants comprise a femoral component made of either stainless steel or chrome cobalt molybdenum alloy, although ceramic heads of aluminium oxide are also used. The acetabular component is generally a cup made of high-density polyethylene, but metal cups can also be used. Implants may be cemented or uncemented. Sometimes a combination is utilized whereby an implant is cemented on one side of the joint, whereas on the other, fixation is dependent on bone growing into the surface of the prosthesis. A coating of hydroxyapatite may stimulate this bone ingrowth.

Over 90 per cent of hip prostheses survive for 10 years after implantation.

In earlier stages of the disease, **osteotomies** of either the pelvis or the femur may be considered,

but these only provide a limited period of symptom relief.

In very advanced disease or after failed surgical intervention, an **arthrodesis** (fusion) of the hip may be performed.

Arthroscopy of the hip is also now being incorporated into orthopaedic practice and this may provide an avenue for future treatment.

INFECTION OF THE HIP

Acute septic arthritis of the hip is an uncommon condition, but must always be considered in the immune compromised patient, e.g. patients with diabetes. The patient will have marked pain, be unable to bear weight on the limb, and have a significantly reduced range of movement. They may also exhibit the systemic features of infection.

Investigation should include routine **blood** investigations, incorporating the markers of infection. An **ultrasound-guided aspiration of the joint** should be undertaken with samples sent for microscopic assessment and **culture**. Once the samples have been taken, **intravenous antibiotics** should be commenced, the antibiotic choice being governed by the sensitivity of the organism. The hip joint should also be explored and **washed out** surgically.

THE KNEE

The knee is a hinge joint. The shape of the bones provides little inherent stability, so the joint's stability relies on its tendons and ligaments and controlling muscles all of which can be injured and cause knee pain and instability.

The patellofemoral complex is essential in both stabilization and controlling extension and flexion.

The problems associated with the knee joint may be:

- traumatic – quadriceps or patellar tendon ruptures
- anterior knee pain
- instability
- inflammation.

TENDON RUPTURES

Investigation

Clinical diagnostic indicators

Rupture of both the quadriceps and patellar tendons is usually associated with sporting activity. An explosive surge may cause the tendon rupture. Steroid use may increase the likelihood of rupture.

Examination shows loss of movement and a gap in the ruptured tendon.

Imaging

An **ultrasound examination** can clearly demonstrate a tendon rupture (Fig 9.6).

Management

Conservative treatment of these tendons is usually inappropriate as retraction of the quadriceps muscle prevents adequate re-alignment of the split tendon ends.

Splinting the knee in full extension does not help.

Surgical repair is the treatment of choice followed by a period of immobilization in a splint and then gradual rehabilitation to strengthen the tendon and restore muscle bulk.

ANTERIOR KNEE PAIN

In addition to osteoarthritis of the patellofemoral joint, anterior knee pain may be caused by

- chondromalacia patellae
- patellar tendonitis
- plica syndrome.

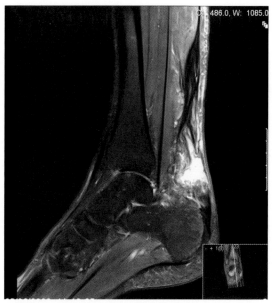

FIGURE 9.6   MRI of ruptured Achilles tendon

Chondromalacia patellae

The cartilage on the posterior surface of the patella is the thickest in the body. If it softens – a change particularly common in teenage girls that may be associated with malalignment of the patella – it can cause anterior knee pain.

Investigation

The diagnosis relies on the history and physical examination.

Imaging

Softening of the articular cartilage is very difficult to identify with current imaging techniques. The most modern MRI scanners may detect oedematous changes but they are not yet a reliable diagnostic tool.

Management

A **conservative approach** with activity modification, physiotherapy, taping of the knee cap and anti-inflammatory drugs is the most appropriate treatment.

Surgical intervention is generally unhelpful except when there is an identifiable malalignment.

Patellar tendonitis (Jumper's knee)

Tendonitis can occur anywhere in the body. When the patellar tendon is affected the patient feels **pain** at the inferior pole of the patella. This problem is often associated with running and jumping sports.

Investigation

An **ultrasound scan** reveals any inflammation in the tendon sheath.

An **MRI** can also show the same but is more expensive and time consuming.

Management

Conservative treatment in the form of activity modification, physiotherapy and non-steroidal anti-inflammatory drugs (NSAIDs) can help in the initial stages.

If the problem becomes chronic, **steroid injection** and **surgical debridement** may be beneficial.

Plica syndrome

Plica are vestigial mesodermal remnants within the knee. If they become scarred or thickened from trauma or overuse, pain and clicking may develop.

Investigation

Imaging

Imaging does not reliably detect plica.

Endoscopy

Plica are usually diagnosed on **arthroscopy** (Fig 9.7).

Management

Arthroscopic **resection** of the plica is appropriate if pain is a significant clinical problem.

LIGAMENT AND MENISCUS DAMAGE

There are four main ligaments around the knee joint: the medial and lateral collateral ligaments and the anterior and posterior cruciate ligaments. They are vital for the stability of the knee joint and are frequently injured in sporting activities.

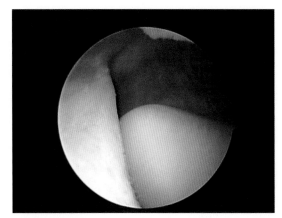

FIGURE 9.7 Arthroscopic photo of plica

Anterior cruciate ligament injury

The anterior cruciate ligament is intra-articular and prevents anterior translation and external rotation of the tibia on the femur. There is often an associated medial meniscal tear. It is frequently injured in footballers who are subject to a sliding tackle, or who suddenly stop running, plant their foot, twist and turn to change direction. There is often an associated medial meniscal tear (see later).

Investigation

Clinical diagnostic indicators

The patient may give a clear history of the type of injury described above and complain of **pain and instability** in the knee. This is particularly apparent when they descend the stairs. Examination will reveal abnormal forward movement of the tibia on the femur.

Imaging

An **MRI scan** should demonstrate a tear or sprain of the anterior cruciate ligament (Fig 9.8), but because of its helical nature, some injuries are missed on the sliced images.

An MRI will also pick up any associated meniscal or other ligamentous injuries.

Management

Conservative management of these ruptures is common because in many cases the stability of the knee can be restored by rehabilitating the quadriceps mechanism. **Physiotherapy is essential.**

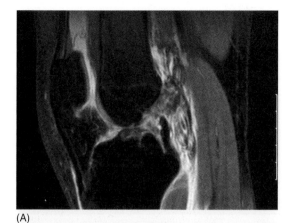

(A)

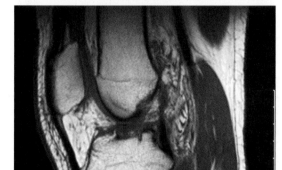

(B)

FIGURE 9.8 (A–B) MRI of torn anterior cruciate

If after a rehabilitation programme the patient is still complaining of instability, then **surgical options** should be considered.

The anterior cruciate ligament can be reconstructed in a number of ways, using both open and arthroscopic techniques.

Grafts can be taken from the **patellar tendon** and **hamstrings**. **Synthetic** grafts are available, fixed in place by screw and buttons.

An intensive period of postoperative physiotherapy is required for full rehabilitation.

Posterior cruciate ligament injury

The posterior cruciate ligament is stronger than the anterior cruciate ligament. It attaches to the posterior horn of the lateral meniscus and prevents posterior translation of the tibia on the femur and hyperextension of the knee. Injuries

to this ligament are less common and harder to identify. They are frequently missed, even by experienced doctors.

Investigation

Clinical diagnostic indicators

The patient may give a history of a direct anterior blow to the tibia – a 'dashboard'-type injury. Examination may reveal abnormal posterior movement and hyperextension of the joint.

Imaging

An **MRI** will pick up most posterior cruciate ligament injuries and show the loss of its 'shepherd's crook' shape (Fig 9.9). It will also identify any associated injury to the posterolateral corner of the knee.

Management

Physiotherapy is always an important part of the treatment regimen but **acute surgical repair** is now being advocated.

Meniscus damage

There are two c-shaped menisci in the knee. They are made of Type 1 collagen fibres, laid radially and longitudinally with proteoglycan interspersed between the fibres. The lateral meniscus is smaller and more mobile than the medial meniscus, with the popliteus muscle attached posteriorly. The c-shaped medial meniscus is larger with the semimembranosus muscle attached to it; it is more likely to be injured. Their blood supply from the geniculate arteries is poor and the menisci have little regenerative capacity.

The menisci are responsible for lubrication and proprioception and, by acting as shock absorbers, distribute the load through the knee joint.

Both menisci can be damaged either in isolation or in association with the cruciate ligaments (see above). The most common injury is a tear and symptoms are usually of **pain, locking and swelling**. They are classified as:

- degenerate
- traumatic.

Degenerate tears become more common with age. There is often no recognized associated episode

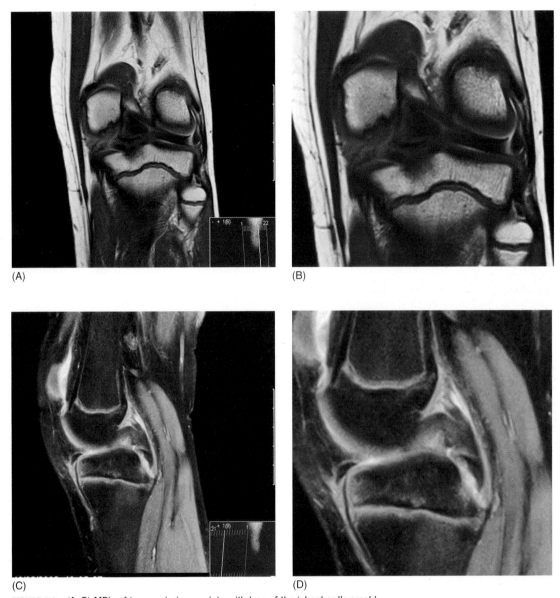

(A)

(B)

(C)

(D)

FIGURE 9.9 (A–D) MRIs of torn posterior cruciate with loss of the 'shepherd's crook'

and they are often symptomless. They are also associated with osteoarthritis of the knee joint.

Traumatic tears occur from adolescence onwards and are often associated with a twisting injury; for example, a running football player stopping on one foot, then twisting to change direction. It is usually the posterior horn of the medial meniscus affected. When there is a large unstable tear, it can fall into the knee joint blocking the movement of the knee, causing 'locking'.

Investigation

Clinical diagnostic indicators

The history of the injury invariably follows one of the patterns described above.

In the acute stage the knee is swollen and may be locked. In the chronic phase there may be intermittent swelling and locking accompanied by pain and limping.

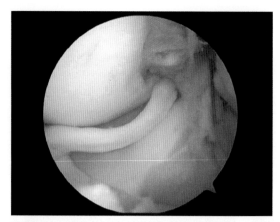

FIGURE 9.10   Arthroscopic photo of meniscus tear

Imaging

An **MRI** is the most effective way of visualizing the menisci but this a costly investigation and has, as far as tears are concerned, a high false negative rate. It is also unable to distinguish between degenerate tears that can be left alone or traumatic unstable tears that may need surgical intervention. **Arthroscopy** may be required for diagnosis and treatment (Fig 9.10).

Management

Conservative treatment is often suitable for degenerative tears in elderly people, helped by changes in lifestyle and physiotherapy.

Arthroscopic menisectomy is more often used in younger patients with traumatic tears that are causing locking. Resecting the torn part of the meniscus is preferable to total menisectomy, as total menisectomy can predispose to the development of osteoarthritis in later life.

In adolescents, **meniscal repair** can be attempted but is controversial.

OSTEOARTHRITIS OF THE KNEE

Osteoarthritis of the knee is one of the commonest conditions causing pain in the joints. The exact aetiology is not known but we do know that certain factors are known to predispose to the development of osteoarthritis, e.g.

- abnormal biomechanics
- fracture.

Osteoarthritis begins when the articular hyaline cartilage lining the joint starts to thin and break down and expose the bony surfaces to wear and tear.

Investigation

Clinical diagnostic indicators

Osteoarthritis is characterized by **pain** in the knee. It may cause pain in its adjoining joints. Night pain and stiffness in the morning are common.

Crepitus, crunching and clicking sounds coming from the joint, are particularly common in the knee joint.

The patient may walk with a limp and use a walking stick. Their restricted mobility may cause them to complain of being unable to put on their socks and shoes.

The legs may develop a varus or valgus deformity (see *Symptoms and Signs*).

Imaging

A **plain weight-bearing X-ray** taken in three planes is required to visualize all the joints of the knee: an **anteroposterior view**, plus **lateral** and **skyline views** of the **patella** to show the patellofemoral joint. The radiograph must be taken with the joint in its functional position, i.e. weight-bearing.

These films will reveal the common signs of osteoarthritis, namely, loss of joint space, sclerosis of the bone and osteophyte formation. Subchondral cysts may be present but are not common in knee osteoarthritis (Fig 9.11).

Management

Conservative treatment of knee osteoarthritis should be attempted first, i.e. activity modification, **weight loss, anti-inflammatory medication, walking aids** and **physiotherapy**.

The role of herbal treatments, for example, glucosamine, remains controversial. Two prospective randomized controlled trials have shown it to produce a significant decrease in pain in the early stages of knee osteoarthritis.

As the disease progresses **surgical intervention** may be required.

An **arthroscopic washout and debridement** of the affected surfaces can bring pain relief for

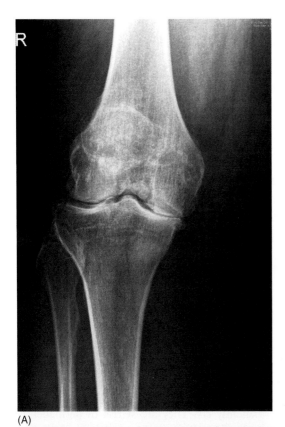

(A)

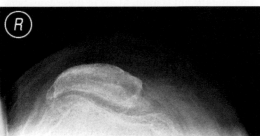

(B)

FIGURE 9.11   (A–B) Osteoarthritis in the knee

some. However, most will progress to further more radical surgery.

Osteotomy of the tibia may allow a redistribution of the load onto the unworn area of the joint if the disease is isolated to one compartment of the knee joint. This treatment is now less popular as its effects are often transient. Most patients opt for a **total knee replacement**, where the joint is replaced with a metallic and polyethylene implant.

Current knee implants survive up to 20 years, in less active older patients, but in younger

active patients they may become loose and need revising.

THE ANKLE

ANKLE ARTHRITIS

Ankle arthritis is less common than hip or knee arthritis. The ankle is a very tight mortice joint so any fracture that has united with a step can lead to abnormal wear of the cartilage.

Investigation

Clinical diagnostic indicators

The majority of cases are post traumatic so it is important to take a detailed history about previous ankle fractures, repeated sprains or significant ankle injuries. The principal problems are **pain, swelling and their effect on walking**.

Imaging

Weight-bearing plain X-rays will show the hallmarks of osteoarthritis: loss of joint space, subchondral sclerosis with cyst formation and marginal osteophytes (Fig 9.12).

The adjacent joints should be included and evaluated from the X-ray.

Management

Initial treatment options include **NSAIDs** or **immobilization** with an ankle brace.

Steroid or viscosupplement injections may produce temporary relief.

Prominent osteophytes at the front of the ankle can be removed arthroscopically or with an **open debridement**.

More advanced cases require **ankle fusion**.

In carefully selected patients there may be a role for **ankle replacement** though the long-term results of this procedure are not as successful as hip or knee replacement.

ANKLE SPRAINS

Ankle sprains are usually caused by an inversion force applied with the ankle in plantar flexion. The commonest ligament to be ruptured is the anterior talofibular ligament, which is part of the lateral ligament complex.

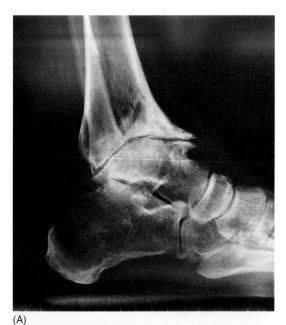

(A)

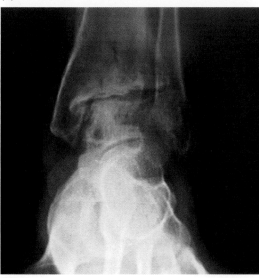

(B)

FIGURE 9.12 (A–B) X-rays of ankle with osteoarthritis

Investigation

Clinical diagnostic indicators

The ankle is **tender** over the anterior part of the lateral ligament. It is essential to palpate three other areas when evaluating an ankle sprain to exclude any associated fractures – the base of the fifth metatarsal, the proximal fibula neck and the medial maleolus.

Imaging

Plain X-rays are indicated if there is tenderness on the bone of the tibia or fibula, or an inability to bear weight, to exclude a fracture.

Symptoms that are still present at six weeks justify an **MRI scan**.

Management

The immediate management of a sprain is **rest, ice, compression** and **elevation** (RICE) plus **compression** with a 'tubigrip' bandage or even in a severe case immobilization with a **plaster backslab**. Rest and elevation are important: the leg must be lifted on pillows so that it is at the same level as the heart.

Most ankle sprains settle with the above regimen.

If the pain and swelling has not settled by 10 days then an X-ray and referral to **physiotherapy** should be requested.

Chronic functional instability occurs if a patient has repeated sprains because of the ligament being permanently lax. They are at risk of permanently damaging the ankle joint. Many of these cases benefit from intensive physiotherapy with strengthening of the antagonist muscles. A small proportion will require surgery to reconstruct the ligament.

ACHILLES TENDON DISORDERS

The Achilles tendon is the strongest, thickest tendon in the body. It is the tendon for the gastrocnemius and soleus muscles, whose primary motor function is plantar flexion of the ankle.

ACHILLES TENDINITIS

Achilles tendonitis, which is seen in athletes, runners and hikers, is caused by local irritation of the paratendon or degeneration within the tendon.

Investigation

Clinical diagnostic indicators

The **pain** may be felt at the site where the tendon inserts into the calcaneus (insertional Achilles

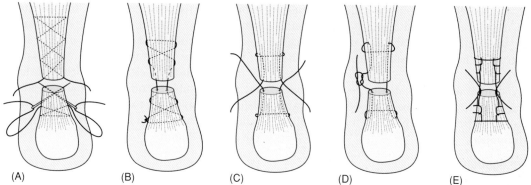

(A)   (B)   (C)   (D)   (E)

FIGURE 9.13 Achilles tendon repairs

tendinosis) or in the watershed area about 3 cm from the insertion (non-insertional Achilles tendinosis). The latter is often associated with a fusiform swelling at this point. The pain is typically exacerbated by activity and sometimes precipitated by a change in training pattern or shoe wear.

Management

Most cases settle with medical treatment with **NSAIDS, eccentric loading exercises and a reduction in activity**.

Surgical decompression of the tendon may be necessary.

RUPTURED ACHILLES TENDON

This is a potentially very serious condition which, surprisingly, is often missed. Its incidence appears to have increased in recent years, a change possibly related to pursuing sports until a later age or more accurate diagnosis.

Investigation

Clinical diagnostic indicators

Patients may or may not have a pre-existing history of pain in their Achilles tendon. They may report hearing a loud noise such as a 'pop' or 'bang', or feel that they had been kicked or shot in the leg.

The diagnosis is clinical. There will be bruising and tenderness at the site of rupture and a step in the tendon.

Simmon's test is a specific test to check for plantar flexion of the ankle when the calf is squeezed. If there is a breach in the continuity of the tendon the ankle will not bend (see *Symptoms and Signs*).

Management

If the rupture presents within 48 hours of the injury then both conservative and surgical treatment is possible. The duration of immobilization is the same.

The ankle is **immobilized** in plantar flexion to allow the tendon ends to approximate and unite. During the healing period the knee must be kept flexed to prevent contraction of the calf muscles. This can be achieved with a splint on wheels on which the patient kneels but can move around.

Surgical repair is associated with extra risks, in particular wound-healing problems, but does offer a reduced risk of re-rupture. After 48 hours, surgical repair is favoured as organization of the haematoma may prevent the tendon ends from coming together, even if the foot is in an equinus position (Fig 9.13).

THE FOOT

CLUB FOOT

Club foot or **congenital talipes equinovarus** is a deformity that is present at birth and can affect one or both feet. The word 'talipes' means simply the foot and ankle and 'equinovarus' refers to the position of the foot, which points downwards and inwards.

It is relatively common, the incidence ranging from 1 to 2 per thousand births. It occurs worldwide. Very little is known about its cause. The condition can be hereditary, and is twice as common in boys as girls.

Where the foot responds well to simple treatment, it is likely to have been caused by a packing problem in the womb. There is a link with **oligohydramnios**.

Investigation

Imaging

Although it can be identified with an **ultrasound** prenatally, it is often not discovered until birth.

Management

Treatment should be commenced soon after birth, and the aim is to achieve functional, pain-free feet.

Initial treatment tends to be conservative, with **physiotherapy and serial corrective casting**. In recent years there have been great improvements in non-surgical treatment with the serial casting technique known as the **Ponsetti technique** and sometimes a **percutaneous lengthening of the Achilles tendon**.

An operation is required if the above method is unsuccessful. The most common is a 'soft tissue release', which involves lengthening the affected tendons, capsule and ligaments. The final outcome is often good, although cosmetically the foot is usually smaller and the calf muscles less developed.

THE TOES

ADULT HALLUX VALGUS

This well-known deformity is more than just a bump or bunion on the medial side of the foot. There is a medial deviation of the first metatarsal leading to an increased laterally directed pressure on the hallux from the shoe. In the initial stages the deformity corrects itself when the shoe is removed but with time the deformity becomes more stuck down and fixed. The phalanx now pushes the metatarsal head even more medially and the deformity can worsen. The medial lump is not just extra bone that forms in reaction to rubbing on the medial side of the toe, its relative

prominence is also caused by the metatarsals becoming less parallel and more divergent. The joint may be congruent in that the articular surface of the phalanx sits on that of the metatarsal head or in more advanced cases the articular surface of the phalanx subluxes off the metatarsal head. This deformity may not be passively correctable and the lack of congruence can lead to arthritic change in the first MTP joint.

Investigation

Clinical diagnostic indicators

A painful bunion can lead to restriction in daily and recreational activity, difficulty in wearing fashionable shoes and decreased quality of life. **Pain in the ball of the foot** may be the primary complaint.

The patient's shoes should be examined. Local stretching of the material of the shoe may be noted.

The deformity is more apparent when the patient stands. An assessment of the width of the forefoot should be made for comparison with the normal side. The presence of a flat foot should be noted. There may be **callosities** under the second or third metatarsal heads. The range of motion of the first MTP joint may be reduced.

Imaging

A weight-bearing AP and lateral plain X-ray of the foot is essential when evaluating foot and ankle problems as it will show what is happening to the foot in its position of function (Fig 9.14).

There may be congruence of the first MTP (metatarsophalangeal) joint. In normal feet the first and second metatarsals are relatively parallel but become more divergent as the hallux valgus deformity progresses. The sesamoid bones normally lie under the metatarsal head. But the sesamoids, which are anchored by the adductor hallucis tendon, stay where they are and appear subluxed.

There may be arthritic changes in the joint and dorsal osteophytes.

Management

The first line of treatment is **shoe wear modification**. Heels are to be avoided as they encourage the foot to slide downhill, squashing the toes into the

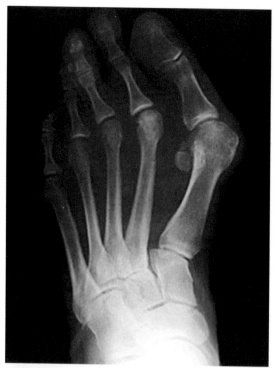

FIGURE 9.14   X-ray of hallux valgus

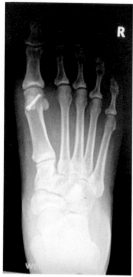

FIGURE 9.15   Hallux valgus operations

toe box of the shoe. Soft lace up leather shoes or trainers may be more comfortable.

A spacer between the first and second toes can ease pressure on the bunion.

Surgery may be indicated if the foot continues to hurt despite the above simple measures (Fig 9.15).

For a mild deformity, simple **shaving off the bunion** and **releasing the deforming adductor tendon** may suffice. Unfortunately the deformity has usually progressed beyond this by the time the patient presents to the doctor.

A moderate deformity can be treated by **breaking the metatarsal close to its head and resetting it** so that the foot is narrower and the metatarsals more parallel.

More advanced deformities need correction at the apex of the deformity, i.e. at the base of the metatarsal.

If the joint is very arthritic then a fusion procedure may be necessary.

Older books describe the **Keller's procedure**. This operation in which part of the proximal phalanx is removed is no longer used and is now of historical interest only.

HALLUX RIGIDUS

Stiffness or 'rigidity' of the first MTP joint can occur at any age from adolescence onwards. In young people it may follow trauma leading to local cartilage damage. In older patients, it may be the result of osteoarthritis or longstanding gout.

Investigation

Clinical diagnostic indicators

Patients complain of pain with activity which they localize to this joint. Inspection of the shoes may show stretching of the leather on the top of the foot and increased wear on the outside of the foot as the patient walks to avoid taking weight through the big toe. There may be a reduction in joint dorsiflexion and plantaflexion. Gout or hallux valgus is the main **differential diagnosis**, although advanced cases of hallux valgus may also have an arthritic component.

Imaging

Weight-bearing plain X-rays will show the hallmarks of arthritis on the AP view. The lateral view may show small osteophytes arising from the metatarsal head. Those on the top are different from those seen with hallux valgus.

Management

Initial treatment includes shoe wear modification. Although soft shoes can ease the discomfort from the dorsal osteophytes, the arthritic pain caused by movement can be relieved by a **stiff soled shoe**, which limits bending at the first metatarsophalangeal joint.

Providing the underlying joint is in reasonable condition, then an **operation** called a **cheilectomy** is indicated. The impinging osteophytes are removed to prevent the pinching of soft tissues.

A **fusion operation** (arthrodesis) may be indicated for more advanced cases. In the fusion operation, the joint surfaces are excised so that the two bones will heal together. If there is no movement there will be no pain.

Joint replacement is possible but lacking in long-term data.

HAMMER TOE/CLAW TOE/MALLET TOE

A hammer toe is a flexion deformity of the proximal interphalangeal joint. A mallet toe is a similar deformity of the distal interphalangeal joint. Claw toe is associated with hyperextension at the MTP joint and flexion at both interphalangeal joints.

Investigation

Clinical diagnostic indicators

Hammer and mallet toes become painful as the deformity causes the affected joint to rub on the shoe. This can lead to excess **callus formation** over the interphalangeal joint and under the metatarsal head.

Claw toes may be associated with **neurological problems** or **rheumatoid arthritis**. A detailed neurological examination is mandatory to exclude such causes.

Management

Conservative treatments include using **silicone sleeves** that roll over the toe. A deep toe box shoe will limit rubbing on the toes.

Surgery may be considered if conservative treatment fails to relieve the pain.

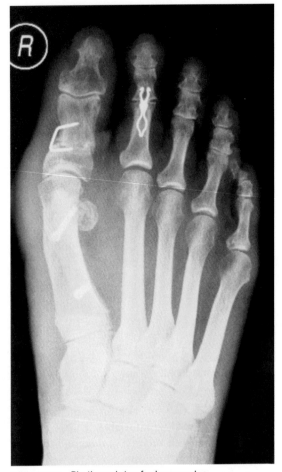

FIGURE 9.16   Pin through toe for hammer toe

If the deformity is passively correctable then **a soft tissue release and temporary pinning of the toe** will suffice (Fig 9.16).

If the deformity is fixed then the joint needs to be **excised or fused straight**. The toe needs to be held with a fine wire to allow healing.

INGROWING TOENAIL

This is a common condition especially in males. The nail rather than growing outwards starts to grow vertically downwards in the nail grove. Once embedded it sets off an inflammatory response with ulceration of the skin and a deep infection.

In initial stages a short course of **antibiotics** may be helpful; but when persistent the portion of germinal matrix from which the ingrowing nail arises needs to be **ablated** chemically, with caustic phenol, or by **curettage**.

Preventative measures include cutting the nail square after lifting the corners up with a cotton bud.

Attempts at hooking out remnants of ingrown nail without anaesthetic can make the pain and infection worse.

THE SOLE OF THE FOOT

PES PLANUS (FLAT FEET)

It is important to differentiate whether this is congenital or acquired. Congenital flat can be flexible or stiff.

Investigation

Clinical diagnostic indicators

The arch of a flexible flat foot can be reconstituted by extending the big toe. It is rarely symptomatic and reassurance is usually all that is required.

A stiff flat foot that cannot be corrected by manipulation suggests a pathological disorder such as a coalition in which the bones of the hind foot are joined abnormally together. This needs specialist investigation.

An acquired flat foot is a separate problem more commonly seen in adults. It can be caused by inflammation in the tibialis posterior tendon – the major support of the medial arch.

Imaging

A coalition may be visible as a bony bar on an **X-ray** (Fig 9.17). A pathognomic sign is the 'anteaters sign' on the lateral X-ray of the ankle.

An **MRI scan** can identify both bony and fibrous tissue bars.

Management

The treatment varies according to the cause.

- Mild cases may be treated by an **insole with a medial arch**.
- More severe cases may require corrective surgery. If the deformities are mild then **tendon transfers** are an option.

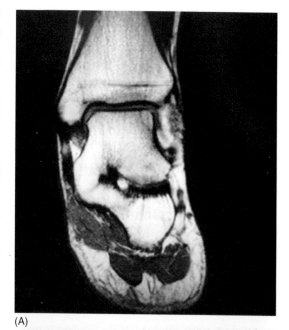

(A)

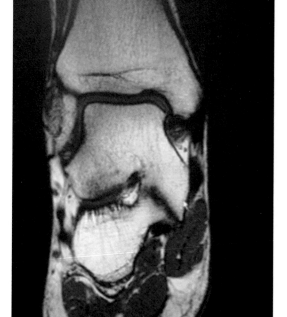

(B)

FIGURE 9.17 (A–B) MRI of coalition bar of flat foot

More fixed deformities may require multiple hind foot joints to be fused, the so-called triple fusion.

PES CAVUS

Pes cavus is a foot with a **higher arch** than normal. It may be associated with **clawing of the toes**. The appearances are similar to those of a neurological foot, suggesting that this condition is related to a muscle imbalance. It is seen in conditions such as hereditary sensory motor neuropathy, spinal cord abnormalities and polio.

Investigation

Clinical diagnostic indicators

The toes are clawed, the metatarsal heads are forced down into the sole causing metatarsalgia, the heel is inverted and the Achilles tendon and calf are often tight.

Neurological abnormalities must be excluded.

Management

Treatment is rarely required. If the forefoot is painful then an **insole** that distributes the weight all over the sole of the foot may be useful.

Surgery is indicated if the foot is still painful.

If the deformities are flexible then **tendon release and lengthening** and **osteotomies** to realign the bones are indicated.

As the deformity becomes more fixed with irreversible damage to the joints, **fusion surgery** may be the only option.

METATARSALGIA

This is a term used to describe general pain in the ball of the foot. It is usually caused by an uneven weight distribution with patients reporting a feeling of walking on marbles or stones. Certain shapes of foot predispose to this, in particular those with relatively long second and third metatarsals. Patients with a high arch foot (pes cavus) load their metatarsals more. Treatment may be **thicker padded insoles** or offloading the painful area with a **felt or silicone metatarsal pad**.

MORTON'S NEUROMA

Repetitive trauma to the interdigital nerves from tight or ill-fitting shoes may lead to the nerve being thickened and inflamed and give rise to a painful

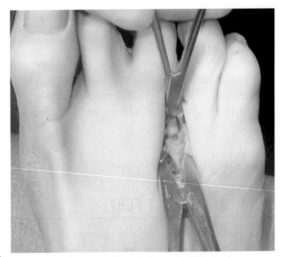

FIGURE 9.18   Intraoperative photograph of Morton's neuroma

neuroma. The ball of the foot is one of the most unpleasant places to have a neuroma as weight is taken at this point.

Investigation

Clinical diagnostic indicators

Patients may complain of numbness or burning, typically in the third webspace, although 10 per cent are found in the second webspace. Pinching pressure at this point recreates the pain, A large neuroma may be associated with a clicking sensation (a 'mulders' click) when the metatarsal heads are squashed together.

Imaging

Ultrasound is the most accurate method of diagnosis. An **MRI scan** may also be used.

Management

A **metatarsal pad** can take pressure off this area.

A **steroid injection** can reduce, temporarily, some of the inflammation and discomfort.

If the pain persists, a more permanent solution is **excision of the neuroma** and affected interdigital nerve (Fig. 9.18). The web space will be permanently numb but not painful.

PLANTAR FASCIITIS

This is the commonest cause of a painful heel. It is caused by inflammation of the plantar fascia.

Patients may report it starting after overuse or a change in shoe wear.

The diagnostic feature of the history is whether the pain is at its worst on getting out of bed in the morning or after having been at a desk or behind a steering wheel for a while, so-called '**start-up pain**'.

The mainstay of treatment is **calf stretching** which indirectly stretches the plantar fascia, if required with physiotherapy supervision.

NSAIDS and **cushioned shoes** can be helpful.

CALLOSITY/CORNS

Callosities/corns appear as areas of hardened, sometimes yellow, skin on pressure points or around bony areas of the foot. Corns form on or between toes; callosities form on the bottom of the feet. They develop to protect the foot from damage but can be a source of pain. Excessive pressure and friction on one area of the foot causes the skin cells to multiply and then die. This leads to a thickened area of skin known as a corn or callus.

Calluses protect bones that don't have natural fat pads to protect them, and develop usually after prolonged wear and tear or rubbing on the shoe. They tend to be a broad area of thickened skin. They are often painless but those that form because of structural problems can become painful on walking. Corns often form as a result of irritation from tight shoes. Hard corns may form on the top of structural problems and at the sides of toes, soft corns form between the toes.

Management

Treatment starts by removing the cause, initially by advising **shoe wear adjustments**. Wider shoes with a shallow heel allow more space for the toes whereas pointed heels make the foot slide downhill into the shoe, cramming the toes into an already narrow toe box.

Redistributing foot pressure away from the area of callus by a custom **insole** may also help.

Corns caused by hammer or claw toes often settle once the bony deformity is corrected.

Plantar callus, which is often seen under the second and third metatarsals, may be treated surgically by a **shortening osteotomy** of the metatarsals to redistribute load around the foot more evenly.

An important exception is the presence of diabetes or peripheral neuropathy. These patients need to be cared for by a specialist podiatrist because any skin break is associated with a higher rate of skin infection and serious complications.

PLANTAR WART

These are often confused with a callus but are generally more painful. They can be differentiated from a corn by being painful, especially if squeezed and if paring down the hyperkeratic skin reveals a papillomatous core dotted with small blood vessels. They are difficult to treat. Corn plasters with salicylic acid may help, but eradication is difficult. Cryosurgery can help as may curettage followed by packing with iodine. Occasionally the whole wart needs to be excised.

FREIBERG'S INFRACTION

This is a crushing type of osteochondritis of the second, and occasionally the third, metatarsal head. It typically affects young adults, mostly women. The metatarsal head becomes enlarged and the joint palpable and painful on stressing. **X-rays** may show the head to be flattened. Initial treatment comprises resting the foot in a boot, hard-soled shoe or a cast. A custom **insole** can take pressure off the joint.

An open **debridement** of the joint and a simple **realignment osteotomy** of the metatarsal head can be performed if these measures fail to relieve the pain. This shortens and decompresses the joint and rotates the good cartilage upwards can treat the pain successfully.

PLANTAR FIBROMATOSIS/ DUPUYTREN'S OF THE FOOT

These are benign growths that occur on the bottom of the foot. A similar condition occurs on the palms of the hands (Dupuytren's contracture) and on the penis (Peyronie's disease).

Its cause is unknown. It may be the result of tiny tears in the plantar fascia which then undergo rapid repair, and actually over-repair the area. Thickened nodules develop along the course of the plantar fascia which may invade the overlying dermis and sometimes the flexor tendons on the bottom of the foot.

The nodules may lay dormant for years only to rapidly increase in size in a very short period of time. It is commoner in men and 25 per cent of cases are bilateral.

Typically, patients present more out of concern about the lump than pain, but the lumps can become painful.

Management

If the nodules are not painful the treatment of choice is to leave them alone. If there is pain, simple care involves padding in the shoe to keep pressure off the lumps.

If conservative measures fail to remove the pain the only other option is **surgical excision**. This is not a straightforward procedure. Recurrence is high as, unlike in the hand, all the diseased tissue cannot be removed as the plantar fascia is critical to normal gait. Also as the incision usually has to be on the bottom of the foot the patient may exchange the fibroma for a painful scar that hurts just as much to walk on as the original lump.

10

The spine

Thomas Ember

INFECTION

Infections of the spine usually affect either the vertebral body or the intervertebral disc, but infections in the epidural space, paraspinal soft tissues and occasionally the posterior elements of the spinal column may also occur.

Spinal infections may be *pyogenic* (bacterial) or *non-pyogenic* (often referred to as atypical and which include tuberculosis and fungal infections).

Pyogenic infections

Most arise following the *haematogenous spread* (a bacteraemia) of a urological, respiratory or skin infection but contiguous (direct) spread can also occur from a penetrating injury or from an adjacent infection, e.g. a retroperitoneal abscess.

Risk factors include diabetes mellitus, alcohol abuse, immunocompromise secondary to HIV infection and organ transplantation, intravenous drug abuse and malignancy.

The commonest infecting organism in more than 50 per cent of cases is *Staphylococcus aureus* but several other organisms may be isolated, including *Pseudomonas* (particularly in intravenous drug users), *Escherichia coli, Klebsiella* and *Proteus* (secondary to genitourinary infections), *Salmonella* (in sickle cell patients) and *Staphylococcus epidermis/streptococcus* (following post-operative metal work infection).

Half of all spinal infections occur in the lumbar spine, 40 per cent in the thoracic spine and less than 10 per cent in the cervical spine. Children and the elderly people being particularly affected.

Because of their disc's rich supply children tend to develop an infection within the disc space itself (a discitis) via haematogenous spread. The adults' less vascular disc is less amenable to the spread of infection via the blood stream and therefore infection typically starts as a **vertebral endplate osteomyelitis** (the endplate of the vertebra is the most vascular part).

As the endplate infection progresses it eventually involves the disc space itself and subsequently causes the typical 'spondylo-discitis' that is seen in adults, i.e. infection of two contiguous vertebral endplate regions and the intervening disc. This may be accompanied by the presence of an epidural abscess (spread of infective material into the spinal canal).

Non-pyogenic infections: tuberculosis

Tuberculosis is increasing in many areas because of the increased incidence of immunosuppression (e.g. secondary to HIV infection), increased immigration and the development of multiple drug-resistant strains.

Mycobacterium tuberculosis is widely distributed in nature and has three microbiologically very distinctive features owing to the complex composition and high lipid content of its cell wall.

(1) It is an acid-fast bacillus and is able to resist decolorization with strong acids.
(2) It stains poorly by Gram's method and hence the special Ziehl–Neelsen stain is required.
(3) It does not grow on ordinary culture media but will grow on Lowenstein–Jensen medium. Incubation takes 2–3 weeks.

The mycobacteria family include *M. tuberculosis* (humans), *M. bovis* (cattle) and *M. leprae* (humans – leprosy). The defining pathological feature of *M. tuberculosis* is that it results in a granulomatous infection. The primary infection is usually caused by inhalation of aerosolized organisms, which results in a primary lung infection. The patient usually quickly recovers from what is often a relatively minor respiratory infection but years later a reactivation may occur with presentation of secondary extrapulmonary metastases, which are most commonly seen in the vertebral bodies. The organisms deposited in the vertebral body precipitate a delayed-type hypersensitivity reaction. The **granulomatous response** involves the **accumulation of monocytes, epitheloid** and **Langerhan's cells**.

Caseation occurs and is surrounded by a **dense fibrosis** that lifts the anterior longitudinal ligament causing cavitation and vertebral body collapse. This may result in a kyphotic deformity and neurological sequelae.

Other non-pyogenic infecting organisms include tuberculosis, brucella, *Actinomyces israelii*, fungi (including aspergillous, *Histoplasma capsulatum*, *Cryptococcus neoformans* and candida species) and yeasts, (*M. tuberculosis* is by far the commonest).

Investigation

Clinical diagnostic indicators

Children usually present with either non-specific back pain or difficulty or refusal to walk.

Adults typically present with non-specific back pain and may also have constitutional symptoms (fevers, night sweats or weight loss).

The symptoms are so non-specific that in over 50 per cent of cases a diagnosis is not made until 3 months after they began.

The presence of neurological abnormalities is a rare mode of presentation (more typically seen with cervical and thoracic infection). Progressive kyphosis can result in neurological sequelae (Pott's paraplegia).

Blood tests

Full blood count, erythrocyte sedimentation rate (ESR) and C-reactive protein (CRP) may indicate chronic infection and inflammation.

Imaging

Plain radiographs are often unhelpful as visible change can take up to 12 weeks to develop.

Magnetic resonance imaging (MRI) is the most useful investigation. There is an increased signal intensity on T2 weighted images caused by the presence of increased water (oedema); a reduced T1 signal intensity as the bone marrow (which is white on T1 as it is mainly made up of fat) becomes replaced by inflammatory and oedematous changes.

Contrast agents (gadolinium) are helpful when identifying the presence of epidural abscess (results in ring enhancement of the abscess).

MRI later shows vertebral body collapse with relative sparing of the disc space, anterior epidural mass with elevation of the anterior longitudinal ligament and skip lesions. With gadolinium there is an absence of rim enhancement as the infecting material is not pus but granulation tissue.

A **bone scan** may reveal a hot spot and is valuable if MRI is contraindicated.

Tissue biopsy and culture

Biopsy can be performed using either fluoroscopic or computed tomography (CT) guidance. It confirms the diagnosis in both pyogenic infections and tuberculosis.

Management of pyogenic infections

The mainstay of treatment is the intravenous administration of an appropriate **antibiotic**. When serial inflammatory markers (in particular the CRP, which is more sensitive than the ESR) have significantly reduced, the antibiotics may be given orally. Adults require longer treatment with antibiotics as their discs are avascular.

The indications for **operative intervention** are the failure of medical management, progressive spinal deformity, neurological compromise or significant epidural abscess.

The principal objectives of surgery are the removal of infected material, decompression of the neural elements and rigid stabilization (pedicle screws and cages).

Management of non-pyogenic infections

The **pharmacotherapeutic treatment** of tuberculosis requires combination chemotherapy for between 6 months and 1 year. Typical regimens include isoniazid, rifampicin, pyrazinamide and streptomycin.

Spinal braces may be used to prevent the formation of kyphotic deformity.

PAEDIATRIC SPINAL DEFORMITY

Spinal deformity can occur in the coronal plane (scoliosis – a lateral curvature of the spine) and the sagittal plane (kyphosis, lordosis and spondylolisthesis).

Scoliosis can be classified as congenital, idiopathic and neuromuscular. Rarer causes include infection, tumour, degeneration and trauma.

Congenital scoliosis

Congenital scoliosis is a lateral curvature of the spine caused by developmental vertebral anomalies that result in an imbalance in the lateral longitudinal growth of the spine. These osteogenic anomalies can be classified as failures of formation (hemivertebrae, see Figure 10.1) and failure of segmentation (bony bar formation) or a combination of the two.

Congenital scoliosis is thought to be caused by **disorders of the homeobox genes** during the first trimester of pregnancy and is associated with a high incidence (up to 60 per cent) of other abnormalities within or outside the spine, particularly in those organ systems that develop in the first trimester, i.e. the genitourinary system and the heart. Up to 15 per cent also have intraspinal anomalies, including cord tethering, syringomyelia or diastematomyelia.

The failure of formation most commonly seen is the hemivertebra (unilateral complete failure of vertebral formation). The hemivertebra may be described as fully segmented (with a disc above and below), semi-segmented (a single disc either above or below) or unsegmented (fused above and below). The potential to cause deformity is related to the asymmetry of active growth plates and therefore the fully segmented hemivertebra has the worst prognosis whereas an unsegmented hemivertebra has limited potential to produce deformity.

A failure of segmentation results in the formation of a bony bar that tethers the growth of a vertebral segment, resulting in differential growth across the spine. A unilateral unsegmented bar with a contralateral segmented hemivertebra has the most severe risk of curve progression.

Idiopathic scoliosis

Idiopathic scoliosis is classified as early onset (less than 5 years old) or late onset (more than 5 years old). Early-onset scoliosis differs from late-onset scoliosis in that it is more common in boys, and left thoracic curves predominate. Some of these children have associated abnormalities, such as congenital heart disease, developmental delay and developmental dysplasia of the hips.

The prevalence of adolescent idiopathic scoliosis is estimated to be two to three per thousand. It is four times more common in girls (and for those requiring intervention the ratio is 9:1).

Management

The management of early and late onset scoliosis differ as the early onset group are too young to undergo definitive fusion (as this would restrict lung development and truncal growth). Treatment is therefore aimed at controlling the curve until such an age where definitive fusion is possible. This is achieved by the use of serial plaster jackets, spinal braces and in the cases that are progressive the use of growing rod constructs that can be lengthened as the child grows.

Plaster jackets are used for progressive cures in the under fives. Older children can have thermoplastic braces to try and control curve progression.

The objectives of **surgery** in these children is to maintain growth and control the curve. Several techniques have been described but none is perfect. Many advocate the use of a **posterior growth rod technique**, which allows for longitudinal growth while maintaining distraction across the curvature in order to try to limit its progression, followed by a definitive **posterior spinal fusion** performed when the child is deemed old enough.

Adolescent idiopathic scoliosis

Adolescent idiopathic scoliosis is much more common in girls, and typically results in the formation of a right thoracic curvature. The prevalence is 3 per cent, and 0.3 per cent go on to require treatment. There is occasionally a **family history**, and various hormonal factors, especially melatonin and calmodulin, have been implicated. These children are essentially normal, but during periods of significant spinal growth the vertebrae rotate resulting in the typical thoracic rib hump deformity.

Investigation

Clinical diagnostic indicators

The two most common classifications of curves are the **King** classification and the **Lenke** classification.

Factors associated with a high risk of curve progression are a young age at diagnosis, female sex, double major curves, left-sided curves and the curve magnitude at diagnosis.

Imaging

When viewing a **plain radiograph**, the curves are described as if one is looking at them from behind in the same way as one views the child clinically.

Management

The treatment options are very much based on the natural history of these idiopathic curves, so regular monitoring is essential.

On reaching skeletal maturity, a curve of less than 40 degrees is unlikely to progress further. Such curves are unlikely to be cosmetically troublesome and therefore can be managed conservatively.

Curves that are greater than 50 degrees on attainment of skeletal maturity have the potential to continue to progress at an expected rate of 1–2 degrees per year. Therefore, curves greater than 50 degrees tend to be treated surgically.

Some curves between 40 and 50 degrees demonstrate late progression. These curves must be managed on an individual basis and the degree of cosmetic deformity also taken into account. If conservatively managed, it is imperative that these curves are monitored for evidence of late progression.

The role of **bracing** is contentious. There is certainly no role for braces in curves that are of a significant magnitude and in children who are approaching skeletal maturity. However, there can be a role for a thoracolumbar support (thermoplastic TLSO brace) in skeletally immature children who have relatively small curves (25–40 degrees) which are progressive on serial radiographs.

The **surgical approach** can be either anterior (via a diaphragm splitting thoraco-abdominal approach) or posterior. The majority of curves are managed via the posterior route using **multisegmental**

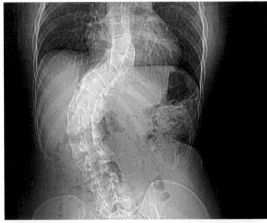

(A)

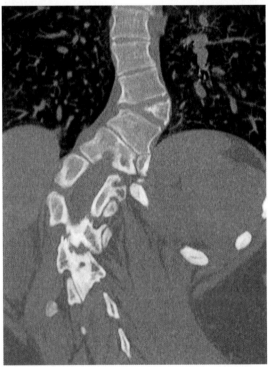

(B)

FIGURE 10.1   (A) Plain X-ray of a congenital scoliosis with a hemivertebra at T9. (B) Coronal CT scan of the same patient

pedicle screw constructs (Fig 10.2). The curves are corrected by a combination of translation, derotation and vertebral body rotation. This is essentially a fusion procedure and meticulous decortication of the posterior elements must be performed prior to laying down of bone graft.

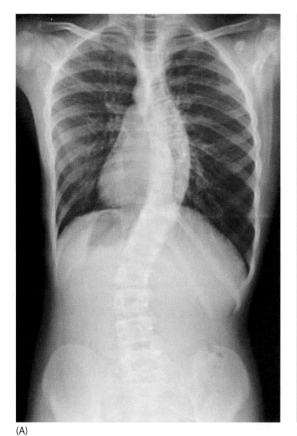

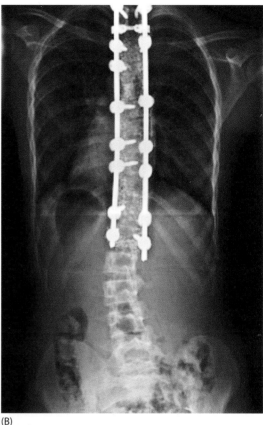

(A)   (B)

FIGURE 10.2   Scoliosis. (A) A whole spine radiograph showing a right thoracic scoliosis. (B) A post-operation radiograph of the same patient showing correction by multi-segmental pedicle screw instrumentation

NEUROMUSCULAR SCOLIOSIS

Neuromuscular curves can be classified as neuropathic or myopathic. The underlying causes of these deformities are set out in Table 10.1.

The risk of curve formation varies according to the underlying condition (cerebral palsy 25 per cent, myelodysplasia 60 per cent, spinal muscular atrophy (SMA) 67 per cent, Freidrich's ataxia 80 per cent, Duchenne's muscular dystrophy 90 per cent, spinal cord injury under 10 years old 100 per cent).

Neuromuscular curves differ from idiopathic curve patterns because they tend to form long C-shaped curves which result in an associated pelvic obliquity. There is rarely any compensatory curve formation. These curves will tend to progress despite attainment of skeletal maturity.

Table 10.1
The causes of neuropathic and myopathic scoliosis

Neuropathic	Myopathic
Upper motor neurone	Duchenne's muscular dystrophy
Rett's syndrome	
Friedrich's ataxia	Congenital myopathies
Hereditary motor and sensory neuropathy	Arthrogryposis
Myelomeningocele	
Lower motor neurone	
Spinal muscular atrophy	
Polio	

Management

Once they reach a significant magnitude, these curvatures can cause pain and discomfort, loss of seating balance, respiratory compromise, sometimes pressure sores and even late neurological deficit.

Treatment should aim to reduce the deformity and arrest progression, thus allowing maximal independence and a stable sitting balance.

Management of these children requires a multidisciplinary approach with treatment modalities including bracing, specialized seating and spinal surgery.

The indications for surgical intervention include progressive scoliosis in spite of bracing, increasing pelvic obliquity, loss of curve flexibility and decreasing independence.

The **surgical options** are similar to those for idiopathic curvatures. The majority are treated by a posterior instrumented spinal fusion. However, in contrast to idiopathic curves where one is trying to fuse the least number of levels possible, the rule with neuromuscular curvatures is to 'go long'. Many of these curves also require fusion to the pelvis in order to correct the associated pelvic obliquity.

SPONDYLOLYSIS/SPONDYLOLISTHESIS

(Greek; Spondylos = vertebrae, lysis = defect). Spondylolysis describes a defect in the pars interarticularis region of the posterior spinal elements. (Greek; Olisthesis = slippage.) Spondylolisthesis, first described by Herbinaux, a Belgian obstetrician, in 1782, describes the forward displacement of one vertebra over the vertebra below it.

Spondylolysis affects 3–6 per cent of the general population. Onset after skeletal maturity is rare. It is commonest in white males and rare in Africans. The highest incidence, which is seen in Alaskan Native Americans (up to 26 per cent), is postulated to be caused by the amount of time spent stooping down while harvesting whale blubber!

The most common level affected is L5 (85–95 per cent). Most of the rest occur at L4.

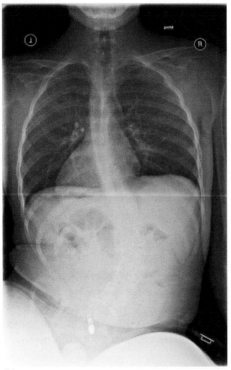

(A)

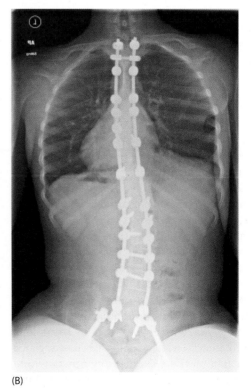

(B)

FIGURE 10.3 (A) A whole spine radiograph showing a long C-shaped curve with pelvic obliquity caused by Duchene's muscular dystrophy. (B) Surgical correction

Table 10.2
The types of spondylolisthesis
(Willtse and Newman)

Type 1 – congenital/dysplastic (a, b, c)

Type 2 – isthmic (a, lytic fatigue fracture of pars;
 b, elongated but intact pars; c, acute pars
 fracture)

Type 3 – degenerative

Type 4 – traumatic

Type 5 – pathological (generalized or local bone
 disease)

Type 6 – post-surgical (iatrogenic)

Dysplastic spondylolisthesis is more common in females (2:1). It is the only true congenital form. The posterior facet complexes either fail to fully develop or are abnormally aligned such that they fail to act as a buttress to the forward slip of L5 on the sacrum. Although the spine is mechanically vulnerable and displacement tends to occur early, the degree of displacement is limited by impingement of the intact posterior neural arch on anterior structures. As the L5 vertebral body slips forward, the movement of the posterior bony arch causes the early symptoms of lumbar spinal stenosis or **cauda equina syndrome**. This is in contrast to the isthmic group (see below), where there is a defect in the pars region which means that when the L5 vertebral body slips forward it does not take the posterior neural arch with it, and therefore the risk of neurological compromise is markedly reduced.

Isthmic spondylolisthesis is by far the commonest group and describes a defect in the pars interarticularis region. There is a 5–7 per cent incidence in the general population, which is often symptomless. It is two times more common in males. The pars defect is thought to be an acquired lesion akin to the stress fracture seen elsewhere in the skeleton. It is postulated to be the result of repetitive hyperextension resulting in the caudal edge of the inferior articular facet of L4 making repeated contact with the pars of L5. This explains why it is seen more commonly in gymnasts, weight lifters and cricket bowlers, all of whom perform repetitive hyperextension type movements. Pars defects have never been reported in non-walking species, suggesting they are secondary to our upright posture.

Investigation

Clinical diagnostic indicators

Eighty per cent of spondylolistheses are symptomless. Of the 20 per cent of patients who develop symptoms, half have a slip that is mild and rarely progresses. Thus the vast majority of patients with spondylolisthesis have a benign clinical course without a significantly increased risk of low back pain.

A minority develop high-grade slips (grade 3 and 4), which may cause low back pain, hamstring tightness, L5 radiculopathy or, in extreme cases, cauda equina syndrome.

The risk factors for progression are onset at a young age, female sex, a high degree of slip at presentation, a slip angle of greater than 40 degrees, and instability on flexion/extension radiographs.

Imaging

(Fig 10.4) The Meyerding classification is used to grade the degree of slippage of one vertebra on another on an X-ray. *Spondyloptosis* is the most severe form and describes the translation of the entire vertebral body in front of the one below.

Management

There are numerous surgical techniques for managing symptomatic high-grade slips using a posterior, anterior or combined approaches. The general objectives are to decompress the neural structures and achieve a solid fusion to prevent further slip progression.

SCHEUERMANN'S DISEASE

Scheuermann's disease (idiopathic adolescent kyphosis) is postulated to be a growth disorder of the vertebral end-plate resulting in wedging that produces a kyphosis.

Although often symptomless, it may present with thoracic back pain and/or an associated deformity – a fixed as opposed to a postural kyphosis.

Imaging

The diagnostic **X-ray** feature is of 5 degrees wedging of at least three contiguous vertebrae and an

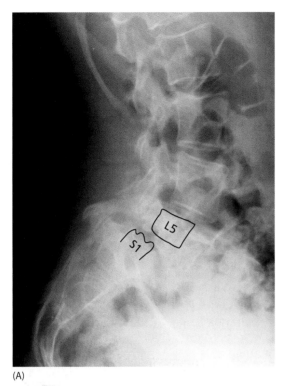
(A)

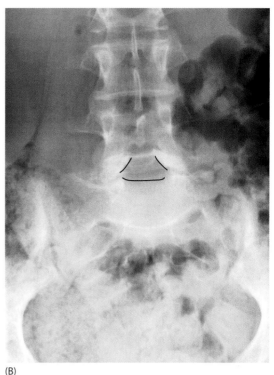
(B)

FIGURE 10.4   (A) Lateral radiograph showing a high-grade isthmic spondilolisthesis with a large pars defect (parallel lines).
(B) AP radiograph of the same patient showing a typical 'Napoleon hat' appearance

overall kyphosis of more than 60 degrees. The vertebral endplates are often irregular with evidence of extrusion of disc material into the vertebral body (Schmorl's nodes).

Management

Conservative treatment modalities include analgesia, physiotherapy and bracing until skeletal maturity is achieved.

Posterior spinal fusion (sometimes preceded by an anterior release of the discs) is reserved for cases of severe progressive deformity.

SPINAL TUMOURS

Spinal tumours are classified as primary (benign or malignant) or secondary (metastases). Spinal metastases are 40 times more common than primary malignant tumours. Primary spinal tumours account for less than 10 per cent of all primary bone tumours.

Benign and malignant primary spinal tumours have differing features. The common primary benign spinal tumours are listed in Table 10.3.

Benign tumours are more common in the young and in the posterior elements of the spine whereas malignant tumours are more common in elderly people and in the vertebral bodies.

Table 10.3
The common primary benign spinal tumours

Haemangioma
Osteochondroma
Osteoid osteoma and osteoblastoma
Aneurysmal bone cyst
Eosinophilic granuloma (Langerhan's cell histiocytosis)
Giant cell tumour

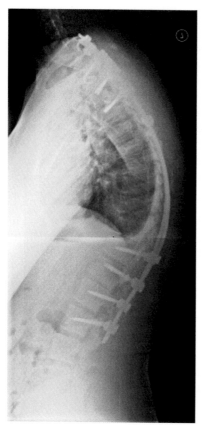

FIGURE 10.5   Control of a global kyphosis by surgical fixation

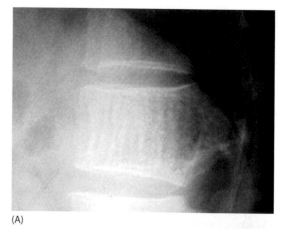

(A)

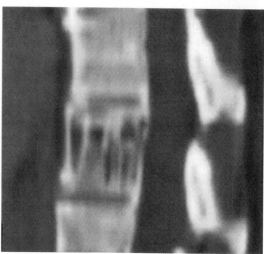

(B)

FIGURE 10.6   Haemangioma. A lateral radiograph (A) and saggital CT scan (B) showing the typical striated appearance

BENIGN SPINAL TUMOURS

Haemangioma

These are the commonest benign spinal tumours (they are not a true tumour but rather dilated venous channels and fat within the vertebral body). They are an incidental finding on an MRI scan and are present in 10 per cent of the population.

Plain radiographs demonstrate thickened trabeculae (jailbar/honeycomb striated appearance).

MRI images demonstrate increased signal intensity on both T1 and T2 images.

They are usually symptomless and rarely require treatment (Fig 10.6).

Osteochondroma

These are benign cartilaginous tumours that are more common in the appendicular skeleton than the spine (less than 5 per cent). They arise from areas of enchondral ossification and result in solitary or multiple bony exostoses (multiple is usually the hereditary form).

Plain radiographs demonstrate sessile or pedunculated osteoblastic lesions.

If they arise in the spine they rarely cause symptoms, but if their slow growth results in neural compression they may have to be **excised**.

Osteoid osteoma and osteoblastoma

These are histologically identical but differentiated by the size of the central lucent nidus (osteoid osteoma <1.5 cm, osteoblastoma >1.5 cm).

In the spine almost all occur within the pedicle.

They typically present with **pain** – especially night pain (which is often relieved by salicylates) – and may produce a painful scoliosis with the tumour at the concavity of the apex of the curve).

Plain radiographs are of little value other than detecting a secondary scoliosis that can be differentiated from structural curves by the absence of rotation.

CT imaging and bone scintigraphy may demonstrate sclerosis around the central lucent nidus (Fig 10.7). The osteoid osteoma demonstrates more sclerosis whereas the osteoblastoma is a more expansile lesion.

The natural history may be of spontaneous resolution, but this can take between 2 and 8 years and therefore intervention is usually required in the form of **radiofrequency ablation** or **surgical excision** (posterior curettage and grafting).

Aneurysmal bone cyst

Aneurysmal bone cysts (ABC) are rare in the spine. Similar to the giant cell tumour, they cause an expansile osteolytic lesion with thinning of the cortex, more often in the neural arch than the vertebral body (Fig 10.8).

Management requires **complete excision**. There is a high recurrence rate after incomplete removal.

Eosinophilic granuloma

This (Langerhan's histiocytosis) is a granulomatous process (an abnormal proliferation of Langerhan's cells in the bone marrow) of unknown cause. It usually affects children between the ages of 5–10 years and is the most common cause of vertebra plana.

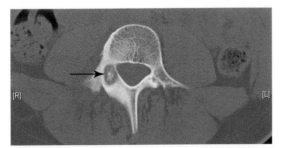

FIGURE 10.7 The typical appearance of an osteoid osteoma >15 cm located in the neural arch with a central nidus and surrounding sclerosis

Plain X-rays or MRI demonstrate wedge-shaped vertebral body collapse (vertebra plana) (Fig 10.9).

Tissue biopsy is often required to confirm the diagnosis.

This is a self-limiting condition which is managed with **analgesia** and occasionally a TLSO brace. Occasionally **curettage and radiotherapy** is required for the more aggressive lesions.

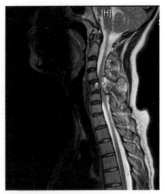

FIGURE 10.8 Aneurysmal bone cyst. A saggital T2 MRI scan showing an aneurysmal bone cyst in a cervical vertebra

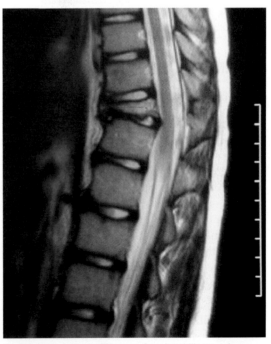

FIGURE 10.9 Lateral MRI scan of eosinophilic granuloma, showing the typical flattened vertebrae (vertebra plana)

Giant cell tumour

This is the most aggressive of all the benign primary tumours and can undergo malignant transformation. It can occur in the sacrum or vertebral body and cause back pain.

Plain radiographs demonstrate an expansile osteolytic lesion similar in appearance to the aneurysmal bone cyst but differentiated by the fact that the ABC tends to occur in the posterior elements rather than in the anterior part of the spine (Fig 10.10).

Management involves **complete excision** plus or minus **adjuvant radiotherapy**. There is a high recurrence rate after incomplete excision.

PRIMARY MALIGNANT SPINAL TUMOURS

Primary malignant spinal tumours are extremely rare. They typically occur in the vertebral body. Eighty-five per cent cause back pain – particularly at night – with associated constitutional symptoms, including weight loss. The three common primary malignant spinal tumours are:

- myeloma (multiple and solitary plasmacytoma)
- chordoma
- sarcoma (osteosarcoma, chondrosarcoma, Ewing's sarcoma).

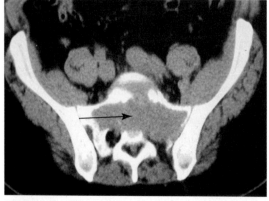

FIGURE 10.10 Giant cell tumour in the sacrum. Its appearance is similar to that of an aneurysmal bone cyst but aneurysmal bone cysts tend to affect the posterior elements rather than the vertebral body

Multiple myeloma

Multiple myeloma is the commonest primary malignant spinal tumour. It is a lymphoproliferative abnormality of the B cells within the vertebral body causing it to collapse. It typically presents in elderly people (60+ years) with back pain and/or a progressive kyphotic deformity secondary to multiple vertebral body collapse.

The presence of **Bence–Jones protein** in the urine and on serum electrophoresis is diagnostic.

Plain radiographs demonstrate multiple lytic lesions with very little surrounding bony reaction. Consequently they are cold on bone scan.

Chemo- and radiotherapy are the treatments of choice. **Surgery** is reserved for progressive deformity, neurological compromise and intractable pain. Vertebroplasty (injecting cement into the vertebral body) has been increasingly used.

Solitary plasmacytoma is of a similar histology but occurring in a single vertebral body. The prognosis is very different – vertebrectomy is potentially curative.

Chordoma

Chordoma is the second most common malignant tumour. It is a malignancy of the notochordal remnants and therefore occurs in the midline (mainly in the sacrum but also cervical spine).

MRI demonstrates a large midline anterior mass, which is often advanced before diagnosis. Complete resection can be curative, but this is often not possible because of adjacent structures.

Sarcoma

This is rare in the spine. *Osteosarcoma* is exceptionally rare. It tends to occur in a young age group. The mainstay of treatment is chemotherapy as it is radio-insensitive.

Chondrosarcoma affects an older age group. It is chemo- and radio-insensitive and thus requires *en bloc* excision.

Ewing's sarcoma affects children and is highly chemosensitive. Chemotherapy is used as an adjunct before and following *en bloc* excision of the affected spinal segment.

SECONDARY MALIGNANT SPINAL TUMOURS

Secondary spinal tumours (spinal metastases) are by far the commonest spinal tumours. The typical primary sites include **breast, lung, prostate, kidney, gastrointestinal tract and thyroid.**

The malignant cells probably travel to the spine via the thin-walled valveless paravertebral venous plexus of Batson.

The **presenting features** include worsening spinal pain (often including night pain), radicular pain (leg/arm), motor weakness, bladder or bowel disturbance and constitutional symptoms (weight loss, anorexia, fatigue).

Investigation

Blood tests

Full blood count, urea and electrolytes, liver function tests, calcium, clotting and tumour markers, and serum electrophoresis.

Urinalysis

Bence–Jones protein is present in patients with multiple myeloma.

Imaging

Small lesions may be missed on X-rays as 50–70 per cent bony destruction must occur before lesions are visible. Lesions that are osteolytic (kidney, lung, colon and melanoma) cause bone destruction with vertebral body collapse. The osteoblastic metastases of carcinoma of the prostate cause bone sclerosis.

CT images of the chest, abdomen and pelvis are needed for staging and detecting other metastases.

Whole spine MRI scan imaging shows a reduced T1 signal if bone marrow is replaced by tumour.

Bone scan

Beware of false negatives, e.g. a cold scan with non-osteoblastic metastases as in carcinoma of the breast.

Tissue biopsy

CT or fluoroscopic guided.

Management

The main treatment modalities available are chemotherapy, radiotherapy and surgery employed in a multimodal combination. A multidisciplinary approach with medical oncologists, palliative care and specialist nurses is essential.

For example, chemosensitive tumours are usually treated by **neoadjuvant chemotherapy** in order to achieve 90 per cent tumour kill prior to surgical resection and then either further chemo- or radiotherapy if the margins are involved.

The *chemosensitive tumours* include small cell lung carcinoma, Ewing's tumour, cancers of the thyroid and breast and neuroblastoma.

Although 80–85 per cent of tumours may be radiosensitive, **radiotherapy** is only of value for reducing soft tissue compression. Renal cell, gastrointestinal tract adenocarcinomata and melanoma are chemo- and radioresistant.

The management of spinal metastases is **palliative rather than curative**. The therapeutic objectives are pain relief and preservation of nerve function. Relative contraindications to surgery include widespread visceral or brain metastases, more than three contiguous spinal levels affected, and an expected survival of less than 3 months.

DEGENERATIVE DISORDERS OF THE CERVICAL SPINE

Cervical spondylosis is a non-specific term that was introduced by Schmorl in 1929 to describe 'chronic degenerative changes caused primarily by intervertebral disc decay'. It must be regarded as a normal 'wear and tear' process because it is seen on plain radiographs in 35 per cent of 41–50 year olds, 80 per cent of 51–60 year olds and 95 per cent of 61–70 year olds, but in most instances it is symptomless (Fig 10.11).

Cervical spondylosis may cause axial neck pain, cervical radiculopathy or cervical myelopathy. Cervical myelopathy is an upper neurone lesion (central compression of the spinal cord itself) whereas radiculopathy is a lower motor neurone lesion (compression of the exiting nerve root).

Both cervical myelopathy and radiculopathy are caused by degenerative changes within any or all of the five articulations that make up a single motion segment of the cervical spine – the interverteral disc, two facet joints and two uncovertebral joints (also referred to as the joints of Luschka). Hypertrophic changes secondary to wear and tear may encroach centrally on the spinal canal (myelopathy) or at the exit foramina (radiculopathy).

The neuro-anatomy of the cervical spine is unique because the nerve roots exit above the pedicle of the same number (e.g. the C5 nerve root exits above the C5 pedicle in the C4/5 interspace and hence a C4/5 disc herniation will result in C5 nerve root compression). This is the opposite to the thoracic and lumbar spine, where the nerve root exits below the pedicle of the same number (e.g. the L4 nerve root exits below the L4 pedicle in the L4/5 interspace).

Investigation

Clinical diagnostic indicators

Cervical myelopathy typically presents with altered sensation, weakness and clumsiness of the hands and eventually legs (the patient often describes a feeling of drunkenness when walking). Sensory disturbances can occur with more severe compression. The neurological findings are those of an upper motor neurone lesion – increased tone, brisk reflexes, clonus and upgoing plantars caused by compression of the corticospinal tracks. Alteration in light touch and pressure sensation may occur with anterior spinothalamic tract compression and changes in temperature sensation if the lateral spinothalamic tract is involved.

Cervical radiculopathy results in pain and sensory changes affecting the distribution of the affected nerve root:

- C3 compression – occipital headaches, pain around the mastoid process and pinna of the ear
- C4 compression – pain/numbness of the base of neck/trapezius muscle
- C5 compression – deltoid region with loss of biceps reflex
- C6 compression – typical brachialgic pain down the arm with loss of brachicoradialis reflex
- C7 compression – brachialgic pain down the forearm with altered sensation running into the middle finger and weakness of the triceps muscle and triceps jerk
- C8 compression – pain/sensory disturbance of the medial forearm and into the ring/little finger with weakness of the intrinsic muscles of the hand.

Imaging

The investigation of choice is **MRI** for demonstrating the location, degree and cause of the compression (Fig 10.12).

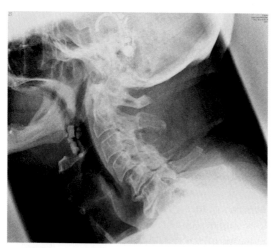

FIGURE 10.11   Cervical spondylosis: a lateral radiograph showing severe multi-level degeneration of the cervical spine

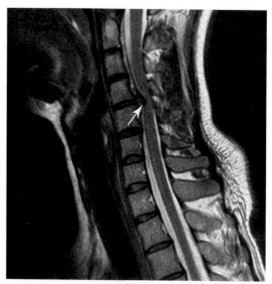

FIGURE 10.12   A sagital T2 MRI scan showing a large C4/5 central disc prolapse compressing the spinal cord

Disc protrusions are often described as 'soft discs' (herniation of nucleus palposus resulting in radiculopathy in much the same way as seen in the lumbar spine) or 'hard discs', which are disc osteophyte bars. Central disc bulges in combination with degenerative changes in the facet joints result in central cord compression with the loss of the cerebrospinal fluid (CSF) water signal on the sagittal and axial images and often evidence of intrinsic cord signal changes suggestive of damage within the spinal cord itself (a prognostic indicator).

Management

The natural history of cervical radiculopathy and myelopathy are different.

Cervical radiculopathy

This is often a self-limiting condition.

Conservative treatment includes anti-inflammatory medication, physiotherapy and selective nerve root block and are often effective.

Cases resistant to conservative treatment may be considered for **surgical intervention**, either in the form of **anterior cervical discectomy** and **fusion** with **decompression of the exiting nerve root** or **posterior decompression** (foraminotomy), depending on the site of maximal compression.

Cervical myelopathy

Numerous natural history studies indicate that some patients improve while others deteriorate slowly or rapidly in a stepwise progression.

The role of surgical intervention is to arrest further neurological deterioration. Several studies indicate that the longer the duration of symptoms the worse the outcome of the decompression, hence surgery should be offered early.

Various **surgical approaches** have been described. The spine can be decompressed anteriorly (**discectomy or corpectomy**) or posteriorly (**laminectomy or laminoplasty**) the approach being tailored to where the maximal compression is located on the imaging.

DISORDERS OF THE THORACIC DISCS

Thoracic disc prolapse is rare. It accounts for less than 4 per cent of all symptomatic disc prolapse. The prevalence is one in a million. It affects the 30- to 50-year-old group with an equal incidence between males and females.

Investigation

Clinical diagnostic indicators

The presentation is very variable. The pain may be axial or radicular in nature (radicular pain results in a band-like sensation wrapping around the chest, which can be mistaken for a myocardial infarction). Sensory complaints are usually in the T10 dermatome regardless of the level of the root compression. The clinical findings will be of an upper motor neurone lesion in the legs. The arms are not affected.

Imaging

The investigation of choice is an **MRI scan** to demonstrate the level and degree of the compression. **CT imaging** is also useful following diagnosis to differentiate between calcified discs (more likely to be symptomatic) and non-calcified discs.

Management

Conservative treatment options include analgesia, physiotherapy and intervertebral nerve blocks.

Surgical decompression can be via an anterior or posterior route directed at the location of the pathology.

DEGENERATIVE DISORDERS OF THE LUMBAR SPINE

Degenerative disease of the lumbar spine is very common and typically presents with activity-related low back pain. The underlying cause is 'wear and tear' but previous injury and genetic predisposition increase the incidence.

A spinal segment is made up of the vertebral body, the intervertebral disc and the posterior elements (laminae, facet joints and spinous process).

The facet joints are true synovial joints and hence develop **osteoarthritic changes** similar to that seen in other joints (e.g. hip/knee). The disc on the other hand is not a true joint and wear and tear changes are better described as '**degenerative disc disease**' rather than osteoarthritis.

Degenerative disc disease and facet complex degeneration are often symptomless. The discs and facet joints are mechanically intrinsically linked and therefore wear is almost always seen in a whole segment. The initial changes occur in the disc. Proteoglycan degradation in the nucleus pulposus reduces the disc's ability to retain water (the proteoglycans are strongly hydrophilic and therefore allow the disc to retain a high percentage of water). The loss of water from the disc alters its mechanical properties and exposes the proteoglycans to increased sheer stresses, resulting in further degradation and loss of water (the degeneration is therefore a self-perpetuating process). Associated degeneration within the annulus of the disc (the tough fibres containing the disc anteriorly and posteriorly) can result in tears within its substance, which can be a potent cause of low back pain. The disc itself has no innervation but the posterior annulus is richly supplied by branches of the sinuvertebral nerve.

Degeneration within the annulus makes it vulnerable to prolapse of the central disc material (a **prolapsed intervertebral disc**). The loss of water within the disc results in a loss of disc height, which then causes increased loading of the facet joints resulting in secondary osteoarthritic changes within these joints (a potential cause of low back pain).

The degenerative changes within the facet joints result in hypertrophy, which combined with loss of disc height, bulging of the posterior annulus, and thickening with infolding of the ligamentum flavum – may cause narrowing of the spinal canal, i.e. **spinal stenosis**.

Disc prolapse

Investigation

Clinical diagnostic indicators

The lifetime risk of a prolapsed intervertebral lumbar disc is 30–40 per cent, occurring at a mean age of 20–40 years. The level most commonly affected is L4/5 followed by L5/S1.

It is important to remember the definitions of the terms used when describing the effect of prolapsed discs:

- sciatica: leg (Latin)
- cauda equina: the continuation of the spinal cord below its termination at L1 as individual spinal nerves bathed in CSF. It is described as resembling a horse's tail
- radiculopathy: leg pain secondary to pressure on a nerve root from a prolapsed intervertebral disc. The pain usually extends below the knee in the distribution of the compressed nerve resulting in sensory disturbance, paraesthesia and occasional motor weakness
- disc bulge: a diffuse, circumferential bulging of disc material (see fig 10.13)
- disc protrusion: asymmetric migration of disc material (typically posterolaterally) with an intact annulus (see fig 10.13)
- disc extrusion: asymmetric migration of disc material through the annulus (see fig 10.13)
- disc sequestration: a migrated disc fragment no longer in continuity with the parent disc that has migrated either caudally or cranially
- cauda equina syndrome: severe compression of the cauda equina caused by a massive central disc prolapse resulting in bilateral sciatica, motor weakness, saddle anaesthesia and bladder or bowel dysfunction. This syndrome presents a surgical emergency.
- anatomical zones of disc prolapse are described as central, posterolateral (commonest), foraminal and extraforaminal
- traversing nerve root: the root that is usually compressed by a disc prolapse. e.g. an L4/5 disc prolapse will compress the traversing L5 nerve root. The exception is a far lateral disc prolapse which may compress the exiting L4 nerve root.

The **presentation of a disc prolapse** varies according to the affected level:

L4/5 disc→compression of L5 root→buttock pain, from lateral calf to big toe, extensor hallucis

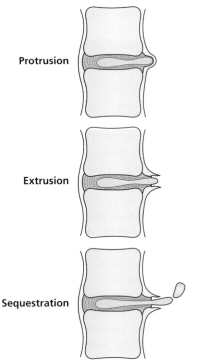

Protrusion

Extrusion

Sequestration

FIGURE 10.13 The three forms of disc prolapse – protrusion, extrusion and sequestration

longus weakness, L5 dermatome sensory disturbance

L5/S1→compression of S1 root→lateral thigh to posterior calf: pain, weakness of ankle plantar flexion, absent ankle jerk, S1 dermatome sensory disturbance

L3/4→compression of L4 root→pain in the posterolateral thigh region and anteromedial aspect of the lower leg, motor weakness of the quadriceps (knee extension) and absence of the knee jerk.

Imaging

The investigation of a patient with sciatic leg pain consists of the following.

Plain radiographs are obtained to assess abnormalities of segmentation (in particular lumbosacral transitional vertebrae) and detect evidence of a spina bifida occulta if surgical intervention is being considered.

MRI scanning is the best method for demonstrating the level, size and morphology of a disc prolapse.

Management

Treatment should be **conservative** whenever possible given the fact that the natural history of the disc prolapse is favourable. Seventy to ninety per cent of cases resolve with conservative treatment measures over an 8- to 12-week period, and of these 90 per cent do not relapse. Of the 10 per cent who relapse, 90 per cent resolve in a further 8–12 weeks but 50 per cent will suffer further relapse.

Conservative treatment consists of **analgesia, anti-inflammatory medication, physiotherapy, selective nerve root injections/caudal epidural**, all of which aim to reduce the inflammation around the nerve root sheath.

There is no role for extended bed rest.

Operative treatment (**open** or **percutaneous discectomy**) is indicated when the symptoms fail to resolve with conservative treatment or there is a progressive neurological deficit or cauda equina syndrome develops.

The risks of lumbar microdiscectomy are small but include infection (wound, pyogenic discitis and epidural abscess), dural tear, vascular injury and recurrent disc prolapse.

LUMBAR SPINAL STENOSIS

Lumbar spinal stenosis is a narrowing of the spinal canal that compresses the neural elements. The causes can be classified as congenital (achondroplasia with short pedicles or other skeletal dysplasia – rare) and acquired (degenerative – common). The narrowing of the spinal canal is described as being either in the central region, the lateral recess or foraminal (neural foramen). The abnormality begins as degenerative changes within the disc cause a reduction of the disc height and posterior bulging of the annulus. The reduction in disc height causes infolding of the ligamentum flavum, which also becomes hypertrophied. Degenerative osteoarthritic changes (hypertrophy and osteophyte formation) result from the increased loading of the facet joints. The combination of these changes results in the typical **trefoil-shaped narrowing** of the cauda equine (Fig 10.14).

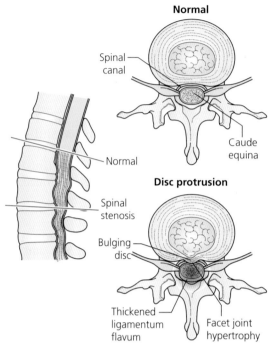

Normal

Spinal canal

Caude equina

Normal

Disc protrusion

Spinal stenosis

Bulging disc

Thickened ligamentum flavum

Facet joint hypertrophy

FIGURE 10.14   Spinal stenosis may be caused by disc protrusion and facet joint hypertrophy

Investigation

Clinical diagnostic indicators

The differential diagnosis of lumbar spinal stenosis includes **osteoarthritis of the hips**, **peripheral vascular disease** (vascular intermittent claudication) and **peripheral neuropathy**. The distinction between neurogenic and vascular claudication can be difficult but there are certain defining differences (see Chapter 11).

Neurogenic claudication is improved by forward flexion so the pain is eased by walking up a hill, whereas vascular claudication gets worse when going up hill. The neurogenic claudication distance is variable but the vascular claudication distance is relatively constant.

There are often few or no other clinical signs in patients with neurogenic claudication, but patients with vascular claudication usually have reduced or absent pulses and other signs of peripheral vascular insufficiency (see Chapter 11).

Imaging

Investigations include **plain radiographs**, **MRI imaging** and occasionally **CT/myelography**.

Ultrasound studies of the circulation may be needed to exclude peripheral vascular claudication.

Management

Conservative treatment including anti-inflammatory medication, physiotherapy, caudal or lumbar epidurals and a TENS machine is the initial treatment of choice.

Severe cases who fail to respond to conservative treatment can be managed **surgically** with **decompression**, which may be either open or distractive.

There is considerable argument within the literature about the role of fusion at the time of an open decompression (fusion may be posterolateral or interbody). The indications for fusion include a degenerative spondylolisthesis, recurrent stenosis and a severe stenosis requiring complete facet joint removal with a resulting potential for instability.

Distractive decompression involves **placing a spacer** between the spinous processes in order to indirectly decompress the canal by distracting the segment. Early results suggest this has a role in patients with mild to moderate compression who are otherwise too unfit to undergo open spinal surgery.

BONE AND CALCIUM METABOLISM

Bone is a reservoir for 99 per cent of the body's calcium and 85 per cent of its phosphate (the rest is found in plasma).

Calcium is absorbed from the gut by an active ATP-driven transport process which is stimulated by 1,25 vitamin D3. Calcium is subsequently excreted in the kidney.

Bone mineral homeostasis is controlled by **vitamin D3, parathyroid hormone (PTH) and calcitonin.**

Vitamin D is acquired via two sources: diet (vitamin D3) and the conversion of 7-dehydrocholesterol by ultraviolet light to cholecalciferol (vitamin D3). Cholecalciferol is subsequently hydralized in the liver into 25-OH-cholecalciferol (25-OH-vitamin D3) and this is then activated in the proximal convoluted tubercle of the kidney into 1,25-dihydroxycholecalciferol (vitamin D3). This active metabolite can then act on the gut to increase calcium and phosphate reabsorption and within bone to cause osteoid mineralization.

Parathyroid hormone is an 84 amino acid polypeptide secreted by the chief cells of the parathyroid glands in response to reduced serum calcium levels. Parathyroid hormone acts to increase reabsorption of calcium in the kidneys and stimulates osteoclastic activity, resulting in release of calcium from bone.

Calcitonin is a 32 amino acid polypeptide from clear parafollicular cells in the thyroid gland. Calcitonin acts to reduce the serum calcium level and is secreted in response to raised serum calcium. Calcitonin directly inhibits osteoclastic activity.

Other hormones that have an effect on bone mineral homeostasis include **oestrogen**, which prevents bone loss by inhibiting bone reabsorption, **corticosteroids**, which increase bone loss by reducing bone formation, **thyroid hormones**, which increase bone reabsorption (hence large doses of thyroxin can cause osteoporosis), and **growth hormone**, which increases serum calcium.

OSTEOPOROSIS

Osteoporosis is a skeletal disorder characterized by a reduction of bone strength predisposing to an increased risk of fractures. It is a quantitative not a qualitative defect.

Risk factors include:

- genetics (ethnicity, family history, low body mass index)
- medical (rheumatoid arthritis, Cushing's syndrome, chronic diseases)
- drugs (corticosteroids, anticonvulsants, chemotherapy, alcohol, smoking).

The pathogenesis is an uncoupling of bone formation by osteoblasts and bone absorption by osteoclasts.

Osteoporosis typically develops in elderly postmenopausal women. It is usually symptomless until a fracture occurs after minimal trauma. Hip and distal radius fractures and vertebral compression fractures are the most common.

Definitions

- Osteopenia: decreased bone mass.
- Osteoporosis: decreased bone mass, normal mineralization.
- Osteomalacia: bone mass variable, decreased mineralization.

Investigation

Screening blood tests

Exclude hyperthyroidism, Cushing's disease, haematological disorders and malignancy: thyroxine, TSH, ACTH and full blood count.

Imaging

Appropriate **plain radiographs** and/or **MRI scan imaging** (Fig 10.15).

DEXA scan is the diagnostic gold standard. It is dual X-ray absorptiometry, which is performed on the spine and the hip.

Management

Prevention is by advising a proper diet and, in appropriate cases, hormone replacement therapy (HRT).

Drug treatment includes **dietary calcium** and **vitamin D supplements. Bisphosphonates,** are

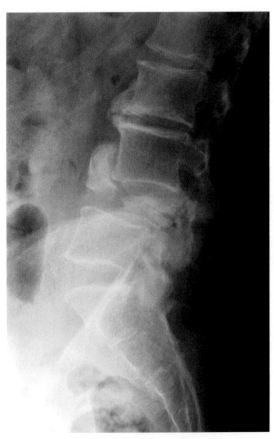

FIGURE 10.15   Severe osteoporosis causing L4 collapse

synthetic analogues of inorganic pyrophosphate and inhibit bone reabsorption by osteoclasts.

SPINAL TRAUMA

Spinal injuries are becoming increasingly common, particularly in developed countries, because of the increasing use of high-speed transportation and recreational activities.

The majority of spinal injuries occur in the thoracolumbar T12–L2 segment, where there is a transition between the rigid thoracic spine and the more mobile lumbar spine.

The differing mechanisms and unique features of the different zones of the spinal column require spinal injuries to be divided as follows:

- fractures of the C1 (atlas) and C2 (axis) segments
- fractures of the subaxial cervical spine (C3–C7)
- fractures of the thoracic spine
- thoracolumbar fractures
- low lumbar fractures.

C1 (ATLAS) AND C2 (AXIS) FRACTURES AND DISLOCATIONS

The first two cervical vertebrae have a unique anatomy.

C1 (**the atlas**) supports the globe of the head. It is a ring structure with anterior and posterior arches and bulky lateral masses to support the weight of the head but has no vertebral body (this has evolved into the peg of the C2 segment.

C2 (**the axis**) forms a pivot on which the C1 vertebra (which is carrying the head) is able to rotate. Its most distinctive feature is the tooth-like process (the odontoid process) projecting from the upper surface of its body. The odontoid process (also known as the dens or peg) has two articulating processes – one anteriorly with the atlas, and one posteriorly with the transverse ligament.

The four injuries/fractures that can occur in the C1/C2 region are:

- atlanto-occipital dislocation
- Jefferson fractures
- odontoid peg fractures
- hangman's fracture.

Atlanto-occipital dislocations are extremely rare injuries and often fatal. They typically occur as a result of a high-speed road traffic accident causing hyperextension and distraction with rotation of the craniocervical junction. They usually result in brain stem and proximal spinal cord injury with loss of the breathing centres and death.

Jefferson fractures involve the atlas and result from compression of the bony ring. They account for 10 per cent of all cervical spine injuries (Fig 10.16).

The typical causal mechanism is axial compression (for example diving into an empty swimming pool), which splits the lateral masses and tears the transverse ligament. These fractures have been classified into three types by Levine and Edwards (type I, posterior arch fracture; type II, anterior arch fracture; type III, the Jefferson burst fracture).

The radiological hallmark of this injury is lateral displacement of the C1 lateral masses as the bony rings splay open. This is best seen on the open mouth (peg) X-ray view and on CT imaging.

The treatment is the **application of a halo** to immobilize the cervical spine.

Odontoid peg fractures are the commonest cervical spine fractures accounting for approximately 18 per cent of all injuries (Fig 10.17). They usually result from a blow to the occiput, either during a fall or a road traffic accident.

They have been classified by Anderson and D'Alonzo into three types:

- Type I is an avulsion fracture of the tip of the peg and can be treated conservatively with a collar.
- Type II is a fracture to the waist of the peg and has a high incidence of non-union as this area is a vascular watershed. In elderly people these are often managed with a collar when painless non-union is acceptable. In younger patients, either a halo or surgical fixation is often indicated.
- Type III is a fracture through the body of the peg. These can be treated in a halo as they have a very high rate of union because there is a large bony surface area for healing.

Hangman's fractures are bilateral fractures through the pars interarticularis region of the axis following a hyperextension distraction injury (Fig 10.18). The typical mechanism is judicial

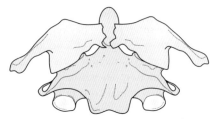

FIGURE 10.16 The Jefferson fracture – a lateral displacement of the bony masses of C1, usually following axial compression

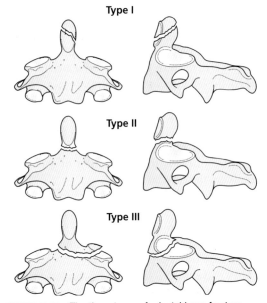

Type I

Type II

Type III

FIGURE 10.17 The three types of odontoid peg fracture

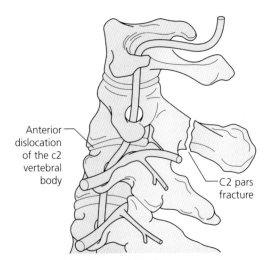

Anterior dislocation of the c2 vertebral body

C2 pars fracture

FIGURE 10.18 The hangman's fracture

hanging but also road traffic accidents where the chin hits the dashboard. This results in a traumatic spondylolisthesis of C2 on C3 with an avulsion injury of the anterior inferior corner of C2. These injuries are rarely associated with neurological injury as the canal is of a wide diameter at this level.

Treatment is typically with a **halo** unless there is dislocation of the facet joints, in which case **reduction and surgical stabilization** is required.

SUBAXIAL CERVICAL SPINE (C3–C6) FRACTURES AND DISLOCATIONS

Subaxial cervical spine injuries have been classified by Allen and Ferguson (Table 10.4). It is a mechanistic classification. Distractive flexion is the commonest injury and often a result of road traffic accidents.

The severity of the injury may be divided into five stages, but in essence they can be regarded as a continuum of increasing severity ranging from the subluxed facets to the facets becoming perched and subsequently dislocated (which may be unifacetal or bifacetal – by far the commonest).

Investigation

Imaging

The investigations of choice for these injuries are **plain radiographs** and **CT imaging** (Fig 10.19).

Table 10.4 Subaxial cervical spine injuries (Alan and Ferguson)	
Movement	**Possible stages (see text)**
Compressive flexion	1–5
Distractive flexion	1–4
Compressive extension	1–5
Distractive extension	1–2
Vertical compression	1–3
Lateral flexion	1–2

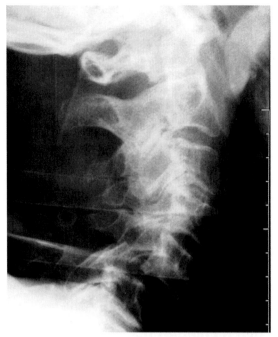

FIGURE 10.19 Lateral radiographs showing a C5/6 bi-facetal dislocation. Note the >50% translation of C5 on C6

The role of **MRI** prior to reduction of these injuries remains controversial. It is valuable to ascertain whether or not there is a disc prolapse (as a result of the injury) prior to reduction. Reduction may result in a large disc injury being prolapsed further towards the spinal cord, resulting in neurological injury. Patients who are unable to respond to regular neurological assessments while attempting a closed reduction warrant urgent MRI.

Management

The treatment of choice is **closed reduction** using Gardner–Wells tongs, starting with 10 lb (4.5 kg) of weight, analgesia and intravenous relaxation followed by 5- to 10-lb increases in weight with a full neurological assessment prior to each increase in weight, plus fluoroscopy to judge the degree of distraction and reduction achieved.

The indications for **operative treatments** are failure of closed reduction or a significant disc prolapse on an MRI scan.

THORACOLUMBAR FRACTURES AND DISLOCATIONS

Thoracolumbar fractures are the commonest of all spinal injuries. Because the segments between T12 and L2 are between the rigid thoracic spine and more mobile lumbar spine, they are biomechanically at greater risk of injury. It is important to remember the relationship between the spinal cord, conus and cauda equina and hence the type and degree of neurological injury that may be associated with fractures at each region.

Always look for a second level injury. Remember that 20–25 per cent of patients with a spinal fracture at one level have a further spinal injury, half of which will be non-contiguous.

The classification of thoracolumbar spinal fractures remains a matter of debate. The Denis classification describes the spine as three columns:

- anterior column: anterior longitudinal ligament, anterior half of vertebral body and disc
- middle column: posterior half of vertebral body and disc and posterior longitudinal ligament
- posterior column: pedicles and laminae.

The fractures are classified as compression, burst, seatbelt and fracture dislocations.

All can affect different columns, have a different axis of injury and varying degrees of stability (Table 10.5).

Investigation

Imaging

The investigation of spinal injuries invariably begins in the Emergency Department with a trauma series of **plain radiographs** (C-spine, chest and pelvis). Spinal imaging should be performed when indicated.

Computed tomography Once a spinal fracture is detected on plain radiographs, there is usually a role for delineating the exact bony anatomy with CT imaging.

MRI scans including STIR sequences have a particular role in determining whether or not there is a posterior ligamentous injury. This is of particular significance when assessing the stability of

Table 10.5
The Denis classification of thoracolumbar spine injuries

Type of fracture	Anterior column	Middle column	Posterior column	Mechanism of fracture	Stability	Treatment
Compression	Compressed	Intact	Intact	Compression about the middle column axis	Stable	Conservative
Burst	Compression	Compression	Intact	Compression about the posterior column axis	Often unstable	Often surgical
Seatbelt	Intact	Distraction	Distraction	Distraction about the anterior column axis	Often unstable	Surgical
Fracture dislocations	Compression plus rotation	Distraction plus rotation	Distraction plus rotation	Translation and distraction about a variable axis	Unstable	Surgical

the posterior tension band in thoracolumbar burst fractures.

Management

Conservative treatment includes analgesia, bed rest and extension braces.

Surgery may involve anterior column reconstruction, posterior pedicle screw instrumentation with distractive decompression by ligamentotaxis and 360-degree fusion techniques. The choice of surgery will depend upon the exact injury anatomy and spine stability.

LOWER LUMBAR (L3–L5) FRACTURES

The management of lower lumbar fractures (L3–L5) is different from that of thoracolumbar junction fractures. They are relatively uncommon.

These segments are stable and there is less potential for post-traumatic kyphotic instability because the vertebral bodies at this level are below the pelvic rim and have the strong iliolumbar ligaments attached to them. These injuries can usually be **managed conservatively**.

11

The arteries, veins and lymphatics

Matthew Waltham and Kevin G. Burnand

Many of the problems caused by diseases of the arteries, veins and lymphatics are common to all of the causative diseases. The problems include:

- pain
- discoloration
- dysfunction
- pulsatile swellings
- visible veins
- swelling
- ulceration of the skin.

Pain

The causes of leg pain can usually be detected by a careful history and examination. Investigations provide only confirmatory information and guidance for further management.

Pain caused by ischaemia may be confirmed by the absence of a blood flow signal on a handheld Doppler flow detector, the measurement of the ankle–brachial pressure indices (ABPIs), and imaging with duplex ultrasound or angiography.

The presence of an acute deep vein thrombosis (DVT) causing pain is usually confirmed by ultrasonography.

Orthopaedic and neurological causes of pain may be confirmed by a combination of plain radiography and more detailed imaging such as magnetic resonance imaging (MRI).

Some of the causes of pain in the lower limb are listed in Table 11.1.

Discoloration

The skin colour may vary between white, blue and red according to the level of skin blood flow.

Venous abnormalities associated with venous hypertension cause intradermal deposition of haemosiderin giving the skin a deep brown colour.

Some of the causes of discoloration are listed in Table 11.2.

Dysfunction

The pain, swelling and deformities caused by the vascular diseases listed in Table 11.1 often interfere with the function of a limb.

Pulsatile swellings

Expansile pulsating swellings – dilated arteries – may develop in any part of the arterial tree but most often occur in the abdominal aorta, iliac, femoral and popliteal arteries. Most are associated with degenerative arterial disease but some are related to

Table 11.1
Some of the causes of acute pain in the lower limb

Arterial	**Acute ischaemia of the leg caused by:**
	Embolism
	Thrombosis
	Thrombosed aneurysm
	Trauma
	Aortic dissection
	Chronic ischaemia of the leg causing:
	Intermittent claudication
	Rest pain
	Ulceration
	Gangrene
Venous	Deep vein thrombosis, acute and post thrombotic
Orthopaedic	Hip/knee/spine
Neurological	Sciatica

Table 11.2
Some of the causes of discoloration

Arterial	Ischaemia
	Gangrene
	Embolism
Venous	Venous obstruction/deep vein thrombosis
	Phlegmasia alba dolens
	Phlegmasia cerulea dolens
	Venous gangrene
Systemic	Pigmentation
	Peripheral cyanosis/hypoperfusion

Table 11.3
The causes of pulsatile swellings

Arterial	Arterial degenerative disease
	Infection – mycotic aneurysms
	Artery wall dissection
	Collagen disorders
	Trauma
	Arteritis

Table 11.4
The causes of dilated (usually varicose) veins

Congenital (primary)

Secondary (to proximal obstruction)

Thrombophlebitis

Haemorrhage

Arteriovenous fistula

Table 11.5
Some of the causes of swelling of the lower limb

Venous	Deep vein thrombosis – post thrombotic
	Venous malformations
Lymphatic	Congenital
	Acquired – metastatic/infections
	Lymphangitis
	Lymphatic reflux
	Lymphangiomata
	Lymphadenopathy
Systemic disease	Heart failure
	Renal failure
	Hypoproteinaemia

haemodynamic factors, e.g. post-stenotic dilatation (Table 11.3).

An ultrasound scan is the quickest and simplest way to confirm that the swelling is an artery and that the pulsations are expansile, not transmitted.

Visible veins

Many patients present complaining about distended visible veins. Although they may have made a correct diagnosis, investigations may be needed to ascertain the cause (Table 11.4) and decide on treatment.

Swelling/oedema

There are many causes of swelling of the lower limb, local vascular and general medical (Table 11.5). The diagnosis of oedema is made by showing that the swelling pits with direct digital pressure. The investigations, which may have to be extensive, should be designed to detect the cause.

Ulceration of the skin

The main causes of ulceration of the skin of the lower limb are listed in Table 11.6.

ACUTE ISCHAEMIA OF THE LOWER LIMB

Acute interruption of the blood supply to the lower limb is caused most commonly by a thromboembolus originating more proximally in the circulation (usually from the heart in atrial fibrillation) or by *in situ* thrombosis on the background of significant peripheral vascular disease. Less commonly, it is the

Table 11.6
The causes of ulceration of the skin

Arterial	Gangrene
Venous	Deep vein thrombosis – post thrombotic
Systemic disease	Diabetes (neuropathic)
Orthopaedic	Osteomyelitis
Malignancy	Squamous or basal cell carcinoma
Autoimmune	Rheumatoid arthritis

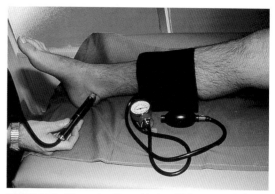

FIGURE 11.1 Measuring the ankle brachial pressure index (ABPI). A cuff is placed around the lower leg and inflated until the Doppler signal disappears in the pedal vessels. The pressure at which this occurs is expressed as a ratio to brachial pressure

result of thrombosis of a popliteal aneurysm, direct trauma, bypass graft thrombosis or iliac branch occlusion in an acute aortic dissection. A reduction in arterial perfusion causes acute pain. When the leg is severely ischaemic there will be progressive loss of nerve function leading to paraesthesia and paralysis, ultimately leading to tissue death.

Investigations

Diagnostic clinical indicators

The presence of the '**6 Ps**' is characteristic (**pain, pallor, pulseless, paraesthesia, paralysis** and **perishing cold**). The limb may be mottled or white. Neurological dysfunction is a late sign and indicates that the viability of the limb is in jeopardy.

Muscle tenderness may indicate local ischaemia, muscle death or a compartment syndrome.

Fixed staining of the skin, muscle rigidity or loss of function are indicators of tissue death.

It is important to seek for a source of an **embolus** by checking the heart rhythm for atrial fibrillation, auscultating for abnormal heart sounds and palpating for an aortic or iliac aneurysm.

A history of previous claudication suggests *in situ* **thrombosis**, whereas the presence of all peripheral pulses in the contralateral limb supports embolism.

A history of a **previous arterial bypass** suggests that the bypass has occluded.

Ischaemia from **trauma** is usually obvious from the history and clinical findings. Arteries may be damaged by blunt or sharp trauma.

Acute aortic dissection is usually accompanied by severe chest, abdominal, and back pain.

Blood flow detection

Examination with a hand-held Doppler probe may confirm absent or reduced blood flow in the peripheral arteries. The ABPI will be significantly reduced (Fig 11.1) (see *Symptoms and Signs*).

In cases where embolism is highly likely on clinical grounds and the limb is threatened, it is reasonable to attempt revascularization without further imaging.

Imaging

Imaging investigations are not always necessary when the survival of the limb is threatened.

Suitable imaging includes **duplex ultrasonography**, **digital subtraction angiography** (DSA) or **computed tomography** (CT) **angiography**. Intra-arterial DSA has the advantage that the imaging can be followed by therapeutic intervention.

The aim of imaging is to establish the site of the vascular occlusion and the presence of distal vessels in case bypass is necessary. Sometimes it confirms that an embolus is the cause by the characteristic angiographic appearance (Fig 11.2). A CT angiography may show an aorto-iliac source of an embolus.

Magnetic resonance angiography with gadolinium contrast is now available in many hospitals and is comparable to CT.

Haematology

A full blood count excludes polycythaemia or thrombocytosis/thrombocythaemia.

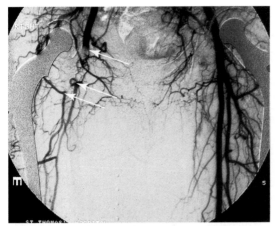

FIGURE 11.2   Digital subtraction angiogram showing a thromboembolus obstructing flow at the bifurcation of the right common femoral artery. The arrows show the top of the embolus. A sharp cutoff is seen

A raised white cell count, C-reactive protein and erythrocyte sedimentation rate suggests a vasculitic cause. A thrombophilia screen should be performed.

Biochemistry

The serum potassium may be raised if there has been significant prolonged ischaemia.

Muscle death and rhabdomyolysis may cause acute renal failure and there may be myoglobinuria. This can be confirmed with a dipstick test.

ECG and echocardiogram

An **electrocardiogram** may show a cardiac dysrhythmia (for example atrial fibrillation). A transthoracic or transoesophageal **echocardiogram** may reveal a cardiac source of an embolus, e.g. intracardiac thrombus or valvular disease.

Emergency care

Patients should receive adequate analgesia and fluid replacement if dehydrated. The circulation should be optimized to maximize perfusion and oxygen delivery to the affected limb. A bolus of 5000–10 000 units of heparin should be given intravenously if treatment is likely to be delayed.

Conservative palliative care

Conservative management of an acutely ischaemic limb is only indicated if the general condition of the patient precludes intervention, for example if the patient is moribund or has severe co-morbidities. Occasionally, if the ischaemia involves the distal circulation, a 'wait and see' approach may be taken. The management should aim to minimize the patient's suffering with appropriate analgesia.

Anticoagulation may be indicated to reduce the progression of a thrombotic vessel occlusion if the extent of limb loss is uncertain.

Complications of palliative care A critically ischaemic limb will become progressively gangrenous and this may lead to a general deterioration, leading to multi-organ failure and death.

Occasionally the condition of the limb and the patient may improve. This should prompt a re-evaluation of the management. In distal ischaemia the tissue may demarcate into viable and non-viable areas.

Complex monitoring should cease if the decision has been made to restrict treatment to palliative care.

Results of palliative care Conservative management of an acutely ischaemic limb results in a high early mortality, from a combination of septicaemia, multi-organ failure and complications of immobility.

Thrombolysis

Thrombolysis may be indicated when acute thrombosis is the cause of the ischaemia but is contra-indicated if there is a specific risk of bleeding, e.g. recent surgery, peptic ulceration or stroke.

Thrombolysis is most successful for **thrombosed prosthetic bypass grafts** (e.g. PTFE grafts) if given within the first couple of weeks, the limb is not too ischaemic and able to survive the 24–48 hours that it often takes to successfully restore circulation (Fig 11.3).

Thrombolysis can be tried for **thrombosed popliteal aneurysm**, especially where the distal vessels are occluded. It may also be used to restore run-off below an occlusion so that bypass surgery can be performed. **The patient must always be told of the risks of bleeding.**

Procedure After angiography has been performed to confirm the site and nature of the occlusion a perfusion catheter is positioned within the vessel or graft adjacent to the thrombus.

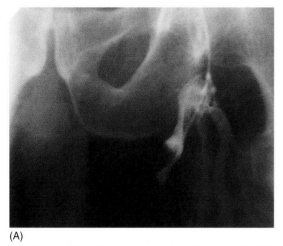
(A)

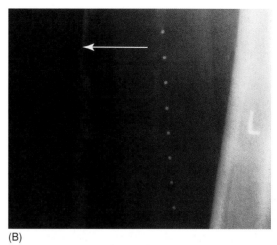
(B)

FIGURE 11.3   Thrombolysis of a prosthetic bypass graft. (A) The catheter tip delivering the lytic agent is just in the thrombus that is occluding the prosthesis. (B) The graft is beginning to clear (arrow)

A bolus of **recombinant tissue plasminogen activator (tPA)** (e.g. 5 mg) is given to lace the thrombus followed by an infusion (e.g. 1 mg/hour).

A **heparin infusion** is given at the same time to prevent rethrombosis. A suction catheter can also be used to attempt to manually remove clot. Angiography is performed at 12- to 24-hour intervals to monitor progress.

Once thrombolysis is successful a cause for the occlusion should be sought and treated, e.g. angioplasty can be performed on a bypass graft stenosis that caused a thrombosis.

Complications

Haemorrhage The patient must be monitored for haemorrhagic complications. Most often this manifests as oozing around the catheter site but may be **intracranial and fatal**.

The thrombolysis must be stopped and the patient resuscitated appropriately if there are any signs of haemorrhage.

Distal embolization During thrombolysis, fragments of the thrombus or clot may embolize into the distal circulation and exacerbate the ischaemia. Although this may make the pain worse, the treatment should be continued to lyse the distal emboli.

Compartment syndrome Once perfusion is restored the patient is at risk of developing a compartment syndrome. Fasciotomies must be performed if a compartment syndrome is suspected after reperfusion (Fig 11.4).

Results

Thrombolysis is most successful when applied to fresh recent thrombus: 70–80 per cent limb preservation, 10 per cent death.

Surgical treatment

Urgent surgical intervention to save the limb is required in many patients with acute lower limb ischaemia.

Depending on the cause and the underlying disease in the vessels, treatment can range from a simple femoral embolectomy to a distal bypass procedure. Careful clinical assessment with appropriate imaging can help predict what procedure will be necessary but the patient should be consented and prepared in the operating room for any of the following procedures.

Femoral embolectomy can be performed under local anaesthetic in frail patients or those with significant co-morbidity. Regional anaesthesia (epidural or spinal) may be considered but may not be possible if anticoagulants have already been given.

An operating table suitable for on-table angiography should be used and radiographers alerted.

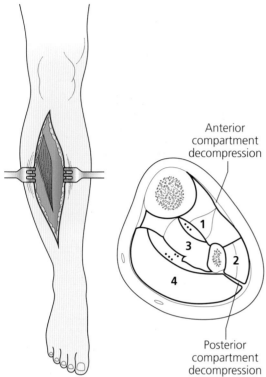

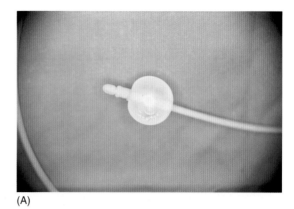

(A)

FIGURE 11.4   The fascial compartments of the lower leg and the site of entry to them

The common femoral artery is exposed and controlled with slings. After giving a bolus of **intravenous heparin** a transverse arteriotomy is made just proximal to the femoral bifurcation. **Fogarty balloon embolectomy catheters** are then used to remove the thrombus from the proximal and distal arteries (Fig 11.5). The embolic material retrieved should be sent for microbiological and histological studies. The arteriotomy is closed with a polypropylene suture.

It may be necessary to explore the below-knee popliteal artery if there is residual thrombus or clot in the distal superficial femoral or popliteal artery that cannot be removed via the femoral arteriotomy. Distal procedures require a general anaesthetic. A bolus of tPA can be given into the distal vessels to attempt to lyse any residual thrombus or clot.

A surgical bypass will be required if it is not possible to remove the thrombus with an embolectomy catheter – usually because of pre-existing atherosclerosis (see below).

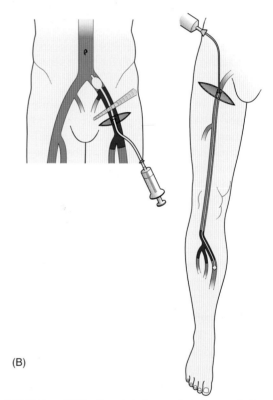

(B)

FIGURE 11.5   (A) The Fogarty balloon embolectomy catheter. (B) The method of using the Fogarty balloon catheter to remove thrombus from the iliac and popliteal arteries

Bypass operations: Aortic or iliac occlusions may be bypassed with an **aortofemoral, femorofemoral or iliofemoral prosthetic graft**. If the patient is unwell, unfit or has had previous abdominal surgery then **axillofemoral bypass** may be considered (Fig 11.6C).

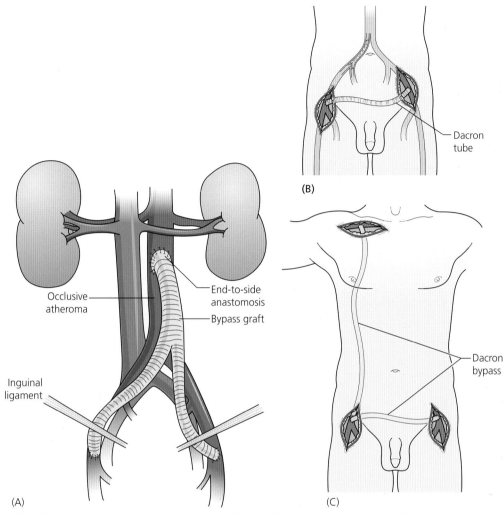

FIGURE 11.6 Types of aortic and iliac bypass operations: (A) aortobifemoral; (B) femorofemoral; (C) axillofemoral

For femoral or distal occlusions a **femorodistal bypass**, preferably using a vein as the conduit rather than a prosthetic graft (Fig 11.7), may be performed after performing pre- or intraoperative angiography to assess run-off and select a suitable distal vessel for the distal anastomosis.

Amputation is likely to be necessary if the limb is not viable or if revascularization fails. The level of the amputation (metatarsal, below knee or above knee) is chosen to preserve as much living tissue as possible without compromising healing (Fig 11.8). A level of demarcation between viable and non-viable tissue may be visible if the patient has been well enough to have been managed conservatively.

The surgical procedure required for acute ischaemia after trauma depends on the type and extent of the injury. Arterial lacerations can sometimes be primarily repaired or patched. Transection or more extensive injuries may require interposition or bypass grafting.

Post-operation care

The limb's general appearance, temperature and pulses (by Doppler ultrasound or palpation) should be frequently checked and recorded.

Anticoagulation is initiated with intravenous unfractionated or subcutaneous low molecular weight **heparin** followed by **warfarin** provided there are no contraindications.

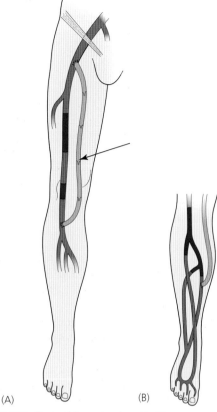

(A)   (B)

FIGURE 11.7   Types of femoral and popliteal bypass operations: (A) femoropopliteal; (B) femorodistal (bypass in blue arrows)

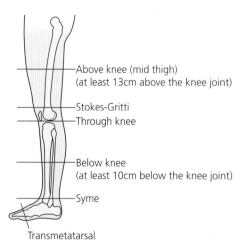

Above knee (mid thigh)
(at least 13cm above the knee joint)

Stokes-Gritti
Through knee

Below knee
(at least 10cm below the knee joint)

Syme

Transmetatarsal

FIGURE 11.8   The levels of lower limb amputation that provide suitable stumps for the fitting of a prosthesis

A source of embolus or a reason for the thrombosis should be sought with echocardiography and imaging of the proximal arterial tree. The source should if possible be treated to prevent recurrence.

Early complications

Compartment syndrome is the progressive increase in pressure in one or several of the muscle compartments. It can be caused by a period of acute ischaemia especially from the tissue swelling that follows revascularization. It causes severe pain, characteristically exacerbated by passive movements, and tense tender compartments.

If a compartment syndrome is suspected it should be surgically decompressed (see Fig 11.4).

Monitoring for late complications

Late complications are related to rethrombosis or restenosis secondary to intimal hyperplasia or progression of the atherosclerosis. Patients present with a recurrence of the symptoms of acute ischaemia or symptoms of chronic ischaemia (see below).

Surveillance of vein grafts using periodic **duplex ultrasound scans** detects restenosis and allows angioplasty with or without stenting to prevent subsequent occlusion.

Prosthetic graft material may become **infected**, either at the time of implantation or much later as a consequence of haematogenous spread. Patients present with the generalized signs of sepsis, erythema, swelling and sometimes anastomotic dehiscence. Imaging with ultrasound or X-rays may show fluid and sometimes gas around the graft.

Graft infection can be treated conservatively with long-term antibiotics if the infection is not aggressive and the anastomosis intact; if not, the graft should be removed and an alternative revascularization procedure performed.

Results

The overall outcome of acute limb ischaemia remains poor because the patients are elderly and many have significant co-morbidity.

Acute ischaemia caused by aortic dissection

Limb ischaemia can occur if the dissection extends into the common iliac arteries or restricts flow through the true lumen. Treatment options include open surgical or endovascular repair of the dissection entry tear (often in the descending thoracic aorta) or extra-anatomical bypass, e.g. axillofemoral bypass or femoro-femoral crossover bypass (see Fig 11.6).

CHRONIC ISCHAEMIA OF THE LEGS

Chronic limb ischaemia is usually caused by a progressive atherosclerotic stenosis or occlusion of the limb's arteries. Occasionally other conditions such as vasculitis can be responsible. The restenosis that may follow therapeutic interventions is often caused by intimal hyperplasia.

Patients with lower limb peripheral arterial disease can be divided into three categories: the asymptomatic; those with intermittent claudication; and those with critical limb ischaemia.

Symptomless peripheral vascular disease

Patients without vascular problems are often found to have evidence of peripheral vascular disease on routine examination. The symptomless limbs may be cooler, have a reduced capillary filling time and impalpable pulses because of a silent arterial stenosis or occlusion.

Management

No specific investigations or treatment are indicated but there is good evidence that these patients should be prescribed **antiplatelet agents and statins** to reduce the chance of cardiovascular events. Management should focus on secondary prevention by minimizing risk factors. Smoking should be stopped and any diabetes, hypertension and hyperlipidaemia treated.

Intermittent claudication

Investigation
Clinical diagnostic indicators
Cramp-like muscle pain that occurs after a relatively fixed amount of exercise and is relieved by rest is usually caused by peripheral vascular disease but may be caused by orthopaedic and neurological disease. A careful examination of the bones, joints and peripheral nerves is essential.

Pressure measurements
The pressures in the peripheral vessels should be measured with the help of an ultrasound flow detector and compared with the brachial pressure by calculating the ABPI (see Fig 11.1). These measurements, especially if performed before and after exercise, are useful not only for diagnosis but for follow-up after treatment.

Imaging
A **chest X-ray** is valuable to exclude a carcinoma of the bronchus and assess the cardiac size.

Duplex ultrasound is useful as an initial non-invasive assessment.

CT angiography images the aorta, iliac and femoral vessels but the distal vessels may be poorly visualized if significantly calcified.

Intra-arterial DSA gives the best distal images and has the advantage that it may provide the option to perform an angioplasty at the same time (Fig 11.9).

Haematology
Anaemia and polycythaemia should be excluded. Inflammatory markers should be checked if there is a suspicion of a vasculitic cause.

Biochemistry
Blood lipids should be measured. The blood urea, creatinine and electrolytes should be checked, particularly if contrast agents are to be used for imaging, as many patients with peripheral vascular disease have significant renal artery disease and poor renal function.

A fasting serum glucose should be checked for undiagnosed diabetes.

Management options
Treatment decisions are based on the balance between the potential benefits and the risks of intervention. Assessment of the impact of the

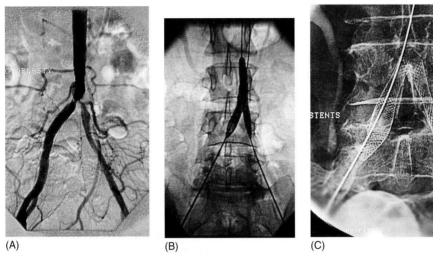

(A)   (B)   (C)

FIGURE 11.9   Intra-arterial digital subtraction arteriographs showing the treatment of an aortic stenosis with angioplasty and stenting. (A) The stenosis; (B) the balloon dilatation; (C) the stent

symptoms on the quality of life is essential to determine whether intervention is appropriate. Treatment should aim to be conservative. Intervention should only be considered for patients with relatively short distance claudication that is having a significant detrimental effect on their quality of life or when there is incipient critical limb ischaemia.

Secondary prevention is paramount.

Conservative treatment

Conservative treatment is indicated if the claudication distance is not significantly interfering with quality of life. Risk factors, especially smoking, should be addressed.

Regular controlled, supervised walking exercises have been shown to improve walking distance, and **raising the heel** of the shoe sometimes helps.

Patients should be told to seek further advice if their walking distance shortens or any symptoms or signs of critical limb ischaemia develop.

Results

The symptoms of approximately one-third of patients with intermittent claudication improve as a result of collateral development. One-third

remain stable. One-third experience a progressive deterioration of symptoms, sometimes in a step-wise fashion as more vessels occlude.

Only about 5 per cent go on to develop critical limb ischaemia, and only 1 per cent eventually come to amputation.

Surgical treatment

This should be considered if the claudication is significantly impairing the quality of life or the walking distance is very short.

Angioplasty is preferable to open surgery because for more proximal vessels (iliac and femoral arteries) or short lesions it carries a lower risk and a long-term patency of 80–90 per cent.

Long or resistant stenoses may require the insertion of stents (see Fig 11.10).

Angioplasty of vessels below the popliteal artery is not indicated for claudication.

Short severe stenoses or occlusions, e.g. in the common femoral or popliteal arteries, may be treated by **endarterectomy** if the vessels above and below it are patent and relatively healthy.

Bypass surgery below the groin should rarely be considered but may be useful for aorto-iliac and common femoral occlusions (see Figs 11.6 and 11.7).

Patients should be counselled about the potential risks of either form of intervention, including limb loss or death.

Post-operation care

Antiplatelet and statin medication is advised unless there are contraindications. **Dual antiplatelet therapy** (for example aspirin and clopidogrel) is indicated after peripheral stent insertion.

Complications

Angioplasty may fail if it is not possible to cross the lesion with a wire or balloon, or if the lesion is resistant to dilation. Arterial wall **dissection** and vessel **thrombosis** may also occur.

Restenosis can occur early, as a result of recoil, or late when it is secondary to intimal hyperplasia or atherosclerotic progression. Bypasses may occlude as a result of poor inflow, graft stenosis or poor outflow.

Vein grafts should be monitored for stenosis with regular duplex ultrasound surveillance. Prophylactic angioplasty should be performed to prevent occlusion if a severe (>50 per cent) stenosis develops.

Results

Aortofemoral bypass has a 90–100 per cent 5-year patency, femoropoliteal vein bypass a 60–70 per cent 5-year patency.

Critical limb ischaemia

Investigation

Clinical diagnostic indicators

Critical limb ischaemia is defined as the presence of **rest pain**, **gangrene** or **tissue loss**, present for more than 2 weeks with an objective measure of reduced tissue perfusion, e.g. a reduced ABPI.

Critical limb ischaemia is a limb-threatening condition and must be treated with immediate revascularization to avoid limb loss. If revascularization is not possible then amputation should be considered, particularly if there is gangrene or infection, as this may be life-threatening.

Flow measurement

Duplex ultrasound can be used as an initial assessment, but more detailed imaging will always be necessary as intervention is obligatory to avoid limb loss.

Imaging

CT or MR angiography is sometimes adequate to assess the possibility of a bypass operation but **formal angiography** is often required to define the distal run-off vessels (Fig 11.10).

Duplex ultrasonography or **saphenography** may be needed to define the suitability of the saphenous or arm veins as conduits for the bypass.

Palliative measures

Conservative treatment of critical limb ischaemia is only indicated if the patient is too unfit to undergo the procedures needed to restore the circulation. Without such measures, the onset of gangrene

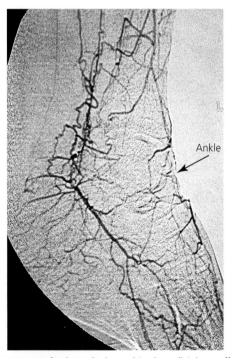

Ankle

FIGURE 11.10 Angiography is used to show distal run-off vessels to demonstrate whether there is a suitable vessel to receive a distal bypass graft

is highly likely, with demarcation of viable from non-viable tissue. Superimposed infection may be life-threatening.

Surgical treatment

Patients with critical limb ischaemia often have multiple co-morbidities, particularly coronary artery, respiratory and renovascular disease. Efforts should be made to optimize the patient's general condition before undertaking any procedures.

Revascularization should be attempted, if possible, to avert limb loss. Critical limb ischaemia is almost always secondary to occlusive or stenotic disease at multiple levels. Each level of disease must be treated either by endovascular or open surgical techniques or a combination, with the objective of establishing an adequate inflow to the limb and the distal run-off.

Any arterial segment from the aorta to the distal vessels can theoretically by treated by **angioplasty** (see Fig 11.10).

A sheath is inserted into the femoral artery using the Seldinger technique either in a retrograde or antegrade direction. A wire is passed across the lesion followed by a balloon, which is inflated to dilate the vessel. **Stents** are placed if indicated. Primary stent placement is more common in the aortic, iliac and tibial arteries, although their use in the femoral arteries is becoming more frequent. Stents can also be placed to deal with complications such as vessel recoil or iatrogenic dissection.

It is not possible to dilate very calcified or fibrotic stenoses.

Long lesions, for example superficial femoral artery occlusions, may be difficult or impossible to cross with the wire or balloon, and the results of dilatation are less favourable than surgical bypass.

The technique of **subintimal angioplasty** involves the passage of the wire and balloon not through the original lumen but through a plane artificially created within the vessel wall. This technique has allowed the treatment or long segments of disease with apparently good results in some centres.

Surgical bypass is necessary if angioplasty is not appropriate or fails. The principle is to deal with more proximal disease first. Operative choices include **axillofemoral, iliofemoral, aortofemoral, femoro-femoral, femoropopliteal** and **femorodistal** bypass (see Figs 11.6 and 11.7).

Prosthetic grafts (Dacron or PTFE) are used for aortic and iliac bypass. The best conduit for long-term patency and resistance to infection for a femoropopliteal or femoral-distal bypass is an autogenous superficial vein.

Post-operation care

The patient should be monitored for any signs of post-operative bleeding or infection. The circulation of the limb should be carefully observed to detect early graft occlusion.

All patients should be given antiplatelet agents. Following the insertion of stents, it is now common to prescribe dual antiplatelet agents.

Complications

Restenosis may occur soon after angioplasty as a result of vessel recoil and later as a result of intimal hyperplasia and recurrent atheroma. Graft occlusion is usually the result of poor inflow.

Late restenosis can be treated with angioplasty and stenting or a bypass graft.

Graft infection can occur soon after surgery or later from haematogenous spread.

Detection and treatment of late complications

Regular **duplex ultrasound surveillance** of vein bypass grafts can be used to detect restenosis. Significant stenoses can be treated by angioplasty to prevent occlusion.

Graft occlusion usually presents with a recurrence of the original symptoms or an acutely ischaemic limb. If there are no contraindications, **thrombolysis** may successfully open the graft if it has thrombosed within a week of presentation. When the cause of the occlusion is a stenosis it can be treated by angioplasty.

Infection may present with pain and erythema over the graft, signs and symptoms of systemic sepsis, or sometimes with anastomotic dehiscence. Imaging will show fluid and possibly gas around the graft. Blood cultures and wound swabs should be taken to attempt to identify the causative organism. Sometimes infection can be kept dormant with antibiotics but prosthetic material is resistant and the graft may need to be removed.

Amputation is indicated for non-viable or gangrenous tissue or intractable rest pain. Small areas of dry gangrene may be allowed to demarcate and auto-amputate, but must be monitored closely for developing infection.

Amputation is performed with the aim of removing all gangrenous or infected tissue while salvaging as much viable tissue as possible. The level of amputation is chosen to ensure wound healing. In the presence of infection it may be appropriate to leave the wound open and allow it to heal by secondary intention. The common levels of amputation are transmetatarsal, below knee, through knee and above knee (see Fig 11.8).

Amputations can be complicated by infection and failure of the wound to heal.

Results

Aortofemoral bypass has a mortality rate of 5 per cent, other bypasses 1–3 per cent, major amputation 10–20 per cent.

DEEP VEIN THROMBOSIS AND PULMONARY EMBOLISM

The formation of thrombosis in the deep veins is precipitated by a combination of low flow, endothelial injury and increased coagulability (Virchow's triad). Triggering of the coagulation cascade results in deposition of alternate layers rich in platelets and erythrocytes embedded in a fibrin mesh giving a characteristic laminated appearance.

Thrombi usually form first in the calf vein sinuses and then propagate proximally. Small thrombi may be removed by the endogenous thrombolytic activity of the blood, but more commonly a process of tissue organization occurs within the thrombus that begins immediately and evolves over several months. An acute inflammatory response in the vein wall is followed by migration of inflammatory cells into the thrombus. Extracellular matrix reorganization leads to replacement of the fibrin, platelets and erythrocytes with collagenous scar tissue that gradually

adheres to and eventually becomes incorporated into the vein wall. As the retraction and neovascularization of the thrombus is variable, the vein lumen may remain totally or partially occluded or become completely recanalized.

Part or all of the thrombus may break off to form an embolus that usually travels to the lungs. **Small pulmonary emboli** may be symptomless, although, if multiple, may result in chronic pulmonary hypertension. **Large emboli** may obstruct the pulmonary arteries and cause acute heart failure and death.

Rarely emboli may pass through a patent foramen ovale and into the peripheral arteries (**paradoxical embolism**).

Investigation

Clinical diagnostic indicators

Classically, deep vein thrombosis (DVT) presents with calf pain which is associated with muscle tenderness, pain on passive ankle movements and swelling.

Extensive iliofemoral DVT may present with a pale swelling of the whole leg ('milk leg' or phlegmasia alba dolens) or a blue swelling of the whole leg caused by severe venous congestion (phlegmasia cerulea dolens) that may progress to venous gangrene.

Most of these clinical symptoms and signs are inaccurate so **the diagnosis must be confirmed with imaging**.

Pulmonary embolism (PE) usually presents with acute pleuritic chest pain and shortness of breath. A large pulmonary embolus may cause cardiogenic shock or sudden death. Small emboli may not cause any symptoms but if recurrent and multiple they may significantly impede pulmonary artery blood flow and cause pulmonary hypertension.

Imaging

Duplex ultrasound of the peripheral veins may show **intraluminal echogenicity**, an **inability to compress** the vein and a **lack of blood flow** (Fig 11.11). It has good sensitivity and specificity for iliofemoral DVT but is less sensitive (70 per cent) for isolated calf thrombi.

CT and MR venography have the advantage of being able to image the common iliac veins and

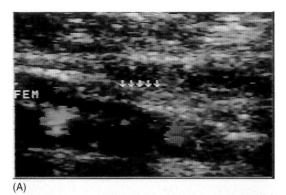

(A)

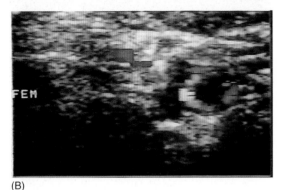

(B)

FIGURE 11.11   (A, B) Longitudinal and transverse duplex ultrasound images of a peripheral vein containing thrombus. Note the intraluminal echogenicity, lack of blood flow and incompressibility

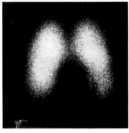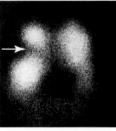

FIGURE 11.12   A ventilation–perfusion scan revealing a large right pulmonary embolus

inferior vena cava, which may be poorly visualized on ultrasound.

Contrast venography has a high sensitivity and specificity for occluded vein segments and is the most accurate method of assessing post-thrombotic changes.

Pulmonary isotope – ventilation scanning (Fig 11.12) will detect small and moderate-sized emboli.

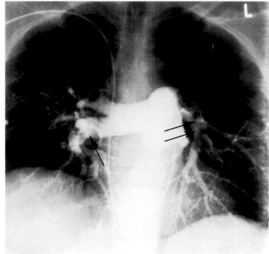

FIGURE 11.13   A pulmonary angiogram showing emboli in both branches of the pulmonary artery seen as filling defects (arrows)

CT and conventional X-ray **pulmonary angiography** (Fig 11.13) detect all but the smallest emboli.

Haematology

Serum D-dimers are usually elevated after an acute DVT. This test is highly sensitive but has low specificity.

A thrombophilia screen should be performed if there are no clear precipitating reasons for DVT. This should include tests for **factor V Leiden mutation** (activated protein C resistance), **prothrombin G20210A mutation**, **MTHFR mutation** (causing high homocysteine levels), antiphospholipid syndrome (**lupus anticoagulant** and **anticardiolipin antibodies**), **protein C and S** and **antithrombin III** deficiencies.

Polycythaemia and thrombocytosis predispose to thrombosis, and must be investigated. Iron deficiency anaemia may indicate the presence of an occult malignancy.

Genetics

Genetic tests may include those for the inherited thrombophilias as above.

Management of deep vein thrombosis

Prophylaxis Low molecular weight heparin (enoxaparin 20–40 mg od) and anti-embolism stockings should be considered for all patients.

Emergency care If the leg is significantly swollen it should be elevated. Antithromboembolism stockings may also be applied to reduce swelling. Pain should be relieved with analgesic drugs.

Conservative treatment Most DVTs are managed medically with anticoagulation in the form of low molecular weight heparin. The initial dose is calculated according to the patient's weight (e.g. enoxaparin 1.5 mg/kg od). **Warfarin** is started with initial loading doses and its effect titrated against the INR.

Anticoagulation carries the risk of **haemorrhage**. This is usually manifest as bruising, particularly at the site of subcutaneous injection, but can be significant. Rarely, heparin induces thrombocytopenia.

Results

In the majority of patients the early symptoms improve as collaterals develop but late chronic post-thrombotic symptoms are common.

Subcutaneous thrombolysis

Catheter-directed thrombolysis should be considered in young patients with large proximal symptomatic DVT. It can reduce the damage to the veins and the incidence of post-thrombotic symptoms but is only effective within the first 2 weeks after thrombus formation.

Thrombolysis is often contraindicated because of specific risks of bleeding, for example recent surgery, major trauma and post partum.

The patient must be counselled regarding the risk of haemorrhage.

An infusion catheter is positioned within the thrombus, usually via the popliteal vein. Phlebography is used to confirm the presence of thrombus and the position of the catheter. The best thombolytic agent is **tPA** (tissue plasminogen activator). The effect of the infusion is monitored with repeated radiographs.

Patients with the **May–Turner syndrome** (partial obstruction of the left iliac vein by the right iliac

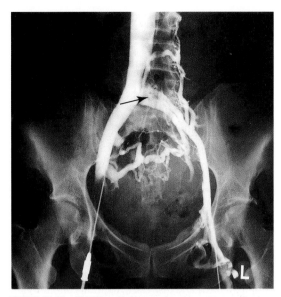

FIGURE 11.14 The May–Turner syndrome – compression and webbing of the common iliac vein that may cause an obstruction and a predisposition to thrombosis

artery) (Fig 11.14) should have a stent inserted after the lysis to prevent recurrence.

The patient should be **anticoagulated**.

During and after the infusion the patient needs to be monitored for haemorrhage, which often manifests itself as oozing around the catheter site but may be intracranial and fatal.

If there are any signs of haemorrhage, the infusion must be stopped, the patient's vital signs monitored and appropriate resuscitation given.

Venous gangrene should be managed conservatively for as long as possible as the necrosis is often superficial and deep tissues will survive. Amputation is an option if gangrene is extensive.

Results

Successful thrombolysis may reduce the incidence of post-thrombotic symptoms.

Many patients with DVT develop the consequences of vein occlusion and valve destruction. Their symptoms include pain, swelling, the skin changes of lipodermatosclerosis, and ultimately ulceration. These may begin immediately after a severe DVT or become apparent many years later.

Class 2 graduated compression stockings will usually ameliorate pain and swelling and reduce the progression of skin damage, thus reducing the incidence of ulceration.

Ulcers are treated with multilayered compression bandaging (see below).

Surgical thrombectomy is rarely performed as the incidence of rethrombosis is high. The common femoral vein is exposed and the thrombus removed with a balloon embolectomy catheter. A temporary arteriovenous fistula can be created to reduce the incidence of rethrombosis.

Management of pulmonary embolism

This is summarized in Table 2.7.

The initial treatment should be full **anticoagulation** with intravenous heparin. If the patient's circulation does not improve within 1 or 2 hours and they remain hypoxic and distressed, methods of removing the embolus should be considered.

Thrombolytic drugs can be administered directly into the embolus via a cardiac catheter. The progress of lysis should be followed by repeat angiography. Instruments are being developed that assist lysis by fragmenting and sucking out the thrombus.

In extreme cases, often when the patient appears to be almost dead, a **pulmonary embolectomy** may be performed. The embolus may be removed via a thoracotomy and incision into the pulmonary artery. This operation is rarely successful but more likely to succeed if the expertise of a cardiac surgeon and cardiopulmonary bypass facilities are available.

Management of recurrent pulmonary embolism

PE may recur in spite of adequate anticoagulation. If these recurrences are life-threatening and/or causing pulmonary hypertension they can be prevented by the insertion of a vena cava filter (Fig 11.15).

ORTHOPAEDIC CAUSES OF LEG PAIN

Orthopaedic causes of leg pain must be differentiated from vascular causes because arthritis of the hip or knee can cause pain referred to the thigh or

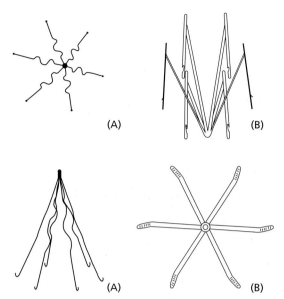

FIGURE 11.15   Types of filter that can be introduced into the vena cava to prevent recurrent pulmonary embolism

lower leg. Degenerative spinal disease can result in nerve root irritation with pain radiating to the leg, sometimes clinically indistinguishable from vascular intermittent claudication (spinal claudication) (see Chapter 9).

Investigation
Clinical diagnostic indicators

A history of arthritis or back pain should be sought. Arthritis tends to cause pain as soon as exercise begins rather than after a distance as in claudication. There may also be pain at rest.

On examination there may be obvious deformities of the joints or tenderness over the spine, knee or ankle. Passive hip, knee or ankle movements may be painful and straight leg raising limited. The gait should be inspected as walking often precipitates the symptoms immediately.

Imaging

Plain radiographs of the lumbar spine, hip, knee or ankle may show characteristic features of degenerative arthritis.

An **MRI** of the lumbar spine may show spinal canal or nerve root compression.

Blood tests

These are needed to exclude serum positive autoimmune causes of inflammatory arthritis, e.g. rheumatoid arthritis.

Management

The management of the common spinal conditions that produce symptoms that mimic intermittent claudication are described in Chapter 10.

NEUROLOGICAL CAUSES OF LEG PAIN

Investigation
Clinical diagnostic indicators

The pattern of neurological symptoms in the legs is not usually the same as that of vascular claudication or critical ischaemia. The pain is often sharp, stabbing, burning or tingling in nature and distributed to dermatomes rather than muscle groups.

The history may reveal co-morbidity associated with neuropathy, for example diabetes or alcoholism.

On examination there may be detectable neurological abnormalities, particularly sensory or proprioceptive loss. The clinical degree of vascular disease is not usually compatible with being a cause for the symptoms.

ABDOMINAL AORTIC ANEURYSM

Intrinsic weakness developing in the wall of the aorta leads to progressive dilation. The morphology of aneurysms is shown in Fig 11.16.

Male gender, smoking, hypertension and genetic factors interplay to cause increased activity of proteinases in the medial layer of the vessel, leading to progressive loss of elastin and collagen.

Specific collagen and elastin defects are associated with certain connective tissue disorders such as Marfan's and Ehlers–Danlos syndromes. Localized infection in the aortic wall can cause a true or false mycotic aneurysm. Occasionally aneurysms develop secondary to aortic dissection or vasculitic disorders (see Fig 11.16).

As the aneurysm expands, the sac often becomes lined with thrombus that has the potential to embolize.

Rupture occurs when the tensile strength of the wall is exceeded. The incidence of rupture

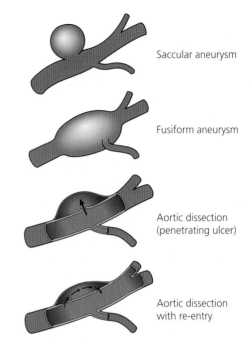

Saccular aneurysm

Fusiform aneurysm

Aortic dissection (penetrating ulcer)

Aortic dissection with re-entry

FIGURE 11.16 The morphology of aneurysms

of abdominal aortic aneurysms less than 5 cm in diameter is low. Once greater than this size the risk increases proportionally.

Investigation
Clinical diagnostic indicators

Patients are usually current or prior smokers and often have a history of hypertension. Most abdominal aortic aneurysms remain symptomless until they rupture, but some are detected incidentally either on examination or when the patient undergoes imaging for other reasons. On examination a pulsatile, expansile central abdominal mass may be detected providing the patient is not grossly obese. The femoral and popliteal pulses should be checked for associated aneurysms.

Pain or tenderness suggests incipient rupture and is an indication for urgent surgical repair. Sudden onset of central abdominal or back pain with signs of hypovolaemic shock is indicative of rupture.

Blood tests

A baseline full blood count and biochemistry should be obtained.

Renal function

Renal function should be checked, as this may be affected by involvement of the renal arteries in the aneurysm or co-existent renal atherosclerosis.

A split renal function study may be useful if one or more renal arteries may be compromised by the surgical repair.

Imaging

Duplex ultrasound can accurately assess the size of the aneurysm (Fig 11.17A). Iliac aneurysms can also be seen and sometimes the relationship of the aneurysm neck to the renal arteries can be determined.

CT angiography accurately defines the anatomy of the aneurysm and gives the information needed to assess whether it is suitable for endovascular repair (Fig 11.17B). The CT angiogram should include the chest to identify any associated thoracic aortic aneurysm and exclude any significant lung co-morbidity.

Management options

Small aortic aneurysms (3–5.5 cm diameter) are kept under surveillance with periodic duplex ultrasound. An abdominal aneurysm is considered for repair once it has reached between 5 and 5.5 cm in diameter.

The patient's fitness for **open repair** should be assessed. The CT angiogram should be reviewed to see whether the aneurysm is suitable for **endovascular repair**. This will be determined by the anatomy of the aneurysm neck and iliac arteries. Once this information has been obtained, the patient should have the risks and benefits of open and endovascular repair explained in order that they can make an informed decision.

The early mortality of endovascular repair is 1–2 per cent compared with open repair of 4–6 per cent. Patients having endovascular repair need lifelong follow-up imaging. There is a re-intervention rate of between 10 and 20 per cent by 3 years compared with less than 5 per cent at 5 years with open surgery.

All patients should be treated with antiplatelet agents, a statin, and blood and diabetes controlled.

Conservative treatment In the presence of significant co-morbidity it may be decided that the

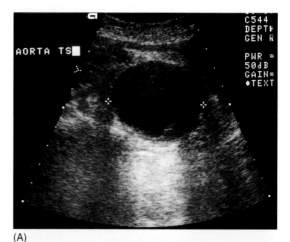

(A)

(B)

FIGURE 11.17   (A) Duplex ultrasound assessment of the size of an aortic aneurysm. (B) CT assessment of an abdominal aortic aneurysm. The lumen is outlined with contrast, thrombus fills the rest of the sac

risk of surgical repair is too great, particularly if the aneurysm is unsuitable for endovascular repair. Sometimes a decision is made to defer treatment until a larger diameter is reached; but if the aneurysm ruptures a choice has to be made between risking a major operation and palliative treatment almost certainly followed by death.

Open surgical repair

This is indicated if the aneurysm is painful or tender, has a diameter greater than 5.5 cm, is causing distal emboli, is rapidly increasing in size (>1 cm per year) and is unsuitable for endovascular repair.

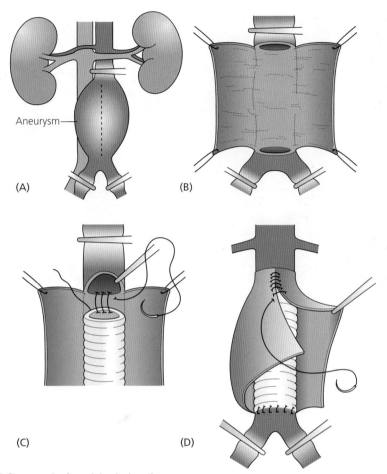

(A)

(B)

Aneurysm

(C)

(D)

FIGURE 11.18   A–D Open repair of an abdominal aortic aneurysm

The cardiac, respiratory and renal function should be assessed and optimized preoperatively. **Antibiotic prophylaxis** should be given.

Technique The aorta is exposed through a vertical or horizontal laparotomy incision (Fig 11.18).

The neck of the aneurysm is located and clamped after giving a bolus of 5000 units of heparin. The iliac vessels are also clamped. The aneurysm sac is opened and back bleeding from lumbar or mesenteric vessels controlled. A Dacron tube or bifurcated graft is sewn within the sac, which is then closed over the graft. The abdomen is closed (Fig 11.18).

Specific postoperative care Patients should be monitored overnight in a high dependency unit. Fluid and blood requirements should be carefully corrected.

Specific complications Postoperative bleeding, renal and respiratory failure, and cardiac events may occur and should be managed appropriately.

Detection and treatment of complications Late complications are rare but include graft infection, false aneurysm formation and development of secondary aorto-enteric fistula.

Results The mortality of open repair is about 5 per cent. Late mortality and morbidity is unusual.

Endovascular repair

Attitudes toward endovascular repair vary because the long-term results are still unknown. Some surgeons will perform an endovascular repair on all patients who are anatomically suitable, whereas others reserve it for the elderly patients or patients unfit for open surgery.

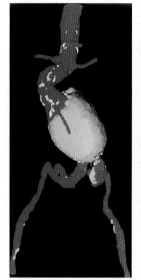
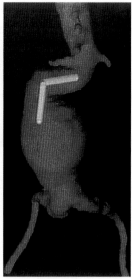

FIGURE 11.19   MRI assessment of the neck of two abdominal aortic aneurysms before endovascular repair

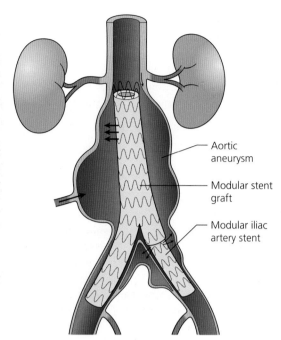

Aortic
aneurysm

Modular stent
graft

Modular iliac
artery stent

FIGURE 11.20   Endovascular repair of an abdominal aortic aneurysm using a stent graft

Preoperative CT angiography is essential to assess the correct size of graft – especially the neck diameter and the angle between the aneurysm and the normal aorta above (Fig 11.19).

Juxta- and suprarenal aneurysms can be treated with custom-made fenestrated or branched devices that must be fabricated in advance.

Technique The femoral arteries are surgically exposed. After heparin administration, the modular parts of the stent graft are introduced and deployed (Fig 11.20). There is usually a main body that is positioned below the renal arteries, and limb extensions that are deployed in the iliac arteries.

Specific complications Small iliac arteries may be injured during graft insertion. Endoleaks (persistent flow into the aneurysm sac) may occur. These need treating if they originate from the landing zones of the graft (Type 1) or from separation of the graft components (Type 3). Endoleak lumbar vessel backflow (Type 2) should be monitored as it often resolves spontaneously.

Detection and treatment of complications The graft should be scanned at 3 months by CT then yearly with ultrasound or CT to detect complications.

Results The mortality of endovascular repair is about 2 per cent. About 10–20 per cent of patients require further interventions to deal with late complications.

RUPTURED ABDOMINAL AORTIC ANEURYSM

Aneurysms that continue to expand eventually rupture. The resulting sudden massive haemorrhage results in the death of half of the patients before they reach hospital. Those who survive to reach hospital usually have a periaortic haematoma confined to the retroperitoneum, rather than a free rupture into the peritoneal cavity. When the combination of systemic hypotension and the pressure within the haematoma reach an equilibrium bleeding stops but the patient remains at risk of sudden exsanguination until the site of the rupture is excluded from the circulation.

Rarely an aorto-enteric or aortocaval fistula can develop, causing massive gastrointestinal bleeding or high output cardiac failure respectively.

Investigation

Clinical diagnostic indicators

There is usually a sudden onset of severe abdominal and back pain accompanied by shock and collapse. The pain is usually central and radiates through to the lower back but may only be experienced in the back or as loin pain when the diagnosis can be confused with renal colic (see Chapter 17).

The presence of a tender, pulsatile, expansile central abdominal mass confirms the diagnosis. There is often pallor, cool sweaty peripheries, restlessness and breathlessness, a rapid pulse and a low blood pressure.

It may be difficult to feel the pulsatile mass in obese patients or in those who are very tender. Hypotension may also make palpation of the pulsatile mass impossible.

The presence of dilated femoral or popliteal arteries strengthens the suspected diagnosis.

It must be assumed that severe abdominal pain in a patient with an aneurysm is the result of rupture or imminent rupture. This is true if the aneurysm is tender even if there are no signs of rupture on CT.

Investigations should be kept to a minimum if the diagnosis is obvious as there is a danger that the patient may exsanguinate.

Imaging

Chest and abdominal X-rays are occasionally useful if other diagnoses are possible. A co-existing thoracic aneurysm may be found and sometimes the calcified outline of an abdominal aneurysm is visible.

Abdominal ultrasonography in the Accident and Emergency Department may confirm the presence of an aneurysm.

Abdominal CT aortography may be performed if the diagnosis is uncertain or if endovascular repair is an option (Fig 11.21). The time taken to perform it needs to be weighed against the risk of clinical deterioration and the clinical circumstances.

Blood tests

A baseline full blood count and **blood grouping** should be obtained. Group specific or O-negative blood may be used for initial transfusion. Appropriate samples should be sent to urgently **cross-match 10 units.** Fresh frozen plasma and platelet preparations may also be required to correct coagulation after transfusion.

The **urea and electrolytes** should be checked. A **serum amylase** should be measured to diagnose or exclude acute pancreatitis if the diagnosis is uncertain. A small rise in the amylase may occur in patients with ruptured aneurysms.

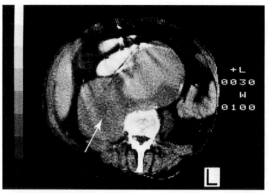

FIGURE 11.21   CT of a ruptured abdominal aortic aneurysm (haematoma arrowed)

Management options

Palliative treatment is indicated if an operation would be futile in view of advanced age, severe comorbidity or loss of cardiac output prior to arriving in the operating theatre.

If the patient is conscious and has a recordable blood pressure, then circulatory resuscitation should be delayed to reduce further bleeding until either the aorta is clamped in a **open procedure**, or the stent graft deployed in **endovascular repair**. A urinary catheter, central venous catheter and arterial line should be placed, but this should not delay transfer of the patient to the operating theatre.

Open operation

When all the above catheters have been inserted, a 'crash' induction of general anaesthesia is performed after the patient is draped and the surgical team is scrubbed and ready to open the abdomen through a long midline incision.

Technique The neck of the aneurysm is located and a clamp applied followed by clamps to the iliac vessels. The repair then proceeds as for an elective procedure.

Specific postoperative care By the end of the operation patients have often lost a large volume of blood, are hypothermic and coagulopathic. They should be sent to intensive care or overnight intensive recovery for careful monitoring and support.

Specific complications These include haemorrhage, ischaemic legs (from thromboembolism), ischaemic bowel, renal failure and multi-organ failure.

Late complications These include incisional hernia, graft infection and secondary aorto-enteric fistula.

Detection and treatment of complications The patient is monitored closely for early complications, particularly ischaemic bowel, which can be difficult to detect. Flexible sigmoidoscopy or laparotomy may be required to make the diagnosis.

Results Death from ruptured aneurysm remains high. Up to half of the patients die perioperatively from bleeding or postoperatively from multi-organ failure.

Endovascular repair

A number of centres now treat ruptured aneurysms with endovascular stent grafts provided they have had a preoperative **CT scan** to determine their suitability for endovascular repair and the size of the required graft is available.

Technique The operation may be performed under local anaesthetic infiltrated in the groin and around the femoral arteries. Guide wires are inserted via the femoral arteries into the aorta and angiographs obtained to locate the renal arteries. The aneurysm and its rupture are excluded with either a bifurcated stent graft or an aorto-uni-iliac device. The latter also requires a femorofemoral cross-over graft be performed.

Specific complications Abdominal compartment syndrome may develop as a result of the retroperitoneal haematoma and ileus. This may require a laparostomy to relieve the pressure. Endoleaks may also occur.

Detection and treatment of complications Patients should undergo the usual surveillance after endovascular aneurysm repair to detect graft migration or endoleak.

Results Early experience suggests that, when possible, endovascular repair may confer a better prognosis than an open operation but will never be applicable to all patients and careful selection is vital.

THORACIC AND THORACOABDOMINAL AORTIC ANEURYSM

These aneurysms account for about 10 per cent of aortic aneurysms. The range of aetiologies is the same as for infrarenal aneurysms with most being degenerative in cause. Aortic dissection is a more common cause of wall weakening and subsequent dilation than in the abdominal aorta.

Investigation

Clinical diagnostic indicators

Many are symptomless and found incidentally on chest radiography or CT. Chest pain may be secondary to compression of surrounding structures or rupture. Recurrent laryngeal nerve or bronchial compression may cause vocal or breathing symptoms.

Risk assessment

The patient should undergo a thorough cardiorespiratory risk assessment if surgery is being considered. This should include **stress testing** and, if available, **aerobic threshold assessment**.

Imaging

CT of the whole aorta will define the diameter and extent of the aneurysm. This may be augmented by **echocardiography** or **angiography**.

Surgical treatment

Surgical repair of thoraco-abdominal aneurysms carries a high risk. In general, the patient should be considered for surgery once the diameter of the aneurysm exceeds 6 cm.

For symptomless aneurysms the operative morbidity and mortality must be weighed against the size and risk of rupture of the aneurysm.

The aneurysm should be repaired once the diameter exceeds 6 cm if the patient is fit enough. Smaller saccular aneurysms should also be treated to prevent rupture.

Open technique Descending thoracic aneurysms are repaired through a left thoracotomy, thoracoabdominal aneurysms through a thoracolaparotomy. Circulatory arrest with bypass may be required.

An inlay graft is sewn in with a patch containing the visceral branches anastomosed to the graft. Major intercostal arteries may be anastomosed to preserve spinal cord blood supply.

Endovascular technique This form of repair is now preferred for uncomplicated descending thoracic aneurysms. Branched device technology is now becoming available allowing endovascular repair of thoraco-abdominal aneurysms.

Patients will usually require intensive care cardiorespiratory support for 2–3 days.

Complications Patients are prone to the usual cardiac and respiratory complications of major surgery. About 10 per cent of patients require dialysis. **Paraplegia** may affect up to 20 per cent of patients after open repair.

Results The mortality after open repair is 20–30 per cent, after endovascular repair it is 5–10 per cent.

POPLITEAL ANEURYSM

The popliteal artery is the commonest site of peripheral arterial aneurysm. The aetiology is usually degenerative, but may be related to trauma, or the popliteal entrapment syndrome.

Investigation

Clinical diagnostic indicators

Popliteal aneurysms may be detected as an incidental finding. Pressure on surrounding structures may cause pain, swelling, or DVT. Peripheral ischaemia is the commonest presentation, either from embolization of clot or thrombosis of the aneurysm itself. Rupture is rare.

Imaging

Duplex ultrasound will confirm the diagnosis and determine whether thrombus is present within the aneurysm.

CT can be useful to define the anatomy prior to repair (Fig 11.22).

Angiography is used after thrombosis as a prelude to thrombolysis and to define distal run-off vessels before bypass surgery.

Surgical treatment

Acute limb ischaemia secondary to thrombosis needs urgent treatment. The aim is to clear the distal circulation, either with thrombolysis or embolectomy and perform a definitive surgical repair.

Small symptomless aneurysms may be monitored with yearly ultrasound.

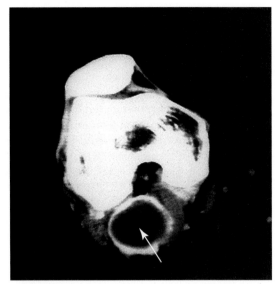

FIGURE 11.22 CT of a popliteal aneurysm filled with thrombus (arrow)

There is no consensus regarding when symptomless popliteal aneurysms should be treated. Most consider a diameter greater than 3 cm, the presence of intraluminal thrombus and the loss of run-off vessels through embolization to be significant indications, but these findings must be balanced against the risk of surgery, particularly if there is associated coronary and cerebrovascular disease.

Technique Surgical repair, whether urgent or elective, consists of exclusion of the aneurysm from the circulation by a bypass or interposition vein graft. Medial or posterior approaches may be used.

Endovascular repair is now possible but there are concerns over the long-term patency of prosthetic grafts in this position.

Results The risk of limb loss is 25 per cent if the presentation is with acute peripheral ischaemia. Short vein grafts rarely occlude but new aneurysms may develop in the remaining native vessel.

PRIMARY AND SECONDARY VARICOSE VEINS

Varicose veins are common in the population and are classified as either primary or secondary (e.g. following a DVT). Primary varicose veins are a result of a congenital, often inherited, valve and vein wall failure. The cause of the underlying physical abnormality is not known.

Secondary varicose veins follow valve destruction by thrombosis and/or valve ring dilatation secondary to proximal obstruction.

The most common site of valve incompetence and reflux is the saphenofemoral junction. Reflux through incompetent valves causes chronic venous hypertension with lengthening, dilation and tortuosity of the upstream tributaries, venular capillary hypertension and changes in the microcirculation.

Investigation

Clinical diagnostic indicators

The presenting problems relate either to the appearance of the veins and/or the skin changes or to symptoms attributed to the veins. The symptoms include pain, heaviness, itching and swelling, superficial thrombosis, haemorrhage and ulceration. There is often a history of previous treatment. Examination should assess the presence and distribution of any dilated veins including an attempt to identify the likely site of reflux and evidence of skin damage and previous surgery. The arterial circulation should always be assessed.

Imaging

Duplex ultrasonography will confirm the prime source of reflux and determine whether there is any evidence of previous deep vein thrombosis.

Phlebography, **saphenography** and **varicography** may by useful, particularly if there is deep venous occlusion, reflux, or complex venous anatomy.

Clinical tests of reflux

The **Trendelenberg test** using a tourniquet can be used to identify the level of reflux, but the results are unreliable.

A hand-held Doppler directional flow detector can also be used to identify the presence of reflux.

Management options

Treatment can be conservative, endovenous or surgical. Varicose veins are a benign condition, and the decision regarding interventional treatment will depend upon the balance of the patient's wishes and the risks of the procedure.

Conservative treatment

Varicose veins are common and do not necessarily require treatment. Class 2 below-knee graduated compression stockings usually relieves many of the associated symptoms.

Reflux in the long or short saphenous veins can be obliterated either by **endo-venous laser ablation** (EVLA), **radiofrequency ablation** or **ultrasound-guided foam sclerotherapy** (UGFS). These techniques can be performed under local anaesthetic. Associated varicosities are treated by foam sclerotherapy or avulsion.

The procedure is performed on an adjustable couch that allows leg elevation or dependency.

EVLA is when a laser fibre or radiofrequency catheter is passed into the vein under ultrasound guidance using the Seldinger technique. After infiltrating dilute local anaesthetic around the vein the laser probe is activated and slowly withdrawn.

For **UGFS** the sclerosant is foamed by mixing with air and passing it back and forth between two syringes and then injected into the vein via a cannula inserted under ultrasound guidance.

Both EVLA and UGFS require **compression** with bandages and then graduated stocking for several weeks to ensure closure of the vein.

Residual varicosities may require one or more local treatments with foam sclerotherapy.

Complications: Deep vein thrombosis (1 per cent), failure and recurrence (25 per cent at 3 years) and skin staining may occur.

Surgical treatment

The long saphenous vein may not be suitable for endovenous procedures when it is large and torturous. Surgical treatment may be more efficient than multiple attempts at sclerotherapy.

Ligation and stripping: The long saphenous vein is exposed in the groin and ligated, together with all its tributaries, at the saphenofemoral junction. The long saphenous vein is exposed just below the knee and after a stripper has been passed through it up to the groin avulsed by gentle traction (Fig 11.23).

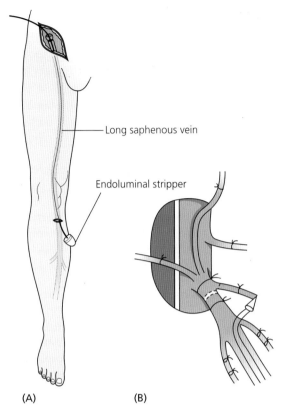

Long saphenous vein

Endoluminal stripper

(A)   (B)

FIGURE 11.23 Surgical treatment of varicose veins of the greater saphenous system

The short saphenous is usually disconnected from the popliteal vein in the popliteal fossa and can be stripped to the ankle.

After surgery an above-knee **compression stocking** should be worn for 2 weeks to reduce bruising.

Complications DVT is a rare but significant complication. Neuropraxias are common. Recurrence is the major problem and affects a third by 5 years.

Results Results of vein procedures are generally good but patients need to be warned that all techniques carry a recurrence rate of 5–30 per cent.

THROMBOPHLEBITIS

Thrombophlebitis is commonly associated with varicose veins. Spontaneous thrombophlebitis in a normal superficial vein in a middle-aged patient is often an indicator of a hidden carcinoma.

Investigations
Clinical diagnostic indicators
The patient presents with a localized inflamed area of skin overlying a tender thrombosed palpable cord of vein.

Imaging
A venous duplex scan should be performed if there are any suspicious features and to exclude DVT.

Management
Thrombophlebitis in a varicose vein should be treated with **non-steroidal anti-inflammatory agents** and **graduated compression stockings**. Heparin and saphenofemoral disconnection are indicated if the thrombosis extends up the thigh.

Once the acute episode has resolved the patient can be assessed for treatment of any varicose veins to prevent recurrence.

Patients with 'idiopathic' superficial vein thrombosis should be investigated to exclude the presence of a hidden carcinoma and have a thrombophilia screen.

VENOUS SWELLING

Chronic venous insufficiency is a common cause of lower limb swelling (see Table 11.5).

Investigation
Clinical diagnostic indicators
Venous disease is often bilateral so venous swelling may be unilateral or asymmetrical. There may be a history of DVT, varicose veins or ulceration.

On examination the limb is swollen and may have a bluish discoloration. There may be dilated veins, thread veins, an ankle flare or the skin changes of venous eczema and lipodermatosclerosis.

Imaging
Duplex ultrasonography should show significant deep or superficial venous reflux and the presence of venous occlusion.

Phlebography may identify post-thrombotic changes (Fig 11.24).

A lymphoscintogram will exclude a lymphatic cause for the swelling.

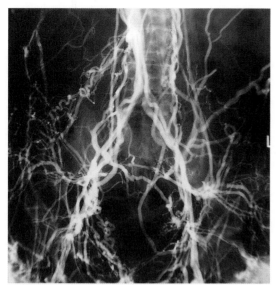

FIGURE 11.24 Venogram showing extensive post-thrombotic changes in the iliac and femoral veins

Management

The majority of patients only need class 2 or 3 graduated **compression stockings**.

Patients with severe symptoms and isolated iliac occlusion or severe stenosis may benefit from either **iliac vein stenting**, a **venous reconstruction** operation or the **Palma operation**.

LYMPHOEDEMA

Lymphoedema is an accumulation of extracellular fluid in tissues as a result of defective lymphatic function. The protein-rich oedema fluid causes a secondary proliferation of fibroblasts and epithelial cells that leads to sclerotic changes in the skin and subcutaneous tissues.

Lymphoedema may be primary (of unknown cause) or secondary. About 30 per cent of primary cases have a family history. In primary lymphoedema there may be fewer or absent lymphatic vessels or they may be dilated with incompetent valves.

Secondary lymphoedema follows obstruction of the lymphatics by conditions such as infection (filariasis, TB), trauma (including surgical lymph node excision), malignancy or radiotherapy damage.

Investigation

Clinical diagnostic indicators

Most patients present with a swollen leg, although the arm, face and genitalia may be affected. The onset can be at any age. True congenital lymphoedema presents in the first year of life but other inherited forms may present later. One or both legs may be affected. A history of attacks of cellulitis, surgery and trauma should be sought.

The oedema will pit on digital pressure, but with chronic lymphoedema this may require prolonged pressure as the subcutaneous tissues become more fibrotic. There may be verrucose skin changes and lymph may leak from lymphocutaneous fistulae.

Imaging

Duplex ultrasonography is useful to exclude a venous cause of the swelling.

Isotope lymphoscintigraphy will usually confirm the diagnosis and show the level of obstruction.

X-ray lymphangiography can be performed if surgery is contemplated, or the isotope test is equivalent.

Management

Compression with stockings or **bandaging** and regular **massage** is adequate for most patients with mild or moderate lymphoedema.

Antibiotics should be prescribed if the patient has recurrent bouts of cellulitis.

Foot hygiene is essential to prevent fungal infection and prevent the development of splits in the skin in the interdigital clefts where infection might enter. Tinia pedis should be treated with Lamisil.

Two to 5 per cent of patients with gross swelling benefit from **surgical procedures** such as reducing operations, bypass procedures and lymphatic ligation to abolish reflux.

VASCULAR MALFORMATIONS

Vascular malformations are inborn errors that occur during the development of the vessels. They can be divided into arteriovenous malformations (AVMs), venous, lymphatic, capillary or mixed abnormalities. Most are sporadic.

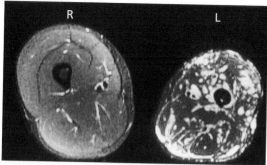

FIGURE 11.25 An MRI with STIR sequence showing an extensive venous malformation of the left limb. The angioma is white against the dark muscle background

Investigation
Clinical diagnostic indicators

Most patients present complaining of the cosmetic disfiguration.

Pain is sometimes a predominant feature, especially in venous malformations, which may also be accompanied by venous eczema and ulceration.

Soft tissue and limb overgrowth may occur.

The nature of the malformation is often apparent from its clinical appearance, consistency, pulsation and compressibility.

Imaging

MRI cross-sectional imaging with vascular enhancement will show the extent of the lesion (Fig 11.25).

Ultrasound and **venography** may give information concerning the lesion's blood supply.

Angiography is useful for defining arteriovenous malformations and can be combined with therapeutic embolization.

Management

Many patients need nothing more than a **diagnosis and reassurance**. Simple treatments such a stocking for a lower limb venous malformation may be useful.

Venous malformations may be treated with direct injection ultrasound-guided **sclerotherapy**. Larger superficial lesions are better **excised**.

AVMs may be **embolized** radiologically, as a definitive treatment or a prelude to **surgical excision**.

ARTERIAL ULCERATION

Ischaemic ulceration is one of the manifestations of critical limb ischaemia. Ulcers may form at the peripheries, particularly over the pressure areas, for example the heel, malleoli and between the toes. The cause is an inadequate blood supply to the tissues.

There may also be a sensory neuropathy, particularly in diabetic patients.

Critical limb ischaemia is limb-threatening and should be treated urgently as described above.

VENOUS ULCERATION

Chronic venous insufficiency describes the condition in the lower limb that follows deep vein reflux and obstruction.

Sustained venous hypertension leads to chronic swelling, pain, eczema, lipodermatosclerosis and ultimately ulceration of the skin.

In most patients the valve damage and obstruction are secondary to a previous DVT, but there is a small group of patients with primary deep venous reflux.

Occasionally severe superficial venous reflux or arteriovenous communications can induce sufficient superficial venous hypertension to cause ulceration.

Investigation
Clinical diagnostic indicators

The patient may have a history of DVT or an unproven episode of leg swelling following a high-risk event, e.g. orthopaedic surgery.

The ulceration usually occurs in the 'gaiter' region of the leg. There is usually evidence of chronic venous insufficiency in the skin surrounding the ulcer – pigmentation and lipodermatosclerosis. There may be varicose veins and scars from previous healed ulcers.

Imaging

Duplex ultrasonography will demonstrate any significant venous reflux or occlusion.

The arterial circulation should be imaged if ischaemia is suspected and the **ABPI** measured.

An **ascending phlebogram** is the best way to demonstrate the presence of chronic obstruction in the iliac veins and inferior vena cava.

Blood tests

A thrombophilia screen should be considered.

Tissue biopsy

A biopsy of the ulcer should be performed if there is a suspicion of malignancy, e.g. an unusual clinical appearance or failure to heal with treatment.

Management

Local compression is the mainstay of treatment with multilayer bandaging.

Most ulcers of a purely venous aetiology will heal with properly supervised compression (80–90 per cent at 1 year).

Surgical treatment The ultimate objective of treatment should be the correction of the causative abnormal venous physiology, as described above, followed by compression therapy.

The local treatment of the ulcer should be followed by correction of the venous abnormality.

Admission for **bed rest**, **excision and skin grafting** should be considered if the ulcer still does not heal with conservative measures. (Biopsies should also be taken to exclude malignancy.)

The ulcer base and edge are excised down to deep fascia. Split skin is applied, usually using the thigh as a donor site.

Once the graft has taken, efforts should be made to prevent recurrence. Twenty to 30 per cent of ulcers recur within 5 years so the patient should wear a **compression stocking** indefinitely.

THE UPPER LIMB, HEAD AND NECK

The main problems caused by vascular disease in the upper limb, head and neck are:

- pain
- discoloration
- dysfunction
- swelling
- transient ischaemic attack, stroke, transient blindness.

The causes of these problems are set out in Tables 11.7–11.

Table 11.7
The causes of pain in the upper limb

Arterial	Acute ischaemia
	Embolism
	Thrombus
	Trauma
	Aortic dissection
	Chronic ischaemia
	Intermittent claudication
	Rest pain
	Ulceration
	Gangrene
Venous	Deep vein thrombosis
Orthopaedic	Shoulder, elbow, wrist
Systemic/neurological	Cervical, thoracic outlet syndrome

Table 11.8
The causes of discoloration of the upper limb

Arterial	Vasospasm
	Ischaemia
	Cyanosis
Venous	Axial vein thrombosis

Table 11.9
The causes of dysfunction in the upper limb

Arterial	Steal syndromes
Neurological	C spine, thoracic outlet syndrome, carpal tunnel syndrome
	Cerebrovascular accident

Table 11.10
The causes of swelling of the upper limb

Venous	Proximal deep vein thrombosis
Lymphoedema	Congenital
	Acquired

Table 11.11
The causes of transient ischaemic attack/stroke/blindness

Arterial	Carotid disease
	Vertebrobasilar insufficiency
	Cerebral haemorrhage
	Cerebral thrombosis
	Vasculitis
	Cardiac embolus
	Cardiac arrythmia
	Subclavian steal syndrome

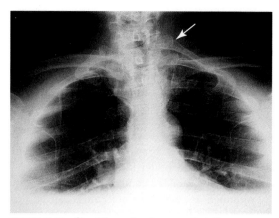

FIGURE 11.26 Chest X-ray showing a cervical rib

ACUTE ISCHAEMIA IN THE UPPER LIMB

Acute upper limb ischaemia can have a number of causes. Embolism is the most common cause. Acute thrombosis *in situ* is rare. Compression of the artery by the bony structures of the thoracic outlet or a cervical rib can lead to local dilation or thrombosis.

Aortic dissection can involve the origin of the branches of the arch of the aorta. The left subclavian artery is more often affected than the right.

Axillary artery thrombosis can occur following trauma, either with a humerus fracture or blunt trauma. Chronic conditions such as Takayasu's disease and giant cell arteritis and thrombosis of a subclavian artery aneurysm are rarer causes.

Investigation

Clinical diagnostic indicators

The patient presents with arm pain, pallor and loss of pulses. A neurological deficit or muscle tenderness indicate a surgical emergency.

As the source of the embolus is usually the heart, there may be a history of fibrillation, heart failure or ischaemic heart disease. The patient must be examined for atrial fibrillation, abnormal heart sounds and other signs of failure.

The level of the arterial occlusion may suggest the cause. Cardiac emboli usually lodge in the upper axillary artery or at the brachial artery bifurcation at elbow level. Digital artery occlusion is more likely to be caused by vasospasm, frostbite or a shower of emboli from infective endocarditis or an axillary artery embolus. There may be a palpable subclavian aneurysm or cervical rib.

Medical assessment

Patients with a cardiac source of emboli should undergo a thorough medical assessment because they often have significant cardiac disease.

Imaging

A hand-held **Doppler flow detector** can rapidly confirm the level of the occlusion.

X-rays of the chest and thoracic outlet may reveal a cervical rib (Fig 11.26).

ECG and **echocardiography** are essential to seek a cardiac cause.

Duplex ultrasonography, **CT angiography** or conventional **digital subtraction arteriography** may be useful in unusual cases where thrombolysis or bypass is being considered.

In cases where the cause is likely to be a cardiac embolus and the site of occlusion apparent on the basis of clinical assessment, arterial imaging may not be necessary.

Blood tests

A full blood count should be performed.

Conservative treatment

Occasionally the symptoms are mild and resolve quickly as collateral vessels open up. In these cases the patient should be **anticoagulated** to stop distal thrombosis, unless there are contraindications. The persistence of arm claudication may be an indication for late revascularization.

Intravenous heparin should be given once the diagnosis is established.

Surgical treatment

Most patients with symptoms and a proven embolus should undergo **brachial embolectomy**. This can be performed under local anaesthetic. Rarely, a bypass using vein as a conduit may be required.

Although a brachial embolectomy can be performed under local anaesthetic these patients are often frail and an anaesthetist should be present to monitor the patient's vital signs with **ECG** and **oximetry** and administer analgesia and sedation as necessary.

The limb is prepared and draped leaving the hand in a transparent plastic bag so that the circulation can be assessed. Embolectomy is performed through a transverse arteriotomy using a 2 or 3 Fr balloon catheter (see Fig 11.5). Following wound closure, a light compression bandage should be applied to prevent haematoma formation.

The anticoagulants should be continued and monitored carefully.

Complications Rethrombosis may occur, particularly if there is an underlying thrombophilia. A significant number of patients may have an occult malignancy. Further emboli can occur if anticoagulation is stopped or a source cannot be treated.

The wound is sometimes complicated by haematoma formation. Amputation may, rarely, be required if the blood supply cannot be restored.

CHRONIC UPPER LIMB ISCHAEMIA

Proximal arterial stenoses or occlusions may be caused by atherosclerosis. This preferentially affects the origins of the innominate and subclavian arteries.

Compression of the artery at the thoracic outlet, either by a cervical rib or a fibrous band, may cause intermittent posture-related symptoms. Post-stenotic dilation may also be the site of thrombosis that subsequently embolizes distally.

Large vessel arteritis such as Takayasu's and giant cell arteritis may be the cause of progressive stenosis, particularly in young females.

Distal vessel vasospasm may be primary (Raynaud's disease) or secondary to a number of conditions including autoimmune disorders, local trauma and cervical rib, when it is called Raynaud's phenomenon.

Investigation
Clinical diagnostic indicators

Patients may present with arm pain on exercise (claudication).

A proximal subclavian stenosis may also result in 'subclavian steal', where blood supply to the arm is provided from retrograde flow down the vertebral artery; use of the arm 'steals' blood from the posterior cerebral circulation and causes vertigo, dizziness or even syncope (Fig 11.27).

In younger patients, **arteritis** should be suspected. Patients with atherosclerotic disease will have vascular risk factors and signs of arterial disease at other sites.

Symptoms of positional arm pain, especially with the shoulder abducted or raised above the head, may be caused by compression of the subclavian artery at the thoracic outlet.

Vasospasm may be triggered by a cold environment and cause the characteristic colour changes of **Raynaud's phenomenon** – pallor, cyanosis and reactive hyperaemia.

In **scleroderma** the digits may have a characteristically tapered appearance.

The supraclavicular fossa should be palpated for a **cervical rib** or **subclavian aneurysm**. Pulses should be checked at all levels and Allen's test performed for palmar arch perfusion. With the arms abducted and externally rotated, slowly clenching the fingers may reproduce the symptoms associated with thoracic outlet compression (Roos test).

A difference between the brachial blood pressures in the arms suggests proximal stenosis.

Imaging

Duplex ultrasonography may locate stenoses or aneurysms, although the intrathoracic portion of the vessels is hard to visualize.

Subclavian blood flow can be measured with the arm in different positions to detect positional occlusion in thoracic outlet syndrome (Figs 11.28 and 11.29).

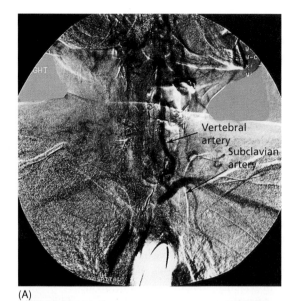

(A)

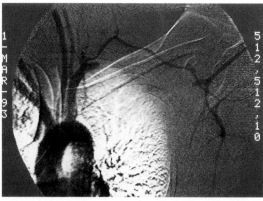

FIGURE 11.28 Angiogram showing arterial thoracic outlet syndrome. The artery is compressed when the shoulder is abducted

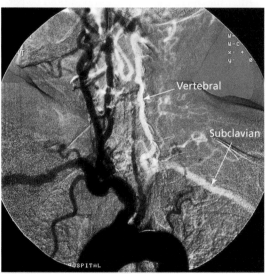

(B)

FIGURE 11.27 (A, B) Angiograms showing cervical steal, with delayed retrograde flow in the vertebral artery filling the occluded subclavian artery

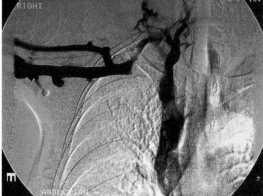

FIGURE 11.29 Compression of subclavian vein at thoracic outlet when the shoulder is abducted

symptoms, for example cervical spine disease, neurological thoracic outlet syndrome or carpal tunnel syndrome.

Management

The aim of treatment should be to relieve the symptoms, as tissue-threatening ischaemia is rare. The patient may be **reassured** and need no further treatment if the symptoms are very mild.

Raynaud's phenomenon is treated by cold avoidance, warm gloves and vasodilators such as calcium blockers. Severe cases may require prostacyclin infusions.

Contrast angiography with intravenous (for proximal causes) or intra-arterial contrast, or **CT angiography** are used to define the disease distribution if intervention is indicated.

A cold provocation test may provoke features of Raynaud's disease.

Electromyography should be used if there is a suspicion of a neurological cause of the arm

Proximal stenoses or occlusions may be treated with **angioplasty and stenting**.

Carotid–subclavian bypass may be performed for proximal disease. Distal disease may be treated with an autogenous vein bypass if the symptoms are severe.

THORACIC OUTLET SYNDROME

The subclavian artery or vein, or the trunks of the brachial plexus, can be compressed at the root of the neck by a cervical rib, a fibrous band, hypertrophy of the scalene muscles or a bony prominence on the first rib or clavicle.

Investigation

Clinical diagnostic indicators

The symptoms may have any combination of arterial, venous or neurological features. They may be related to the position of the arm – often being exacerbated by abduction and external rotation.

Venous thoracic outlet syndrome (TOS) may present with congestion, swelling or venous thrombosis, and often occurs in body builders or those who perform repetitive arm movements.

Arterial TOS usually presents as arm ache or ischaemia, especially on elevation or, occasionally, Raynaud's syndrome. Post-stenotic aneurysm formation may result in thrombosis or embolism. Neurological TOS usually affects the lower roots (C8, T1) of the brachial plexus and presents with paraesthesiae, pain or wasting of the intrinsic hand muscles.

Imaging

X-rays of the thoracic outlet will demonstrate a cervical rib (see Fig 11.26).

A **duplex ultrasound** with the arm in different positions will show flow disturbance in the artery or vein.

Phlebography and **digital subtraction angiography** have the advantage over CT in that flow may be assessed with the arm in different positions.

MRI can be used to distinguish degenerative cervical spine disease as a cause of nerve root dysfunction.

Function studies

Electromyography will confirm nerve dysfunction and may indicate alternative or coexisting pathology, for example carpal tunnel syndrome.

Management

Symptomless cervical ribs or patients with mild symptoms may be treated conservatively.

Cervical or **first rib resection** should be performed on those with symptomatic arterial or nerve compression and following venous thrombolysis.

A cervical rib can be removed through a supraclavicular incision. First rib resection can be performed through supra- and/or infraclavicular incisions or from an axillary approach. The scalenus anterior muscle and any fibrous bands constricting the neurovascular structures must be divided.

After the operation a chest X-ray should be performed to exclude a pneumothorax.

Complications Damage to the brachial plexus, phrenic nerve and vascular structures needs to be avoided.

Results Recurrence of the symptoms is rare. The persistence of neurological symptoms is most often a result of an incorrect original diagnosis.

Subclavian vein thrombosis

Subclavian vein thrombosis should be treated with **thrombolysis** if there is significant swelling.

Following confirmatory phlebography, a catheter is placed into the thrombus via the brachial vein and tPA infused as a 5-mg bolus and then at 1 mg/hour until there is radiographic clearance.

The patient should be warned of the potential haemorrhagic complications of thrombolysis. If the thrombus is old it will not lyse.

If successful the patient should be anticoagulated until the cause, e.g. a cervical rib, is treated.

A follow-up phlebogram should be performed and any residual stenosis dilated with a balloon angioplasty.

CAROTID ATHEROSCLEROSIS

Atherosclerosis affects the carotid artery, predominantly around the carotid bifurcation. Unstable carotid plaque can be the source of emboli to the

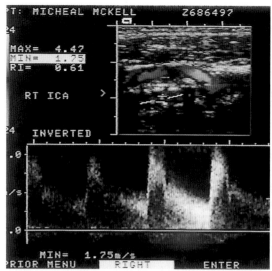

FIGURE 11.30 Duplex ultrasound of the carotid bifurcation showing significant stenosis. Increased velocity and widening of the spectral band indicates stenosis

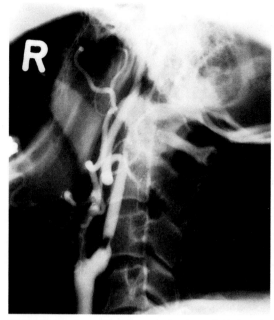

FIGURE 11.31 A carotid angiograph showing a tight stenosis

cerebral circulation causing transient ischaemic attacks (TIAs) or stroke. Occasionally a stenosis resulting from the plaque may cause symptoms of hypoperfusion, particularly if the contralateral or vertebral arteries are also affected.

Investigation

Clinical diagnostic indicators

Patients may be symptomless. Disease in the carotid artery may be detected on auscultation, on imaging for contralateral symptomatic disease or during work-up for coronary surgery.

Symptomatic patients present with focal motor or sensory deficits or amaurosis fugax.

The presence or absence of a carotid bruit is a poor indicator of carotid disease.

Imaging

Duplex ultrasound is able to image the bifurcation to assess the extent of disease and degree of stenosis in most patients (Fig 11.30).

As ultrasonography is user-dependent. **CT angiography**, **DSA** or **MRI** may be required to confirm the diagnosis. These methods also allow imaging of the aortic arch, proximal common carotid and distal internal carotid and intracranial vessels.

Formal **angiography** can be useful particularly if there is significant calcification of the carotid artery, which can obscure imaging by other methods (Fig 11.31).

Management

All patients with carotid atherosclerosis should be treated with optimal medical care – the control of hypertension, hyperlipidaemia and diabetes, stopping smoking, an antiplatelet agent and a statin.

Patients presenting with severe (>70 per cent) stenosis and ipsilateral carotid territory symptoms should be treated by carotid endarterectomy, which significantly reduces the risk of subsequent stroke.

Symptomless patients with >60 per cent stenosis have a low annual risk of stroke but this can be reduced by carotid endartectomy. Local policies vary on when operation is offered, but careful counselling of the patient regarding the risks and benefits is essential.

The place of carotid **angioplasty** and **stenting** has yet to be demonstrated in trials and is reserved for patients with surgically 'hostile' necks, for example after previous surgery or radiotherapy.

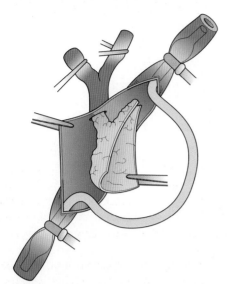

FIGURE 11.32 Carotid endarterectomy showing shunt in place and removal of atheroma

Patients with <70 per cent stenosis should be managed **conservatively** with best medical therapy. All patients should be on an antiplatelet agent and a statin if there are no contraindications.

Carotid endarterectomy should be reserved for symptomatic patients with >70 per cent stenosis and severe symptomless stenoses associated with significant contralateral disease prior to coronary artery bypass surgery.

The operation can be performed under local or general anaesthetic.

Cerebral perfusion during the operation can be monitored with a transcranial Doppler flow detector to determine whether any emboli are occurring and whether a shunt is required during carotid clamping.

The carotid artery and the carotid bifurcation are exposed through an incision anterior to the sternomastoid muscle, preserving the vagus and hypoglossal nerves.

Following the administration of 5000 units of heparin the artery is clamped and a longitudinal arteriotomy performed. During the endarterectomy cerebral perfusion can be maintained with a shunt. The atheroma is removed and the artery closed primarily or with a patch. Quality control with an intra-operative completion duplex scan or angiograph is recommended to exclude technical errors.

The patient should be closely monitored during early recovery for the appearance of neurological complications.

Complications Wound haematoma sometimes requires evacuation. Emboli causing minor cerebral symptoms may be treated with heparin or dextran infusions to reduce the risk of postoperative stroke. Carotid artery occlusion by thrombosis causing a stroke requires an urgent reoperation.

Patch infection is a rare late complication, and can be treated with excision and interposition vein grafting.

Results The 30-day mortality of carotid endarterectomy should be no more than 1 per cent, and the stroke rate 2–4 per cent.

The majority of strokes occur intraoperatively.

12

The mouth, tongue and lips

Jeremy Collyer

The problems caused by abnormalities and disease of the mouth, tongue and lips can be grouped together into the following categories:

- cleft lip and cleft palate
- facial asymmetry
- coloured skin lesions
- ulcers on the lips
- swellings of the lips
- pigmented lesions in the mouth
- swellings within the mouth
- coloured patches within the mouth
- ulcers on the tongue.

On many occasions the patient will not only complain about their problem but also know the diagnosis because many of the conditions of the mouth, tongue and lips are common, well known and easily recognized by both the patient and the surgeon.

This chapter discusses the investigation and management of the above problems.

CONGENITAL ABNORMALITIES OF THE LIPS, PALATE AND JAW

Cleft lip and palate

Cleft lip and palate has an incidence of 1.5 in 1000 live births in Europe. The incidence is higher in Native Americans and lowest in Africans. Cleft lip is more common in boys and cleft palate more common in girls.

The lip and primary palate begin to develop at 4–5 weeks' gestational age. The two medial nasal swellings and the maxillary swellings fuse to form the upper lip. The nasal swellings also merge at deeper levels to form the primary palate, which is the premaxilla in the adult, so for embryological reasons clefts of the lip are almost invariably associated with clefts of the primary palate.

The secondary palate develops at approximately 9 weeks of developmental age. It is formed by medial growth of the palatal shelves of the maxilla – which normally fuse together – and with the nasal septum as the tongue is pushed down during development.

Cleft lip and cleft premaxilla may be associated with chromosomal defects such as **trisomy 13 (Patau)** and **trisomy 21 (Down's) syndromes** but many cases are isolated abnormalities. If one child has a cleft lip subsequent siblings have a higher than average risk of being similarly affected.

By contrast isolated cleft palate is more commonly associated with other congenital deformities, such as Treacher Collins syndrome, velocardiofacial syndrome and Stickler syndrome.

Investigation

Clinical diagnostic indicators

The diagnosis of these abnormalities is obvious at birth to the mother and the physician, but nowadays with the general introduction of antenatal ultrasound scanning the prenatal diagnosis of cleft lip and palate is becoming increasingly common. This allows the mother to be prepared for the problems the child is likely to encounter and for the surgeon to arrange appropriate multidisciplinary team management.

A careful postnatal clinical examination is important to look for any of the other congenital abnormalities mentioned above.

Genetic counselling should be arranged if a specific syndrome is detected.

Diagnostic pitfall: the submucous cleft

Most cleft deformities are diagnosed at or before birth. A submucous cleft is an incomplete cleft of the hard palate in which there is a defect in the bone and muscles of the palate beneath an intact mucosa, so the condition may not be noticed. Patients may be symptomless or have signs of **velopharyngeal insufficiency** (VPI). This indicates an inability to separate the nose from the mouth during speech leading to an abnormal voice. A submucous cleft is diagnosed by looking for a cleft uvula or feeling for a notch in the hard palate. Adenoidectomy can precipitate VPI in these patients.

Immediate management

The immediate management priorities for a newborn with a cleft palate are:

Maintain an airway. Dyspnoeic infants should be nursed prone so that the tongue falls out of the airway.

Ensure that feeding can take place. Feeding is difficult as the lack of a lip seal causes difficulty in suckling. Those with a cleft palate and a cleft lip have problems caused by milk escaping into the nose. **These babies are best fed sitting upright.** Special teats and bottles are available for those who cannot breast feed.

Surgical repair

The surgical management of cleft lip and palate is aimed at restoring normal facial appearance and function as soon as possible so that the child can develop normally.

   Repair of the lip and anterior palate should be performed between 6 weeks and 3 months after birth. The musculature must be repaired as well as the skin and mucosa of the lip.

   Repair of the palate is carried out at 6 months. Palatal repair is timed to allow speech to develop normally and to minimize interference with the growth of the maxilla. **Grommets** are usually inserted at the same time because there is often Eustachian tube dysfunction.

   Bone grafting to bridge the cleft in the pre-maxilla to aid eruption of the upper canine tooth should be performed around 9 years of age.

   As the child approaches skeletal maturity it may be necessary to reposition the maxilla with **maxillary osteotomy or distraction.**

Hemifacial microsomia

Investigation

Hemifacial microsomia (HFM) is a rare asymmetrical congenital deformity affecting the lower half of the face, most commonly the ears, mouth and mandible, with an incidence of 1 in 5600 live births. There may be respiratory obstruction. Most cases are sporadic.

Imaging

The diagnosis of hemifacial microsomia can be confirmed with **X-rays** and a **CT scan**.

Management

Emergency tracheostomy may be necessary after birth. Major **corrective surgery** is often deferred until the patient has grown enough.

Treacher Collins syndrome

This is an autosomal dominant inherited condition, affecting males and females equally, with an incidence of 1 in 10 000 births. It is caused by a defect in the development of the first branchial arch.

Investigation

Clinical diagnostic indicators

The first branchial arch defect causes a small mandible, poor zygomatic development leading to downward slanting eyes and abnormal or absent ears. Some of these abnormalities may be obvious to the surgeon but are not always noticed by the mother.

Management

Tracheostomy may be required soon after birth. Any associated cleft palate should be repaired at 6 months.

   Mandibular elongation is achieved by **distraction osteogenesis** using a variety of external and internal devices. The principle is to fracture the bone, allow a primary callus to form, and then gradually move the ends apart so that the callus is stretched to fill the gap.

   The orbits are repaired with bone grafts and the soft tissue defects corrected at 5–6 years of age.

PIGMENTED LESIONS OF THE LIPS
Oral melanotic macules

These brown spots consist of normal melanocytes that produce excessive amounts of melanin. The cells are mature and are therefore incapable of transformation into malignant melanoma.

Investigation

Clinical diagnostic indicators

These lesions are most common on the lips, but can occur anywhere on the oral mucosa. They are small, usually less than 5 mm across, evenly pigmented, and are seen in small numbers.

Diagnostic pitfall: malignant melanoma

Even though **malignant melanoma of the lip is a rare condition**, more likely to be seen in the nasal cavity and palate than the lip and usually presenting with the same features as malignant melanomata elsewhere, it is the most important differential diagnosis. Any suspicious lesion should be fully investigated.

Tissue biopsy

If there is doubt about the diagnosis a biopsy must be performed.

Ancillary investigations

Multiple melanocytic macules occur in Peutz–Jegher syndrome and Addison's disease, so both these alternative diagnoses should be excluded.

Peutz–Jegher syndrome is an autosomal dominant congenital condition of intestinal polyposis with a possibility of malignant change. It is associated with oral melanocytic macules. This diagnosis should be excluded by investigating the alimentary tract.

Melanocytic macules are also found in **Addison's disease** because high ACTH (adrenocorticotrophic hormone) levels stimulate the melanocytes. If it is suspected, biochemical tests will reveal hyponatraemia and hyperkalaemia, and the diagnosis confirmed by demonstrating a failure of cortisol levels to rise after an ACTH infusion.

Management

The only indication to remove an oral melanotic macule is when there is diagnostic doubt.

Vascular malformations

Vascular malformations can be venous, capillary, arterial, lymphatic or mixed (see Chapter 5), and are clinically and histologically distinct from the haemangiomata that affect neonates. They are classified as high- or low-flow malformations.

Investigation

See Chapter 5.

Ancillary investigations

Patients with high-flow lesions may have clinical and haemodynamically measurable evidence of high-output cardiac failure. Adequate volumes of blood should be cross-matched before surgery.

Management

Bleeding from a high-flow lesion in the oral cavity is a **surgical emergency** and can be precipitated by the extraction of a tooth. Emergency management is appropriate: blood and fluid resuscitation with the simultaneous arrest of haemorrhage usually by packing.

Treatment of these lesions and associated swelling may require management of the airway.

Symptomless lesions of both high- and low-flow subtypes can be managed **conservatively** with reassurance and cosmetic advice.

The indications for emergency treatment are:

- airway compromise
- bleeding (more common with high-flow lesions).

Low-flow lesions may be **excised** but recurrence is common because of the pathological factors discussed above.

Sclerosant injection and compressive suturing are alternatives, but recurrence is also frequent.

High-flow lesions are considerably more difficult to treat. They are best managed by **embolization of the feeding vessels followed by immediate surgical excision**. Even radical surgery may not provide long-term cure.

Squamous cell carcinoma

Benign ulcers of the lip caused by trauma or a virus such as herpes simplex are characterized by rapid healing within 14 days. The commonest cause, in an adult, of a non-healing ulcer of the lip is a squamous cell carcinoma. Aetiological factors include exposure to sunlight, immunosuppression and pipe smoking. The main **differential diagnosis** is a basal cell carcinoma.

Investigation

Clinical diagnostic indicators

The diagnosis may be obvious from clinical examination. The sites are:

- lower lip – 95 per cent
- upper lip – 5 per cent
- oral commissure – 5 per cent.

The ulcer usually has a thick rolled edge.

Metastatic disease is uncommon but when it does occur it involves the lymph nodes in the submental triangle and then the jugular chain. If the ulcer is infected these lymph nodes may be enlarged by inflammation.

Tissue biopsy

A simple punch biopsy is usually sufficient to confirm the diagnosis.

Imaging

Small lesions do not require any imaging. Larger lesions and more aggressive histological subtypes should have **CT imaging** of the regional lymph nodes, as this is more sensitive and specific than clinical examination alone.

The tumour should be staged before planning treatment. Clinical staging employs the TNM system (Table 12.1).

Management

Surgical excision with a 5-mm margin of normal tissue taken in all dimensions around the palpable tumour is the first line treatment (Fig 12.1).

The surgical defect is then reconstructed to maintain the muscular and sensory function of the lip. The mouth is in the centre of the face and it is essential that the lip be restored with tissues that match both the colour and the contour of the nearby tissues. Small defects can be closed primarily. Larger defects may need local flap reconstruction.

Metastatic lymph nodes in the neck can be treated by block dissection with or without radiotherapy.

Squamous cell carcinoma of the lip can be treated by external beam **radiotherapy** using a lead shield to protect the rest of the oral cavity. However, the best results require fractionated treatments, which means many hospital visits. There may also

Table 12.1
TNM classification of carcinoma of the lip

T for tumour

T1	T2	T3	T4
Lesion less than 2 cm	Lesion greater than 2 cm, less than 4 cm	Lesion greater than 4 cm, does not involve adjacent structures	Lesion invading adjacent structures, e.g. soft tissue of chin or nose, bony involvement

N for lymph node involvement

N0	N1	N2	N3
No detectable lymph node involvement	Single ipsilateral node less than 3 cm	N2a: Single ipsilateral node between 3 and 6 cm N2b: Multiple ipsilateral nodes less than 6 cm N2c: Contralateral or bilateral lymph node involvement less than 6 cm	Any lymph node greater than 6 cm

M for metastases

M0	M1
No evidence of distant metastasis	Evidence of distant metastasis

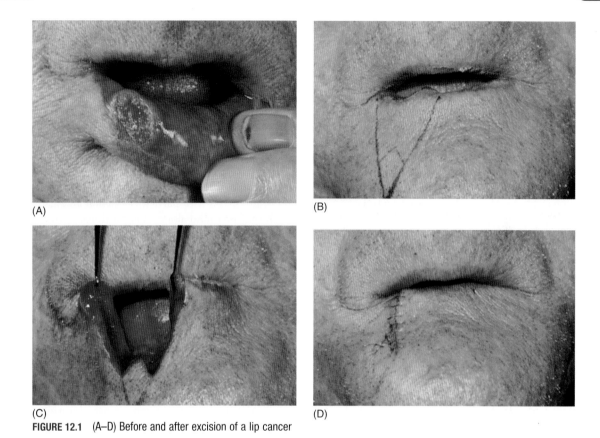

(A)

(B)

(C)

(D)

FIGURE 12.1 (A–D) Before and after excision of a lip cancer

be unpredictable scarring causing problems with lip function. Radiotherapy is usually reserved for an adjunctive role in combination with surgery for the treatment of aggressive tumours.

Mucocele

A mucocele results from the extravasation of mucin into the submucosal tissues following trauma to the fine ducts of the many minor salivary glands within the lower lip. This triggers an inflammatory reaction which walls off the mucin with a fibrous lining, so forming a cyst. They are very rare in the upper lip.

Investigation

Clinical diagnostic indicators

The diagnosis is clinical. Mucoceles present as a localized lower lip swelling which varies in size depending on the leakage of its mucus. The swelling is blue or grey, soft and smooth and transilluminates. No special investigations are necessary.

Diagnostic pitfall: salivary gland tumour

If there is no history of intermittent swelling, or if the lesion is hard and not cystic on palpation, and particularly if it is in the upper lip, the swelling may be a minor salivary gland tumour.

Management

Mucoceles can be **excised** through the mucosal surface of the lip, taking care to avoid any fibres of the mental nerve. Salivary gland tumours require a wider margin of surgical excision to ensure complete removal.

Fibroepithelial polyp

Fibroepithelial polyps are benign hamartomata. They consist of all the normal components of oral mucosa in a pedunculated lesion. They are thought to be caused by trauma as most arise on the lateral borders of the tongue, lips and cheeks, areas prone to being accidentally bitten, but they can occur anywhere in the oral mucosa and without a history of trauma.

The lesion is a rubbery pedunculated polyp. The clinical appearance is usually sufficient to make the diagnosis.

If symptomless they can be left *in situ*. Symptomatic polyps can be removed by simple **surgical excision** with local anaesthesia. Recurrence is unusual.

Orofacial granulomatosis

Orofacial granulomatosis is diagnosed by finding giant cell granulomata in a biopsy of a swollen lip. It is an allergic condition related to various food allergens including cinnamon and benzoates. It is more common in the upper lip. The swelling varies but hardly ever resolves completely, and may be accompanied by aphthous ulcers.

Investigation

Blood tests

It is associated with inflammatory bowel disease so it is important to obtain a **full blood count** and estimate **serum folate, vitamin B12 and systemic inflammatory markers**.

Tissue biopsy

The histological diagnosis is made from a biopsy of the mucosal surface of the lip, deep enough to sample the full depth of the submucosa.

Diagnostic pitfall: angio-oedema

Angio-oedema is acute-onset swelling after contact with an allergen. It is associated with the rare condition of complement deficiency.

Management

If inflammatory bowel disease is revealed and treated the oral symptoms will usually improve.

A **cinnamon-** and **benzoate-free diet** should be tried if there is no obvious cause.

Corticosteroids and other immune modulators have a role in refractory cases.

It is possible to reduce the bulk of the lips surgically (cheiloplasty) if the medical approach fails.

PROBLEMS ON THE FLOOR OF THE MOUTH, GUMS AND PALATE

PIGMENTED LESIONS

Amalgam tattoo

This condition results from staining of the gums and oral mucosa with particles of dental amalgam, which may be found along collagen fibres or in the walls of blood vessels.

The process is most common in the mucosa lining the buccal aspect of the dento-alveolar processes of the mandible and the maxilla. The lesion is blue-grey with an indistinct border. The palate is less commonly affected, and it is rare to find lesions on the tongue.

The proximity to current or previous dental restorations indicates the diagnosis.

It does not show on X-ray.

Conservative management is appropriate unless there is doubt about the diagnosis, when **surgical excision** may be used for the purpose of obtaining histological confirmation of the diagnosis and treatment.

Malignant melanoma

The oral mucous membranes are thinner than skin and lack the thick layers of epidermis and dermis. As a consequence the rich lymphatics of the submucosa are relatively superficial and mucosal melanoma tends to enter the vertical growth phase earlier than its cutaneous equivalent (see Chapter 5). Satellite tumours are common, and the regional lymph nodes must be assessed carefully. Melanoma of the oral mucosa has a worse prognosis than cutaneous melanoma – a 5-year survival rate of only around 20 per cent.

Investigation

Clinical diagnostic indicators

Mucosal melanoma most commonly affects the palate. It displays clinical features similar to those of the cutaneous tumour. The ABCD mnemonic is a useful way of remembering the features of a pigmented lesion that suggest it is or is becoming malignant:

A   asymmetry
B   border irregularity
C   colour black and variable with darkening of pigmentation
D   diameter enlarging

Tissue biopsy

A biopsy, preferably excisional, should be obtained from any suspicious lesion to confirm the diagnosis.

Fine needle aspiration cytology can be used to confirm the presence of lymph node metastases.

Imaging

The staging investigations required are similar to those needed to stage a squamous carcinoma of the oral cavity, namely **CT or MRI scanning of the primary site and neck**, along with **CT scanning of the chest and upper abdomen**.

Management

Surgical treatment of these difficult tumours should be planned at a meeting of the appropriate surgical disciplines.

Excision of the tumour with a wide surgical margin is essential and may require major reconstruction. Regional lymph node metastases are treated by **block dissection**.

There is no cytotoxic drug regimen of any value. Surgery is the only effective treatment.

SWELLINGS
Ranula

A ranula is a mucus-containing cyst in the floor of the mouth, usually in young people, caused by damage to the ducts of the sublingual salivary gland.

Clinical diagnostic indicators

A ranula has the same bluish tinge as a mucocele of the lip. The swelling is soft and fluctuant. Diagnosis is clinical.

Diagnostic pitfall: tumour of the sublingual gland

Tumours of the sublingual gland are rare and present as a **solid mass** in the floor of the mouth. Unlike the ranula they do not vary in size. A significant proportion of sublingual tumours are malignant.

Management

If the ranula is symptomless it does not need treatment.

Partial excision or deroofing, a simple procedure that can be carried out with a local anaesthetic, will reduce its size but cannot guarantee a permanent cure.

Persistent recurrent lesions are best treated by **excision of the sublingual gland**. This requires a general anaesthetic, and familiarity with the structures of the floor of the mouth to avoid damage to the submandibular duct and the lingual nerve.

Exostosis

An exostosis is a bony hard swelling arising from the cortex of the mandible or maxilla, of no known cause and consisting histologically of normal bone. They are commonly found in the midline of the hard palate (**torus palatinus**) and on the lingual aspect of the mandible (**torus mandibularis**) where they may be bilateral and symmetrical.

Their bony hard consistency is diagnostic and X-rays are rarely indicated.

Conservative treatment is appropriate for the majority as they are usually symptomless and present as incidental clinical findings.

Large masses interfering with chewing can be removed.

Odontogenic cysts

A wide variety of the pathological abnormalities that affect the mandible and maxilla arise from the teeth.

Dental cysts are relatively common and produce radiolucent swellings within the jaws. Their cause is chronic infection around the root structure of damaged and decayed teeth.

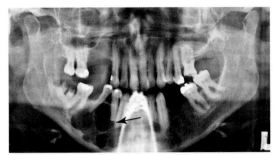

FIGURE 12.2 An orthopantomograph of an ameloblastoma showing 'soap bubbles'

Dentigerous cysts arise from the follicle that surrounds the enamel of unerupted teeth. They have an epithelial lining that sheds cells into the cyst cavity, which then degenerate to produce a cholesterol-rich content.

Odontogenic keratocysts arise from the oral epithelium that gives rise to the dental follicles. They are lined with keratinized epithelium based on a flat basement membrane. They are likely to recur after simple enucleation.

The presence of multiple keratocysts is a cardinal feature of **basal cell naevus syndrome** (an autosomal dominant condition which is characterized by keratocysts, calcification of the falx cerebri, frontal bossing, basal cell carcinomata, epidermoid cysts and rib anomalies). Life expectancy is normal.

Investigation
Imaging
Many odontogenic cysts present as incidental findings on dental and facial **X-rays**. They appear as radiolucent areas greater than 1 cm in diameter.

Tissue biopsy
Larger swellings should be biopsied as they might be keratocysts that require definitive excision.

Diagnostic pitfall: ameloblastoma
Ameloblastoma can be misdiagnosed as a dental cyst.

Management
Infection is treated initially with **antibiotics**. **Surgical drainage** is indicated if an abscess forms outside the confines of the mandible spreading into the fascial planes of the neck.

Odontogenic cysts require surgical treatment, except in older or unfit people. The operation is done through the mouth. The cyst may be **excised**, or **marsupialized**, i.e. the removal of the roof of the cyst leaving the remaining cyst lining open to drain into the oral cavity.

Odontogenic tumours

Ameloblastoma is the commonest odontogenic tumour to cause swelling of the jaw. Metastases are rare but it is prone to recur if not adequately excised.

Investigation
Imaging
Plain radiographs may show the multilocular 'soap bubble' appearance of an ameloblastoma (Fig 12.2).

CT scanning will demonstrate the full extent of the lesion and help to plan surgical treatment.

Management
Surgical excision is the preferred treatment. The entire lesion with a surrounding cuff of normal bone must be removed. In the mandible, reconstruction may be required.

Lichen planus (white and red patches)

Lichen planus may be found anywhere in the mouth without associated skin desease. Malignant transformation is rare.

Investigation
Clinical diagnostic indicators
Lichen planus frequently appears as **lacy white patches on a red background** (striate type). There are atrophic and ulcerative variants, which can co-exist in the same patient.

It may be symptomless or be painful after eating spicy food.

Although the clinical appearance of lichen planus is often diagnostic, particularly when the lesions are symmetrical, the variability of the lesions often means that full thickness incisional biopsy may be required to exclude other important differential diagnoses, including squamous cell carcinoma.

Tissue biopsy

Incisional biopsies are for diagnosis not treatment, but if there is doubt about the true diagnosis it may be more appropriate to **excise the whole patch**. This situation arises most often with an asymmetrical area on the tongue, where there is a high possibility of cancer.

Diagnostic pitfall: squamous cell carcinoma

Squamous cell carcinomata can arise in any type of lichen planus lesion, although most do not.

Management

Topical steroids are employed in a variety of ways to treat the affected area of oral mucosa. More potent immunosuppressive agents such as **cyclosporin** and **tacrolimus** should only be used in severe cases, as they are associated with the induction of oral cancers.

Leukoplakia and erythroplakia

Investigation

Clinical diagnostic indicators

Leukoplakia means 'white flat area', erythroplakia means 'red flat area' and erythroleukoplakia means 'red and white flat area'. Each is a descriptive term, not a pathological diagnosis. These lesions are important as a few will undergo malignant transformation. Nodular growth or areas of mixed colour are suggestive of malignant change.

Tissue biopsy

Incisional biopsy is quite often indicated to prove that the lesion is leukoplakia and not a squamous cell carcinoma. Biopsy may also show candidal infection.

Management

Lesions need to be treated in the context of the patient's overall risk of developing oral malignant disease. Smoking and excessive alcohol consumption are potentially **reversible risk factors**, particularly in combination, and should be stopped if possible.

Lesions found on biopsy to contain *Candida* should be treated with **antifungal agents**. It is also important to make sure that the patient has good oral hygiene and does not wear any removable dental prosthesis at night.

Excision is indicated if cancer is suspected. Lesions on the tongue have the highest risk. Surgical excision has the advantage that the whole lesion is available for histological analysis.

CONDITIONS AFFECTING THE TONGUE

ULCERS

Squamous cell carcinoma

In North America and Europe the commonest site for oral squamous cell carcinoma to develop is the tongue and the floor of mouth. In the Indian subcontinent, tobacco is chewed not smoked, which makes cancer in the buccal sulcus and cheek more common.

The clinical features are described in detail in *Symptoms and Signs*.

Investigation
Biopsy

Incisional biopsy is essential.

Imaging

MRI or CT scanning of the neck to detect occult metastases in lymph nodes should be routine. Although distant metastasis in the lung or liver is rare, it is appropriate for staging to have a **CT scan of the thorax and upper abdomen**.

The stage of the disease is classified as for carcinoma of the lip (page 269).

Management

Radiotherapy or surgery can be curative for small tongue cancers. As a rule surgery is preferred because external beam radiotherapy causes permanent damage to salivary glands. The subsequent dry mouth can result in long-term difficulty with chewing, swallowing and speech.

The primary tumour must be removed with an adequate margin of normal tissue. If patients have lymphatic metastases at presentation or are thought to be at high risk, neck lymph node excision is performed at the same time. The wide excision of larger tumours can leave a considerable defect, requiring complex reconstruction.

Patients with untreated or untreatable oral cancer face a bleak existence and an unpleasant death, so treatment should be given whenever possible. In patients with advanced disease the **palliative effect** of surgery and/or radiotherapy is better than any other modality. Current chemotherapy regimens have little effect.

Aphthous ulcers

The cause of recurrent aphthous stomatitis is unknown but it is likely that the aetiology is immune mediated. The exact mechanism remains unclear. Aphthous ulceration is commonly associated with giving up smoking, and other forms of stress. It also occurs in immunodeficiency states.

Investigation
Clinical diagnostic indicators
The diagnosis can usually be made from the history of small painful recurrent ulcers with an area of surrounding erythema on the tongue, floor of mouth and buccal mucosa.

Blood tests
Up to 20 per cent of patients will have iron, folate or vitamin B12 deficiency. Patients should therefore have a full blood count and measurement of serum iron, folate and vitamin B12 levels.

Tissue biopsy
Biopsy is only indicated for ulcers that are unusually large or take longer than 2 weeks to heal.

Management
Some patients find local anaesthetic gels helpful, but the mainstay of treatment of troublesome recurrent aphthous ulcers is **topical steroids**.

Traumatic ulcer of the tongue

A traumatic ulcer is caused most frequently by the tongue rubbing on a sharp tooth.

Investigation
Clinical diagnostic indicators
The clinical appearance of an ulcer with smooth keratotic edges is usually diagnostic. These ulcers are usually painful, and lack of pain should alert the clinician to an alternative diagnosis. The lesions tend to be small, and careful examination of the mouth should reveal the cause of the injury.

Tissue biopsy
If there is the slightest doubt about the diagnosis a biopsy should be performed.

Diagnostic pitfall: squamous cell carcinoma
The most significant differential diagnosis is squamous cell carcinoma. It is usually possible to make the diagnosis on the basis of clinical examination alone, but **when in doubt perform a biopsy**.

Management
The sharp tooth should be dealt with and the patient followed up to make sure that the ulcer has healed.

Drug-induced ulceration

A number of drugs may cause ulceration of the oral cavity, especially nicorandil and methotrexate.

The clinical appearance of nicorandil-induced ulceration is often dramatic – large irregular painful ulcers which can look very similar to malignant disease. However, the lesions are rarely indurated.

Biopsy may be required to exclude cancer.

Nicorandil-induced ulceration is managed by reducing the dose of nicorandil or stopping the drug altogether.

Similar problems with methotrexate can be helped by prescribing folic acid with the methotrexate.

Tongue-tie

This condition, more properly called **ankyloglossia**, is caused by a congenital shortening of the lingual frenulum. Diagnosis is clinical and obvious.

In few conditions is there less agreement on management! Many believe that the only consequence is cosmetic, while others are convinced that it may interfere with feeding in babies and with speech in older children.

Should treatment be deemed necessary, simple surgical division is curative, and certainly allows the young patient to put out their tongue.

13

The neck and the salivary glands

S.P. Balasubramanian and William E.G. Thomas

Diseases in the neck include a wide variety of pathological conditions, some of whose symptoms and signs are confined to the neck, e.g. thyroglossal cyst and carotid body tumours, to diseases that originate in the neck but present with the symptoms of dysfunction in organs outside the neck, e.g. the systemic symptoms caused by a toxic goitre, and to diseases that originate outside the neck but present with neck symptoms, e.g. cancers that spread to and enlarge the lymph glands of the neck.

Patients with neck problems may be referred to different specialists – general surgeons, endocrine surgeons, ENT surgeons and physicians.

Because the diagnosis can often be made from the symptoms and signs, the family doctor often initiates the initial diagnostic workup – blood tests and simple imaging – leaving the specialist to order the more complex haematological and imaging investigations required to help choose the best management.

Patients with neck diseases commonly present with the following problems:

- localized or diffuse swelling
- pain or discomfort
- deformity
- voice change
- stridor
- dysphagia
- clinical syndromes associated with hormone dysfunction.

A complete history and examination will often indicate the source of the symptoms and signs, commonly the lymph nodes and the thyroid gland. Neck symptoms can, however, arise from any of the structures in neck: from the musculoskeletal system (cervical spine spondylosis, osteophytes, cervical rib), from the vascular and lymphatic structures (carotid body tumour, subclavian aneurysm, cystic hygroma), from the pharynx (pharyngeal pouch), from the nervous system (neuralgia, neurogenic tumours), from the skin and soft tissues (lipoma, sebaceous cyst) and from congenital lesions (thyroglossal tract, branchial clefts).

Conditions which are not specific to the neck, i.e. those affecting the spine, nerves, skin and soft tissue, are not discussed in this chapter.

To help clinicians describe the exact anatomical location of any abnormality, the neck is subdivided into several compartments. For example, the anterior border of the sternocleidomastoid muscle is used to divide the neck into anterior and posterior triangles, a distinction particularly relevant to the definition of the site of lymph node disease and lymph node dissection.

If the exact location of the disease and its nature is ambiguous, two simple investigations, an **ultrasound scan** of the neck and **fine needle aspiration or core biopsy**, can usually speedily reveal the source of the patient's problems, confirm the clinical diagnosis and expedite management. Biopsy should never be used before excluding lesions such as a **carotid body tumour**, an **aneurysm** or a **pharyngeal pouch** because a needle inserted into these swellings can be fatal.

Diseases of the larynx (laryngocele), hypopharynx (globus, pharyngeal pouch) and the cervical oesophagus (tumours, dysmotility) are discussed in other chapters.

CERVICAL LYMPHADENOPATHY

Lymphadenopathy presents in the neck more often than elsewhere because the cervical lymph nodes are close to the skin and receive lymph from the structures of the upper airway, the mouth and pharynx, the limbs and all the organs in the chest abdomen.

The common causes of cervical lymph node enlargement are listed in Table 13.1.

Table 13.1
Causes of cervical lymphadenopathy

Reactive or inflammatory

Viral illness – Epstein–Barr virus, cytomegalovirus, human immunodeficiency virus, hepatitis B virus

Acute suppuration in the head and neck

Granulomatous diseases such as tuberculosis, syphilis and sarcoidosis

Other infections – toxoplasmosis, cat scratch disease, lymphogranuloma venereum, chancroid, typhoid, brucellosis, plague, tularaemia, measles, rubella, lyme disease

Systemic lupus erythematosis, rheumatoid arthritis, Kawasaki disease,
Still's disease, dermatomyositis

Malignant disease

Primary – lymphoma, leukaemia

Secondary – metasteses from primaries in the head and neck, breast, lungs, abdomen and testes

Drug induced

By allopurinol, carbamazepine, hydralazine, phenytoin and certain antibiotics

Miscellaneous

Amyloidosis

Investigation

Clinical diagnostic indicators

A detailed history and physical examination of a patient with cervical lymphadenopathy often reveals not only the underlying diagnosis but also the optimum management pathway.

A history of blood transfusions or intravenous drug abuse should alert the clinician to a possible viral cause.

A history of **tuberculosis** may point to tubercular lymphadenitis.

Travel to certain tropical countries or specific occupations can suggest specific chronic infections such as trypanosomiasis, leishmaniasis and tularaemia.

The presence of **other associated conditions** such as upper respiratory tract infection, pharyngitis, conjunctivitis, periodontal disease, insect bites and dermatitis are obvious pointers to the source of a reactive lymphadenopathy.

The physical features of the lymph nodes such as their size and location can point to the underlying diagnosis. Multiple small lymph nodes tend to be reactive, while large, matted nodes that may occasionally be fluctuant are likely to be caused by an acute bacterial infection or tuberculosis with cold abscess formation.

Diseases such as lymphoma and certain systemic autoimmune conditions can present with a generalized as well as cervical lymphadenopathy which are large and rubbery.

Hard enlarging cervical lymph nodes often contain carcinoma originating in the organs the nodes drain. Identification of the specific groups of lymph nodes enlarged should indicate to the clinician which drainage areas to examine and investigate.

Lymph nodes greater than 1 cm diameter, nodes that are increasing in size and nodes that persist for more than a month should be considered significant and investigated.

The investigations of a patient with significant lymphadenopathy can be used just to screen for the various conditions listed in Table 13.1 or designed, with the clinical features already established, to be diagnostic.

Blood tests

A full blood count and erythrocyte sedimentation rate (ESR) is almost always helpful but rarely identifies the cause of the lymphadenopathy unless a marked leucocytosis indicates leukaemia.

Imaging

An ultrasound scan of the neck often helps reveal the origin of the lymphadenopathy and establish its extent. It will also identify or exclude associated lesions in the neck such as thyroid lumps and facilitate an image-guided biopsy or needle aspiration.

An **ear, nose and throat examination, an upper gastrointestinal (GI) endoscopy and CT scans** of the chest and abdomen may be needed if metastatic lymphadenopathy is suspected to identify the primary tumour before considering an excision biopsy.

Tissue biopsy

Fine needle aspiration (FNA) is often the test that reveals the diagnosis, but if it does not and if a detailed pathological examination of the lymph node is essential for accurate classification, as in suspected lymphoma, an **excision biopsy** may be required.

Fine needle aspiration has a good chance (85 per cent) of revealing caseation and epithelioid cells if tuberculosis is suspected, but acid-fast bacilli will only be seen in 50 per cent. If pus is aspirated it must be sent for culture and tested for antibiotic sensitivity.

It is important to exclude a metastatic neck malignancy before performing an open biopsy, to avoid compromising a subsequent block dissection.

Management

The management of cervical lymphadenopathy depends on the underlying cause. If the cause is reactive or inflammatory, treatment of the underlying or associated illness is all that is required.

Combined drug therapy for tuberculosis may be started on the basis of a positive FNA with further supervision by a surgeon and physician.

If an abscess develops it should be drained by aspiration or incision while medical therapy continues.

Occasionally, after successful medical treatment, a large residual fibrotic mass of glands may need excision.

The treatment of other serious underlying illnesses, such as malignancy, requires discussion with a specialist team to review and choose the best oncological and surgical options.

THYROID SWELLINGS

Investigation

Clinical diagnostic indicators

A neck swelling is considered to arise from the thyroid gland if it is in the region of the thyroid gland (front of the neck) and **moves on swallowing**. Rarely a solitary colloid cyst arising from one of the lobes may lie in a more lateral position.

A centrally placed swelling just below or above the hyoid bone that moves with protrusion of the tongue is suggestive of a **thyroglossal cyst**.

The examination of a patient with a thyroid lump should be aimed towards obtaining answers to the following questions.

▨ Is the lump solitary, multi-nodular or diffuse?
▨ Is the patient clinically euthyroid, hypothyroid or hyperthyroid?

▨ If a thyroid cancer is suspected, is there associated lymphadenopathy or evidence of distant disease in the lungs, bones etc?

Although the clinical features may not accurately distinguish between specific diseases of the thyroid, they provide valuable clues about the possible diagnosis. For example, a diffuse goitre in a patient with obvious hyperthyroidism suggests Graves' disease, whereas a long-standing nodular goitre in a patient living in an endemic area suggests a benign multinodular goitre.

Table 13.2 lists the various possible causes of goitre and relates them to the patient's thyroid functional status and their presentation in the neck.

The investigations used to identify thyroid function, in addition to clinical examination, are mostly blood tests. Imaging is used for establishing the anatomical abnormality and guiding tissue biopsy.

Blood tests

Thyroid function tests evaluate thyroid function and determine whether the cause of any thyroid dysfunction originates within the thyroid or the pituitary gland.

The tests of function include measurements of the levels of **TSH** (thyroid-stimulating hormone), **free T4** (thyroxine) and occasionally **free T3** (tri-iodothyronine). Normal T3 and T4 levels with abnormal TSH levels indicate subclinical dysfunction. High and low TSH levels indicate subclinical hypothyroidism and hyperthyroidism respectively.

Antithyroid antibodies may be present in patients with suspected autoimmune thyroid disorders.

Serum calcium levels should be checked to confirm normal parathyroid function.

Calcitonin levels should be performed in patients with a family history of **medullary thyroid carcinoma** and are increasingly being recommended in all patients with thyroid nodules for the early detection and appropriate treatment of sporadic medullary thyroid cancer.

Imaging

An ultrasound scan of the neck is performed as routine by many surgeons on patients with thyroid

Table 13.2
Relationship between clinical features, function and pathology

Clinical features	Function and pathology		
	Hypothyroid	Euthyroid	Hyperthyroid
Diffuse	Thyroiditis	Iodine deficiency Enzyme defects Goitrogens Thyroiditis Amyloid Pregnancy, puberty	Primary hyperthyroidism (Graves' disease)
Multinodular enlargement	Multinodular goitre with gross degeneration	Multinodular goitre Anaplastic carcinoma Medullary carcinoma Lymphoma	Secondary hyperthyroidism (Plummer's syndrome)
Solitary nodule	Coincidental nodule with myxoedema	Cyst Dominant nodule Adenoma Follicular or papillary carcinoma	Autonomous toxic nodule
No goitre	Thyroiditis Primary myxoedema Post-thyroidectomy Post-radioiodine	Normal gland	Primary hyperthyroidism Thyroxine overdose

lumps (Fig 13.1). It has several uses: it can confirm the presence of thyroid enlargement, differentiate between solitary and multiple nodules, differentiate between solid and cystic lumps, identify retrosternal extension and any associated cervical lymphadenopathy, and be used to target FNA or biopsy.

Recent advances in technology also allow the ultrasonographer to distinguish between benign and malignant lumps.

CT or MRI scans of the neck should be performed in patients with large thyroid masses with suspected retrosternal extension (Fig 13.2), tracheal deviation and compression or locally advanced malignancy (Fig 13.3).

Thyroid scintigraphy is occasionally undertaken to look for ectopic thyroid tissue and in those with subclinical hyperthyroidism to identify functioning (hot) nodules.

Laryngoscopic vocal cord examination is performed routinely in most centres before thyroid

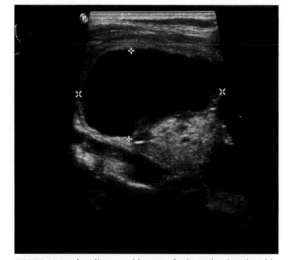

FIGURE 13.1   An ultrasound image of a large benign thyroid cyst arising in the left lobe of the gland with multinodular change

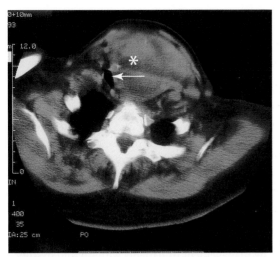

FIGURE 13.2   CT scan of a retrosternal goitre (∗) compressing the trachea (arrow)

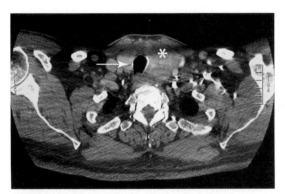

FIGURE 13.3   CT scan of the neck showing a large heterogeneous thyroid mass (∗) arising mainly from the right lobe and displacing the trachea (arrow) to the left. Biopsy showed a poorly differentiated thyroid cancer

surgery to establish a pre-operative baseline of recurrent laryngeal nerve function against which any postoperative vocal disturbance may be compared and as a medico-legal precaution.

Tissue biopsy

Fine needle aspiration (either free hand or ultrasound guided) should be performed on all solitary or dominant nodules to determine their morphology (Fig 13.4).

Ultrasound-directed FNA provides a more accurately defined source and representative specimen.

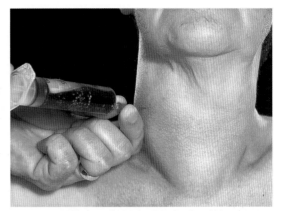

FIGURE 13.4   Fine needle aspiration of a thyroid lump

FNA cannot differentiate between a follicular adenoma and a follicular carcinoma as the latter is distinguished from a benign adenoma by the presence of vascular and/or capsular invasion, something which can only be identified on histological examination.

Fine needle aspirations can and often are repeated if the aspirate is inadequate/insufficient or if a benign result does not corroborate with clinical suspicion. **FNA can be therapeutic for thyroid cysts.**

An **ultrasound-guided core biopsy** or an **open incisional biopsy** is occasionally performed on tumours of uncertain origin and anaplastic cancers.

Patients with **medullary thyroid cancer** should undergo investigations to exclude hyperparathyroidism and phaeochromocytoma in case they have the MEN II (multiple endocrine neoplasia) syndrome and be offered genetic screening for RET mutations irrespective of family history.

Management

The results of thyroid function tests, ultrasound imaging and FNA cytology help determine the management options of a thyroid nodule as set out in Fig 13.5.

EUTHYROID BENIGN NODULES

Surgical excision (partial thyroidectomy) is indicated for benign nodules, single or multiple, that are increasing in size, causing pressure effects or are causing cosmetic concern.

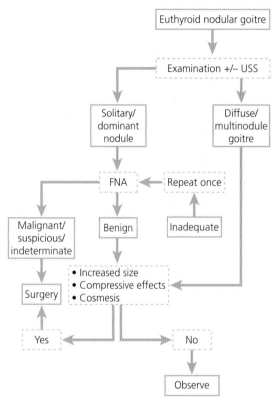

FIGURE 13.5 Key steps in the management of a thyroid nodule

EUTHYROID MALIGNANT NODULES

Surgical excision is recommended for all thyroid lumps that are malignant on cytological examination, whether definite, suspicious or indeterminate, except in cases of lymphoma, secondary deposits or anaplastic cancer.

For a well-differentiated thyroid cancer of less than 1 cm diameter, a **lobectomy** may be sufficient treatment, provided there is no family history of thyroid cancer or a history of neck irradiation.

Large (>1 cm diameter) malignant tumours are treated with a **total thyroidectomy**.

Masses that are suspicious or indeterminate on preoperative cytology such as follicular neoplasms may be offered a **hemi-thyroidectomy**, but if the lesion is found to be malignant and of more than 1 cm diameter a second operation should be performed to complete the **total thyroidectomy**, often accompanied by a **central lymph node dissection**.

Lateral lymph nodal excision is recommended in patients with palpable lymph node disease.

Radio-iodine ablation and TSH suppressive doses of thyroxine are recommended as adjuvant treatments for differentiated thyroid cancer of >1 cm diameter, while thyroxine replacement is sufficient in medullary thyroid cancer.

External radiotherapy and chemotherapy may be required in advanced disease and in those with anaplastic cancer. All such treatment options should be considered at a multidisciplinary team meeting.

DIFFUSE OR NO ENLARGEMENT WITH DISORDERED THYROID FUNCTION

The management of patients with thyroid dysfunction (hypo- or hyperthyroidism) with or without enlargement of the gland or benign lesions such as nodules, without pressure effects or cosmetic concerns, is usually referred to an endocrinologist for long-term medical management.

Thyroxine replacement is given for hypothyroidism.

Anti-thyroid drugs, such as carbimazole or propylthiouracil, and/or radio-iodine are given for hyperthyroidism. The risk of hypothyroidism after radio-iodine may be as high as 30 per cent 3 years after treatment and then increases steadily thereafter.

Local problems are dealt with once the patient has been rendered euthyroid.

Total thyroidectomy (with careful preservation of the parathyroid glands) may be offered to patients with hyperthyroidism caused by recurrent or poorly controlled Graves' disease who are young, female or have a large toxic goitre, as an alternative to long-term anti-thyroid drugs or radio-iodine.

For many years the standard operation for hyperthyroidism was **subtotal thyroidectomy**, an operation that preserves just 2–10 g of thyroid tissue; but because the results of pharmacological and radio-iodine treatment are now so good, and because this operation has a 5 per cent recurrence of hyperthyroidism at 5 years and a slowly increasing rate of hypothyroidism, it is rarely practised

Before the operation all patients with hyperthyroidism should receive a course of anti-thyroid drugs to establish a euthyroid state – a prerequisite for a successful surgical intervention.

All patients need thyroxine after total thyroidectomy, as do some after subtotal thyroidectomy.

BENIGN SOLITARY TOXIC NODULE

Patients with a toxic autonomous nodule should be offered **thyroid lobectomy** after being rendered clinically euthyroid with anti-thyroid drugs.

SOLITARY THYROID CYSTS

Thyroid cysts are usually managed by **aspiration**. **Excision** is reserved for those cysts which are large, symptomatic or recurrent.

THYROGLOSSAL CYST

The thyroglossal tract is the remnant of the diverticulum that develops in the floor of the primitive embryonic pharynx at the base of the tongue (foramen caecum) which, after extending caudally, develops into the isthmus and pyramidal lobe of the thyroid gland. The tract normally disappears but occasionally part of it can persist to become a cyst.

Investigation
Clinical diagnostic indicators
A thyroglossal cyst usually presents early in life, but may appear in adult life, as a **midline swelling**, most often **in front of or below the hyoid cartilage**. However, it can develop anywhere from the base of the tongue to the manubrium sterni.

In addition to moving upwards during swallowing, as other thyroid swellings, the thyroglossal cyst also **moves upwards with protrusion of the tongue**.

Differential diagnoses include a mid-line lymph node, an enlarged pyramidal lobe of the thyroid gland, a dermoid cyst and a sebaceous cyst. Very occasionally, the cyst wall contains the patient's only functioning thyroid tissue (an ectopic thyroid) and so the demonstration of a normal thyroid gland by ultrasound imaging is an important precaution.

Imaging
An ultrasound scan will confirm the diagnosis.

Table 13.3
Causes of hypercalcaemia

Malignancies – primary solid tumours, metastases and haematological malignancies

Hyperparathyroidism

Other endocrine diseases – hyperthyroidism, Addisonian crises

Drugs – thiazide diuretics, lithium, vitamin A and vitamin D toxicity, aluminium toxicity

Miscellaneous – immobilization, laboratory error, milk alkali syndrome, granulomatous diseases, e.g. sarcoidosis

An **isotope scan** should be performed before excising the cyst if there is doubt about the presence of normal thyroid tissue in the orthotopic location.

Management

Surgical excision with the tract above it including the central portion of the hyoid bone (Sistrunk's procedure) is indicated for infection, cosmetic reasons, pressure effects or malignant change (rarely diagnosed before definitive histology is available).

Recurrence is possible if the tract is not completely excised.

THE PARATHYROID GLANDS

The four parathyroid glands (a superior and an inferior on either side) normally lie close to the thyroid gland. The clinical manifestations of parathyroid diseases are invariably the result of abnormal levels of serum calcium caused by pathologically high or low levels of parathyroid hormone (PTH).

Hypercalcaemia is often a chance finding detected during the screening investigations for gastrointestinal, cardiovascular, renal and neuro-psychiatric disorders and other symptom patterns such as myalgia, lethargy, visual changes and pruritus.

The causes of hypercalcaemia and the disorders of the parathyroid glands that cause it are listed in Tables 13.3 and 13.4.

Patients with *hypo*parathyroidism are managed by endocrinologists with calcium and vitamin D supplementation.

Table 13.4
Disorders of the parathyroid glands

Hyperparathyroidism

Primary hyperparathyroidism
  Single adenoma (89 per cent)
  Double adenoma (4 per cent)
  Hyperplasia (6 per cent)
  Parathyroid cancer (1 per cent)
Secondary hyperparathyroidism
  Associated with renal failure
  Associated with vitamin D deficiency
Tertiary hyperparathyroidism
  Autonomous function after long-standing
  secondary hyperparathyroidism
  Familial hypocalciuric hypercalcaemia
  Idiopathic hypercalcaemia
  Lithium

Hypoparathyroidism

Anatomical damage – post surgery, radiotherapy,
autoimmune
Reduced function – hypomagnesaemia, PTH and
calcium sensing receptor gene defects
Parathyroid agenesis

Table 13.5
Biochemical characteristics in hyperparathyroidism

Test	Primary HPT	Secondary HPT	Tertiary HPT
Serum PTH	High	High	High
Serum calcium	High	Low/normal	High
Serum phosphate	Low	High/normal	High
Vitamin D	Normal/low	Low	Low/normal

HPT, hyperparathyroidism.

The investigation and management of patients with an autoimmune hypoparathyroidism are beyond the scope of this book.

The following paragraphs focus on the investigation and management of *hyper*parathyroidism.

The results of thyroid function tests, ultrasound imaging and FNA cytology that help determine the management options of a thyroid nodule are set out in Fig. 13.5).

Investigation

Clinical diagnostic indicators

Clinically detectable parathyroid gland enlargement is extremely rare.

Symptoms such as myalgia, lethargy, visual changes and pruritus should alert the clinician to the possible presence of hyperparathyroidism.

The presence and type of hyperparathyroidism and, when appropriate, the necessary imaging tests to localize the parathyroid glands must be performed before considering surgical treatment.

Blood and urine tests

The serum calcium, phosphate, PTH and vitamin D levels and 24-hour urinary calcium excretion should be measured.

Table 13.5 shows the various biochemical results found in the different types of hyperparathyroidism.

In patients with suspected primary hyperparathyroidism, determination of the 24-hour urinary excretion of calcium is essential to confirm high levels and thus rule out the autosomal dominant benign disorder called *familial hypocalciuric hypercalaemia* (FHH). In this condition, PTH levels may be elevated but urinary calcium levels are typically low because of an inability of the kidneys to secrete calcium. These patients do not benefit from a parathyroidectomy.

Imaging

Imaging for localization of the abnormal parathyroid gland/s is currently undertaken in patients with primary hyperparathyroidism (and by some surgeons in secondary/tertiary hyperparathyroidism) to facilitate the performance of a **unilateral or focused parathyroidectomy**.

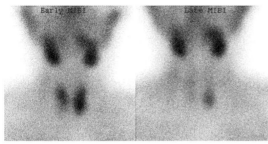

FIGURE 13.6   A parathyroid MIBI scan showing, in the early phase MIBI images, a prominent area of tracer activity in relation to the inferior aspect of the left thyroid lobe. This persists on the late phase images while the rest of the thyroid activity washes out. This is consistent with a parathyroid adenoma in the left inferior position

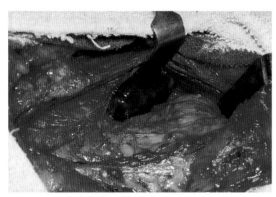

FIGURE 13.7   A methylene blue adenoma

The tests used to identify an abnormal gland include a combination of **a preoperative ultrasound scan** and a **^{99}Tc sestamibi radionuclide subtraction scan (MIBI)** (Fig 13.6).

Intraoperative localization techniques such as an **intraoperative ultrasound**, **radio-guided surgery** and **methylene blue injection** may improve the success of the primary operation, and facilitate a focused approach and thus avoid extensive dissection and the risk of damaging the normal parathyroid glands in patients with a single parathyroid adenoma (Fig 13.7).

An intraoperative PTH assay may be used to confirm successful excision of the overactive parathyroid tissue.

CT or MRI scanning may be required for patients with recurrent disease prior to re-operation, with or without **selective venous sampling for PTH levels**.

Management of primary hyperparathyroidism caused by an adenoma

Parathyroidectomy is the gold standard in the treatment of symptomatic primary hyperparathyroidism.

The indications for parathyroidectomy in symptomless hyperparathyroidism include patients at high risk of developing complications, i.e. those with high calcium levels (>2.85 mmol/L), high urinary calcium (excretion of >10 mmol/day), reduced creatinine clearance (<70 per cent of normal), significant osteoporosis (bone density T score less than −2.5), young patients (<50 years of age) and patients in whom surveillance is not possible.

Lithium therapy can increase both calcium and PTH levels and should be excluded as a cause of hyperparathyroidism before surgery.

Thiazide diuretics can exacerbate hypercalcaemia in primary hyperparathyroidism. Patients on these medications should be taken off these drugs if possible, and the levels of calcium and PTH rechecked.

As the majority of cases of primary hyperthyroidism are caused by a solitary adenoma, preoperative localization with or without intraoperative localization facilitates unilateral exploration. If the preoperative imaging is inconclusive, as is often the case with glandular hyperplasia, bilateral neck exploration is needed.

The success of a focused parathyroidectomy is thought to be equivalent to a formal bilateral neck exploration in terms of resolution of hypercalcaemia.

Management of primary hyperparathyroidism caused by general hyperplasia

Parathyroid hyperplasia can be familial and can occur as part of the MEN syndromes (MEN I and MEN IIa). Other endocrine abnormalities (especially a co-existing phaeochromocytoma) should be excluded by biochemical testing in all patients with suspected hyperplasia (young patients with a family history) prior to parathyroidectomy.

Excision of three glands and one-half of the fourth gland, leaving the remaining half gland carefully marked, or else autotransplanted, is the most common surgical treatment for patients with primary general parathyroid hyperplasia.

Management of secondary and tertiary hyperparathyroidism

This condition is usually associated with renal failure and patients on haemodialysis. It occurs in renal transplant patients and in those with long-standing end-stage renal disease, where one or more of the glands assume autonomous function following chronic stimulation by hypocalcaemia.

Medical management consists of **calcium supplements, vitamin D analogues and phosphate binding agents** in an attempt to regulate the levels of calcium, phosphate and vitamin D.

New organic agents (**calcimimetics**) are now being used to increase the sensitivity of calcium receptors to extracellular calcium and suppress PTH secretion.

Surgery is occasionally required; but as only a small proportion of these patients have single gland disease, and even though this can be localized preoperatively by imaging and excised, the traditional treatment in these patients is a **full neck exploration** with either **subtotal excision of the parathyroid glands (three and a half glands) or total parathyroidectomy** with autotransplantation of some parathyroid tissue into either the sternocleidomastoid muscle or the forearm muscles.

Many surgeons perform a **thymectomy** in addition to excision of the parathyroid glands as these patients can have accessory parathyroid tissue within their thymus.

Complications of parathyroidectomy

Specific complications of parathyroid surgery include **persistent or recurrent hypercalcaemia** needing further treatment, **hypoparathyroidism** and the uncommon possibility of **recurrent laryngeal nerve damage**. Short-term **hypocalcaemia** is common and requires intravenous calcium.

Hypoparathyroidism in patients with renal transplants can contribute to worsening of graft function.

Prognosis Failure to control hyperparathyroidism is usually the result of a failed surgical exploration. Recurrence after two explorations is over 10 per cent. Hypoparathyroidism is treated with vitamin D and calcium supplements.

CAROTID BODY TUMOUR

A number of different tumours of neuro-ectodermal tissue origin can develop in the neck, including neuroma, neurofibroma, neurilemmoma, carotid body tumour and glomus tumour. The last one develops from paraganglionic cells in close anatomical association with the carotid artery bifurcation and occasionally from cells adjacent to the jugular bulb, the middle ear cavity and the ganglion nodosum of the vagus nerve.

Carotid body tumours may be associated with other parangliomata in the neck, chest and abdomen and with *phaeochromocytomata*. This is especially true in 10 per cent of familial cases where around 30 per cent are also bilateral.

These tumours are very vascular and approximately 10 per cent are malignant.

Investigation
Clinical diagnostic indicators
The presence of a relatively long-standing painless firm mass below the angle of the mandible should raise the suspicion of a carotid body tumour. The swelling is often associated with a **transmitted pulsation** and a **bruit** and occasionally with pressure effects on adjacent vital structures. It is easily compressible and refills on release. It can be moved from side to side but not vertically.

Imaging
A CT scan, MRI or duplex scan can provide accurate localization and define the tumour's relationships to adjacent structures while excluding bilateral disease (Fig 13.8).

Screening
The family members of patients with a family history should be screened in view of the conditions autosomal dominant mode of inheritance.

Tissue biopsy
Percutaneous aspiration or biopsy can be hazardous and **should not be attempted**.

Management
Surgical resection should be carried out through the same incision as a carotid endarterectomy. The

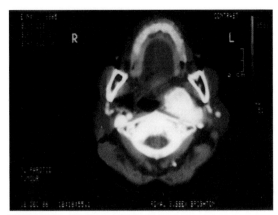

FIGURE 13.8   CT of a carotid body tumour

tumour, which is very vascular, needs to be dissected off the artery. It is rarely necessary to resect the artery unless the tumur is malignant.

Damage to the cranial nerves in the neck is a potential complication. Stroke is rare.

Radiotherapy may be considered in patients with inoperable malignant tumours, incomplete resections, recurrent disease or metastases but is rarely effective.

BRANCHIAL SINUS AND BRANCHIAL FISTULA

These abnormalities arise from the embryological remnants of the branchial arches.

A branchial sinus is a blind epithelium-lined tract extending inwards from an external opening in the skin of the lower third of the neck just anterior to the sternocleidomastoid muscle. A branchial fistula is similar to a sinus but has an internal opening on the pharyngeal wall. Its lining epithelium is either respiratory or squamous in type and its wall may contain muscle fibres and lymphoid tissue.

Investigation

Clinical diagnostic indicators

The patient is usually the first to notice the external skin opening.

Both a sinus and fistula may be associated with an intermittent mucoid discharge. Both may become infected to form an abscess with or without purulent discharge.

Imaging

The only investigation required before surgery for a symptomatic sinus/fistula is a **fistulogram** to help determine the extent of the tract and ensure complete removal.

Management

A complete surgical excision of the tract is required, extending if necessary from the skin, through the deep cervical fascia, between the internal and external carotid vessels – anterior to the IX and X cranial nerves – to its deepest extent which may be at the internal opening on the pharyngeal wall.

BRANCHIAL CYST

Branchial cysts may be present at birth or appear later in life (commonly in the third decade). They are thought by some to be unrelated to branchial abnormalities and arise in the lymphatic tissue of the neck.

Investigation

Clinical diagnostic indicators

A typical branchial cyst lies beneath the anterior border of the sternocleidomastoid muscle at the junction of its upper third and middle third. It is smooth and fluctuant.

Other neck swellings that need to be considered in the **differential diagnosis** include lymphadenopathy (in all age groups), cystic hygroma (in the young) and occasionally cystic secondary lymph node deposits of a papillary thyroid cancer.

Imaging

An **ultrasound scan** will confirm the presence and extent of the cyst. **Fine needle aspiration cytology** often helps to confirm the swelling's cystic nature.

Management

Surgical excision is recommended both for treatment and for confirmation of the diagnosis.

If the cyst is infected it should be aspirated under the cover of a course of antibiotics and excision delayed until the infection has resolved.

CYSTIC HYGROMA

A cystic hygroma is a collection of dilated lymphatic sacs that develop and fill during prenatal life from sequestered (unconnected) embryonic lymph vessels. They usually present before the second year of birth and can sometimes be diagnosed prenatally by antenatal ultrasonography, but they may appear in adult life.

Investigation

Clinical diagnostic indicators

Cystic hygromata present as a **brilliantly translucent, fluctuant mass**. Although commonly found in the posterior triangle of the neck, they can often extend across the boundaries of the neck compartments. They occasionally cause compression of the oesophagus, trachea or the great vessels. In a neonate a complication such as haemorrhage into the cyst or acute infection can be fatal.

The **differential diagnoses** include other causes of cystic neck masses such as branchial cysts, thyroglossal cysts, thymic cysts, cervical bronchogenic cysts, dermoid and epidermoid cysts.

Imaging

Ultrasound scanning will confirm the cystic nature of the mass and determine its extent and relationship to other neck structures.

A **CT scan or MRI** provides superior resolution and is very helpful in planning the excision of an extensive hygroma especially in young children or neonates (Fig 13.9).

Management

Surgical excision is the appropriate treatment of symptomatic or large hygromas at any age. Small cystic lesions in children can be left until the child is 3–4 years old.

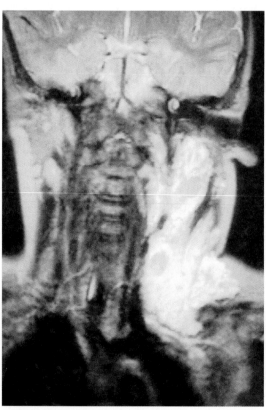

(A)

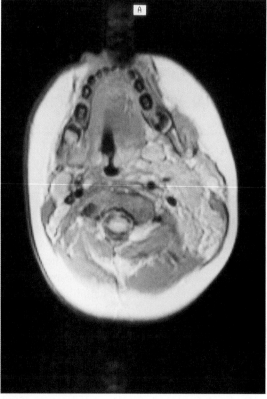

(B)

FIGURE 13.9   Nuclear magnetic resonance scans of a large lobulated cystic hygroma in the neck. (A) Axial STIR scan showing the cyst surrounding the major neck vessels and extending down below the clavicle. (B) Coronal STIR scan showing the cyst extending medially deep to the mandible and displacing the pharynx to the right. Reproduced by kind permission of the Department of Paediatric Surgery, Queen's Medical Centre, Nottingham.

Although a complete excision is usually possible, technical difficulties caused by the adherence of the cyst to nearby nerves and vessels and the weak friable cyst wall are not uncommon, making the chance of an incomplete removal and subsequent recurrence not insignificant.

Obliterative sclerosis is an alternative to surgery. Intralesional injections of compounds such as *Ethibloc* or *OK 432* have been used with variable results.

CERVICAL RIB AND THORACIC OUTLET SYNDROME

One per cent of the population have an accessory rib at the level of the seventh cervical vertebra which can be the cause of the thoracic outlet syndrome, i.e. upper limb symptoms caused by compression of nerves and/or blood vessels at the thoracic outlet.

Compression of the brachial plexus and subclavian vessels occurs in the triangle bounded by the scalenus anterior and scalenus medius muscles and a cervical rib or the first rib, but can also be caused by accessory muscle bands and tendons, fibrous bands and hyperextension neck injury.

Investigation and management

See Chapter 11.

PHARYNGEAL POUCH

See Chapter 18.

THE SALIVARY GLANDS

Salivary glands are traditionally classified as being major (the parotid, submandibular and sublingual glands) and minor (those widely distributed below the mucosa of the lips, palate, pharynx and larynx). The following only discusses problems in the parotid and submandibular glands because they are the commonest sites of salivary gland pathology. Many of the problems described can be encountered in the sublingual and minor salivary glands.

Table 13.6 gives a comprehensive list of salivary gland pathology and the distribution of the different diseases in the different glands.

Infective, inflammatory and neoplastic conditions occur more frequently in the parotid gland; the submandibular gland is more often the site of obstructive calculus disease. This is attributed to the increased mucin content in the secretions of the submandibular gland and the ascending course of its duct.

Investigation

Clinical diagnostic indicators

The commonest presenting symptoms in patients with salivary gland pathology are **pain and swelling.**

Patients with Sjögren's syndrome may present with dry mouth and eyes.

Examination of these patients should not be limited to the symptomatic gland but include an examination of all the major salivary glands, the seventh cranial nerves and the neck.

Blood tests

Blood tests demonstrating the presence of **antinuclear factor (ANF), rheumatoid factor (RF)** and raised **gamma globulin levels** can be useful in providing corroborative evidence of Sjögren's syndrome.

Serum angiotensin-converting enzyme levels (SACE) may be useful in suspected sarcoidosis.

Imaging

A **chest X-ray** may reveal sarcoidosis.

An **X-ray of the floor of the mouth and cheek** may reveal stones in the salivary ducts and in the glands (Fig 13.10).

An **ultrasound scan** is often employed to confirm that the swelling is in a salivary gland and exclude other swellings such as dental and branchial cysts and abnormalities of the masseter muscle and the mandible.

Although further investigations are rarely required, **CT scanning** and **MRI** are now replacing plain X-rays, **sialography** and **radionuclide scanning**.

If a neoplastic lesion is suspected, MRI can provide more information than CT about the involvement of the deep lobe, the extent of invasion and any associated soft tissue abnormalities.

Cytology

Fine needle aspiration is of variable value in benign conditions. It is used routinely by some and rarely by others but can be helpful in ruling out conditions such as lymphadenopathy, lipoma, neuroma and non-salivary gland cysts, and, when the nature of the pathological change is in doubt, malignant change.

Table 13.6
Conditions of the salivary glands

Infections	Carcinoma in a pleomorphic adenoma
Acute bacterial infection – e.g. suppurative parotitis	Acinic cell carcinoma
Viral – mumps (commonest) and other viruses including coxsackie, influenza and herpes	Squamous cell carcinoma
Other – tuberculosis, syphilis, cat-scratch disease, toxoplasmosis, actinomycosis	*Miscellaneous rare tumours (benign and malignant)*
Obstructive salivary disease	Haemangioma
Sialectasis (recurrent parotitis)	Lymphangioma
Calculus disease	Lipoma
Inflammatory and autoimmune diseases	Sarcoma
Sarcoidosis	Lymphoma
Sjögren's disease	Secondary deposits
Tumours	**Sialomegaly associated with chronic disease**
Benign	Endocrine diseases – Myxoedema, Cushing's disease and diabetes mellitus
Pleomorphic adenoma	Cirrhosis
Warthin's tumour	Alcoholism
Oncocytoma	Gout
Malignant	Bulimia
Mucoepidermoid carcinoma	HIV
Adenoid cystic carcinoma	Drugs – thiouracil, phenylbutazone, isoprenaline, dextropropoxyphene, oral contraceptive pill
Adenocarcinoma	

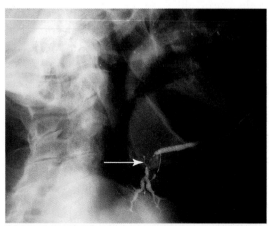

FIGURE 13.10   A sialograph showing a sub-mandibular stone in floor of mouth

Figure 13.11 shows how the combination of clinical features and investigations can lead to a diagnosis.

Management

Infection: bacterial and viral

Institute adequate analgesia and hydration, and give antibiotics for bacterial infections. Investigate other sites for chronic infections such as tuberculosis and granulomatous diseases such as sarcoidosis and institute specific treatment as appropriate.

Sjögren's disease

Lubrication of the oral cavity and eye and pilocarpine to stimulate residual function are required.

Sialectasis

Institute analgesia and hydration during acute episodes.

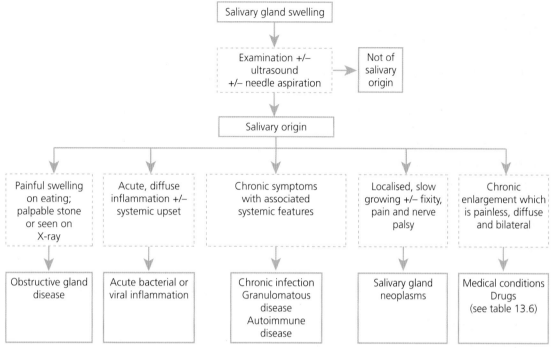

Salivary gland swelling

Examination +/–
ultrasound
+/– needle aspiration → Not of salivary origin

Salivary origin

| Painful swelling on eating; palpable stone or seen on X-ray | Acute, diffuse inflammation +/– systemic upset | Chronic symptoms with associated systemic features | Localised, slow growing +/– fixity, pain and nerve palsy | Chronic enlargement which is painless, diffuse and bilateral |

| Obstructive gland disease | Acute bacterial or viral inflammation | Chronic infection Granulomatous disease Autoimmune disease | Salivary gland neoplasms | Medical conditions Drugs (see table 13.6) |

FIGURE 13.11   A plan for the investigation of a salivary gland swelling

Sialography can help in confirming the diagnosis, and may also help in relieving symptoms.

Duct dilatation may improve flow, while very occasionally radiotherapy and **division of parasympathetic nerve** supply may help.

Total parotidectomy is the last resort and is fraught with complications.

Salivary gland calculi

The treatment is **stone removal** from the duct via the oral cavity or **elective excision** of the gland for intraglandular calculi or recurrent disease. These can also now be treated by lithotripsy (as for urinary calculi).

Pleomorphic adenoma

Pleomorphic adenoma is the commonest salivary gland tumour and occurs predominantly in the superficial lobe of the parotid gland. **Local excision of the involved lobe (superficial parotidectomy)** or **total parotidectomy** are the treatments of choice (Fig 13.12). Malignant transformation is very rare, but local recurrence is common.

Warthin's tumour

Warthin's tumour (papillary cystadenoma lymphomatosum) often occurs in older people and can be multiple or bilateral in up to 10 per cent. It occurs in the parotid gland usually in the superficial lobe. **Superficial parotidectomy** (Fig 13.12) is the treatment of choice. Local recurrences after excision are rare.

Oncocytoma

Oncocytoma (oxyphil cell adenoma) often occurs in minor salivary glands. It is often seen in older people as a slow-growing soft tumour and rarely turns malignant. **Complete excision** usually requiring no more than a **superficial parotidectomy** (Fig 13.12) is the treatment of choice.

Mucoepidermoid carcinoma and other malignant conditions

Malignant salivary gland tumours are rare. The commonest type is mucoepidermoid tumour; the other types are listed in Table 13.6.

Fortunately, the vast majority are amenable to surgical excision but the proximity of the major

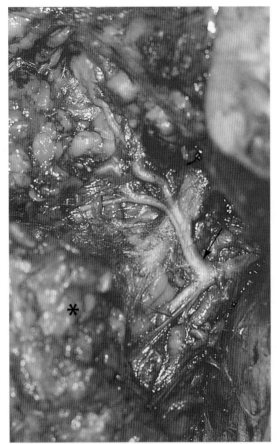

FIGURE 13.12 Operative photo showing tumour (∗) and preservation of VII nerve (arrow)

salivary glands to important nerves and vessels significantly influences the extent of radical resection. Nevertheless, surgery is often the only curative option for overtly malignant tumours.

There is no alternative effective treatment although radiotherapy may be a useful adjunct.

Preoperative imaging with **MRI** is useful to stage the local extent of the disease and is helpful in preoperative planning.

Radical excision of the tumour, including sacrificing the facial nerve if necessary, is the only treatment likely to succeed.

Lymph node dissection is indicated only if the nodes are involved.

Postoperative radiotherapy is often used after surgery for mucoepidermoid and adenoid cystic carcinoma. This serves to reduce local recurrence especially after incomplete excision.

The facial nerve, if excised, can be bridged by a nerve graft. Alternatively, the corner of the mouth can be pulled up with a facial sling. This can be combined with a lateral tarsorrhaphy to protect the eye from exposure damage.

Complications of parotid gland surgery

Damage to the facial nerve, salivary fistula and paraesthesia of the ear lobe (from damage to the greater auricular nerve) is possible.

Frey's syndrome is discomfort, sweating and redness of the skin overlying the parotid gland – related to the innervation of the skin by the parasympathetic secretory nerve fibres that normally supply the parotid gland.

Complications of submandibular gland surgery

Damage to the mandibular branch of the facial nerve, the hypoglossal nerve and the lingual nerve is possible.

TRACHEOSTOMY

A tracheostomy is an artificial opening between the cervical trachea and the external air. It may be made to assist inadequate natural ventilation and/ or provide mechanical ventilation, to protect the lungs from regurgitated gastric contents, secretions and blood and to provide access for bronchial toilet. These and other indications are listed in Table 13.7.

Investigation
Clinical Diagnostic Indicators

A patient's inability to inhale is usually obvious from their gasping struggles to breath and in extreme circumstances the rapid development of acute cyanosis, collapse and death.

Consequently it is always better to anticipate the need for and to perform a tracheostomy before the situation becomes an acute life threatening emergency.

Management
Surgical technique

Except in extreme circumstances perform the procedure in an operating room together with an anaesthetist.

Table 13.7
Indications for tracheostomy

To bypass acute upper airway obstruction by:

  Foreign body

  Infection (Diptheria, Acute epiglossitis, Acute laryngitis)

  Oedema

  Haemorrhage

  Tumours

  Bilateral vocal cord paralysis

To assist natural respiration or facilitate artificial ventilation, as in:

  Unconsciousness associated with head injuries

  Neurological conditions causing coma, e.g. bulbar palsy

  Chest injuries (such as flail chest)

  Fulminating bronchopneumonia

  Severe emphysema

  By reducing the dead space

To protect the airway

  from e.g. blood, gastic reflux, secretions

For bronchial toilet

  e.g. in bronchiectasis and encrustations

Following laryngeal excision

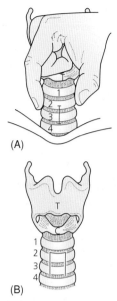

(A)

(B)

FIGURE 13.13　(A–B) Surgical technique of a tracheostomy

Place the patient supine with a firm pillow between the shoulder blades to make the neck extend.

If time allows, infiltrate the skin incision midway between the larynx and the suprasternal notch) with a local anaesthetic but if the patient is becoming unconscious make the incision without any anaesthesia.

Identify the position of the trachea by palpating the larynx between two fingers and moving them downwards. Then hold the trachea still. Fixing the trachea between the fingers prevents the incision slipping lateral to the trachea (Fig 13.13).

In a dire emergency, a vertical incision is made through the skin and all the underlying structures right down to and through the second, third tracheal rings. This may involve cutting through the thyroid isthmus which will bleed profusely, but the bleeding will diminish rapidly once the trachea is open and the cervical venous congestion and cyanosis relieved. Attention may be paid to any continuing haemorrhage later.

If a tracheostomy tube is unavailable, any hollow tube, such as the plastic tube of a pen, will suffice. If a hollow tube is unavailable a rigid structure must be pushed between the divided tracheal rings to hold them apart and allow the ingress of air until a proper tracheostomy tube is obtained.

In less urgent circumstances, a transverse incision is made midway between the cricoid cartilage and the suprasternal notch. This leaves a better scar and should be at the level of the 2nd and 3rd tracheal rings. Divide and ligate or retract any tissues such as the thyroid isthmus before opening the trachea.

In children, make a vertical incision in the trachea. In adults remove a square of trachea between the second and fourth rings large enough to admit the tracheostomy tube.

In both situations, insert a silastic tracheostomy tube with an inflatable balloon (Fig 13.14) and connect it to the ventilation mechanism of an anaesthetic machine.

It is better to make the incision in the trachea in the form of an inverted **U**, the top lying just above the second ring and the sides cutting through second and third rings, to form a flap of trachea

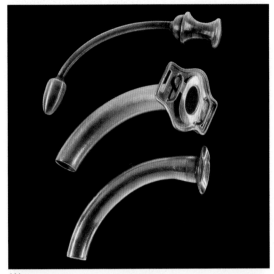

(A)

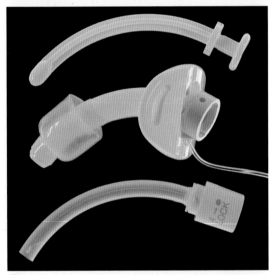

(B)

FIGURE 13.14 (A) Silver tracheostomy tube. From above: introducer, outer tube and inner tube. (B) Modern plastic tracheostomy tube with introducer, low-pressure cuff and inner canula. (With permission from Bailey and Love's Short Practice of Surgery, 25th edition).

that can be sutured to the lower edge of the skin incision. This is known as a Bjork flap. Its advantage is that it forms a smooth surface on which a replacement tube can be slid into the trachea.

The securing tapes should be tied with the neck flexed, to avoid the tube falling out when the neck is flexed.

Most tracheostomies in intensive care are now performed using a percutaneous closed insertion under local anaesthetic. A gide wire is inserted into the trachea, the trachea is dilated and an endotracheal tube is inserted.

After care

Keep a suction device, a sterile catheter, tracheal dilator and a spare tube beside the bed at all times.

Ensure that the inhaled air is warm and humidified to stop the encrustation of bronchial secretions. Commercial humidifiers are available.

Clean the incision and suck out the bronchial tree regularly.

Try not to replace a silastic tube for 48hours, i.e. until the track has started to organise and become fixed, but deflate the balloon at regular intervals to prevent the development of pressure necrosis in the tracheal endothelium.

A silver tube with a talking piece can be inserted when positive pressure ventilation is no longer required. The inner speaking tube of a silver tracheostomy tube must be removed and cleaned at regular intervals – at least every 24 hours.

Complications

- Accidental dislodgement or obstruction.
- Haemorrhage, from the wound or the trachea.
- Surgical emphysema in the neck and mediastinum.
- Pneumothorax.
- Rarely a fistula may develop between the trachea and the oesophagus .
- The trachea may become permanently stenosed at an angle of 5–10 degrees.

OTHER METHODS OF EMERGENCY VENTILATION

There are a number of other methods of assisting ventilation when the airway is obstructed. These include:

- cricithyroidotomy
- fibroptic endotracheal intubation
- the laryngeal mask
- transtracheal ventilation.

14

The thoracic cage, lungs and heart

Timothy J.P. Batchelor and Chris Munsch

The thoracic cage, bounded by the thoracic inlet superiorly, the diaphragm inferiorly, the sternum anteriorly, the vertebral column posteriorly and the chest wall laterally, forms an airtight cage whose continuous movements and subsequent intrathoracic pressure changes ventilate the lungs. In addition to this vital role, its walls protect the organs and structures it contains – the lungs, trachea, heart, great vessels, thymus and oesophagus.

Surgical procedures on the structures within the thoracic cage (with the exception of drainage of empyema necessitates) began in the twentieth century. Previous attempts to enter the thoracic cavity invariably proved fatal because of the pneumothorax that quickly developed as a result of the negative intrathoracic pressure present in a spontaneously ventilating patient. Furthermore, surgeons were frightened to touch the heart. In 1883 Theodor Billroth said that 'a surgeon who tries to suture a heart wound deserves to lose the esteem of his colleagues'. Intrathoracic surgery (including cardiac surgery) has developed over the last 100 years, mainly as a result of the advance of anaesthetic techniques, particularly positive pressure ventilation.

CHEST WALL AND LUNGS

The principal problems caused by diseases of the chest wall and lungs are:

- chest pain
- difficulty with breathing (dyspnoea)
- haemoptysis
- cough and expectoration
- dysphagia
- an abnormality on a chest X-ray or CT scan in a patient without symptoms
- swelling of the neck and congestion of the neck veins

- excessive muscle fatigue, droopy eyelids
- chest wall deformities.

Pain and breathlessness are common symptoms of many of the conditions described in this chapter so a clinical diagnosis of the underlying disease, especially if it does not have any distinctive physical signs, is often not possible. The diagnosis of most intrathoracic problems depends on diagnostic imaging, endoscopy and tissue biopsy.

Chest pain

Pain in the chest is a very common presenting symptom. It can arise from the heart, pericardium, mediastinum, oesophagus, pleura, spine or chest wall. The causes are listed in Table 14.1.

Difficulty with breathing (dyspnoea)

Breathlessness is usually caused by the lung and heart diseases listed in Table 14.2, but there are also some non-thoracic causes such as anaemia.

Dyspnoea, the sensation of breathlessness experienced by the patient, is usually first noticed during exercise but may progress to be present at rest and become a most disabling and frightening symptom.

Haemoptysis

The causes of haemoptysis are listed in Table 14.3. Although small-volume haemoptysis in a smoker may be a symptom of lung cancer, massive haemoptysis is more commonly caused by an inflammatory process. The management of haemoptysis is summarized in Revision panel 4.

Table 14.1
The causes of chest pain

Heart	Angina
	Acute coronary syndromes
	ST elevation myocardial infarction
	Aortic dissection
	Aortic aneurysm
Pericardium	Pericarditis
	Pericardial cyst
Mediastinum	Mediastinitis
	Oesophagitis
	Oesophageal tumour (rare)
	Oesophageal motility disorders
	Ruptured oesophagus
	Other mediastinal masses (e.g. thymoma, lymphadenopathy, teratoma, neurogenic tumour, foregut cysts)
	Spontaneous pneumomediastinum (Hamman's syndrome)
Pleura	Pneumonia
	Pulmonary embolus
	Pneumothorax
	Pleural effusion
	Empyema
	Tumour (e.g. invasive lung cancer, mesothelioma, metastatic disease)
Chest wall	Trauma (e.g. rib fractures)
	Tumour (e.g. invasive lung cancer, secondary bony deposits, mesothelioma, primary chest wall sarcomas)
	Costochondritis
	Tietze's syndrome
	Osteomyelitis
Spine	Degenerative disease

Table 14.2
The causes of breathlessness

Asthma

Chronic obstructive pulmonary disease (COPD)
Obstructing lesion (e.g. tumour of the trachea or major bronchi, inhaled foreign body, sputum retention)

Lung parenchyma

Pulmonary embolus
Pulmonary oedema
Pneumonia
Interstitial lung disease
COPD/emphysema/bullous lung disease
Pulmonary contusion
Pulmonary haemorrhage

Pleural space

Pleural effusion
Pneumothorax
Pleural tumour (e.g. mesothelioma)
Haemothorax
Empyema

Chest wall and diaphragm

Trauma with associated pain
Flail chest
Diaphragmatic hernia
Diaphragmatic paralysis

Mediastinum

Intrinsic obstruction
Primary lung cancer
Metastatic cancer
Direct invasion by other cancers (e.g. oesophageal)
Other primary tracheal or bronchial tumours

Extrinsic compression

Mediastinal lymphadenopathy
Retrosternal goitre
Thymoma
Germ cell tumours
Bronchogenic cyst
Great vessel arterial aneurysm

Other

Tracheomalacia (usually following removal of mass)
Anaemia
Hyperthyroidism

Cough and expectoration

Cough is an extremely common problem. Cough with expectoration indicates the presence of a significant problem somewhere in the lungs, bronchi and upper respiratory passages. A cough without expectoration may be caused by conditions such as pharyngitis, laryngitis and external irritation, but if

Table 14.3
The causes of haemoptysis

Inflammation and infection (e.g. tuberculosis, aspergillosis)

Bronchiectasis

Lung cancer

Trauma (e.g. pulmonary artery catheter, penetrating trauma)

Pulmonary embolus

Pulmonary arteriovenous malformations

Table 14.4
Some causes of cough and expectoration

Acute bronchitis

Chronic bronchitis (smoking)

Bronchiectasis

Lung abscess

Viral pneumonia

Bronchopneumonia

Acute pleurisy

Influenza

Upper respiratory tract infections

Tuberculosis

Measles

Whooping cough (pertussis)

Psittacosis

Heart failure

Mediastinal masses

Table 14.5
Non-oesophageal causes of dysphagia in the mediastinum

Retrosternal goitre

Mediastinal lymphadenopathy

Thymoma or thymic hyperplasia (with associated myasthenia gravis)

Enlarged left atrium

Thoracic aortic aneurysm

Aberrant right subclavian artery ('dysphagia lusorum')

Bronchial and tracheal tumours

Bronchogenic cyst

Pericardial cysts

Neurogenic tumours

Fibrosing mediastinitis

Opacity on a chest X-ray or CT scan

There are many causes of an opacity in the lungs revealed by a chest X-ray (Table 14.6).

The difficulty lies in distinguishing a benign lesion that requires no intervention from one that is malignant or could cause harm, such as a massive haemoptysis or airway obstruction.

Although the radiological features of the opacity sometimes suggest its pathological nature, most cases require blood tests, further radiological investigation, attempts at histological diagnosis using bronchoscopy, CT-guided or open surgical biopsy and staging. These are discussed in detail in the sections on the solitary pulmonary nodule and lung cancer.

Distended neck veins

The conditions that may obstruct the upper mediastinum and thoracic inlet and cause venous distention in the neck are listed in Table 14.7.

Muscle weakness and droopy eyelids

These are the problems caused by myasthenia gravis.

it persists the mucosa lining the airways becomes irritated, secretes excess mucus and the cough becomes wet. Some of the causes of a cough are listed in Table 14.4.

Dysphagia

The non-oesophageal causes of dysphagia are listed in Table 14.5. Most are much less common than the oesophageal causes, which are discussed in Chapter 18.

Table 14.6
Causes of a radiologically detected lung mass

Infective

Area of consolidation/pneumonia

Lung abscess

Tuberculosis

Aspergilloma

Histoplasmosis

Inflammatory

Scar tissue

Rheumatoid arthritis

Sarcoidosis

Wegener's granulomatosis

Benign tumours

Hamartoma

Solitary fibrous tumour

Other rare benign tumours

Malignant tumours

Non-small cell lung cancer

Small cell lung cancer

Metastatic disease (e.g. colorectal cancer, renal cell carcinoma, melanoma, osteosarcoma)

Carcinoid tumours

Lymphoma

Miscellaneous

Arteriovenous malformation

Bronchogenic cyst

Lung sequestration

Pulmonary infarct

Round atelectasis

Table 14.7
Causes of superior vena cava obstruction

Benign

Fibrosing mediastinitis

Great vessel arterial aneurysm

Retrosternal goitre

Malignant

Lung cancer

Mediastinal lymphadenopathy (e.g. lymphoma, metastatic disease)

Mediastinal masses (e.g. thymoma, germ cell tumours)

Iatrogenic

Thrombosed neck lines

Primary spontaneous pneumothoraces occur in young adults and are caused by a ruptured apical subpleural bleb or bulla. The affected individual is typically tall and thin. Smoking is a risk factor, especially for recurrence.

Secondary spontaneous pneumothoraces are the result of underlying lung disease and therefore tend to occur in late-middle and old age. The most common cause is a ruptured bulla on a background of **emphysema**.

Other rarer predisposing conditions include cystic fibrosis, cavitating infections and tumours (e.g. tuberculosis), *Pneumocystis carinii* pneumonia in AIDS patients, alpha-1 antitrypsin deficiency, connective tissue disorders and catamenial pneumothorax (associated with menstruation).

Traumatic pneumothorax may be iatrogenic in nature (e.g. during CVP catheter insertion) or the direct result of chest trauma, penetrating and blunt.

Tension pneumothorax is a condition in which air continues to enter during inspiration. As it expands it compresses the heart, the mediastinum and the contralateral lung, preventing proper ventilation and embarrassing the circulation and eventually death.

Investigation

Clinical diagnostic indicators

The common symptoms are shortness of breath, chest pain, an ipsilateral hyper-resonant percussion

PNEUMOTHORAX

A pneumothorax is a collection of air within the pleural space. This allows the lungs to collapse and, depending on its size and type, causes respiratory and eventually haemodynamic distress.

Pneumothoraces can be classified according to their aetiology. They have a bimodal age distribution.

note and an ipsilateral reduced air entry (see *Symptoms and Signs*).

A tension pneumothorax can cause distension of the neck veins, deviation of the trachea and heart to the contralateral side, shock and eventually death.

Note that if suspected on the basis of the symptoms and signs, decompression must be performed immediately before any further investigations.

Imaging

The diagnosis can be confirmed with a **chest X-ray**. A **CT scan is** only used to define the anatomy of the lung in cases of secondary pneumothorax (Fig 14.1A).

Management

Immediate care

All patients who are symptomatic should be given **supplemental oxygen**. If a tension pneumothorax is suspected the chest should be **decompressed** as a matter of urgency by inserting a large bore cannula through the second intercostal space in the midclavicular line (see Chapter 6).

Conservative management

A small, symptomless primary pneumothorax – less than 2 cm from the lung edge to the chest wall on chest X-ray – should be observed. It should resolve spontaneously.

Larger (>2 cm) or symptomatic pneumothoraces may be treated by **simple aspiration**.

If this fails to achieve satisfactory lung re-expansion or if symptoms persist, repeated aspiration should be considered but it is likely that intercostal catheter drainage will be required.

The **intercostal chest drain** should be inserted through the fifth intercostal space in the anterior axillary line, within the 'triangle of safety', an area bounded by *pectoralis major* anteriorly and *latissimus dorsi* posteriorly, and connected to an **underwater seal**.

The drain can be removed when:

- the lung has re-expanded on chest X-ray
- the patient is asymptomatic
- there is no evidence of a persistent air leak (bubbling) or excessive fluid drainage (>200 mL/day).

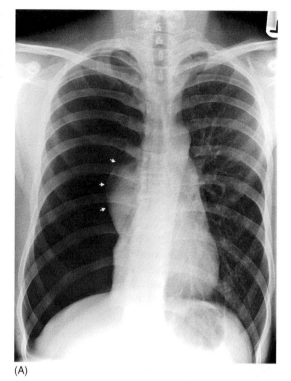

(A)

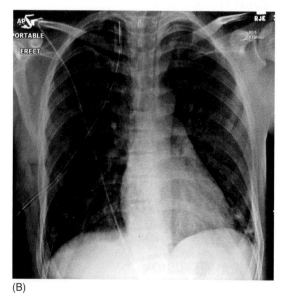

(B)

FIGURE 14.1 (A) Chest X-ray of a primary spontaneous pneumothorax. The right lung has completely collapsed (the white arrows indicate the lung edge). (B) Immediately following a VATS bullectomy and pleurectomy, the right lung has almost completely re-expanded. The chest drain is ideally positioned at the apex

Surgical management

The indications for surgery are:

- recurrent pneumothorax (i.e. a second ipsilateral or first contralateral episode)
- bilateral pneumothorax
- tension pneumothorax
- complicated pneumothorax (e.g. as a result of a torn adhesion between the lung and the chest wall)
- failure of conservative treatment after 5 days of drainage (persistent air leak or failure of lung to re-expand)
- professional necessity (e.g. fighter pilots, divers).

The aim of surgery is twofold: first, to **resect** the underlying **subpleural blebs** or **bullae**; and second, to **obliterate the pleural space** by pleurectomy, pleurodesis or pleural abrasion (Fig. 14.1B). Although the standard operation involves a **thoracotomy and pleurectomy**, a minimally invasive approach (video-assisted thoracoscopic surgery, or **VATS**) is more acceptable to the patient as it is associated with less pain and a shorter hospital stay. Endoscopic mechanical stapling devices may be employed to resect the blebs or bullae.

Complications

Complications include bleeding (more often after pleurectomy), chest infection and empyema. Acute respiratory distress syndrome (ARDS) has been reported after pleurodesis.

Results

The long-term results of open surgical management are better than those following minimally invasive procedures. Recurrent pneumothorax occurs in 1 per cent following thoracotomy and in 5 per cent following a VATS approach.

PLEURAL EFFUSION

A pleural effusion is defined as fluid in the pleural space. Normally the pleural space contains about 5 mL of pleural fluid. The normal flux of fluid into the pleural space is 0.01 mL/kg/hour. It comes from three sources: the pleural capillaries (governed by Starling forces), the interstitial spaces of the lung, and the peritoneum via small connecting holes

Table 14.8
The causes of a pleural effusion

Transudates (protein <30 g/L, LDH <200 IU/L)
Congestive heart failure
Renal failure
Liver failure
Hypothyroidism
Exudates (protein >30 g/L, LDH >200 IU/L)
Pneumonia (may lead to empyema)
Other infection (e.g. tuberculosis)
Malignancy (e.g. mesothelioma, lung cancer, metastatic disease)
Collagen vascular disease (e.g. rheumatoid arthritis, systemic lupus erythematosus, Wegener's granulomatosis)
Pulmonary embolus
Trapped lung
Haemothorax
Chylothorax
Post surgery (e.g. CABG, liver transplant)
Pancreatitis
Subphrenic abscess
Oesophageal perforation
Meig's syndrome (associated ovarian tumour)
Iatrogenic (e.g. radiation therapy)
Idiopathic

[CABG-coronary artery bypass grafting; LDH-lactate dehydrogenase]

in the diaphragm. It is removed by the pleural lymphatics. A pleural effusion will form when the rate of fluid production associated with conditions such as inflammation and congestive heart failure exceeds the rate of fluid resorption or when conditions such as a pleural tumour decrease resorption.

Whether an effusion is an exudate or transudate is dictated by the underlying cause (Table 14.8).

Investigation

Clinical diagnostic indicators

Patients with a pleural effusion complain of shortness of breath and chest discomfort/pain. Examination

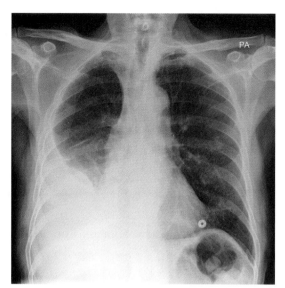

FIGURE 14.2 Chest X-ray of a large right-sided pleural effusion, in this case secondary to malignant mesothelioma

will reveal a dull percussion note (typically described as 'stony dull'), reduced vocal resonance, reduced air entry and possibly the stigmata of the underlying cause (e.g. rheumatoid arthritis).

Imaging

Chest X-ray The only sign of an early effusion (around 500 mL) may be blunting of the costophrenic angle (Fig 14.2).

Larger effusions may have a fluid level or show a complete whiteout of the whole lung field.

An **ultrasound scan** of the chest is more sensitive and specific than an X-ray.

A **CT scan** will demonstrate the size and anatomical characteristics of an effusion. It may also provide diagnostic information regarding any underlying thoracic pathology.

Examination of pleural fluid

Thoracocentesis, ultrasound or CT guided, or performed blind, is the single most useful test and the fluid should be sent for **microbiological, biochemical** and **cytological examination**.

Microbiology

The fluid may be purulent if infected. Gram stain and culture will help diagnose an empyema.

Cytology

Cytology is diagnostic in 45–50 per cent of malignant effusions. Blood-stained fluid is an ominous sign.

Biochemistry

The **protein** and lactate dehydrogenase (**LDH**) levels differentiate a transudate from an exudate (Table 14.8). LDH is very high ($>1000\,\text{IU/L}$) in empyema.

Glucose Low levels ($<2.2\,\text{mmol/L}$) are seen in empyema and malignancy.

pH A low level (<7.20) suggests infection.

Triglycerides A high level and the presence of chylomicrons are diagnostic of a chylothorax.

Pleural biopsy

A biopsy can be achieved by the bedside with an Abram's needle, percutaneously under radiological guidance, or surgically. The diagnostic yield is greatest with surgery.

Blood tests

White blood cell and **C-reactive protein** (CRP) may help in the diagnosis of infection. **Autoantibodies** (e.g. rheumatoid factor) are indicated if a collagen vascular disease is suspected.

Endoscopy

Bronchoscopy should be performed to exclude endobronchial disease.

Management
Immediate care

Oxygen should be administered if the patient is symptomatic. Pain relief may be required. If a chest drain is to be inserted, intravenous access should be established first.

Conservative treatment

A transudate should resolve following treatment of the underlying condition. This may also apply to some exudates, e.g. rheumatoid arthritis, systemic lupus erythematosus (SLE).

Repeated aspiration may be used for symptomatic relief. However, in these circumstances, insertion of an **intercostal drain** may be more appropriate.

Pleurodesis for recurrent effusions can be performed at the bedside via the drain using various agents such as talc, tetracycline and bleomycin. Talc slurry is the most effective, with a response rate of up to 90 per cent. Side-effects include pain, fever and infection. A pleurodesis should not be performed in the presence of an infected pleural space.

A **long-term indwelling pleural catheter** can be placed percutaneously in patients who cannot tolerate pleurodesis, in those who have already had a failed pleurodesis, and in those with trapped lung (see below).

Further investigation is essential if there is any doubt about the diagnosis or if conservative treatment fails to control the effusion.

Surgical treatment

The role of surgery is to establish a diagnosis and prevent reaccumulation of pleural fluid.

Open pleural biopsy can be performed via a mini-thoracotomy with or without resection of a rib, but **minimally invasive methods** are now more commonly used (often through a single port) to drain the effusion, biopsy the pleura and perform a pleurodesis The diagnostic yield for malignancy is 95 per cent.

The pleurodesis success rate of talc poudrage is 90 per cent.

Complications include empyema, death and tumour seeding in the surgical wounds or drain sites.

Palliation is the goal when treating malignant effusions, as the majority of patients do not survive longer than a year.

The use of the more radical surgery sometimes appropriate for empyema and pleural malignancy is controversial.

TRAPPED LUNG

The phenomenon of *trapped lung* describes the situation in which *the lung fails to re-expand after drainage of a pleural effusion*. This is usually secondary to malignancy, pleural infection (empyema) or chylothorax. The cause is a thick layer of tumour, fibrin or fibrotic tissue overlying and incorporating the visceral pleura that encases the lung. Management strategies are based on the underlying cause and the prognosis of the patient (see the sections 'Mesothelioma' and 'Empyema').

MESOTHELIOMA

This is a rare malignant tumour arising from the mesothelial layer of the pleura. The aetiolo-gical factor in almost all cases is exposure to asbestos inhalation, typically 30–40 years prior to presentation with the disease. The incidence in the UK is around 2000 cases per year, a number which is expected to continue rising for another 10 or 15 years.

Investigation

Clinical diagnostic indicators

There is chest pain and dyspnoea usually caused by a pleural effusion.

Imaging

A chest **X-ray** will usually reveal a pleural effusion with pleural thickening. Contraction of the hemithorax may be present.

In addition to confirming the X-ray findings, a **CT scan** will provide more information on the anatomy and stage of the disease (Fig 14.3).

Cytology of pleural effusion

Cytological examination of the pleural effusion if present is diagnostic in 40 per cent of cases.

Tissue biopsy

A CT-guided **core biopsy** may be diagnostic but a video-assisted thoracoscopy or open larger pleural

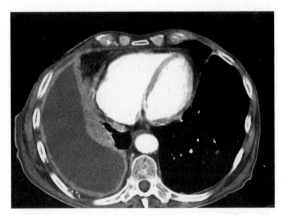

FIGURE 14.3 CT scan of the patient in Fig 14.2 confirms the presence of a right-sided pleural effusion. In addition, there is associated gross pleural thickening

biopsy is often required as histological interpretation can be difficult (Fig 14.4).

Management

Treatment is generally aimed at symptom control, as the disease is incurable. Median survival is 8–9 months. However, there are reports of long-term survivors following radical surgical treatment combined with chemoradiotherapy.

Conservative treatment

Chest pain should be managed with **analgesics**. A pleural effusion should be managed by **talc pleurodesis** or a long-term indwelling pleural catheter.

Surgical treatment

As with other malignant pleural effusions, the role of the surgeon in the management of this dreadful disease is to achieve both a diagnosis and prevent effusion recurrence if this has not been possible by less invasive means. This is usually possible with video-assisted thorascopic techniques.

Several enthusiasts around the world have advocated a more radical approach with the hope of prolonging survival.

An **extrapleural pneumonectomy** (*en bloc* resection of the lung, visceral and parietal pleura, diaphragm and pericardium) combined with preoperative chemotherapy and postoperative radiotherapy has produced encouraging results in some

case series. The disadvantage is an operative mortality of around 10 per cent.

The mortality is lower with a lung-preserving **radical pleurectomy/decortication**.

Chemotherapy

A combination of **cisplatin** and **pemetrexed** can prolong survival and is indicated in patients with a good performance status.

Radiotherapy

Drain-site and operation-site prophylactic radiotherapy is still advocated by some centres to prevent tumour growing through the chest wall. Radiotherapy can be useful in palliating symptomatic chest wall involvement.

EMPYEMA

Empyema is pus in the pleural space. It can be a life-threatening condition, even in young people, and typically develops from a para-pneumonic effusion. An iatrogenic empyema may complicate chest surgery or chest drain insertion.

It is estimated that over 50 per cent of patients with pneumonia develop a para-pneumonic effusion but only a small proportion of these effusions become infected.

There are three stages in the development of an empyema.

1. *Exudative.* A simple effusion becomes complicated by infection.
2. *Fibrinopurulent.* A macroscopically purulent effusion develops with fibrin deposition. Fibrin strands may cause the effusion to become loculated.
3. *Organizing/chronic.* Both the visceral and parietal pleura become thickened and the lung is encased by a fibrous peel or cortex. The pus is extremely thick.

Streptococcus pneumoniae and *Staphylococcus aureus* are the main causes of community-acquired pneumonia. Gram-negative bacteria (e.g. *Escherichia coli*, *Haemophilus influenzae* and *Klebsiella pneumoniae*) and anaerobes (e.g. *Bacteroides fragilis*) are also commonly isolated. Hospital-acquired empyemas (both iatrogenic and para-pneumonic) are

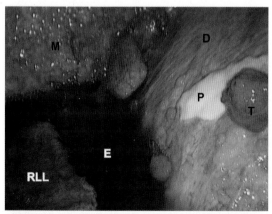

FIGURE 14.4 At surgical thoracoscopy in a patient with a right-sided pleural effusion it is clear there is an underlying malignant cause. D, diaphragm; M, mediastinum; T, tumour nodule; P, benign asbestos pleural plaque; E, blood-stained effusion; RLL, right lower lobe of lung

often caused by *Staphylococcus aureus* (including methicillin-resistant *Staphylococcus aureus* (MRSA)), enterococci and *Pseudomonas aeruginosa*.

Untreated, an empyema can become complicated by:

- invasion into the bronchial tree (bronchopleural fistula)
- invasion through the chest wall with spontaneous external drainage (empyema necessitatis)
- chronic lung fibrosis with hemithorax contraction
- osteomyelitis.

Investigation

Clinical diagnostic indicators

Patients with an empyema develop shortness of breath, chest discomfort, pain, fever and a productive cough with a dirty sputum. The percussion note over the empyema will be dull and the vocal resonance and air entry reduced.

Patients with empyema can be extremely unwell. There may be respiratory compromise secondary to both the causative pneumonia and the compression of underlying lung by the effusion/pus. The general signs of sepsis and haemodynamic compromise are also present.

Blood tests

The **white cell count** and **C-reactive protein** will usually be elevated.

Imaging

A **chest X-ray**, an **ultrasound scan** of the chest and a **CT scan** will each confirm the diagnosis

Bacteriology

Fluid from the empyema should be sent for culture and biochemical analysis (pH <7.2, high LDH).

Management

The patient's respiratory and cardiovascular systems should be carefully assessed and the appropriate resuscitative measures implemented. This may involve the administration of oxygen, respiratory support, intravenous fluid and/or vasoactive drugs.

Conservative treatment

The goals of treatment are to drain the pus and treat the underlying cause.

Antibiotic therapy should be dictated by Gram stain and culture results.

An **intercostal drain** should be inserted in a dependent position. It is a widely held, but unsubstantiated belief, that a large-bore drain should be used.

This treatment if employed at an early stage is often curative. Drains should remain in place until there is radiological and clinical improvement and the draining fluid minimal and sterile. The correct duration of antibiotic treatment is unknown but 3 weeks appears to be an appropriate length of time.

Although trials are still ongoing, the use of intrapleural fibrinolytic agents (e.g. streptokinase) to break down fibrin strands and encourage complete empyema drainage cannot be recommended.

Surgical treatment

The indications for surgery include the failure of conservative measures, the presence of a multiloculated pleural collection, and the presence of a thick cortex 'trapping' the lung.

A **rib resection and drainage procedure** is a quick, uncomplicated and safe method of treating many empyemas. The resection of a small portion of rib in a dependent position allows the manual breakdown of loculations, the evacuation of fluid, pus or debris and the accurate placement of large drains.

A **decortication and drainage** is a more complex, time-consuming operation with a mortality of around 2 per cent. It is indicated in those patients in whom either a rib resection has failed or who clearly have a trapped lung from the outset. A **thoracotomy** is performed. Any pus is evacuated and the fibrous cortex peeled off the lung to allow it to expand and fill the pleural space.

LUNG ABSCESS

A lung abscess is a localized collection of pus in a cavity formed by the disintegration of the lung parenchyma. Immunocompromised patients may have multiple abscesses.

A **primary lung abscess** is either caused by aspiration or is a complication of pneumonia.

Secondary lung abscesses occur as a result of another pathology such as metastatic septic emboli, an obstructing bronchial carcinoma or an infected bulla.

Anaerobic bacteria (particularly the *Bacteroides* species) are commonly isolated from the pus. Aerobic bacteria such as *Staphylococcus aureus* and *Streptococcus pneumoniae* (and occasionally coliforms) are sometimes found.

Investigation

Clinical diagnostic indicators

Patients with a lung abscess usually have a cough that becomes productive of pus later in its natural history, especially if the abscess drains spontaneously into the bronchial tree. They have a fever, night sweats and weight loss.

There may be a history of aspiration or a risk factor thereof (e.g. alcohol abuse, bulbar palsy), of recent dental work or pneumonia.

Blood tests

White cell count and **C-reactive** protein may be elevated.

Sputum culture and antibiotic sensitivities

Full bacteriological studies are essential and may demonstrate a heavy growth of a single organism.

Imaging

Chest X-ray and **CT scan** can help to exclude the other diseases that can cause a cavitating lesion (Table 14.9).

Endoscopy

Bronchoscopy can exclude causative diseases in the bronchial tree.

Management

Conservative treatment

The majority of lung abscesses can be treated without surgical intervention especially since the advent of radiologically guided percutaneous

Table 14.9
The causes of cavitating lung lesions

Lung abscess

Lung cancer (especially squamous cell carcinoma)

Tuberculosis

Fungal infection (e.g. *Aspergillus*, *Histoplasmosis*)

Hydatid cyst (caused by the *Echinococcus* tapeworm)

Empyema with bronchopleural fistula

Bronchogenic cyst

drainage techniques. The essentials of conservative treatment are:

- a **prolonged course of antibiotics** (6–8 weeks) dependent on repeated bacterial cultures
- **drainage of the abscess**: internal drainage can be achieved by chest physiotherapy or by bronchoscopy. If this is unsuccessful, then a percutaneous drain should be inserted under CT guidance to drain the pus externally
- **nutritional support**.

Surgical treatment

Only approximately 10 per cent of cases now require surgical intervention. In the acute phase, surgery is indicated for complications of the abscess such as a bronchopleural fistula, empyema or bleeding (haemoptysis).

After the initial illness, surgery should be performed if:

- there are persistent symptoms and signs despite medical therapy
- there is a suspicion of an underlying carcinoma of the lung
- a large abscess (>6 cm) persists radiologically despite a full course of treatment
- complications develop such as a bronchopleural fistula or an empyema.

Surgical treatment entails a **thoracotomy** and **resection of the abscess**, often with the affected lobe of lung. However, if the patient has been unwell and is not a suitable candidate for such major surgery, it may be safer to exteriorize the abscess cavity and allow external drainage.

BRONCHIECTASIS

Bronchiectasis is a chronic condition character-ized by the permanent dilatation of the subseg-mental airways. It may be congenital or acquired (Table 14.10). Its development requires the pres-ence of infection and one of the following:

▨ impairment of bronchial drainage
▨ airway obstruction
▨ a defect in the host defence.

The result is transmural inflammation, mucosal oedema and bronchial neovascularization.

Investigation
Clinical diagnostic indicators
The common symptoms of bronchiectasis are repeated respiratory tract infections, haemoptysis (which may be massive), shortness of breath and chest pain. Coughing may produce large amounts of foetid sputum – sometimes triggered by a change of posture and a bout of coughing. Auscultation reveals wet sounds (coarse crepitations) over the affected segment. There may be cyanosis and finger clubbing.

Blood tests
Markers of inflammation (e.g. WCC, CRP) are often raised and useful for monitoring the disease and the response to treatment.

Table 14.10
Aetiology of bronchiectasis

Congenital

Cystic fibrosis

Hypogammaglobulinaemia

Alpha-1 antitrypsin deficiency

Sequestration of the lung

Kartagener's syndrome

Acquired
Infection

Bronchial obstruction: intrinsic (e.g. foreign body, obstructing tumour); extrinsic (e.g. lymphadenopathy)

Tuberculosis

Bacteriology of sputum
Imaging
A **CT scan** will show the characteristic appearances of bronchial dilatation and peribronchial inflam-mation. The lung parenchyma may be diseased.

CT also provides information as to whether the disease is operable or not (localized or multifocal) and may, in addition, reveal an underlying cause.

Bronchoscopy
Pus may be seen originating from the affected lobar segment(s). It should be subjected to bacteriological analysis.

Management
Bronchiectasis is a chronic condition. The main indi-cation for urgent treatment is massive haemoptysis.

Conservative treatment
The majority of bronchiectasis cases are managed conservatively. The appropriate antibiotics should be administered during flare-ups. Repeated courses may be required. Chest physiotherapy and postural drainage help to clear out the dirty secretions.

Surgical treatment
The indications for surgery are persistent symp-toms with recurrent infections and haemoptysis.

To be amenable to **lobectomy** (resection of one lobe of lung) or **sublobar resection** (segmentectomy, or resection of one lobar segment) the disease should be

▨ unilateral
▨ localized to one lobe or segment
▨ completely resectable.

Surgery for bronchiectasis is often more dif-ficult than surgery for lung cancer because of the presence of chronic inflammation, but its mortality is much the same (2–3 per cent). The operation immediately relieves patients of their symptoms.

THE SOLITARY PULMONARY NODULE

This is defined as a discrete mass in the lung measur-ing less than 3 cm in diameter. There are many pos-sible diagnoses (Table 14.6) but malignant disease must always be excluded. The features that make malignant disease more likely are the following.

- *Size*. The majority of nodules greater than 2 cm in diameter are malignant.
- *Growth rate*. Any increase in size suggests malignant change. The doubling time for a non-small cell lung carcinoma is 100 days: for a small cell lung cancer it is 30 days.
- *Appearance*. A spiculated mass is likely to be a primary lung cancer. Calcification is usually seen only in benign nodules.
- *Past history*. A smoking history greatly increases the chance of a nodule being a cancer. The presence or history of an extrathoracic malignancy makes it likely that it is a metastasis.

Investigation
Imaging
Chest X-rays and CT scans. Lung nodules are often picked up incidentally.

Positron emission tomography (PET) scan. A 'hot' nodule is likely to be malignant.

Endoscopy
Bronchoscopy (for central lesions) can be diagnostic if tumour is seen and biopsied.

Tissue biopsy
CT-guided biopsy is used for peripheral lesions.

Excision biopsy. Surgical removal, either via a thoracotomy or using a VATS technique may be the only way to achieve a diagnosis. Histological examination of a frozen section of the removed tissue at the time of surgery allows the surgeon to progress to a more formal cancer operation (e.g. lobectomy) if a primary lung cancer is confirmed.

Management
If the lesion is less than 8 mm in diameter on CT, then **radiological follow-up** with repeated monthly scans is indicated. Any increase in size normally mandates **surgical excision**.

Any nodule larger than 8 mm should be fully investigated as described above, further management depending upon the histological diagnosis.

BENIGN LUNG TUMOURS

Benign lung tumours are rare, although they are being diagnosed with increased frequency as CT scanning becomes a more common routine investigation.

Hamartoma

This, by far the most common tumour, accounts for almost 80 per cent of cases. It has a characteristic calcified 'popcorn' appearance and consists of cartilage and fat.

Solitary fibrous tumour

These tumours which arise from the visceral pleural surface rather than the lung parenchyma may occasionally be malignant.

Other rare tumours

Adenoma, clear cell tumour, fibroma, haemangiopericytoma, inflammatory pseudo-tumour, leiomyoma, lipoma, sclerosing haemangioma and teratoma have all been reported.

Investigation

Most of these tumours are symptomless and are discovered incidentally. The investigations required are the same as those for a solitary pulmonary nodule (see above).

Management

Repeated CT scans or chest X-rays may be reassuring by demonstrating that the lesion is static. Attempts at obtaining a tissue diagnosis by CT-guided needle biopsy may suggest a benign aetiology or fail. A definitive diagnosis can only be made following surgical excision and therefore a thoracotomy (or VATS) becomes both diagnostic and curative.

TUBERCULOSIS

Mycobacterium tuberculosis is a virulent anaerobic bacillus. The incidence of tuberculosis is increasing worldwide. In developed countries, it is often associated with immunosuppressed individuals.

It causes cavitating lung disease that is usually amenable to drug therapy (although multi-resistant strains have developed). Despite being of historical importance, the surgical methods for treating pulmonary tuberculosis are now rarely used.

Investigation
Clinical diagnostic indicators

Patients develop a cough, fever and night sweats and haemoptysis (which may be massive), accompanied by constitutional symptoms – lethargy, anorexia and weight loss.

Skin tests

Tuberculin skin testing has a significant false-negative rate in immunosuppressed individuals.

Blood tests

The **interferon-γ assay** (e.g. ELISPOT) is now preferred to skin testing as a screening tool.

Sputum microscopy and culture

Organisms may be visible with microscopy using a Ziehl–Neelsen stain.

The culture of infected **sputum**, **bronchial washings** or **lymph node biopsies** takes several weeks to yield results.

Imaging

Chest X-ray and **CT scanning** are useful diagnostic adjuncts.

Tissue biopsy

A diagnostic wedge excision may be needed to confirm the cause of the nodule.

Management

Medical therapy with multiple **anti-tuberculous drugs** is the first-line treatment.

Surgery is now rarely used except for the management of complications such as:

- **empyema** (may require drainage or decortication)
- **bronchiectasis** (may require lung resection)
- massive or troublesome **haemoptysis** (may require lung resection or bronchial artery embolization).

ASPERGILLOSIS

Aspergillus fumigatus is an opportunistic fungus found in soil and decaying vegetation that may infect immunocompromised patients.

It can also affect immunocompetent individuals with underlying lung disease or cavities (e.g. old tuberculosis).

The aspergilloma (or fungus ball) is a matted sphere of hyphae, fibrin and inflammatory cells, usually found in a pre-existing upper lobe cavity, and has the capacity to erode the surrounding lung parenchyma.

Fungal infection may manifest itself in four different clinical syndromes:

- aspergillus hypersensitivity lung disease
- aspergilloma
- invasive pulmonary aspergillosis
- empyema.

Investigation
Clinical diagnostic indicators

The main symptoms are cough, haemoptysis (which may be massive), dyspnoea and chest pain.

Blood tests

Aspergillus immunoglobulin (Ig)G antibodies indicate past or present infection if elevated.

Imaging

Chest X-ray and **CT scan** show a solitary pulmonary nodule.

Endoscopy

Bronchoscopy and washings confirm the diagnosis.

Bacteriology

Culture of sputum and bronchial washings may also confirm the diagnosis.

Tissue biopsy

Histopathology should demonstrate the characteristic hyphae.

Management
Conservative treatment

Antifungal agents such as **amphotericin B** and **itraconazole** have been used in symptomatic patients with varying degrees of success. These drugs may be given intravenously or locally (i.e. intracavity or intrapleural).

Surgical treatment

A simple aspergilloma may be **excised** as part of the investigation and treatment of a solitary pulmonary nodule.

In more complex cases with local parenchymal destruction, *excision is controversial* because of a perceived high mortality and morbidity and no guarantee of a cure. Thoracotomy and surgical resection (e.g. **lobectomy**) should probably be reserved for those whose symptoms of cough or haemoptysis are troublesome enough to justify the risk.

NON-SMALL CELL LUNG CANCER

Lung cancer is the cause of more cancer deaths than any other cancer in the UK. Smoking is the main risk factor. Around 40 000 new patients are diagnosed each year, of whom less than 5 per cent will survive 5 years. As patients with lung cancer tend to present late, treatment options are limited and less than 10 per cent are currently offered surgery.

Lung cancers can be broadly divided into two groups depending on their histology – **small cell lung cancer** (SCLC, discussed later) and **non-small cell lung cancer** (NSCLC), which can be further divided into **adenocarcinoma**, **squamous cell carcinoma** and **large cell carcinoma**.

The distinction between small and non-small cell cancer has been made because the treatments available are different. Essentially, NSCLC (which makes up 80 per cent of cases) is amenable to radical treatment provided there is no metastatic spread. The diagnostic, investigative pathway is necessarily complex and reflects the need to exclude metastatic disease and assess the patient's physiological fitness before offering surgery or radical radiotherapy.

Lung cancer commonly metastasizes to the mediastinal lymph nodes, the liver, the adrenal glands, bone and the brain. Patients with symptoms generally have metastases at presentation.

Investigation
Clinical diagnostic indicators
Patients with operable disease are often symptomless, their lung cancer having been picked up

incidentally on a routine chest X-ray. In others, the symptoms may include cough, chest pain, recurrent chest infections, haemoptysis, constitutional symptoms (weight loss, malaise) and symptoms from local and distant spread.

Symptoms from local spread include:

- **stridor** from involvement of the major airways
- **superior vena cava obstruction** secondary to mediastinal lymphadenopathy or right hilar tumour invasion
- **dysphagia** from direct spread into the oesophagus
- **arrhythmias** or signs of **cardiac tamponade** from direct spread into the pericardium
- **hoarseness** from invasion of the recurrent laryngeal nerve (usually the left)
- **Horner's syndrome** from invasion of the stellate sympathetic ganglion
- **arm pain** (brachial plexus invasion by a Pancoast tumour)
- **dyspnoea** and **chest pain** (phrenic and intercostal nerve invasion).

Symptoms from distant spread include:

- **bone pain** caused by metastases and pathological fractures
- **headache, nausea and central nervous system signs** caused by brain metastases
- **abdominal pain and jaundice** if there are liver metastases
- **para-neoplastic syndromes** (Table 14.11).

The aims of the investigation of a patient with probable lung cancer are threefold: to establish the diagnosis; to accurately stage the disease; and to assess the patient's pulmonary and general physiological fitness.

Imaging
A **chest X-ray** is an important screening tool. It may show a lung mass, lobar collapse, pleural effusion, mediastinal lymphadenopathy, diaphragmatic paralysis or bony destruction (Fig 14.5).

CT scan In the presence of an abnormal chest X-ray, a CT scan of the thorax and abdomen is the single, most useful investigation. Not only does it suggest a diagnosis, but can be used to stage the cancer and direct the most appropriate method of biopsy.

Table 14.11
Paraneoplastic syndromes associated with lung cancer

Endocrine/metabolic

Inappropriate acute diuretic hormone secretion

Hypercalcaemia (parathormone-like hormone)

Cushing's syndrome (ACTH)

Gynaecomastia

Neurological

Peripheral neuropathy

Polymyositis

Eaton–Lambert syndrome

Skeletal

Finger clubbing

Hypertrophic pulmonary osteoarthropathy

Cutaneous

Hyperkeratosis

Hyperpigmentation

Dermatomyositis

Acanthosis nigricans

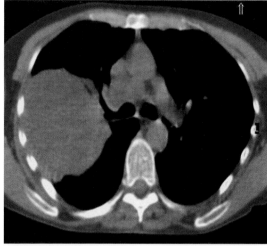

(A)

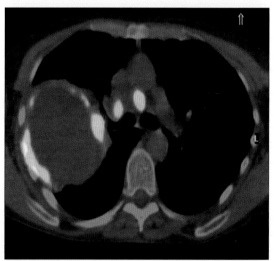

(B)

FIGURE 14.6   (A) CT-PET scan of the chest demonstrates a large right upper lobe lung mass with possible chest wall involvement. (B) There is avid uptake of labelled fluorodeoxyglucose (FDG) in the periphery of the tumour suggesting a necrotic centre (typical of a squamous cell carcinoma). Furthermore, two mediastinal lymph nodes are also 'hot', precluding radical treatment if confirmed as metastatic disease. The clinical tumour stage is T3N2

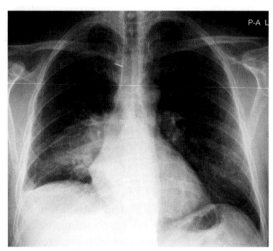

FIGURE 14.5   Chest X-ray of a right central tumour. There is loss of the right heart contour. The patient subsequently underwent a pneumonectomy for confirmed non-small cell cancer (see Fig 14.7)

A **PET scan (or combined CT-PET)** may be useful in assessing the probability of malignancy in a solitary pulmonary nodule in the absence of a histological diagnosis. However, false positives are seen with infection, inflammation, rheumatoid nodules, sarcoid, tuberculosis (TB) and aspergillomas. Furthermore, as the spatial resolution of PET is 8 mm, a negative scan does not exclude cancer (Fig 14.6).

PET is more useful as a staging tool in those patients who do not have obvious metastatic disease on CT and who are fit for radical treatment (be it radiotherapy or surgery). A CT-negative mediastinum normally excludes mediastinal lymph node involvement, with certain caveats (see Mediastinoscopy below).

PET is 93 per cent sensitive and 96 per cent specific at detecting extrathoracic metastases. All possible metastases detected by PET should be further investigated, ideally by tissue biopsy.

Endoscopy

Awake flexible bronchoscopy is the procedure of choice for obtaining a histological diagnosis in central lung tumours, especially when combined with **endobronchial brushings** and **washings**, but the sensitivity of bronchoscopy in obtaining a tissue diagnosis in peripheral tumours is poor.

Tissue biopsy

CT-guided needle or core biopsy is recommended for peripheral tumours. Post-procedure pneumothoraces occur in 30 per cent of cases.

Endoscopic oesophageal ultrasound (EUS) and transbronchial needle aspiration (TBNA). Suspicious subcarinal and paraoesophageal lymph nodes may be biopsied using these techniques. Similarly, paratracheal and subcarinal nodes are accessible using a transbronchial approach with or without endobronchial ultrasound.

Invasive staging of the mediastinum. Mediastinoscopy, anterior mediastinotomy or a VATS approach, under general anaesthesia, may be needed to biopsy PET-positive mediastinal lymph nodes if less invasive techniques fail.

Even if there are no PET-positive N2/3 nodes, mediastinoscopy should still be performed if there is a central tumour, N1 disease or enlarged mediastinal nodes (larger than 1.6 cm).

Blood tests

Raised **serum calcium** and **alkaline phosphatase** may indicate the presence of bony metastases, whereas liver involvement may produce deranged liver function tests.

Lung function tests

Postoperative morbidity and mortality is dependent on the predicted postoperative pulmonary function and the peri-operative cardiovascular fitness.

Spirometry The forced expiratory volume in 1 second (FEV1) helps to determine whether a patient will tolerate having all or a part of their lung removed. An FEV1 of more than 1.5 L would suggest a lobectomy can safely be performed, whereas an FEV1 of greater than 2 L is required before performing a pneumonectomy. However, these are crude raw values and do not take into account a patient's age or size.

The FEV1 expressed as a percentage of the predicted value for age and size is more meaningful. It can be used to estimate the per cent predicted post-operative FEV1 (%ppoFEV1) by determining the number of lung segments to be removed. A %ppoFEV1 of more than 40 per cent indicates operability.

Transfer factor

The **transfer factor** (or diffusing capacity of the lung for carbon monoxide, DLCO) should be measured in cases where there is some doubt whether a patient's lung function is good enough to tolerate lung resection, A %ppoDLCO of less than 40 per cent in combination with a %ppoFEV1 of less than 40 per cent indicates a prohibitive operative risk.

Cardiopulmonary exercise testing (CPEX)

A more sophisticated method of determining fitness for lung resection involves the calculation of peak oxygen consumption during exercise (VO_2max). Surgery should probably not be performed if the VO_2max is less than 15 mL/kg/minute.

Echocardiography

All patients undergoing pneumonectomy should have an echocardiogram to determine both left and right ventricular function.

Management

The management of a patient with NSCLC is determined by the stage of the disease, the fitness of the patient and the patient's wishes. Surgery offers by far the best chance of long-term survival.

Conservative treatment

Best supportive care is reserved for those patients with a performance status so poor that they would not tolerate even palliative therapy.

Surgical treatment

Any NSCLC with a tumour (T) stage of 1–3 and a nodal (N) stage of 0–1 and with no evidence of distant metastases is potentially curable by surgical resection. Ultimately, however, this depends on the fitness of the patient (see above). Ideally, all patients should have an anatomical **lung resection with lymph node sampling** of the mediastinum.

This usually involves a **posterolateral thoracotomy** and a **lobectomy** (removal of an entire lobe of lung).

Some central tumours will require a **pneumonectomy** (removal of the entire lung) (Fig 14.7).

In patients with borderline respiratory function and a small peripheral tumour, a lesser resection such as a **segmentectomy** (anatomical removal of a lung segment) or **wedge resection** may suffice. However, the chance of local recurrence is greater with nonanatomical wedge resections.

Postoperative pain is relieved by a continuous epidural or paravertebral infusion of local anaesthetic. A prophylactic mini-tracheostomy is useful for elective postoperative suction in those at high risk of retaining secretions (e.g. smokers, and those requiring a combined chest wall resection).

Early mobilization and chest physiotherapy should be encouraged in all.

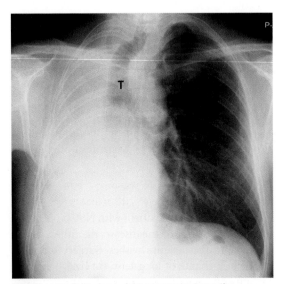

FIGURE 14.7 Following a right pneumonectomy, the trachea (T) and mediastinum shift to the right. The right hemidiaphragm is elevated and the remaining space has filled with fluid

Chest drains are removed once there is no air leak and minimal fluid drainage.

Complications

The peri-operative mortality is 2–3 per cent for a lobectomy and 7 per cent for a pneumonectomy. Early complications also include wound infection, empyema, respiratory failure (secondary to retained secretions, pneumonia or ARDS), supraventricular tachycardia, bleeding and prolonged air leakage.

One of the dreaded complications of a pneumonectomy is **dehiscence of the bronchial stump** staple/suture line and the formation of a **bronchopleural fistula**. This may occur in the first 2 weeks as a simple mechanical breakdown, resulting in aspiration of the fluid in the pneumonectomy space into the good lung and respiratory failure. Immediate treatment is an intercostal drain to remove the pleural fluid and protect the contralateral lung before returning the patient to the operating theatre to refashion and close the bronchial stump.

Late bronchopleural fistulas can occur secondary to an infected space. Treatment is usually chronic chest drainage, although some surgeons attempt staged procedures to clean the pneumonectomy space and close off the fistula.

Long-term survival is stage dependent (particularly nodal stage) and is summarized in Table 14.12. An incomplete resection will adversely affect survival and these patients should be offered adjuvant radiotherapy.

Radiotherapy

Adjuvant radiotherapy should only be offered in cases of incomplete surgical resection. Neoadjuvant treatment is of no benefit except for

Table 14.12
Relationship between stage of non-small cell lung cancer and prognosis

Stage	5-year survival
1 (T1 or 2, N0, M0)	75–85%
2 (T1 or 2, N0, M0)	40–55%
3 (T1 to 4, N0 to 3, M0)	10–45%
4 (T1–4, N0–3, M1)	<5%

Pancoast tumours (usually in combination with chemotherapy), where tumour size is reduced and resection rates are improved.

Radical radiotherapy is indicated for T1 and small T2 tumours in patients whose co-morbidities preclude surgical treatment. Results are inferior to surgical resection with a 5-year survival of around 20 per cent. Palliative treatment is reserved for those patients with symptomatic inoperable primary disease (e.g. haemoptysis, chest wall pain) or with symptomatic metastases (e.g. bone, spine, brain).

Chemotherapy

Adjuvant chemotherapy has been demonstrated in several recent big trials to confer a survival advantage in patients with fully resected disease and is now the standard care of many patients. However, there is no advantage in giving it to patients with early cancers, i.e. T1N0 and T2N0.

Palliative chemotherapy is offered to patients with inoperable NSCLC with a view to extending life rather than attempting a cure.

SMALL CELL LUNG CANCER

Around 20 per cent of patients with lung cancer have small cell lung cancer (SCLC). This form of cancer, *previously known as oat cell cancer*, metastasizes early and presents late. Para-neoplastic syndromes are not uncommon, especially Cushing's syndrome and SIADH.

Investigation

Imaging

A **CT scan** will help provide the diagnosis and allows staging.

Tissue biopsy

Histological confirmation of the disease may be obtained by bronchoscopy, CT-guided biopsy (of the primary lung tumour or metastatic deposits) or mediastinal lymph node biopsy.

In general, there is little point in staging SCLC using the TNM system. Instead, staging is classified according to whether the disease is *limited* (to one hemithorax) or there is *extensive* (spread beyond the hemithorax).

Management

Platinum-based **chemotherapy** is the mainstay of treatment for both limited and extensive disease. Patients with limited SCLC may also be offered **thoracic irradiation**.

In addition, those who respond to chemotherapy may also benefit from prophylactic cranial irradiation.

Surgery is occasionally performed for solitary pulmonary nodules.

Overall survival is poor, with less than 5 per cent surviving beyond 5 years. For extensive disease, median survival is less than a year.

METASTATIC LUNG DISEASE

The lungs are a common site for metastases from many primary malignant tumours. Although it might appear counterintuitive to resect metastatic disease, there are enough case series to suggest that long-term cures are possible. Most of the published studies have been about surgery for metastatic colorectal cancer, but metastases of osteosarcoma and renal cell carcinoma have also been resected. The rationale is that some malignancies have a stepwise spread between the liver and lung, whereas other lung metastases are a marker of widespread disease.

Investigation

Isolated pulmonary metastases amenable to surgical resection are usually symptomless and detected on routine surveillance scans following the surgical treatment of the primary tumour.

Blood tests

The relevant **tumour markers** should be measured for initial assessment and post-operation follow-up.

A high level of carcino-embryonic antigen (CEA) in presumed metastatic colorectal cancer is a poor prognostic sign.

Imaging

A solitary pulmonary nodule on the background of previously treated cancer is a metastasis until proven otherwise. A **whole-body CT scan** is useful in detecting other extrapulmonary metastases and ensuring there is no local recurrence at the primary site.

A **PET scan** may detect extrapulmonary metastases and mediastinal lymph node involvement which would preclude surgery.

Tissue biopsy

Histological confirmation is not strictly speaking necessary; but if there is concern that a pulmonary nodule may represent a primary lung cancer rather than a metastasis, efforts should be made to obtain a preoperative tissue diagnosis with a **CT-guided biopsy**.

Mediastinoscopy

Routine mediastinoscopy is advocated by some surgeons as 10 per cent of patients will have other metastases in the mediastinal lymph nodes.

Management

The indications for surgery are a low operative risk control of the primary tumour site, and the absence of extrapulmonary metastases. Many surgeons prefer to perform a **thoracotomy** rather than using a VATS approach so that the rest of the lung can be manually palpated (despite there being no difference in long-term survival).

The aim of surgery is to remove the metastasis while preserving as much lung parenchyma as possible to allow for future resections. A **stapled wedge resection** or **diathermy excision** is therefore the treatment of choice, greater resections (e.g. lobectomy) being avoided if possible.

The overall 5-year survival following resection of colorectal pulmonary metastases is 40 per cent (this compares to a 5-year survival for Duke's D colorectal cancer of 5 per cent). Factors which indicate a poor prognosis include:

- more than one metastasis
- original Duke's stage B, C or D
- a raised CEA
- positive mediastinal lymph nodes.

Patients with multiple poor prognostic factors should probably not be offered surgery.

OTHER RARE LUNG MALIGNANCIES

Rare lung malignancies include carcinoid tumours (typical and atypical), adenoid cystic carcinoma, mucoepidermoid carcinoma and sarcoma. Carcinoid tumours, which account for less than 5 per cent of lung cancers, are occasionally associated with the carcinoid syndrome or Cushing's syndrome. Surgical resection is the mainstay of treatment as other treatment modalities are relatively ineffective.

THE MEDIASTINUM

The mediastinum is the space between the thoracic inlet and the diaphragm, bounded laterally by the left and right medial pleura. Anatomically, it is often divided into superior, anterior, middle and posterior compartments but a more useful surgical description is to divide it into three compartments: anterior, visceral and paravertebral.

The **anterior compartment** extends from the innominate (left brachiocephalic) vein to the diaphragm and from the underside of the sternum to the anterior surface of the pericardium.

The **visceral compartment** extends from the thoracic inlet to the diaphragm and from the pericardium – inferior to the innominate vein or underside of the sternum – superior to the innominate vein to the anterior surface of the vertebrae.

The **paravertebral compartment** is not a true mediastinal space but a potential space lateral to the vertebral column.

MEDIASTINAL MASSES

Primary mediastinal masses may arise in any compartment. They are rare. Most common is mediastinal lymphadenopathy, often secondary to metastatic cancer (usually lung cancer) or infection but sometimes caused by other diseases such as sarcoidosis, tuberculosis or lymphoma (Fig 14.8A).

The causes of anterior compartment masses can be remembered as the 'four 'T's': thymoma, thyroid, teratoma and 'terrible' lymphoma.

The causes of mediastinal masses are summarized in Table 14.13.

Investigation

Up to half of all mediastinal masses are symptomless and discovered incidentally on a chest X-ray or CT scan. The presence of symptoms or signs is likely to represent a sinister pathology.

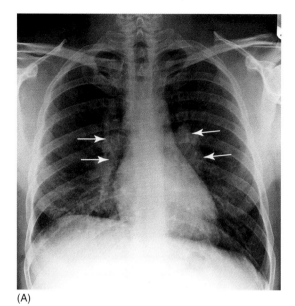

(A)

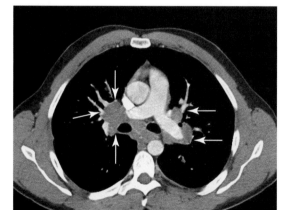

(B)

FIGURE 14.8 (A) Chest X-ray demonstrating the bilateral hilar lymphadenopathy characteristic of sarcoidosis. (B) A CT scan confirms enlarged hilar and mediastinal lymph nodes. The diagnosis was proven at mediastinoscopy

Clinical diagnostic indicators

Symptoms may include dyspnoea, cough, dysphagia, chest or back pain, malaise, fevers and night sweats.

Blood tests

Full blood count. Anaemia is sometimes seen in thymomas (secondary to red cell aplasia). A grossly

Table 14.13
The causes of mediastinal masses

Anterior compartment (contains thymus gland, fat and lymph nodes)

Thymoma or thymic hyperplasia

Thyroid (retrosternal goitre)

Germ cell tumours

Lymphadenopathy

Visceral compartment (contains trachea and main stem bronchi, lymph nodes, heart, pericardium, great vessels, oesophagus and thoracic duct)

Tracheal and bronchial tumours (e.g. lung cancer, benign tracheobronchial tumours)

Lymphadenopathy

Foregut cysts (bronchogenic, oesophageal)

Pericardial cysts

Heart: enlarged chambers (e.g. enlarged left atrium in mitral valve disease), cardiac tumours

Aortic aneurysm

Oesophageal tumours

Hiatus hernia

Paravertebral compartment (contains sympathetic chain, thoracic spinal ganglia and azygous and hemiazygous venous system)

Neurogenic tumours (e.g. neurofibroma, schwannoma, ganglioneuroma, phaeochromocytoma)

Lymphadenopathy (e.g. lymphoma, tuberculosis, sarcoidosis, metastatic cancer)

elevated white count may occasionally accompany a lymphoma.

Germ cell tumour markers and lactate dehydrogenase. Raised levels may be diagnostic for some germ cell tumours.

Heaf test. Tuberculosis is unlikely in the presence of a negative test.

Imaging

PA and **lateral chest X-rays** are useful in localizing the mass.

A **CT scan** is often the single most useful test (Fig 14.8B). The location of the mass and its CT appearances may be diagnostic or indicate a very short list of differential diagnoses.

An **MRI scan** may be indicated for paravertebral masses when there is a suspicion of foraminal extension into the spinal canal.

Endoscopy

Bronchoscopic examination of the tracheobronchial tree is important whenever there is an endobronchial tumour, local invasion or extrinsic compression. Biopsies can be taken directly or by transbronchial needle aspiration. This latter technique can be helped by the use of endobronchial ultrasound (see below).

Oesophagoscopy is indicated for oesophageal tumours. Biopsies can be taken using endoscopic oesophageal ultrasound (see below).

Tissue biopsy

Not all mediastinal masses require surgery. Histological diagnosis is, therefore, often crucial. This can be achieved in several different ways of varying invasiveness.

Fine needle aspiration or core biopsy

This is usually ultrasound- or CT-guided and is operator dependent. Fine needle aspiration may be inadequate for making a definitive diagnosis.

Mediastinal lymph nodes and oesophageal tumours can be visualized and biopsied using **EBUS or EUS**. Transbronchial or transoesophageal fine needle aspiration guided by these images can avoid more invasive procedures.

Mediastinoscopy

Under general anaesthetic, an incision is made just above the suprasternal notch and the mediastinoscope inserted into the pretracheal plane. Paratracheal and subcarinal lymph nodes and masses can then be biopsied under direct vision. Although there is a small risk of major vascular injury, the mortality rate is less than 1:1000.

Anterior mediastinotomy

This is performed through an incision made just lateral to the midline after removing the second costal cartilage. This provides access to the anterior mediastinum and the hilum of the lung. It is most commonly performed on the left side for masses in the aortopulmonary window. Refinements in CT-guided biopsy techniques mean that this is now rarely performed.

VATS

If less invasive methods fail, most intrathoracic masses can be biopsied using a VATS approach.

Thoracotomy is usually a last resort when acquiring a tissue diagnosis is essential.

THYMOMA

A thymoma is a tumour arising from thymic tissue. Although rare, it is the most common tumour occurring in the anterior mediastinum. Histologically they vary from being relatively benign to frank thymic carcinoma (Table 14.14).

Thirty to 50 per cent of patients with a thymoma will have myasthenia gravis. Twelve per cent of patients with myasthenia gravis will have a thymoma.

Investigation

Clinical diagnostic indicators

Thirty per cent are symptomless. The non-specific symptoms include vague respiratory symptoms, chest pain and anaemia (secondary to the paraneoplastic syndrome of red cell aplasia).

Those with myasthenia gravis present with an abnormal degree of fatigue after repetitive exercise and often complain of drooping eyelids.

Table 14.14
Staging of thymoma (Masaoka)

I	Capsule intact
IIa	Microscopic invasion through capsule
IIb	Macroscopic invasion through capsule ± invasion of pleura or pericardium
III	Direct invasion of surrounding structures (e.g. vessels, lung)
IVa	Pleural or pericardial dissemination
IVb	Lymphatic or blood-borne metastases

Imaging

Chest X-ray should reveal an enlarged thymus. On a **CT scan** an isolated anterior mediastinal mass with no associated lymphadenopathy is often diagnostic. CT is also useful for staging and assessing operability (Fig 14.9).

Tissue biopsy

Biopsy of the mass is controversial as seeding of the needle tract and in the mediastinum has been reported. If the presumed thymoma is operable, surgical excision is preferable. Biopsy should be reserved for inoperable tumours.

Blood tests

Full blood count and **germ cell tumour markers** should be obtained. Investigate for myasthenia gravis (see later).

Management

The majority of thymomas are found to be at stages I or II on presentation and are therefore operable. The approach is usually via a median sternotomy. The thymoma and all the thymic tissue should be removed (i.e. **total thymectomy**).

Stage III tumours may be operable, depending on the nature of the local invasion.

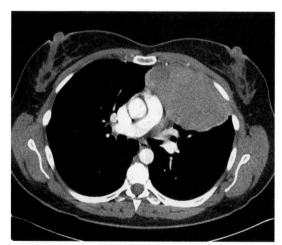

FIGURE 14.9 A large anterior mediastinal mass extending into the left chest is seen on the CT scan of a patient with myasthenia gravis. A left thoracotomy was performed and a large thymoma (stage IIb) excised completely

En bloc resection of lung or pericardium should be considered but involvement of vital structures (e.g. aorta, pulmonary artery, heart) often precludes surgery.

Stage IV tumours are inoperable.

Complications

Operative complications include phrenic nerve and vascular injury. Postoperatively, the complications tend to be related to the median sternotomy (atelectasis, pneumonia, sternal dehiscence).

Myasthenia gravis may emerge for the first time in a minority of patients following resection and should be suspected if symptoms of muscle fatigue develop.

Results

Prognosis depends on the stage of the tumour, the histological classification and the completeness of the resection. The 5-year survival in stage I fully resected type A or AB thymomas approaches 100 per cent.

Radiotherapy

Thymomas are very radiosensitive. The use of adjuvant radiotherapy is controversial if resection margins are clear. Although it may reduce recurrence rates, radiotherapy has no impact on long-term survival.

Postoperative radiotherapy can only be recommended for incomplete resection at present.

In patients with inoperable tumours or the lack of physiological reserve to undergo surgery, radiotherapy may be given following treatment with chemotherapy.

Chemotherapy

The majority of thymomas are chemosensitive and some patients achieve complete remission from cytotoxics. Tumours previously deemed inoperable may be down-staged to the point where surgery or radical radiotherapy becomes feasible.

MYASTHENIA GRAVIS

Myasthenia gravis is an autoimmune neuromuscular disorder. The production of antibodies to the acetylcholine receptors at the neuromuscular junctions causes complement-mediated damage and a reduction in the number of receptors.

There is an association with thymomas and thymic hyperplasia.

Investigation

Clinical diagnostic indicators

These patients suffer from:

- abnormal fatigability on repetitive exercise
- ptosis
- dysphagia and dysarthria (bulbar symptoms)
- shortness of breath on exertion (respiratory involvement)

Imaging

On a **CT scan** a thymoma will be present as a mediastinal mass in 12 per cent of cases (see Fig 14.9). Thymic hyperplasia may be visible in up to 70 per cent of cases.

Function tests

There are characteristic changes on electromyography (EMG).

Diagnostic test

When using the 'Tenilon test', symptoms, remit with the injection of anticholinesterases.

Management

Medical management

Myasthenia gravis is usually managed with a combination of anticholinesterases and steroids.

Thymectomy

The indications for surgery are:

- the presence of a thymoma
- generalized symptoms
- failure of medical treatment in patients with ocular symptoms only.

Almost all patients, therefore, are potential candidates for thymectomy.

Surgery involves a **total thymectomy**. It was originally believed that the procedure should be as radical as possible and involve excision of all thymic tissue, mediastinal fat and the pericardium from one phrenic nerve to the other. This could only really be achieved via a median sternotomy. However, many surgeons now believe that excision of the thymus gland alone gives adequate control of the symptoms and consequently adopt less invasive procedures. These include VATS techniques (usually through the right chest) and transcervical approaches.

During the preoperative preparation of the patient, the dose of steroids should be reduced to the lowest the patient can tolerate in order to reduce postoperative infection.

Postoperatively, the most feared complication is a **myasthenic crisis** and **respiratory arrest**. For this reason, many patients are recovered on an intensive care unit.

Results

Results are good for patients without thymomas and 60–95 per cent will achieve either complete remission or an improvement in their symptoms. Symptom control is less successful in patients with a thymoma.

A minority will experience worsening of their symptoms.

GERM CELL TUMOURS

Extragonadal germ cell tumours are most commonly found in the anterior mediastinum and usually present in young men (median age 24 years). Thymomas tend to occur in middle-aged people.

The three main tumour types are listed below.

- **Teratoma** A benign tumour composed of tissue foreign to the anatomical site in which it arises. Tumour markers are normal.
- **Seminoma** A malignant germ cell tumour.
- **Non-seminomatous tumours** This describes a group of malignant tumours that include yolk sac tumours and choriocarcinomas. They grow more quickly than seminomas and metastasize early. There is an association with Klinefelter's syndrome.

Investigation

Clinical diagnostic indicators

The symptoms of these tumours can be divided into their

- mass effects, e.g. chest pain and dyspnoea
- constitutional effects, e.g. tiredness and weight loss

hormonal effects, e.g. gynaecomastia if the β-human chorionic gonadotrophin (β-HCG) levels are high.

Blood tests

The **lactic dehydrogenase** is elevated in seminoma and non-seminomatous malignant tumours.

β-**HCG** is elevated in non-seminomatous malignant tumours and some seminomas. α-fetoprotein (AFP) is only elevated in non-seminomatous malignant tumours.

Imaging

A **CT scan** will show an anterior mediastinal mass. Such a finding in association with high levels of tumour markers and LDH is virtually diagnostic of a non-seminomatous malignant tumour.

Tissue biopsy

CT-guided biopsy or aspiration.

Management

Seminoma and non-seminomatous malignant tumours are not primarily managed with surgery whereas teratomas should undergo complete surgical resection.

Chemotherapy

Seminomas are usually treated with a combination of **chemotherapy** and **radiotherapy**. The prognosis is good.

Non-seminomatous malignant tumours are also chemosensitive. The 5-year survival is less impressive (50 per cent).

Surgery

Teratomas should be completely excised. This can be achieved via a median sternotomy or thoracotomy. VATS has been used for smaller tumours. Long-term survival approaches 100 per cent if the resection margins are clear.

Following non-surgical treatment for seminomas and non-seminomatous malignant tumours, any residual tumour should be excised provided the tumour markers have returned to normal. The presence of raised markers indicates residual malignant disease and further chemotherapy should be considered.

MEDIASTINAL CYSTS

Mediastinal cysts may be congenital or acquired. They can occur in any mediastinal compartment depending on the structure or organ of origin (Table 14.15). Bronchogenic cysts are the most common.

Investigation

Clinical diagnostic indicators

The usual symptoms of chest pain, dyspnoea, cough and dysphagia are not diagnostic.

Sixty-six per cent of patients with the common bronchogenic mediastinal cyst have symptoms.

Imaging

Chest X-ray and **CT scan** are often diagnostic (Fig 14.10).

Needle aspiration

Water-like fluid is often aspirated, hence the alternative name for pericardial cysts – 'spring water cysts'.

Management

Conservative management

Congenital mediastinal cysts are benign and simple observation is often all that is required.

Surgical treatment

Oesophageal cysts should be **excised**. Excision is indicated if symptoms develop (usually caused by

Table 14.15
The causes of mediastinal cysts

Congenital
Foregut (bronchogenic, oesophageal)
Mesothelial (pericardial, pleural)
Lymphatic (lymphangiomatous, thoracic duct)
Acquired
Inflammatory
Infective
Thymic
Thyroid
Teratoma

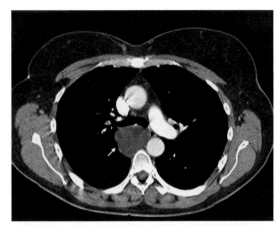

FIGURE 14.10 The CT scan of a patient with chest pain demonstrates a bronchogenic cyst arising from the carina (arrow)

the mass effect), if the cyst enlarges on serial scans, or to establish a tissue diagnosis. The aim is to completely excise the cyst. The surgical approach is dictated by the location of the cyst and may involve thoracotomy, median sternotomy or a VATS procedure.

NEUROGENIC TUMOURS

Within this group is a mixture of benign and malignant tumours. They are the most common cause of a mass in the paravertebral region.

Schwannoma This is usually a well-encapsulated benign tumour of nerve sheath origin, e.g. the intercostal nerve. Malignant schwannomas make up just 1–2 per cent of cases.

Neurofibroma This is also a benign tumour of nerve sheath origin. The tumour capsule tends to be less distinct. There is an association with von Recklinghausen's disease.

Neuroblastoma This is a malignant tumour arising from sympathetic ganglia. It usually occurs in infants and young children.

Phaeochromocytoma This rare tumour is a paraganglioma or functionally active tumour of the sympathetic nervous system, secreting catecholamines. Around 20 per cent of thoracic phaeochromocytomas are malignant.

Occasionally, a paravertebral neurogenic tumour grows through the intervertebral foramen and into the spinal canal – a 'dumb-bell' tumour.

Investigation

Clinical diagnostic indicators

Many neurogenic tumours are symptomless. Some patients have symptoms related to nerve compression (e.g. intercostal nerve pain, Horner's syndrome, hoarseness) and/or spinal cord compression (in 'dumb-bell' tumours).

Phaeochromocytoma may present with hypertension (paroxysmal or persistent).

Urine analysis

A 24-hour urine collection is needed to detect the metabolites of the catecholamines produced by a phaeochromocytoma, i.e. meta-nephrines and vanillylmandelic acid.

Imaging

Chest X-ray shows a mass (Fig 14.11A).

CT scan of the thorax gives anatomic detail (Fig 14.11B).

The majority of paravertebral masses are neurogenic tumours.

MRI is useful in delineating any intraspinal extension of a tumour.

A **CT of the abdomen** is needed for staging of malignant tumours.

Tissue biopsy

CT-guided biopsy is usually diagnostic.

Management

All suspected neurogenic tumours should be surgically removed if the anaesthetic risks are acceptable.

Conservative treatment

If a phaeochromocytoma is deemed inoperable, then lifelong treatment with both alpha- and beta-blockade is essential.

Surgical excision

Most lesions can be removed via a **posterolateral thoracotomy** (or a VATS approach if the tumour is small enough). Schwannomas can be **enucleated**

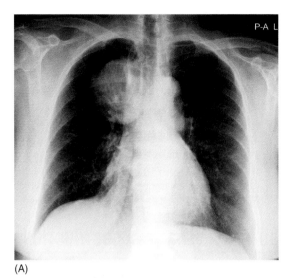

(A)

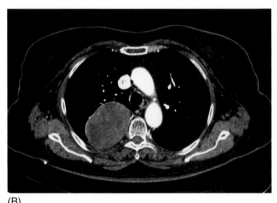

(B)

FIGURE 14.11   (A) The chest X-ray of a patient with chest pain shows a large mass in the right upper zone. Visualization of the more anterior mediastinal structures suggests a posterior mediastinal mass. (B) A CT scan of the chest confirms a mass in the right paravertebral region. Subsequent excision revealed a benign neurogenic tumour

but neurofibromas and malignant tumours require a more **extensive dissection** and **resection of the associated nerve**.

The excision of 'dumb-bell' tumours requires a neurosurgical approach (a **laminectomy**) prior to mobilization and the removal of its intrathoracic portion to reduce the complications of spinal cord injury (possibly Brown–Séquard syndrome) and intraspinal haemorrhage.

The peri-operative **medical management** of phaeochromocytoma is of utmost importance in preventing extremes of hypertension and hypotension. **Both alpha- and beta-blockade is required** together with an expert anaesthetic technique and blood volume control.

Results

The long-term results for the surgical management of benign tumours are excellent. There is a small risk of recurrence, particularly in von Recklinghausen's disease. Five-year survival following malignant schwannoma resection is less good –50 per cent.

DYSPHAGIA (see also Chapter 18)

Symptomatic masses in the mediastinum (excluding intrinsic oesophageal lesions) can cause dysphagia by extrinsic compression of the oesophagus (see Table 14.5). In addition, the muscle weakness associated with myasthenia gravis can extend to the bulbar muscles and result in swallowing difficulties (see later). Malignant tumours of the mediastinum may directly invade the oesophagus and occasionally cause a fistula (e.g. tracheo-oesophageal fistula).

Investigation

Imaging

Chest X-ray, **CT scan** of the thorax and **contrast swallow** are indicated.

Endoscopy

Oesophagoscopy is also usually diagnostic.

SHORTNESS OF BREATH

A mediastinal mass may cause dyspnoea on exertion or at rest by compressing the major airways. Stridor may also be evident in severe airway obstruction. Primary tracheobronchial masses (e.g. lung cancer) and invasive mediastinal malignancies can also compromise the airway by obstructing its lumen.

A mediastinal mass compressing the trachea (e.g. a retrosternal goitre) may cause tracheomalacia (disruption of the normal supporting cartilaginous structure of the trachea). Once the mass is removed the trachea may collapse during expiration and the patient experience acute dyspnoea.

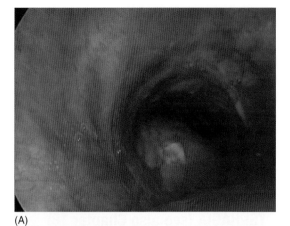

(A)

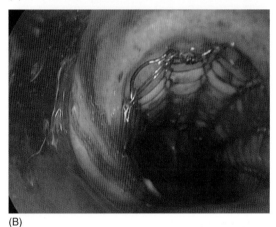

(B)

FIGURE 14.12   (A) Rigid bronchoscopy under general anaesthetic in a patient with stridor and shortness of breath reveals an obstructing tumour of the distal trachea. (B) Debulking of the tumour and insertion of a self-expanding metallic stent has restored the patency of the airway with immediate symptomatic relief. The carina is just visible distally

Investigation

Imaging

Chest X-ray and **CT scan** of the thorax should be obtained in patients with dyspnoea (Fig 14.12A).

Endoscopy

Bronchoscopy may be helpful in diagnosing tracheobradial disorder.

Function studies

Spirometry and flow-volume loops. Lung flow-volume loops may show characteristic flattening of the expiratory curve as the intra-thoracic airway collapses.

Management

Treatment of the mass (with surgery, chemotherapy or radiotherapy, depending on the histological diagnosis) often dramatically relieves the symptoms.

Endobronchial treatment is sometimes more appropriate for **palliation**.

Rigid bronchoscopy allows visualization of the airways and permits endobronchial therapies such as **tumour debulking** (Fig 14.12B).

SUPERIOR VENA CAVA OBSTRUCTION

The superior vena cava (SVC) is a short wide-bore vein between the junction of the left and right brachiocephalic veins and the right atrium. It carries blood from the arms, head, neck and upper thorax. It is a thin-walled, low-pressure conduit and susceptible to external compression. Causes of compression are lung cancer in the right upper lobe (usually of the small cell variety), right hilar tumours and metastatic mediastinal lymphadenopathy.

Other causes are listed in Table 14.7.

Investigation

Clinical diagnostic indicators

The clinical features of SVC compression and obstruction are dyspnoea, swelling of the arms and face and distension of the veins of the head, neck, arms and anterior chest wall.

Imaging

Chest X-ray and **CT scan** of the thorax demonstrate any predisposing conditions (Fig 14.13). **Phlebography** shows the occlusion.

Tissue biopsy

SVC obstruction is not a contraindication to CT-guided biopsy, bronchoscopy and mediastinoscopy. Previously it was considered a contraindication to major invasive tests.

Management

The symptoms of patients with lymphomas or germ cell tumours with a good prognosis improve with

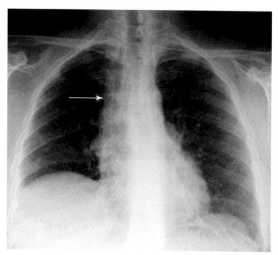

FIGURE 14.13   The chest X-ray of a patient with superior vena cava (SVC) obstruction following radiological intervention shows an SVC stent *in situ*. Also evident is the underlying cause (a right hilar lung cancer) and a raised right hemidiaphragm secondary to invasion of the phrenic nerve

the appropriate treatment of the primary cause. Other patients require palliation. A tissue diagnosis is, therefore, vital in most cases.

Radiotherapy to the affected site can often produce relief of symptoms in patients with advanced malignant disease.

Chemotherapy may produce dramatic results in diseases such as small cell lung cancer, lymphoma and germ cell tumours.

The above treatment modalities are sometimes complemented by **intravenous stents** to produce a rapid relief of symptoms. Stents can also be employed for treating benign SVC obstruction (Fig 14.13).

Surgical management is usually limited to obtaining tissue for diagnosis.

Occasionally, a surgical **venous bypass** procedure may be helpful in benign disease.

En bloc **resection** of an invaded SVC during right upper lobectomy for lung cancer has a 5-year survival of around 20–30 per cent.

CHEST WALL DEFORMITIES

The causes of chest wall deformities are listed in Table 14.16.

Table 14.16
The causes of chest wall deformity

Congenital

Pectus excavatum

Pectus carinatum

Acquired

Trauma (e.g. rib fractures, sternal fracture)

Iatrogenic (e.g. thoracoplasty)

Large chest wall tumour

PECTUS EXCAVATUM AND PECTUS CARINATUM

The aetiology of pectus excavatum (depressed sternum or 'funnel chest') and pectus carinatum (protruding sternum or 'pigeon chest') is not known but both are thought to be caused by abnormal growth patterns of the costal cartilages. They usually occur in isolation but may be associated with Marfan's syndrome and scoliosis.

They may not become apparent until the adolescent growth spurts begin.

Management

Neither needs to be treated. The usual indication for surgical treatment is cosmesis.

Surgical correction

In the **Ravitch procedure** the sternum and costal cartilages are approached through either a midline or submammary incision and the costal cartilages excised. The sternum is then manipulated into a cosmetically acceptable position (which may require a wedge osteotomy) and supported using a metal bar.

Complications are infrequent but include bar migration. There is a low incidence of recurrence.

The **Nuss procedure** can be performed for pectus excavatum using a minimally invasive VATS. A large metal bar is shaped to the chest and then passed from one hemithorax to the other via the anterior mediastinum. The bar is then rotated and fixed to the chest wall laterally to push the sternum forward. This technique was first developed for children but can be used for less malleable adult chest walls. Complications are rare but include bar migration and mediastinal injury.

CAUSES AND INVESTIGATION OF HEART DISEASE

The investigation and management of cardiac disease may at first glance appear to be heavily dependent on sophisticated technology and complex techniques. Although this is to some extent true, there is no substitute for a carefully taken history and an accurate clinical examination. A detailed description of the specific symptoms and signs of cardiac disease are not within the remit of this chapter, but it is vitally important to retain a sense of perspective when interpreting investigations and to put the results of sophisticated tests into the context of the patients' symptoms and lifestyle. The temptation to treat the investigation rather than the patient should be resisted.

The common problems associated with cardiac disease are:

- chest pain
- breathlessness
- blackouts/collapse
- palpitations
- ankle swelling and abdominal distension
- fatigue
- few or no symptoms.

The initial investigation of these problems is described below.

CHRONIC CHEST PAIN: STABLE ANGINA

The causes of chronic stable chest pain, angina, are listed in Table 14.17.

Investigation

Clinical diagnostic indicators

Although there are many potential causes of chest pain, enumerated in Table 14.1, a careful history and examination will rarely leave little doubt that the patient is suffering from angina pectoris – a dull constricting substernal pain that often radiates to the arms and neck associated with exercise.

Table 14.17
Non-cardiac causes of chronic stable chest pain

Chest wall pain, e.g. Tietze syndrome

Pulmonary disease

Pleural disease

Disease of the cervical and thoracic spine

Gastrointestinal pathology (oesophageal pain)

Table 14.18
The investigation of chronic chest pain

Resting ECG

Chest radiograph

Exercise stress ECG

Coronary arteriography

Echocardiography

Stress echocardiography and radionuclide scan

Investigations are required to confirm the diagnosis, defining the anatomical and functional extent of the condition and to ensure appropriate treatment is offered (Table 14.18).

Electrocardiograph

The **resting ECG** is often normal but may show signs of pre-existing myocardial infarction.

A more relevant investigation for exertional angina is the **treadmill stress ECG**, using a recognized exercise protocol such as the modified Bruce protocol. The development of ST segment changes and the time taken for them to appear not only establishes the diagnosis of exercise-induced myocardial ischaemia but also informs decisions about further investigation and management.

Imaging

A **chest X-ray** is often normal.

Coronary angiography is used to define coronary anatomy and coronary artery disease as well as left ventricular function. Although this is an invasive procedure, usually performed retrogradely via the femoral artery, it has a very low risk and is the crucial

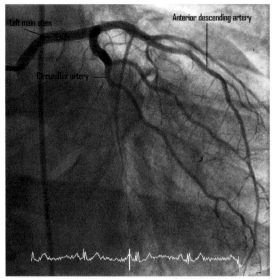

(A)

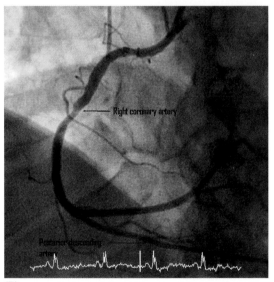

(B)

FIGURE 14.14 Selective coronary angiography showing (A) normal left and (B) normal right coronary arteries

investigation in ischaemic heart disease (Fig 14.14). It is not that unusual for coronary angiography to be the first and only investigation of patients with angina.

Stress echocardiography and **radionuclide scanning** may be required if the diagnosis is still uncertain or more information is required concerning myocardial function or reserve. These tests can also be used to differentiate between reversible and irreversible myocardial ischaemia, which may

Table 14.19
Causes of acute chest pain and the differential diagnosis of myocardial infarction

Aortic dissection

Acute pericarditis

Acute pulmonary embolism

Chest wall pain

Gastrointestinal disorders

Table 14.20
Investigation of acute chest pain

Resting ECG

Chest radiograph

Cardiac enzymes (troponin I or T)

Coronary angiography

Echocardiography

CT scan

D-dimers

be important if surgical revascularization is being considered.

Echocardiography is indicated if the patient has signs of valvular heart disease. For example, aortic valve stenosis may produce typical angina symptoms in the presence of normal coronary arteries because of the combination of left ventricular hypertrophy and reduced coronary perfusion.

ACUTE CHEST PAIN

Some of the causes of acute chest pain are listed in Table 14.19.

Investigation
Clinical diagnostic indicators

The diagnosis of acute chest pain depends on a combination of clinical acumen and the targeted investigations listed in Table 14.20.

Although the clinical pattern of acute myocardial infarction is well recognized, there is a need to establish the diagnosis definitively and rapidly.

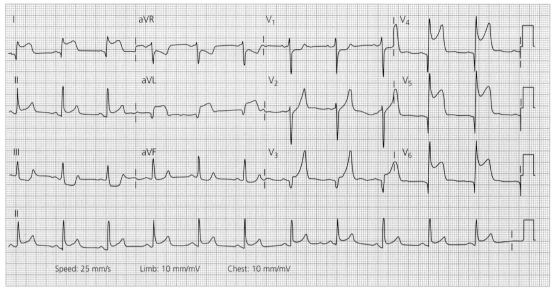

FIGURE 14.15   ECG during ST segment elevation myocardial infarction (STEMI)

Early diagnosis and treatment of myocardial infarction has a significant impact on survival, and misdiagnosis in the presence of another condition such as aortic dissection can be disastrous.

ECG and blood tests

The **ECG** and **biochemical markers of myocardial damage**, such as **troponin**, are the cornerstones of diagnosis.

Recent changes in the terminology of acute coronary syndromes reflect the importance of these two investigations. An elevated troponin confirms the presence of myocardial infarction; the ECG is used to distinguish between ST elevation and less severe non-ST elevation infarcts (Fig 14.15).

The diagnosis of pulmonary embolism may be helped by determination of **D-dimers** (see Chapter 10).

Imaging

It is now usual for patients with troponin-positive infarction to undergo **urgent (same admission) coronary angiography**, for diagnosis, and, if indicated, coronary angioplasty. Many patients are now receiving angiography soon after admission with a view to acute angioplasty in efforts to salvage ischaemic myocardium.

Echocardiography and radionuclide scans are not routinely performed in acute myocardial infarction but may be indicated if the diagnosis is not certain.

The so-called 'triple rule out' emergency **CT scans** are not yet commonplace in the UK. A CT scan may reveal the presence of an aortic dissection.

BREATHLESSNESS

Some of the causes of breathlessness are listed in Table 14.21. For a more comprehensive list see Table 14.2.

Investigation

Clinical diagnostic indicators

Breathlessness is an extremely common symptom and it can be difficult to determine whether and to what extent cardiac disease is responsible. An extensive battery of investigations may be needed, not only to arrive at the diagnosis, but also to determine the functional significance of the cardiac disease and the appropriate management (Table 14.22).

Imaging

A **chest X-ray** is the key initial investigation for breathlessness. Signs of pulmonary congestion or

Table 14.21
Some of the causes of breathlessness

Cardiac causes

Impaired cardiac function owing to myocardial ischaemia and infarction

Valvular heart disease

Congenital heart disease

Arrhythmias

Cardiomyopathy

Pericardial disease

Some non-cardiac causes

Airway obstruction

Pulmonary disease, e.g. chronic obstructive pulmonary disease

Pleural disease, interstitial lung disease e.g. pneumothorax, pleural effusion

Obesity

Anaemia

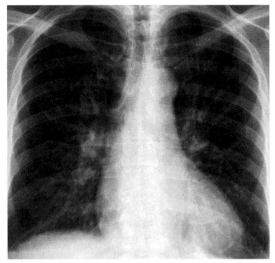

FIGURE 14.16   Chest X-ray showing pulmonary congestion and cardiomegaly in heart failure

Table 14.22
Investigation of breathlessness

Chest radiograph

Transthoracic echocardiography

Transoesophageal echocardiography

Cardiac catheterization including coronary angiography

Stress echocardiography

MRI scan

Investigation of non-cardiac causes of breathlessness

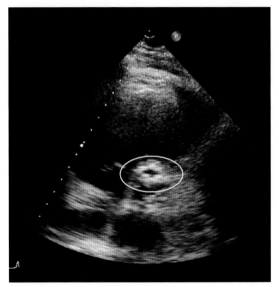

FIGURE 14.17   Two-dimensional transthoracic echo: short axis (end on) view of calcific aortic stenosis, demonstrating echobright calcification of the valve and severely restricted valve opening

oedema, together with the configuration of the cardiac silhouette, are important indicators of cardiac disease (Fig 14.16).

Transthoracic echocardiography is a convenient, non-invasive technique for evaluating valvular, congenital and pericardial disease. As well as providing two-dimensional images of cardiac structure, echocardiography can be used to determine abnormal patterns of blood flow, both qualitatively and quantitatively (Figs 14.17 and 14.18).

Enhanced echo images may be obtained by **transoesophageal echocardiography**. This is particularly useful in mitral valve disease (Figs 14.19 and 14.20).

The excellent detail obtained from echocardiography has reduced the need to use cardiac

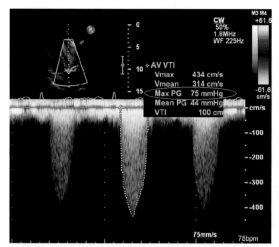

FIGURE 14.18   Pulsed wave Doppler of aortic stenosis demonstrating peak transvalvular gradient of 75 mmHg

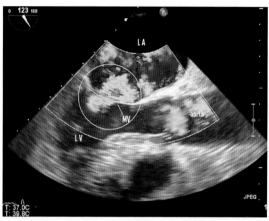

FIGURE 14.20   Colour flow mapping showing the mosaic turbulent jet of mitral regurgitation (LA, left atrium; LV, left ventricle; MV, mitral valve)

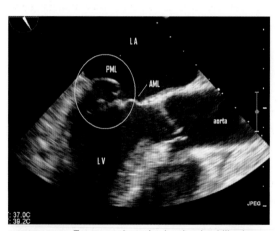

FIGURE 14.19   Transoesophageal echo showing billowing and prolapse of the posterior leaflet of the mitral valve (LA, left atrium; LV, left ventricle; AML, anterior leaflet of the mitral valve; PML, posterior leaflet of the mitral valve)

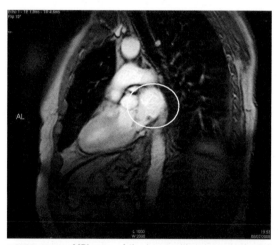

FIGURE 14.21   MRI scan of the heart with tumour in the left atrium (myxoma)

catheterization to reach a diagnosis, but many patients require coronary angiography to determine the presence of concomitant coronary artery disease.

Stress echocardiography (either exercise or dobutamine induced) can clarify the functional significance of valve lesions.

MRI scanning provides excellent imaging and functional data (Fig 14.21). Unfortunately, cardiac MRI scanning requires the patient to lie flat, so not all cardiac patients can tolerate it.

Pulmonary function tests

Pulmonary and cardiac disease often coexists and a full assessment of pulmonary function may be required including **CT scanning**, **V/Q scan**, **spirometry** and **transfer factor**.

PALPITATION

Palpitation is awareness of the heart beating and is typically, although far from always, associated with an abnormality of cardiac rhythm. In fact, many people with palpitation have no significant abnormality and investigation is often aimed at confirming the absence of serious pathology.

Electrocardiogram

Although the standard **resting ECG** may often reveal the underlying abnormality, **ambulatory ECG** recording may be needed in paroxysmal arrhythmias, sometimes linked to remote patient-activated recorders.

Electrophysiology (EP) study is an invasive mapping technique used to assess inducibilty and the mechanism of the tachycardia. It is usually reserved for those patients with serious arrhythmias for whom intervention is planned.

Echocardiography may be required to determine whether or not there is a structural cardiac abnormality underlying the arrhythmia.

BLACKOUTS/COLLAPSE

Most blackouts are not related to cardiac disease. Cardiac blackouts may be linked to abnormalities of heart rhythm, cardiac valve pathology or cardiac thromboembolic disease. Simple investigations such as **ECG** and **transthoracic echocardiography** usually identify a cardiac cause, if present.

ANKLE SWELLING AND ABDOMINAL DISTENSION

Signs of fluid retention usually signify **congestive cardiac failure** with right heart decompensation, with or without tricuspid regurgitation. Primary right ventricular failure is not common and investigation is aimed at determining the underlying cause, which is frequently pulmonary hypertension secondary to mitral valve disease or to pulmonary pathology.

FATIGUE

Fatigue and lethargy are very common symptoms, but are also common in heart disease. Clinical evaluation will usually determine whether or not cardiac investigation is required and what form it should take. Cardiac cachexia may be a feature of advanced heart disease.

Table 14.23
Investigation of symptomless cardiac disease

ECG
Echocardiography
Coronary angiography
Exercise and or stress testing

FEW OR NO CARDIAC SYMPTOMS

Some patients with significant heart disease do not present with overt cardiac symptoms. Cardiac abnormalities may be detected during routine medical or preoperative examination.

Patients with diabetes are notorious for 'silent' myocardial ischaemia and infarction. Investigation of these patients (Table 14.23) is a matter of clinical judgement but is of relevance not only in making an accurate diagnosis but also in determining a management strategy. For example, patients with symptomless mitral regurgitation but with enlarged left ventricular dimensions are at high risk of developing irreversible heart failure if surgery is left until symptoms do develop. On the other hand, patients with critical aortic stenosis or silent myocardial ischaemia present increased risk if undergoing major non-cardiac surgery and require modified intra- and postoperative care. By contrast, the majority of heart murmurs detected incidentally turn out to be innocent, but reassurance is often needed.

MANAGEMENT OF HEART DISEASE
USE OF CARDIOPULMONARY BYPASS AND MYOCARDIAL PRESERVATION

Cardiac surgery is distinguished from other forms of surgery by its routine use of extracorporeal circulation or cardiopulmonary bypass (CPB), without which the majority of heart operations could not take place. Although the details and refinements of CPB are sometimes complex, the principles are straightforward (Fig 14.22). *Deoxygenated venous blood is drained from the right atrium into a reservoir and then delivered to an artificial oxygenator. The oxygenated blood is then pumped back into the aorta, and hence into the arterial circulation. The heart and lungs are thus bypassed and the patient's*

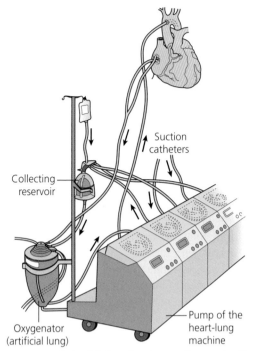

Collecting reservoir

Suction catheters

Oxygenator (artificial lung)

Pump of the heart-lung machine

FIGURE 14.22   A simplified cardiopulmonary bypass circuit

Table 14.24
Medical management of ischaemic heart disease

Symptomatic control

Beta-blockers, e.g. bisoprolol

Long-acting nitrates, e.g. isosorbide

Calcium-channel blockers, e.g. diltaizem

Potassium-channel activators, e.g. nicorandil

Short-acting nitrates, e.g. glyceryl trinitrate spray

Risk adjustment

Platelet inhibition, e.g. aspirin

Cholesterol lowering, e.g. simvistatin

Hypertension management, e.g. ramipril

Lifestyle issues:

   Cessation of smoking

   Weight loss

   Diabetic management

   Regular moderate exercise

oxygenation and circulation supported entirely by the CPB circuit.

Under these circumstances, the heart continues to beat and the coronary arteries remain perfused with blood.

In order to create an environment that allows complex and accurate surgery the heart needs to be quiescent and coronary blood flow stopped. This can be achieved by clamping the aorta proximal to the arterial inflow from the CPB to render the heart globally ischaemic. But the myocardium is exquisitely intolerant of ischaemia and a strategy of myocardial preservation needs to be employed during cardiac ischaemia. The most commonly used technique of myocardial preservation is **hypothermic cardioplegia**. This is a combination of low temperature and potassium-induced diastolic arrest which preserves myocardial energy supplies and ensures recovery of function.

STABLE ISOLATED ISCHAEMIC HEART DISEASE

As with all conditions, the management of ischaemic heart disease (IHD) may be either conservative or interventional.

Conservative/medical management (Table 14.24) is aimed not only at symptomatic relief but also at adjusting risk factors for IHD, and reducing the risks of progressive disease and death. It goes without saying that **lifestyle adjustment** is often indicated.

Interventional techniques are aimed at directly restoring myocardial blood supply either by **percutaneous coronary intervention (PCI)** (also known as **angioplasty**), or by **coronary artery bypass grafting (CABG)** (Fig 14.23).

Coronary artery bypass grafting (CABG) is one of the most commonly performed surgical procedures. A total of 23 000 were performed in the UK in 2005.

Reversed saphenous vein is used to construct bypass grafts between the ascending aorta and stenosed coronary arteries. Although extremely effective in the medium term, long-term patency rates for the saphenous vein have been less good, although it is worth noting that the reported patency rates of 50 per cent at 10 years pre-date the routine postoperative use of aspirin and statins.

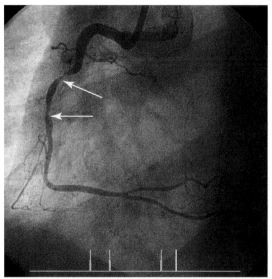

(A)

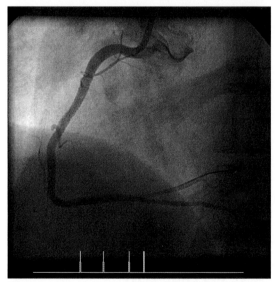

(B)

FIGURE 14.23 Coronary arteriogram showing critical right coronary stenosis (A) before and (B) after deployment of an intracoronary stent

Table 14.25
The evidence base for coronary artery bypass grafting (CABG)

CABG is the most intensively studied surgical procedure with over 30 years of detailed follow up

CABG is highly effective in relieving the symptoms of ischaemic heart disease

CABG improves life expectancy in certain anatomical subsets such as left main stem and triple vessel disease

This benefit is increased in patients with poor left ventricular function

CABG is a safe procedure with a hospital mortality of approximately 1%

CABG is extremely cost effective in the long term.

There has been much debate (some of it heated) about the relative merits of the two interventions in the treatment of stable IHD. CABG has a strong, well-established evidence base (Table 14.25), but the low impact nature of **angioplasty** (PCI), combined with technological advances such as **drug-eluting stents**, has led to PCI becoming increasingly prevalent. PCI is an extremely valuable and effective treatment in appropriately selected patients, but is associated with high reintervention rates, and in the longer term is probably less effective than CABG.

ACUTE MYOCARDIAL INFARCTION

In recent years, an aggressive approach to the management of acute myocardial infarction has developed, initially with the early administration of **thrombolytic drugs** such as streptokinase and now followed by **primary angioplasty** targeting the culprit coronary lesions.

Surgical myocardial revascularization by CABG in the first few days after an infarction was associated with a prohibitively high operative mortality and has largely been abandoned.

COMPLICATIONS OF ISCHAEMIC HEART DISEASE

Aggressive interventional management of myocardial infarction has significantly reduced the

Improved long-term graft patency is achieved using the pedicled *in situ* **left internal mammary artery (LIMA)** as a conduit. There are some reported advantages to complete arterial revascularization (using bilateral mammary and radial arterial grafts), but a combination of a single LIMA and vein grafts remains the conventional choice of many surgeons.

Table 14.26
Complications of myocardial infarction

Acute mitral regurgitation due to rupture of a papillary muscle

Post-infarction ventricular septal defect

Rupture of infarcted left ventricular free wall

Systemic thromboembolism from mural intraventricular thrombus

Pericarditis and post-myocardial infarction (Dressler) syndrome

Left ventricular aneurysm.

Table 14.27
Aetiology of heart valve disease

Congenital abnormality, e.g. bicuspid aortic valve

Collagen degeneration, e.g. 'floppy' mitral valve, Marfan's disease

Senile degeneration, e.g. calcific aortic stenosis

Rheumatic valve disease

'Functional' regurgitation, e.g. tricuspid regurgitation in mitral stenosis

Infection: infective endocarditis

Table 14.28
Medical management of heart valve disease

Fluid retention (pulmonary and peripheral oedema): diuretics, e.g. furosemide

Heart rate and rhythm (e.g. atrial fibrillation): digoxin, amiodarone, beta-blockers

Thromboembolic disease: anticoagulation, e.g. warfarin

Heart failure: angiotensin-converting enzyme inhibitors, e.g. ramipril, and nitrates, e.g. isosorbide

incidence of the acute complications of myocardial infarction, i.e. acute mitral regurgitation, ventricular septal defect and free-wall rupture (Table 14.26).

These complications have traditionally been regarded as 'surgical' and although operative mortality is uniformly high, survival without surgery is unlikely.

Full thickness infarction when it does occur may lead to fibrosis, thinning and localized dilatation of the left ventricle leading to aneurysm formation, with dyskinetic wall motion and thrombus formation. A wide range of surgical techniques have been described to treat this complication.

VALVULAR HEART DISEASE

There is a wide range of causes of heart valve pathology (Table 14.27), but it is the consequences of that pathology that determine the management strategy.

Stenotic valves promote an increase of *pressure* upstream of the obstruction which, transmitted backwards, leads to venous hypertension, oedema and usually compensatory myocardial hypertrophy.

Regurgitant valves typically cause upstream *volume* overload with cardiac chamber dilatation and dysfunction.

The management of heart valve disease is determined not only by the symptoms but by the myocardial consequences of the valve dysfunction.

Many of the patients that present with mild disease can be managed by **medical treatment** at least initially (Table 14.28), but continued surveillance with repeated echocardiography is advisable in all but those with the most benign heart valve disease. It is all too easy to 'miss the boat' surgically. *Late surgery carries a significantly increased risk of operative mortality with limited prognostic benefit.*

When contemplating surgery for heart valve disease it is often a case of '*not if – but when*'.

VALVE REPLACEMENT

Modern prosthetic heart valves (Figs 14.24 and 14.25) offer excellent haemodynamic performance. In this regard there is little to choose between the mechanical and the biological prostheses. The arguments relate to the risks, with mechanical valves, of thromboembolism and the need for lifelong anticoagulation; and the risks, with biological valves, of structural deterioration and further surgery. There are no hard and fast rules but biological valves are generally recommended for elderly patients (>70 years) and for those who cannot or refuse to take warfarin.

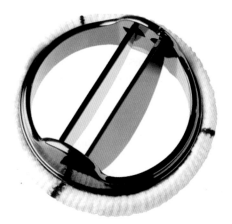

FIGURE 14.24   Mechanical valve prosthesis

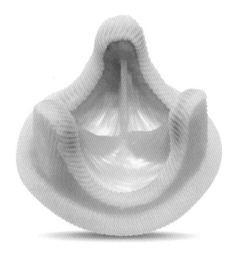

FIGURE 14.25   Biological valve prosthesis

VALVE REPAIR

An often preferable alternative to valve replacement is valve reconstruction or repair. This is particularly applicable to certain types of **degenerative mitral valve disease**, where redundant tissue can be excised and the remaining valve reconstructed to provide a competent valve with good long-term durability, which avoids the need for anticoagulation (Fig 14.26). *In some circumstances the aortic valve may also be repaired.*

Functional valve regurgitation occurs when the valve annulus dilates and otherwise normal leaflets no longer co-apt. It can often be managed by the implantation of a remodelling annuloplasty ring that restores normal annular geometry and dimensions.

INFECTIVE ENDOCARDITIS

The majority of cases of infective endocarditis (IE) occur in situations where **the valve is already abnormal** (Fig 14.27). The classical *Streptococcus viridans* infection following dental treatment is less common than supposed (around 15 per cent). *The National Institute for Clinical Excellence (NICE) no longer recommends antibiotic prophylaxis for high-risk dental patients.* Almost any organism can be acquired through almost any portal of entry. Despite the myriad of eponymous physical signs, the clinical features of infective endocarditis are often non-specific and difficult to interpret. Consequently, the diagnosis is often missed, especially after repeated doses of community-administered antibiotics.

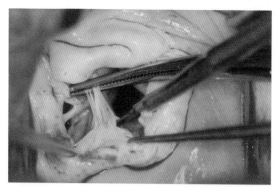

FIGURE 14.26   Intraoperative picture of mitral valve repair – the posterior leaflet chordae are being assessed

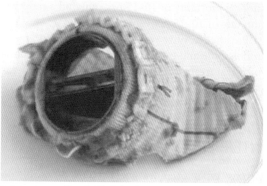

FIGURE 14.27   Prosthetic infective endocarditis affecting a previously implanted aortic valve conduit

Table 14.29
Indications for surgery in infective endocarditis (IE)

Conventional indications

Congestive heart failure which accounts for 90% of all deaths

Structural complications or intracardiac extension (e.g. development of heart block)

Embolic events

Persistent infection or failure to respond to appropriate antimicrobial therapy

More controversial indications

Staphylococcal infection

Large, 'asymptomatic' vegetations

Recent cerebral embolic event

Late-presentation, culture-negative infective endocarditis is not uncommon, is associated with a less favourable outcome and continues to have a high mortality. With appropriate antimicrobial therapy, approximately 75 per cent of cases can be cured provided there is a high level of **surveillance** by a multi-disciplinary team and repeated **echocardiography**.

Surgery is only recommended in certain high-risk circumstances (Table 14.29) and is often difficult. The principles of surgery are to remove *all* infected material and to reconstruct the heart while preserving its function. Avoidance of prosthetic material is a common mantra of any surgery in an infected field, but once complete debridement has taken place, there is usually no alternative but to implant a prosthetic valve. This is followed by a surgical mortality of 10–15 per cent and a reoperation rate of 10–15 per cent.

Prosthetic valve endocarditis is even more troublesome and typically does not respond to anti-microbial treatment. Early surgery is the only therapeutic option but carries a predictably high mortality.

VALVE DISEASE AND PERCUTANEOUS INTERVENTION

Certain types of mitral stenosis are amenable to **percutaneous balloon valvuloplasty**, a process analogous to the long-established but now largely abandoned surgical technique of **closed mitral valvotomy**.

Recent developments have produced **stented aortic valve bioprostheses** that can be introduced retrogradely via the femoral artery. Currently this technique is reserved for patients who would otherwise be denied conventional surgery on the grounds of excessive risk, but judging by past experience it is only a matter of time before it becomes widespread.

Specific valve disease

Table 14.30 summarizes in a simplified manner the salient points of the individual valve lesions.

CARDIAC RHYTHM DISTURBANCES

The majority of cardiac rhythm problems are managed by cardiologists. **Pacemaker implantation** for bradycardia and heart block is long established, and **automatic implantable cardioversion devices** (AICDs) are now commonly used to treat malignant ventricular arrhythmias. In addition, the vast majority of troublesome supraventricular arrhythmias can be successfully treated by **catheter ablation of abnormal pathways**.

Atrial fibrillation is difficult to manage conventionally and is associated with a previously unrecognized high incidence of complications and death. A simple technique of **intraoperative ablation** has been developed based on the principles of the adventurous Cox maze procedure.

Currently restricted as an adjunct to a primary cardiac procedure such as mitral valve replacement, future developments will see stand-alone atrial fibrillation (AF) ablation using thoracoscopic techniques. The mid-term results are encouraging with approximately 75 per cent of patients returned to sinus rhythm following ablation.

DISEASE OF THE INTRATHORACIC AORTA

Acute aortic dissection is frequently fatal if not managed appropriately.

Accurate and early diagnosis by **CT scanning** (Fig 14.28) is essential. Other investigations are

Table 14.30
Valvular heart disease

	Pathogenesis	Clinical features	Investigations	Management
Aortic stenosis	Secondary calcification of congenitally bicuspid valve Senile calcification Rheumatic valve disease (rare)	Angina Syncope Breathlessness Sudden death Harsh systolic murmur Slow rising pulse	LVH on ECG 2D echocardiography Doppler measurement of transvalvar gradient Coronary arteriography	Valve replacement for symptomatic patients Valve replacement if gradient >70 mmHg Percutaneous valve implantation in high-risk patients
Aortic regurgitation	Infective endocarditis In association with aortic root disease, e.g. Marfan's disease, annulo-aortic ectasia Syphillis Rheumatic valve disease	Fatigue Breathlessness Orthopnoea Paroxysmal nocturnal dyspnoea Early diastolic murmur Wide pulse pressure	Repolarization changes on ECG Enlarged cardiac shadow on chest radiograph 2D echocardiography – LV (left ventricular) dilatation, aortic root abnormalities	Often conservative if mild disease Diuretics and angiotensin-converting enzyme (ACE) inhibitors Follow up of asymptomatic patients Surgery if LV dilatation or reduced LV function Aortic valve replacement Aortic root replacement if aortic dilatation present
Mitral stenosis	Rheumatic valve disease	Fatigue and cachexia Breathlessness Orthopnoea Paroxysmal nocturnal dyspnoea Palpitation (atrial fibrillation) Peripheral embolus (thromboembolic disease) Mid-diastolic murmur Opening snap Atrial fibrillation Mitral facies Pulmonary congestion	Atrial fibrillation (AF) on ECG Chest radiograph – small cardiac shadow with prominent left atrium and pulmonary artery Pulmonary congestion 2D echocardiography Doppler transvalvar gradient Transoesophageal echocardiography Pulmonary artery pressure measurement by echo or catheter	Drug therapy to control heart rate, reduce fluid overload and prevent thromboembolism (digoxin, diuretics and warfarin) Percutaneous valvuloplasty if suitable Mitral valve repair or replacement preferably before development of pulmonary hypertension, atrial fibrillation or thromboembolism Ablation surgery for atrial fibrillation

(Continued)

Table 14.30 (Continued)

	Pathogenesis	Clinical features	Investigations	Management
Mitral regurgitation	Myxomatous degeneration (floppy valve prolapse)	Asymptomatic Fatigue Breathlessness Palpitation Pan systolic apical murmur Hyperdynamic apex Atrial fibrillation	Enlarged heart on chest radiograph 2D echocardiography Transoesophageal echocardiography Doppler colour flow mapping for quantitative assessment	Often conservative if mild disease Diuretics and ACE inhibitors Follow up of asymptomatic patients Surgery if LV dilatation or reduced LV function even in asymptomatic patients Mitral valve repair if suitable Mitral valve replacement Ablation surgery for AF
Tricuspid regurgitation	'Functional' regurgitation secondary to right ventricular dilatation in mitral valve disease or cor pulmonale Infective endocarditis in intravenous drug abusers	Fluid retention and peripheral oedema Abdominal pain (hepatic congestion) Cachexia Systolic murmur Elevated JVP Atrial fibrillation	AF on ECG Enlarged right atrial shadow on chest radiograph 2D echocardiography Doppler echo assessment of severity	Mild cases treated with diuretics Management of underlying left heart problem Tricuspid valve annuloplasty if severe and in combination with mitral surgery Endocarditis treated by repair or valve excision

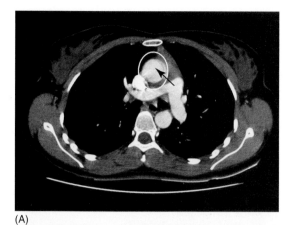

(A)

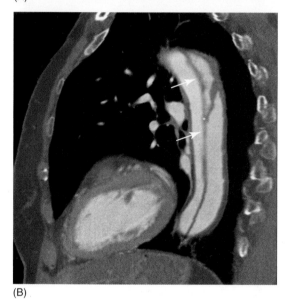

(B)

FIGURE 14.28   (A) CT scan of type A dissection of the aorta of the ascending aorta. (B) Sagittal CT reconstruction of complex type B dissection of the descending aorta

either less reliable or too difficult and/or time-consuming to perform in seriously ill patients. Management is based on whether or not the ascending aorta is involved. The Stanford classification simply divides aortic dissection into two categories:

▪ type A involves the ascending aorta
▪ type B does not involve the ascending aorta.

Type A dissection is managed as a surgical emergency. There is a 25 per cent mortality rate for

each of the 24 hours that pass with the condition left untreated.

The surgical strategy is often complex and involves replacing any or all of the aortic root with or without coronary artery implantation, aortic valve replacement, arch replacement and 'elephant trunk' implantation with staged stent graft deployment to the descending aorta. Not surprisingly, the operative mortality is high, but far less than the mortality that follows medical management.

Type B dissections do better with initial medical management, although some will go on to need a staged **aortic stent graft** (see Chapter 11).

Emergency medical management is based on pharmacological **control of the blood pressure** and **reduction of aortic wall tension** with **beta-blockers and vasodilators**.

PENETRATING WOUNDS OF THE HEART

Death rates following penetrating wounds to the heart vary. They can be as high as 85 per cent, with many victims dying at the scene of the incident, but are much lower in situations where the victim is in a stable condition and the correct treatment can be given.

Most penetrating trauma to the heart has to be dealt with by non-cardiothoracic surgeons at the time of their presentation by the application of relatively straightforward surgical techniques.

Haemodynamically normal patients who have stab wounds with the anatomical potential to injure the heart need careful evaluation. Investigation by **CT scan** or **echocardiography** may be performed, but should not delay surgical intervention if it becomes necessary.

Controversy surrounds the role of the Emergency Department thoracotomy in an *apparently* dead patient. The difficulty during triage is to decide whether the patient is actually dead on arrival or potentially treatable. A commonly adopted strategy is to assume that a patient who has no signs of life during 5 minutes of observation (in the absence of endotracheal intubation) or 10 minutes (if intubated) is not likely to respond to resuscitative thoracotomy and not attempt it (see Chapter 6).

Table 14.31
Risk stratification and analysis of surgical outcomes

The *Euroscore* is a simple, additive and accurate risk stratification model, providing patients and relatives with a reasonable estimate of the operative risk

Variable life-adjusted display (VLAD) plots can be used to track unit or individual surgeon outcomes over time, and are useful performance indicators

Monitoring of performance, as part of an integrated package of quality improvement, leads to improved surgical outcomes

Individual surgeon profiles and outcomes are publicly available, enhancing the patient's ability to make informed treatment decisions

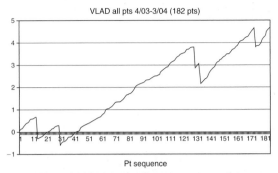

FIGURE 14.29   VLAD plot using Euroscore as a predictor of risk for a series of 182 consecutive operations by one surgeon in a single year

BLUNT TRAUMA OF THE HEART

Cardiac blunt trauma is usually related to high-speed traffic accidents. It is now less common since the compulsory introduction of seatbelts and airbags. Cardiac contusion leads to impaired function and heart failure.

Management is supportive with cardioactive drugs and, if necessary, mechanical circulatory support in the hope that cardiac function will eventually recover.

MEASURING SURGICAL OUTCOMES

Crude mortality data does not paint the whole picture and adjustments need to be made for case mix. The relevant factors that need to be taken into consideration include the type of operation, age, urgency, left ventricular function, gender and a wide range of co-morbidities. Risk stratification systems such as the *Euroscore* have been developed to account for the relevant risk factors and provide a numeric score that can be used to predict the risk of death (Table 14.31). The variable life-adjusted display (VLAD) is a plot of actual outcome against predicted outcome, and is a useful indicator of surgical performance (Fig 14.29).

15 The breast

John Black

More than a quarter of the patients referred to a general surgical outpatient department are females with breast symptoms. Only a small proportion of these have cancer. Less than 10 per cent of general surgical operations are for breast disease.

Breast cancer properly treated has by far the best prognosis of the common solid organ malignancies. With constantly improving assessment and treatment, up to 80 per cent of sufferers are alive and well 10 years after diagnosis.

In many cases, a careful history and painstaking examination will reveal the diagnosis. On other occasions, the history and physical signs may be misleading, and this has led to the universal introduction of **triple assessment** (Table 15.1) (Revision panel 5 in the appendices).

The **clinical problems** produced by diseases of the breast are:

- a painless lump
- a painful lump
- pain and tenderness without a lump
- nipple discharge
- changes in the nipple or areola
- changes in breast size and shape.

DISCRETE BREAST LUMPS

Investigation

Every discrete breast lump should be investigated in three ways, by history and examination, diagnostic imaging and histology (Table 15.2).

Clinical diagnostic indicators

The history and clinical signs that indicate the diagnosis underlying the problems listed above are described in full in *Symptoms and Signs*. In many cases the diagnosis will be obvious by the end of the examination but it is, nevertheless, **always essential to perform a full triple assessment**.

Table 15.1
Triple assessment in breast disease

1. History and examination
2. Diagnostic imaging by mammography or ultrasound scanning
3. Histology or cytology

Table 15.2
Causes of a breast lump

Painless lump
Carcinoma
Cyst
Fibroadenoma
An area of fibroadenosis
Painful lump
An area of fibroadenosis
Cyst
Periductal mastitis
Abscess (usually postpartum or lactational)
Sometimes a carcinoma

Imaging

Mammography is a well-established low-dose X-ray technique (Fig 15.1). The breast is compressed between Perspex plates in two planes and the images are usually stored digitally. The standard planes are the mediolateral oblique (MLO) and craniocaudal (CC) views. The oblique view includes the axillary tail, a common site for cancer. Interpretation of the images is sometimes straightforward but often subtle and requires the

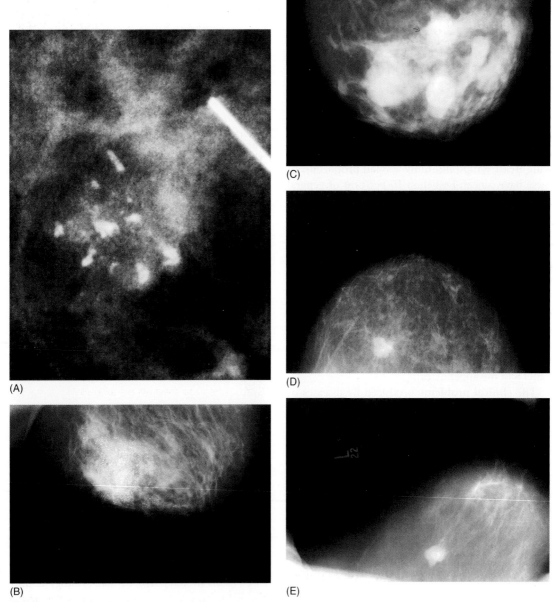

FIGURE 15.1 (A) Multiple areas of calcification, with a marker. (B) Typical ductal carcinoma in situ (DCIS) with associated mass. (C) Multiple breast cysts. (D and E) A typical carcinoma viewed in two planes

opinion of *a skilled radiologist*. Students should not become downhearted by finding it difficult to interpret mammographs.

The X-ray abnormalities fall into four main categories:

- asymmetric density
- a mass, of which the clarity of its margins provides important diagnostic information

- architectural distortion
- calcifications: clusters of fine calcification are especially suspicious of cancer.

Fibroadenomata and cysts appear as well-circumscribed masses with smooth borders.

Mammography fails to detect at least 10 per cent of breast cancers, including some that are palpable, particularly the lobular type.

Mammography is less reliable in younger women with dense breast tissue, is unsuitable for the very large breast where peripheral lesions may be outside the field, and is impracticable in women who cannot tolerate the compression required.

Mammography is widely used in screening for breast cancer (see page 351).

Ultrasound scanning has the advantages of not employing ionizing radiation and, unlike mammography, being free from discomfort. Modern machines are mobile and can be used in the outpatient department. However, the technique is operator-dependent and requires experience to achieve a high diagnostic accuracy.

If an abnormality is seen, it is possible to proceed immediately to an image-guided core biopsy.

Ultrasound scanning is particularly helpful in detecting breast cysts (Fig 15.2).

Magnetic resonance imaging (MRI) has a developing role in the diagnosis of breast pathology. It is particularly good at delineating lobular carcinoma, which is easily missed by mammography and cytology. It may also have a role in the assessment of ductal carcinoma *in situ* (DCIS).

Tissue biopsy

Before considering the treatment of a palpable lump the clinician must have a definitive 'tissue diagnosis' **by core biopsy**. Various needles are available which enable the surgeon to obtain a **core of tissue** from a lump using local anaesthesia, in the outpatient department, for immediate dispatch to the laboratory for **histological** analysis (see Fig 1.2).

Overall diagnostic accuracy, even when the swelling is readily palpable, is significantly improved by the use of image guidance, commonly with ultrasound scanning.

Results are classified as follows. Students need not memorize these but will pick them up quickly if they attend multidisciplinary team meetings.

- B1: normal breast or inadequate sample
- B2: benign tissue
- B3: abnormality with uncertain malignant potential
- B4: suspicious of cancer
- B5a: *in situ* malignancy
- B5b: invasive cancer
- B5c: malignant but uncertain whether 5a or 5b.

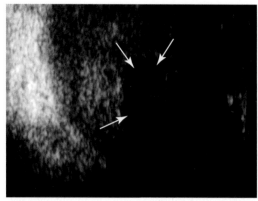

FIGURE 15.2   An ultrasound of a breast cyst

Fine needle aspiration is an alternative technique to core biopsy which provides a **cytological** diagnosis (see Fig 1.1). It does not require local anaesthesia. The material aspirated from the swelling, through a fine-bore needle, is smeared on to a slide and fixed immediately. Interpretation of the nature of the aspirated cells must be made by an experienced pathologist.

Specimens are classified as follows:

- C1: insufficient cells for diagnosis
- C2: benign cells
- C3: atypical cells probably benign
- C4: atypical cells probably malignant
- C5: malignant cells.

It should be noted that a C5 result does not necessarily indicate invasive cancer, as malignant cells can be aspirated from a DCIS.

A C1 report means that the procedure has failed and must be repeated or a core biopsy obtained. It must also be remembered that cytology is only reliable if the tip of the needle enters the actual pathological abnormality being investigated. *It is easy to miss the target!*

In all cases where fine needle aspiration reveals atypical cells a histological (tissue) diagnosis must be obtained.

The lobular carcinoma, mentioned above because of its diagnostic elusiveness with mammography, is also notorious for producing false-negative cytology. This is because this tumour consists mostly of fibrous stroma with relatively few malignant cells, which, consequently, are not readily aspirated.

Image-guided biopsy. When an impalpable abnormality has been detected by diagnostic imaging, either when investigating symptoms or for screening purposes, the biopsy device must be guided to the abnormality by **ultrasound scanning**, **X-rays** or **MRI scanning**.

Once the radiologist locates the abnormality, a core biopsy needle is inserted into it to obtain a specimen for histology, or a fine aspiration needle inserted to obtain cells for cytology.

Open surgical biopsy is nowadays a rare event except in countries without scanning facilities. It is possible, using modern methods, to obtain a definite diagnosis of a breast swelling in nearly every case without admission to hospital.

PAIN AND TENDERNESS WITHOUT A LUMP

Investigation

Clinical diagnostic indicators

The patterns of breast pain and tenderness are described in *Symptoms and Signs*, where it is stressed that **cyclical breast pain**, which has various clinical features and is exceedingly common, is almost never a symptom of cancer (Table 15.3). Consequently, if there is no palpable lump the full routine triple assessment is not always required.

Very occasionally, particularly when the pain is described as '**prickling**', there may be an underlying carcinoma, so it is always important to carry out a careful clinical examination of the breasts in all patients with breast pain. If a swelling is found it must be investigated in the usual manner.

Imaging

Patient's concerns may dictate that it is appropriate to arrange some form of imaging, even when there is no palpable lump, because this may be the only way the patient will accept reassurance and discharge

Table 15.3
Causes of pain and tenderness without a lump

Cyclical breast pain

Non-cyclical breast pain

A carcinoma (uncommon)

from the clinic. In these circumstances, most clinicians choose to employ ultrasound scanning rather than mammography to avoid unnecessary use of X-rays.

NIPPLE DISCHARGE

Investigation

Clinical diagnostic indicators

Nipple discharge (Table 15.4) is a common symptom and usually has a benign cause – most often duct ectasia. Remember that the breast is designed to produce fluid!

If the discharge contains blood it is more likely to be caused by significant disease such as **carcinoma, DCIS or a duct papilloma**.

Some benign conditions may be associated with production of an apparently blood-stained dusky fluid. **Testing the discharge for the presence of blood** in the outpatient department with the same reagent strips used to test urine will resolve the uncertainty.

Imaging

Imaging may be carried out by **ultrasound scanning** or **mammography.** The former is preferable in younger women.

Occasionally a patient presents with a blood-stained discharge from a single duct orifice, without a palpable swelling and with normal imaging. This may be caused by an **intraduct papilloma** or a **carcinoma**. It is possible to insert a narrow cannula into the discharging duct, inject contrast material

Table 15.4
Causes of nipple conditions

Discharge

Duct ectasia

Intraduct papilloma

Ductal carcinoma *in situ*

Associated with a cyst

Changes in the nipple or areola

Duct ectasia

Carcinoma

Paget's disease

Eczema

and obtain an X-ray termed a **ductogram**. This may demonstrate a papilloma.

Another new technique is the insertion of a miniature **fibreoptic endoscope** (less than 1 mm in diameter) into the discharging duct to visualize any pathology and obtain samples for cytology or histology.

Cytology of discharging fluid

Patients presenting with nipple discharge without an obvious benign cause or lump should be submitted to a modified triple assessment. **Cytology of the fluid** from the nipple should replace the core biopsy or aspiration cytology.

In **duct ectasia**, the discharge contains **macrophages** and **chronic inflammatory debris. Red blood cells are suspicious of a carcinoma**, and the finding of **malignant cells indicates ductal carcinoma**, either *in situ* or invasive.

CHANGES IN THE NIPPLE OR AREOLA

Investigation
Clinical diagnostic indicators

Nipple inversion in post-menopausal women is a symptom that is quite likely to be caused by **cancer**. In younger women the commonest cause is **duct ectasia**.

With duct ectasia the clinical appearance of the **transverse slit-like nipple**, frequently **bilateral**, is highly characteristic.

Imaging

Imaging is mandatory for all patients with **nipple inversion**, even if there is strong clinical evidence of duct ectasia. **Mammography** is the preferred method in the post-menopausal woman as it detects the calcification found with intraduct or invasive cancer.

Tissue biopsy

A **core biopsy** or **fine needle aspiration** should be used to ascertain the nature of any abnormality detected by the imaging.

PAGET'S DISEASE

Suspected cases of Paget's disease are investigated with another variant of triple assessment, which after **mammography** includes a **punch biopsy of the areolar skin** using a specially designed instrument.

CHANGES IN BREAST SIZE AND SHAPE

In many cases, for example pregnancy, the diagnosis may be made on clinical grounds alone (Table 15.5). In post-menopausal women, imaging with **mammography** is essential.

CARCINOMA OF THE BREAST

Carcinoma of the breast is the commonest cancer in women. Approximately 45 000 new cases are diagnosed each year in the UK, but breast cancer produces fewer cancer deaths each year than the less common lung cancer.

Only 0.7 per cent of breast cancers occur in males, i.e. in the UK approximately 330 each year.

The lifetime risk of a woman developing breast cancer is one in nine.

Almost 80 per cent of women with carcinoma of the breast are alive 5 years after diagnosis.

Investigation

Investigations are required to plan management after diagnosis.

Blood tests

Preoperative investigation will normally comprise of a chest X-ray and:

- a full blood count
- liver function tests
- measurement of serum calcium level.

Table 15.5
Causes of changes in breast size and shape

Pregnancy
Carcinoma
Benign hypertrophy
Rare large tumours

Staging investigations

If the tumour is removable with no symptoms or signs suggestive of metastases, there is no value in carrying out staging investigations. Staging investigations are carried out if:

- the primary tumour is inoperable
- distant metastases are suspected on clinical grounds
- neoadjunctive treatment is being considered (see below).

The usual staging investigations are based on the common pattern of metastatic spread associated with breast cancer:

- **isotope bone scan** looking for bone metastases
- **ultrasound scan of the liver** for liver metastases
- **CT scan of the thorax and upper abdomen** for lung and liver secondaries.

Management

The treatment of breast cancer falls into two main categories: **primary treatment by surgery** with or without radiotherapy, and **adjunctive therapy** by hormone manipulation, chemotherapy and immunotherapy.

The aim of treatment is to achieve local control of the primary tumour in the breast and the axillary lymph nodes and maximize survival prospects by employing the most appropriate adjunctive treatments. This aim is nowadays directed by a multidisciplinary team (MDT), which meets regularly to discuss the detailed management of each patient. The core members of the MDT are:

- surgeon
- radiologist
- pathologist
- oncologist.

Selection of the most appropriate primary and adjunctive treatment requires knowledge of the prognosis.

Prognostic factors

Size

The bigger the tumour the worse the prognosis.

Axillary lymph node status

Prognosis declines in proportion to the number of lymph nodes containing metastatic tumour.

Type

Most cancers (85 per cent) are described as 'of no special type'. These are invasive ductal carcinomas. The others have distinguishing histological features and are described as lobular, mucinous, papillary, tubular and medullary. Some of these have a better prognosis than invasive ductal carcinomas.

Histological grading

This is based on the assessment of nuclear pleomorphism, mitotic counts and tubule formation. Each is scored to produce a numerical grading:

- Grade 1: low grade
- Grade 2: intermediate grade
- Grade 3: high grade.

Vascular invasion

The presence of tumour cells invading blood vessels indicates a worse prognosis.

Hormone receptor status

Tumours containing oestrogen and progesterone receptors respond to hormone manipulation. This gives more treatment options and hence a better prognosis.

Hormone receptor status is not always absolute and clear-cut. Breast tumours contain multiple clones of cells some of which may contain hormone receptors and others which do not. It is possible to assess the range of receptivity by various methods of scoring using immunohistochemical techniques such as the Quick Score, which rates oestrogen receptivity on a scale of 1 to 7.

Hormone receptor status may alter after adjunctive treatment if the initial treatment suppresses the growth of sensitive cells but not of resistant cells, which continue to grow.

HER2 status

HER2/neu is an epidermal growth factor receptor associated with the HER2 gene found in a quarter of breast cancers. It is associated with a poor prognosis, but can be treated with a monoclonal antibody.

Prognostic indices

By quantifying some of the risk factors, it is possible to construct indices of likely survival. A method in common use is the Nottingham Prognostic Index (NPI), which is the sum of:

> One-fifth of the tumour size in centimetres, plus the lymph node stage (1 = no nodes involved; 2 = one to three nodes; 3 = four or more nodes) plus the histological grade (1, 2 or 3). (There is no need for the student to memorize how to calculate the NPI.)

An NPI of 3 or less indicates a good prognosis and conversely a score above 6 suggests a significantly lower chance of long-term survival. It must be remembered that a prognostic index gives a statistical probability of survival based on a population. Although the predicted outlook for an individual patient may be poor or uncertain, it should never be considered hopeless.

The value of calculating a prognostic index in breast cancer is that it helps the clinician to tailor the treatment to the needs of the individual patient. A patient with a small grade 1 node-negative tumour has a prognosis very little different from the population as a whole and, once the breast has been treated adequately, may not need any adjunctive treatment. Increasingly toxic measures are reserved for those who will benefit.

Relative and absolute benefit from treatment

When planning treatment, relative and absolute benefit must be considered. If a woman with a 90 per cent chance of survival, i.e. a 10 per cent chance of dying, is given a treatment which reduces her chance of dying from breast cancer over the next 5 years by one-tenth (10 per cent to 9 per cent), its use would only increase her chance of survival from 90 per cent to 91 per cent. If the treatment is arduous or has significant side-effects, an absolute benefit of only 1 per cent might not be acceptable.

Whereas for a patient with a poor prognosis tumour with only a 50 per cent chance of survival, the reduction in the chance of dying produced by the same treatment would be 10 per cent of 50 per cent, i.e. 5 per cent. Few patients would wish to forgo the chance of an increase in survival from 50 per cent to 55 per cent, however unpleasant the treatment might be.

This simple calculation illustrates why it is so important to know the prognosis when selecting the most appropriate treatment for those with breast cancer.

SURGICAL TREATMENTS

The first effective treatment for carcinoma of the breast was the **radical mastectomy**, introduced in the USA by Halstead at the end of the nineteenth century. It involved removal of the breast, the pectoral muscles and all the axillary lymph nodes. The cosmetic appearance afterwards was poor and, when followed with radiotherapy, massive lymphoedema of the arm was not uncommon. As it became apparent that prognosis depended on the biological features of the tumour and the likelihood of fatal metastases rather than the radical excision of the breast, more conservative surgical procedures were introduced, usually followed by local radiotherapy. The results of this approach, in terms of survival, were the same as with radical surgery, so surgeons now aim for the minimal excision consistent with achieving local control.

WIDE LOCAL EXCISION (WLE)

Wide local excision aims to resect the tumour with a margin of normal breast around it.

A clearance of as little as 5 mm (when the specimen is fixed in the pathology laboratory) may be enough if followed with radiotherapy to the breast and chest wall. This usually achieves an acceptable cosmetic result but occasionally the defect in the breast is unsightly and reconstruction is needed.

The surgical specimen must be properly oriented to allow the pathologist to identify the *in vivo* position of the specimen's margins. Not infrequently, further surgery is required to excise cancer left at one of the margins. This is disheartening for the patient and the surgeon, but is the price to be paid to avoid mastectomy.

MASTECTOMY

The breast is removed in its entirety down to the pectoral fascia, with excision of part of the pectoral muscles if the tumour is deeply situated and invading into them.

Mastectomy is needed in at least a third of all women presenting in the UK, for the following reasons.

- **The tumour is large in relation to the size of the breast**, the excision of which would either not be possible or would leave an unsightly remnant. Women with small breasts are more likely to come into this category.
- **The tumour is situated close to or invades the nipple or areola.** If the nipple/areola complex is removed, the breast looks unsightly so the preferred cosmetic solution is to complete the mastectomy.
- **Multifocal disease**, as is frequently found with lobular carcinomata.
- **A second metachronous cancer** in a breast that has previously been irradiated.
- **The patient prefers mastectomy**, sometimes to avoid the need for radiotherapy after wide local excision and sometimes in the belief that they will experience less long-term anxiety if the whole breast is removed rather than conserved.

MANAGEMENT OF THE AXILLA IN PATIENTS WITH BREAST CANCER

Axillary lymph node status is the most important prognostic factor in breast cancer and some form of surgical assessment is carried out in most patients. This is done first to assess the prognosis, but the axilla must then be properly treated to avoid the very unpleasant situation of uncontrollable axillary metastases. The surgical options are discussed below.

Axillary block dissection is a formal removal of all the lymph nodes *en bloc*. It is the best method of investigating the axillary nodes, as it allows full histological assessment, and also the most effective treatment. If the nodes contain tumour it provides excellent long-term control with a recurrence rate of less than 2 per cent. However 60–70 per cent of patients do not have axillary metastases and unfortunately the operation is associated with some morbidity, in particular **lymphoedema of the arm** (see Chapter 11) and **numbness** and **paraesthesia** in the area supplied by the intercostobrachial nerves, which are inevitably sacrificed.

If the axillary nodes are *palpable*, it is very likely that they contain tumour. In this event most surgeons will proceed directly to axillary block dissection.

Axillary node sampling. The surgeon explores the axilla through a smaller incision and locates four nodes by palpation, which allows calculation of the NPI. This may not be as straightforward as it sounds in a fat patient. If there is tumour involvement, the options are to proceed to a block dissection or to consider radiotherapy to the axilla.

Sentinel node biopsy is when an isotope and/or blue dye which will travel to the lymph nodes is injected into the breast (Fig 15.3). The first node the tracer reaches is located and removed through a small incision. Known as the sentinel node, it is the node most likely to contain tumour. If the sentinel node is positive, it is followed by either axillary dissection or radiotherapy. Although currently fashionable, this technique has to demonstrate a sensitivity of over 90 per cent before it becomes acceptable for general use. It is now in widespread use in the UK.

In the future, **positron emission tomography (PET scanning)** and other radiological techniques may replace surgical procedures for axillary staging.

A promising recent advance is to employ **DNA technology** in the operating theatre to determine whether the sentinel node contains cancer. The results are almost immediate, and if the node is positive, axillary dissection can be done as part of the same operation.

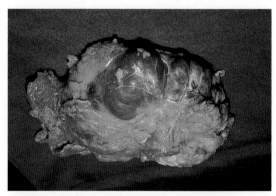

FIGURE 15.3 A surgical specimen of axillary dissection showing selective uptake of blue dye by lymph nodes

RECONSTRUCTION OF THE BREAST AFTER MASTECTOMY

Reconstruction is usually performed some time after surgery, when adjunctive radiotherapy or chemotherapy has been completed. It can, however, be carried out synchronously with mastectomy. There are many techniques (Fig 15.4).

Breast implants – usually made of silicone – are widely used for augmentation of the normal breast for cosmetic purposes. Insertion is often preceded by the use of a *tissue expander*, which is a balloon inserted into a pouch made in the tissues of the chest wall, connected to a subcutaneously placed separate small chamber. Fluid is repeatedly injected over several weeks to expand the pouch to the size of the removed breast. Finally, the expander is replaced with a prosthesis.

There is no evidence of long-term harm from silicone implants but there may be local problems with the formation of a pseudo-capsule of dense fibrous tissue.

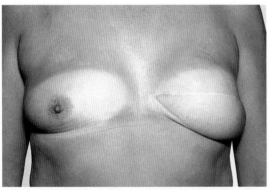

(A)

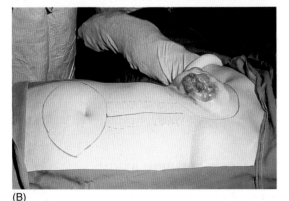

(B)

FIGURE 15.4 Examples of reconstruction: (A) a latissimus dorsi flap; (B) a rectus abdominis flap

A more realistic reconstruction is achieved by the use of autologous tissue transferred either from an adjacent area on a vascular pedicle or moved as a free transfer requiring micro-anastomosis of its blood supply. The commonest techniques are discussed below.

For the **latissimus dorsi flap**, a portion of this muscle with its overlying skin and fat is tunnelled into the breast area. The tissue available is limited and will not replace a large breast.

For the **transverse rectus abdominal muscle (TRAM) flap**, a portion of abdominal skin with subcutaneous fat is taken in continuity with a section of the rectus abdominalis muscle. It may be possible to move this on its vascular pedicle or as a free transfer with vascular anastomosis. An advantage is loss of any 'spare tyre' carried by the patient, but the abdominal wall may be weakened.

The **deep inferior epigastric perforator (DIEP) flap** is named from the vessel supplying the skin and fat transferred as a free flap. There is little or no muscle loss, so there is no threat to the integrity of the abdominal wall.

It may well be impossible to find the amount of tissue necessary to replace a large breast. A good balanced cosmetic result may then be achieved by a simultaneous reduction procedure on the remaining breast.

DUCTAL CARCINOMA *IN SITU*

In ductal carcinoma *in situ* (DCIS) the malignant cells are confined to the ducts and there is no invasion of adjacent tissue. Therefore, there is no risk of metastasis. The importance of the condition lies in the fact that it carries a high risk of transformation to invasive cancer. This risk is difficult to quantify, but may be as high as 30 per cent over 10 years.

Investigation

Clinical diagnostic indicators

DCIS presents as follows:

- as a palpable lump noticed by the patient
- with nipple discharge or bleeding
- as Paget's disease of the nipple
- via breast screening – it has a highly characteristic mammographic appearance.

It is classified by its *architecture* into four types, **papillary**, **cribriform**, **solid** and **comedo**, and by *nuclear grading* into low, intermediate and high grades. Its architecture is not related to its progression to invasion, but its nuclear grade is.

Imaging

DCIS is associated with characteristic **mammographic** appearances: calcification confined to the ducts producing a fine linear or branching pattern.

Tissue biopsy

A preoperative histological diagnosis is essential, i.e. **a core biopsy**. A diagnosis based on cytology cannot indicate the presence of invasion.

Management

DCIS must be **excised** with an adequate margin of at least 10 mm.

As this is not an invasive cancer, axillary staging is not necessary.

Mastectomy is required if the lesion is large, multifocal or associated with Paget's disease and involves the nipple.

If it is screen detected and impalpable, localization is needed before excision.

There is an unresolved debate about the place of radiotherapy and adjunctive tamoxifen after a wide local excision, particularly for high-grade lesions.

BREAST CANCER IN THE MALE

Breast cancer in males is similar to that in females. Pathology, hormone receptor status, symptoms, diagnosis and treatment are the same. All varieties occur in males, including DCIS and Paget's disease. The prognosis, depending on the stage of the disease, is the same as for females.

Presentation is often late because of a lack of awareness of this unusual condition. Screening of the male breast is unlikely to be introduced.

As there is only a rudimentary breast, the tumour is close to and often involves the pectoral muscles. This requires mastectomy with excision of a cuff of muscle.

Surgical clearance will rarely if ever be adequate and radiotherapy will be needed in almost every case.

RADIOTHERAPY IN PRIMARY TREATMENT

Radiotherapy has a major role in the primary treatment of breast cancer.

Irradiation is indicated in the following circumstances.

- Radiotherapy should follow a wide local excision of a carcinoma of the breast *in every case*. Without it, recurrence rates in the breast reach 40 per cent. After radiotherapy, the chance of tumour recurrence in the breast is low, approximately 6 per cent.
- Radiotherapy to the chest wall is indicated after a mastectomy performed in the presence of risk factors for local recurrence, namely:
  - a large tumour over 4 cm in diameter
  - a grade 3 tumour
  - axillary lymph node involvement
  - the presence of vascular invasion.
- Radiotherapy to the axilla is controversial although widely used. There is a very significant risk of lymphoedema of the arm and there may even be damage to the brachial plexus. In terms of survival and recurrence, it is as effective as block dissection.
- Radiotherapy should also be given to the supraclavicular nodes if there is massive axillary lymph node involvement because in this situation these nodes are also likely to be involved.

ADJUNCTIVE TREATMENTS

The 5-year survival after treatment of breast cancer by surgery alone is around 70 per cent. Use of the best and most appropriate adjunctive treatment increases the 5-year survival to around 80 per cent. Hormone manipulation is the biggest contributor to this improved survival, followed by chemotherapy, but there is a synergistic effect if both are used.

HORMONE MANIPULATION

About three-quarters of breast tumours test positive for oestrogen receptors and, of these, about two-thirds also contain progesterone receptors.

Treatment attempts either to reduce the production of oestrogen or to block its effects.

OOPHORECTOMY

Removal of the ovaries appears a logical treatment for an oestrogen-sensitive tumour, but it must be remembered that there are other endogenous sources of oestrogen-like hormones, particularly the adrenal glands. At one time surgical adrenalectomy was often employed in the treatment of advanced breast cancer.

Surgical removal of the ovaries has been largely replaced by drugs but is still occasionally used in younger women. A laparoscopic approach is highly appropriate. Ovarian function may also be destroyed by irradiating the ovaries (Table 15.6).

PHARMACOLOGICAL HORMONE MANIPULATION

Tamoxifen (Table 15.7) is an oral anti-oestrogen drug that is the single most important factor in the improvement in breast cancer survival seen over the last 20 years. It has contributed to the treatment of oestrogen-sensitive tumours in women of all ages, both as an adjunctive agent and in the treatment of advanced disease. Serious side-effects are rare. There is an undoubted risk of **thromboembolic** episodes and the drug should not be used in patients with a history of deep vein thrombosis or pulmonary embolism. A few patients experience a vaginal discharge caused by endometrial hypertrophy, with possible progression to endometrial carcinoma.

Aromatase inhibitors work by preventing the enzyme aromatase converting circulating hormone precursors, largely androgens produced by the adrenal glands, to oestrogens. The effect would therefore be expected in post-menopausal women who are no longer producing ovarian oestrogen. This has been confirmed in clinical trials where aromatase inhibitors appear to be more effective than tamoxifen in terms of preventing relapse of the disease. No difference in survival has yet been shown.

Three drugs are currently in use, **anastrazole** and **letrozole**, which inhibit aromatase for the duration of the treatment only, and **exemestane**, the action of which appears to be permanent. There is no evidence that any of them is more effective than the others. **An important side-effect is osteoporosis**. Aromatase inhibitors should not be used in women with, or who have a high risk of, this condition.

Progestogens such as **megestrol** have an action on oestrogen receptor-positive cancers, and have a role in premenopausal women unable to tolerate tamoxifen.

Luteinizing hormone-releasing hormone (LHRH) agonists, such as **goserelin**, are used similarly. The surgical equivalent, removal of the pituitary gland (hypophysectomy), is now obsolete.

There is some evidence that the combination of **tamoxifen for 2 or 3 years followed by long-term treatment with an aromatase inhibitor** may have advantages over the use of either therapy alone. The field is complex, with numerous ongoing clinical trials of new drugs and different regimens. The

Table 15.6
Hormone manipulation for oestrogen-sensitive breast cancers

Remove the source of oestrogens by:
  Surgical oophorectomy, open or laparoscopic
  Radiotherapy to the ovaries
Block the effect of circulating oestrogens by:
  Anti-oestrogen agents, e.g. tamoxifen
  Preventing the synthesis of oestrogen by use of aromatase inhibitors, e.g. anastrazole
  Progestogens
  Luteinizing-hormone releasing hormone analogues

Table 15.7
Tamoxifen: key facts

Treatment should go on for 5 years
A dose of 20 mg daily is adequate
Mild menopausal symptoms are to be expected, which may include vaginal discharge and even endometrial carcinoma
Occasional nausea is overcome by taking the drug at night
There is an increased risk of thromboembolism

breakthrough in the use of hormonal manipulation in women with oestrogen receptor-positive breast cancer came about through the introduction of tamoxifen. All subsequent improvements are marginal when compared with its benefits (Revision panel 6).

CHEMOTHERAPY

Cytotoxic chemotherapy given as adjunctive treatment for breast cancer prolongs survival, particularly in patients with oestrogen receptor-negative tumours. The improvement is of the same order as that achieved by hormone manipulation in those with oestrogen receptor-sensitive tumours. There is also a small additional effect from adding chemotherapy to hormone manipulation for oestrogen receptor-positive tumours.

Combinations of drugs are always used, for example **cyclophosphamide**, **methotrexate and 5-flourouracil** (**CMF**), or regimens including **anthracycline**, which may be more effective. The treatment is given in monthly cycles, usually for 6 months. Adjunctive chemotherapy is far more effective in younger women, with an absolute improvement of about 7–11 per cent in 10-year survival for women aged below 50, and of about 2–3 per cent for those aged 50–69. There is little evidence of benefit in women over 70, in whom the side-effects are also more dangerous.

Chemotherapy and hormonal therapy are complementary, not competing, adjuvant treatments. However, it might be expected that agents, such as tamoxifen, which slow cell division will reduce the effectiveness of chemotherapy which acts on the rapidly dividing cell. For this reason it is common practice not to commence hormone manipulation until any chemotherapeutic regimen is completed. There is no evidence base for this intuitive approach.

ADJUNCTIVE IMMUNOTHERAPY

Patients with tumours testing positive for HER2 overexpression may be treated with **trastuzumab** (Herceptin), a monoclonal antibody. The drug has been shown to prolong survival in women with advanced disease. It is given intravenously and is **cardiotoxic.**

Trials are in progress to test its efficacy in primary treatment, but because of public demand it is increasingly used as an adjuvant agent.

NEOADJUNCTIVE TREATMENT

When **hormone manipulation and/or chemotherapy** are employed as the first treatment, this is termed **neoadjunctive therapy**. Staging investigations are undertaken before it is used, as the presence of systemic disease will affect the management of the primary lesion in the breast. The purpose of this treatment is:

- to shrink a large tumour so that wide local excision rather than mastectomy is possible
- to render a large fixed tumour operable.

These objectives are achieved in about two-thirds of cases. Sometimes neoadjunctive treatment is so successful that the primary tumour apparently disappears. However, unless there are distant metastases, surgery will still be necessary, as microscopic disease will invariably be present in the breast.

HORMONE MANIPULATION AS SOLE TREATMENT

The incidence of breast cancer increases with age. It is not uncommon for a frail elderly breast cancer patient to present with significant co-morbidity and any operation would best be avoided. Triple assessment should be carried out in the usual way, and if a core biopsy is taken, **oestrogen receptor status** can be determined.

Primary treatment with an **aromatase inhibitor** (or **tamoxifen** if there is evidence of osteoporosis) may be appropriate. Long-term survival may be marginally impaired if no surgery is performed, but there is no difference until at least 3 years after starting treatment. Long-term survival is unlikely in this group. Careful monitoring is essential to avoid loss of local control.

Some patients will refuse surgery but accept hormone manipulation.

FOLLOW-UP AFTER TREATMENT

There is no evidence that early detection of recurrent disease, local or systemic, affects survival. Therefore, no harm is done to the patient by discontinuing clinic attendances after active treatment is completed. There is also no evidence in favour of repeated routine investigations.

Patients who have breast-conserving surgery have a small but significant (6 per cent) risk of developing recurrent disease in the residual conserved breast. This invariably occurs within the first 5 years after primary treatment, with a peak incidence at between 2 and 3 years. It is therefore logical in these patients to carry out annual mammography for 5 years.

Patients who have undergone mastectomy have a 1 per cent per year risk of developing disease in the remaining 'normal' breast. For this reason **mammography screening at 2-year intervals** has become routine, although without an evidential base.

RECURRENT DISEASE

Breast cancer may recur locally or systemically. Locally the patient may notice another lump in the breast, on the chest wall or in the axilla.

Systemic disease usually affects bones, lung or liver but no site is exempt, each site presenting with its appropriate symptoms. There is often a 'tip of the iceberg' effect, i.e. local recurrence is often associated with disease elsewhere in the body.

Treatment depends very much on whether there is systemic disease requiring systemic treatment, or a purely local recurrence. It is therefore essential to carry out staging investigations, usually an **isotope bone scan and a CT scan**.

Recurrent disease is treated with the same methods employed in primary treatment.

- **surgery**, for localized recurrence in the breast or the axilla after wide local excision
- **radiotherapy**, for chest wall and skeletal recurrence (It is particularly effective for relieving the pain that comes from bony metastases.)
- **hormone manipulation**: a change of the type used is often surprisingly effective
- **chemotherapy**, which must be tailored to the pattern and symptoms of recurrence
- **immunotherapy**, for the HER2-positive tumour.

Although recurrence of breast cancer usually indicates that the patient will ultimately die from the disease, patients may survive for many years or die of something else. This distorts breast cancer mortality statistics based on the death certificates, because when a patient is known to have been treated for breast cancer the breast cancer tends to be given as the cause of death whatever the real cause.

Curiously, those with recurrent breast cancer rarely feel ill or lose weight, and can often function normally until shortly before death.

SCREENING FOR BREAST CANCER

As the prognosis of breast cancer depends on the stage of the disease it is an attractive concept to try to detect it before the onset of symptoms, namely before the lesion becomes palpable to the patient. Neither regular clinical examination by a health professional nor teaching patients to examine their own breasts has been shown to have any clinical value.

Screening with mammography is widely used. There is no evidence of value in women under the age of 40, a fact that has not prevented its use in this age group in the USA. Using two-plane views and reducing the interval between examinations to 2 years rather than 3 increases screening's sensitivity.

In the UK, mammography detects an abnormality requiring some form of further investigation in approximately 5 per cent of women between the ages of 50 and 70. Of these, 0.8 per cent have a malignant lesion, a fifth a carcinoma *in situ*.

Screen-detected invasive cancers are less aggressive than symptomatic cancers based on size, lymph node status, type, histological grade, and the NPI.

A proportion of screen-detected cancers are palpable by the clinician even though not noticed by the patient, and are assessed and treated in the standard way.

The **impalpable lesion** requires special measures.

- **Guided core biopsy** provides a preoperative histological diagnosis. This allows appropriate management of the axilla at a single definitive operation.
- **Preoperative marking** of the lesion by the insertion of a hooked wire under X-ray control requires a skilled radiologist.
- **X-ray of the operative specimen** during the operation seeks to make sure that the lesion has been excised with an adequate margin. If not, the surgeon must excise the margins of the residual cavity.

It is not always possible to get a full histological diagnosis before surgery, particularly if the lesion is small. It is then necessary to carry out an **open biopsy with guide-wire localization**. The minimum amount of tissue is excised, as the abnormality may be benign, followed by definitive surgery if it turns out to be malignant.

EFFECTIVENESS OF BREAST CANCER SCREENING

Screening detects a population of breast cancers at an early stage. The 5-year survival of women in the UK with screen-detected breast cancer is 94 per cent. Adding this cohort to those women presenting with symptomatic disease will result in an overall reduced chance of death from breast cancer in that population. However, a significant proportion of the screen-detected cases have *in situ* disease or small grade 1 tumours with an excellent prognosis. It is not known if they would have eventually become symptomatic before dying of other causes, and consequently their treatment may have been unnecessary. Breast screening has yet to be shown to reduce overall mortality anywhere in the world.

The topic remains controversial. A Cochrane systematic review in 2006 concluded that:

> for every 2000 women invited for screening throughout 10 years, one will have her life prolonged. In addition, 10 healthy women, who would not have been diagnosed if there had not been screening, will be diagnosed as breast cancer patients and will be treated unnecessarily. It is thus not clear whether screening does more

good than harm. Women invited to screening should be fully informed of both benefits and harms.

PREVENTION OF BREAST CANCER

About 1 per cent of the population carry a mutation on one of the breast cancer genes (BRCA1, BRCA2 and TP53), associated with an 85 per cent risk of developing breast cancer by the age of 70. They also have a high risk of developing ovarian cancer. A strong family history of breast cancer without a detectable gene mutation is also associated with an increased risk of developing the disease.

More intensive mammographic surveillance of this group has been suggested, but there is no evidence of its effectiveness in women under 40 years of age, and controversy over its role after that.

Definitive **preventative** treatments involve the pre-emptive use of proven modalities.

- **Bilateral mastectomy** (with immediate reconstruction), usually only for those with a proven very high risk, reduces the chance of developing breast cancer by 90 per cent. Failure is caused either by cancer arising in breast tissue left on the chest wall or in the axilla, or by micrometastases from an occult primary already present at the time of surgery.
- **Oophorectomy** (see page 349) reduces the risk of ovarian cancer in those with gene mutations and also provides endocrine therapy against oestrogen receptor-positive breast cancer.
- **Tamoxifen** is effective, at the cost of thromboembolic episodes and a small risk of endometrial carcinoma.
- **Aromatase** inhibitors have also been employed, at the cost of osteoporosis.

BENIGN DISEASES OF THE BREAST

Any swelling in the breast should be investigated with triple assessment as described in Table 15.1.

FIBROADENOMA

This diagnosis may often be made with confidence on the clinical signs, e.g. a mobile lump, a **'breast mouse'**, in a young woman. Nevertheless, it is mandatory to complete **triple assessment** and obtain a histological diagnosis.

Management

Until the development of triple assessment, it was standard practice to recommend surgical removal of all fibroadenomata as this was the only way to confirm that the lump was benign. Since it became possible to obtain a definite histological diagnosis using a simple **tissue biopsy** technique, their natural history has been investigated. It has been found that they do not become malignant, half do not alter in size and a few regress. Enlargement to a diameter of more than 2–3 cm is unusual.

Increase in size is more common in adolescents. Some become calcified with time.

The choice of treatment may be left to the patient. Most women wish to lose an easily palpable breast lump.

Excision through the smallest and most cosmetic incision requires a short general anaesthetic. If feasible, an incision at the areolar margin gives an excellent result with a hardly detectable scar.

Minimally invasive methods are under development. The **mammotome** is a large-bore version of a core biopsy needle. With ultrasound control, the lump is drawn by vacuum aspiration into a side chamber and sliced off with a cylindrical knife. *It seems likely that this approach will become the treatment of choice.*

PHYLLOIDES TUMOUR

The treatment of this rare lesion is adequate **surgical excision**, which may occasionally mean **mastectomy**. These tumours have a histological spectrum from clearly benign to potentially malignant, although lymph node metastasis is rare.

INTRADUCT PAPILLOMA

This lesion is a papillary neoplasm and must be treated by surgical excision. If it presents with nipple discharge coming from a single duct orifice, it can be **localized radiologically** or **endoscopically**.

Treatment options are:

- **open surgical excision**, involving removal of the affected duct system via an incision at the areolar margin
- **endoscopic excision**, which is still experimental.

Surgical excision must be complete to avoid recurrence, but there is no risk of malignant change.

LIPOMA

Lipomata of the breast may be ignored or removed by simple local **excision**.

LUMPS, NODULARITY AND PAIN

Five treatment option are set out below.

Reassurance

Many women with benign breast disease are worried that they might have cancer. Once this possibility is excluded and they are reassured, they should not want or need any treatment.

Modification of life style

There is conflicting information on the effect of wearing a brassiere. Some women with painful lumpy breasts are better if they stop wearing one. Others are improved by properly fitted support.

Diet

Avoiding coffee, tea and chocolate sometimes results in the relief of symptoms.

Drugs

Simple **analgesia** and the use of **non-steroidal anti-inflammatory agents** may relieve breast pain, even though there is no inflammatory process involved in either breast pain or nodularity.

Many breast symptoms are related to the menstrual cycle and are clearly related to circulating endogenous oestrogens. Manipulation by various drugs is therefore logical.

Some premenopausal women with cyclical pain are better when taking the contraceptive pill. Conversely, for others, the pain is associated with taking oral contraception, and in this event it may be worthwhile changing to another type of contraception.

Anti-oestrogen agents may be effective.

- **Tamoxifen** relieves symptoms in almost all those suffering from breast pain. There is concern over using this highly effective adjunctive treatment for breast cancer for a benign condition. It should only be used in refractory cases and as a short course.
- **Danazol** is an anti-oestrogen drug that is effective for breast pain but may cause menstrual irregularity and masculinization.
- **Bromocriptine** and **LHRH antagonists** have also been used, but have significant side-effects.
- **Evening primrose oil** is a herbal remedy available 'over the counter' in pharmacies. Its weak anti-oestrogen effect explains why it helps many patients with breast pain if taken in adequate doses.

Surgery

There is **no role for surgery** in the management of breast pain and nodularity.

BREAST CYSTS

Cysts may often be diagnosed with reasonable confidence by clinical examination. Many develop around the menopause, are often multiple and appear anywhere in the breasts over a period of several years. They are sometimes seen in an older age group taking oestrogens as hormone replacement therapy.

Management

The treatment is simple **aspiration** of the fluid. Individual cysts do not usually refill, but further cysts may develop until the underlying hormone environment alters.

After aspiration, it is important to confirm that the lump has disappeared. The presence of a residual swelling or obvious blood in the aspirate suggest the rare possibility that the lesion is a partly cystic carcinoma.

If aspiration leads to complete disappearance of the lump, several large studies have shown that it is not necessary to request cytology examination of the cyst fluid.

The only complication of aspiration is **refilling of the cyst cavity with blood**, caused by the aspirating needle damaging a vessel. When the blood clots it leaves a hard lump, which takes several weeks to resolve. Application of external pressure for a few minutes after aspiration reduces the chance of this happening.

A protocol for the management of breast cysts is given in Revision panel 7.

A **galactocele** is a cyst containing milk, associated with lactation. It is reasonable to make the diagnosis directly by aspiration. Galactoceles usually refill but, once diagnosed, should only be re-aspirated if they become uncomfortable because they resolve when lactation stops.

NIPPLE INVERSION

Nipple inversion is commonly associated with **duct ectasia** and has characteristic clinical features. When the underlying cause is a carcinoma, it will be unusual to be able to avoid mastectomy.

The condition may also be idiopathic. Various cosmetic plastic procedures are available.

DUCT ECTASIA

Duct ectasia is treated by the options listed below.

Reassurance

Most women with this common condition are happy to live with the symptoms of nipple inversion and a mild discharge provided there is no periductal mastitis. Symptoms usually improve at the menopause. It has been suggested that there are two disease processes, one with infective complications in younger woman, and another causing nipple inversion and a discharge in older women.

Modification of life style

Nipple inversion is three times more common in those who smoke, probably because of a direct effect of nicotine on the ducts and the skin commensal organisms responsible for periductal mastitis. All patients should be advised to stop smoking.

Diet
There are no known dietary factors.

Drugs
Antibiotics may be required to treat episodes of periductal mastitis, but there is no evidence that long-term treatment has any effect on the course of the disease.

Surgery
Surgery may be required for:

- drainage of periductal abscesses
- cure of a mamillary fistula. This can be achieved either by laying open the fistula and allowing it to heal by granulation, or by excising the fistulous track (with antibiotic cover).

It is possible to excise the major duct systems through an incision in the areolar margin, with the intention of relieving the symptoms of the disease and everting the nipple. Because the surgery involves cutting across dilated ducts containing easily infected inspissated material, postoperative infection is common even with antibiotic cover.

Long-term results are poor. Reinversion of the nipple and recurrence of pain and infection are common. Excision should be reserved for severe cases.

Although duct ectasia is a benign disease, it can be debilitating and patients will occasionally request mastectomy.

BREAST ABSCESS

There are two varieties of breast abscess, the acute abscess associated with **lactation** and the chronic abscess which results from **periductal mastitis associated with duct ectasia**.

Abscesses in the breast may be treated by:

- **serial aspiration**, often aided by ultrasound guidance, plus antibiotic cover
- **incision and drainage** in a way that allows dependent drainage.

Lactating patients who develop a tender area in the breast perhaps with a fever and malaise are commonly prescribed antibiotics in the hope of

aborting the formation of an abscess. This may succeed if there is cellulitis without an abscess, but it may result in a chronic abscess, palpable as a hard lump, which is termed an **antibioma**. This condition takes a long time to resolve as the hardness is caused by fibrous tissue that will remain after the fluid is drained.

BENIGN HYPERTROPHY

The female breast has many shapes and sizes. The 'ideal' form alters with fashion. Patients may wish to have the size of their breasts reduced for cosmetic reasons. Such surgery is associated with significant complications.

There is a group of women with breasts large enough to produce genuine morbidity such as:

- **skeletal pain** in the neck and back
- **deep grooves in the shoulders** from brassiere straps
- **fungal infections of the skin** under the breasts, known as intertrigo.

If not associated with general obesity, **breast reduction** is indicated in these patients. The surgery is major and carries the complications of bleeding, haematoma, infection and necrosis of skin flaps.

GYNAECOMASTIA

Investigation
Clinical diagnostic indicators
Gynaecomastia presents in adolescent and elderly men.

The vast majority of cases in adolescents are idiopathic or have an obvious cause, such as **puberty**. Gynaecomastia in elderly men is usually a side-effect of **drug ingestion**.

There are, however, some very rare endocrine causes. The investigations will depend on what cause is suggested by the history and clinical examination.

Blood tests
There is no need for any special investigations in most cases, but it is important to consider **endocrine causes** and order the necessary blood tests

needed to exclude them during the general assessment of the patient.

Tissue biopsy

If there is a discrete palpable lump, **triple assessment** is essential. Carcinoma of the male breast is uncommon but not unknown.

Management

Most patients require only **reassurance**. An obvious cause may be removed, e.g. stopping the use of anabolic steroids.

Drug therapy

Treatment with **anti-oestrogen agents** is effective. **Danazol** has significant side-effects. **Tamoxifen** appears to be more effective and better tolerated.

Subcutaneous mastectomy

Surgical treatment depends on the age and build of the patient. Persistent adolescent-type gynaecomastia is associated with a hard, sometimes tender, disc of breast tissue behind the nipple. This is best dealt with by subcutaneous mastectomy.

An incision is made in the areolar margin and the **breast tissue is excised preserving the nipple**. It is important to save a layer of breast tissue under the nipple to preserve its blood supply and to avoid an unsightly depression.

In older patients the swelling is likely to be bilateral, fatty and more diffuse. **Liposuction** is the method of choice. A 3-mm diameter open-ended tube is inserted through a small incision and the fatty element sucked out. Results are dependent on the skill of the operator. Haematoma formation is common.

16

The abdominal wall and groin

John Black

Most conditions affecting the abdominal wall and groin can be diagnosed by taking a full history and carrying out a careful examination. There are few things more satisfying to the surgeon than to make a precise diagnosis based on anatomical and clinical knowledge alone. Special investigations are rarely required.

The surgical problems of the abdominal wall and groin may be subdivided into:

- swellings arising in the rectus sheath and abdominal wall fasciae (Table 16.1)
- herniae (Table 16.2)
- disorders of the umbilicus (Table 16.3).

SWELLINGS IN THE RECTUS SHEATH AND SWELLINGS ARISING FROM THE ABDOMINAL WALL FASCIA

Investigation

Clinical diagnostic indicators

The diagnosis of swellings in the rectus sheath rarely requires anything more than a careful clinical examination.

Painful swellings Rupture of the inferior or superior epigastric arteries will usually be diagnosed by the appearance of a tender swelling shortly after a bout of coughing or after heavy exercise. There is often discoloration of the overlying skin.

Painless swellings If the swelling is painless it is probably a lipoma or a chronic rectus sheath haematoma – the acute phase having been forgotten or not noticed.

A lipoma may be diagnosed clinically with confidence, as careful examination will usually reveal that it is in the subcutaneous fat rather than in the rectus sheath. However, a lipoma may also lie under the deep fascia, when it will display the

Table 16.1
Causes of a swelling in the rectus sheath

Rupture of the inferior or superior epigastric arteries

Chronic rectus sheath haematoma

Benign tumour

Malignant tumour

Table. 16.2
Varieties of abdominal hernia

Common

Inguinal

Umbilical

Incisional

Femoral

Epigastric

Rare

Spigelian

Obturator

Lumbar

Gluteal

Table 16.3
Disorders of the umbilicus

Exomphalos

Umbilical fistula

Other umbilical swellings:

    Granuloma, adenoma, ompholith,

    Secondary carcinoma, endometrioma

characteristic features of an intramuscular swelling (see *Symptoms and Signs*).

If the swelling is truly in the abdominal wall it may be a malignant tumour such as a desmoid tumour or a sarcoma; in this event accurate histological diagnosis and staging is required before treatment (Table 16.4).

Imaging

A **CT or MRI scan** will reveal the extent and consistency of a malignant lesion.

A **chest X-ray, bone scan and/or PET scan** may be needed to detect distant metastases.

Tissue biopsy

A histological diagnosis by **core biopsy or an incisional biopsy** must be obtained if the swelling is thought to be malignant.

Table 16.4
Investigation of a suspected sarcoma of the abdominal wall

- Obtain a histological diagnosis by multiple core or a small incisional biopsy
- Assess the extent of the primary tumour by computed tomography and/or magnetic resonance imaging
- Look for distant metastases with a chest X-ray, an isotope bone and/or positron emission tomography

---

Table 16.5
Treatment of a sarcoma in the abdominal wall

In the absence of distant metastases

Radical surgery removing the tumour with a wide margin

Appropriate reconstruction, which may be major

Adjunctive treatment tailored to the tumour type with radiotherapy and/or chemotherapy

If there are metastases

Radiotherapy and/or chemotherapy

Palliative excision of the primary tumour

Management

Haematomata in the rectus sheath

No treatment is necessary for a rupture of the inferior or superior epigastric arteries. The patient should be told that the pain will diminish over a few days, given mild analgesia and reassured that the swelling will resolve in a few weeks.

A chronic rectus sheath haematoma, once diagnosed, also requires no treatment other than to await resolution.

Sarcoma of the abdominal wall

The management of this uncommon condition is beyond the scope of this book but follows the principles set out in Table 16.5. Treatment depends on the tumour's histological type and its size. Inadequate surgery must be avoided at all costs to prevent disastrous untreatable local recurrence. Patients with a swelling in the abdominal wall that might be a sarcoma should be referred to a unit with experience in treating these rare tumours.

SWELLINGS IN THE GROIN

An inguinal hernia and the other causes of groin swelling (Table 16.6) can usually be diagnosed and treated with confidence on the history and physical signs alone.

Investigation

Clinical diagnostic indicators

The clinical features of the many varieties of hernia listed in Table 16.2 are described in detail in

---

Table 16.6
The differential diagnosis of a lump in the groin

Inguinal hernia

Femoral hernia

Enlarged lymph node(s)

Sapheno varix

Ectopic testis

Femoral aneurysm

Hydrocele of the cord or canal of Nuck

Lipoma of the cord

Psoas bursa or abscess

Symptoms and Signs. The most significant clinical sign is an expansile cough impulse. Occasionally, particularly in an obese patient, the diagnosis may not be obvious and in these circumstances the presence of a hernia may be confirmed by herniography, laparoscopy, CT or MRI scanning; but once the diagnosis has been made, with or without special local investigations, there is no need for more investigations other than those indicated by the type of anaesthesia to be employed.

Imaging

Herniography involves the instillation of a radio-opaque fluid into the peritoneal cavity which, when it runs down into the pelvis, makes the sac of the suspected hernia visible on fluoroscopy or a plain X-ray (Fig 16.1). This technique is only required when diagnosis is difficult and is not entirely reliable. It is indicated when:

- the patient has groin pain or localized tenderness without a lump
- the patient has a history of an intermittent lump, not detected by the surgeon after repeated examinations
- there is a cough impulse of uncertain significance.

Herniography is particularly useful when there is suspicion of a recurrent hernia, when scarring may obscure the physical signs and when diagnosis is important if strangulation is a significant possibility.

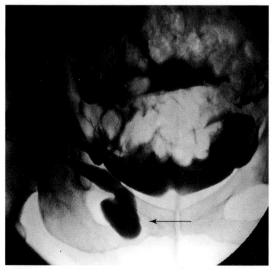

FIGURE 16.1   An X-ray herniograph sac filled with contrast medium

Although **laparoscopy** requires a general anaesthetic it is a very sensitive method of detecting an occult hernia. It also allows the surgeon to proceed directly to a laparoscopic repair.

Open exploration for diagnostic purposes, often employed in the past, is now obsolete.

CT or MRI scanning may be useful in the diagnosis of rare and complex herniae.

GENERAL PRINCIPLES OF HERNIA MANAGEMENT
Observation and reassurance

Many herniae do not require treatment, particularly if they are symptomless and have a low risk of complications. An example would be a small direct inguinal hernia, or an incisional hernia that consists of a general bulge of the wound area without a sharp-edged defect. In assessing the need for definitive treatment the following factors should be considered.

- **The age of the patient.** A small hernia in a young patient will enlarge and cause problems whereas a similar hernia in an older patient may not produce problems within the patient's likely life expectancy.
- **The degree of co-morbidity.** The risks of surgery in a frail elderly diabetic patient may be greater than the risk of future complications. Surgery in the morbidly obese patient carries an increased risk. Some patients are so obese that a large hernia is impossible to repair.
- **The chance of an operation providing a long-term cure.** The recurrence rate after repair of an inguinal hernia in a child is virtually zero but the result of surgery for a complex incisional hernia in an elderly adult is uncertain.

Modification of life style

A physically active patient is more likely to have symptoms from a hernia than, for example, a patient confined to a wheelchair.

Avoiding certain forms of exercise may render a hernia symptomless. Minor discomfort from a small inguinal hernia would not bother most people but could prevent a professional sportsman from earning a living.

Smoking and its associated coughing is a cause of many herniae. Treatment is more likely to be successful if the patient stops smoking.

Diet

Herniae often have fatty sacs, contain omentum or consist solely of extraperitoneal fat. Loss of weight usually makes a hernia smaller. Surgery is more difficult and has more complications in obese patients so these patients should be advised to lose weight preoperatively. Few patients succeed in both stopping smoking and losing weight.

External support

External pressure devices to reduce and control herniae have been employed for centuries. There is consensus that they do not prevent complications but they may ease discomfort and pain.

There are many varieties of **truss** for inguinal herniae. They rarely function properly and it is not uncommon to see an elderly male patient very pleased with the effect of his truss when it is pressing firmly alongside an unreduced hernia!

Abdominal support belts are useful for patients with incisional herniae. They need to be carefully and individual fitted.

Surgery

A hernia is a mechanical problem whose cure requires a mechanical solution, namely a surgical repair. Herniae are repaired electively for two reasons:

- to relieve symptoms
- to prevent complications, especially intestinal obstruction and bowel strangulation.

GENERAL PRINCIPLES OF HERNIA REPAIR

There are two stages in the repair of a hernia: the herniotomy and then the herniorraphy.

Herniotomy

Herniotomy is literally the opening of the hernia sac so that the contents of the sac can be restored to whence they came, usually the abdomen, followed

by its removal. No hernia repair will succeed unless the sac is excised, or inverted, and its neck ligated or oversewn.

Herniorraphy

Herniorraphy means repairing the abdominal wall defect through which the hernia appeared. There are two complementary means of achieving this.

- **Anatomical repair**. The surgeon restores the anatomy to normal as far as is possible. However, if the tissues in the area had not failed, a hernia would probably not have developed so it is usually necessary to reinforce the local tissues with a natural or synthetic material.
- **Synthetic reinforcement**. This was done traditionally with fascia or nylon using a variety of complex suturing and darning techniques. Nowadays it is achieved by covering the weak area with a synthetic material commonly, but not exclusively, in the form of a mesh. A repair using a synthetic material is sometimes called a **hernioplasty**.

The cardinal rule for success in hernia surgery is to keep the repair tension free. If there is tension the stitches holding the reinforcing materials in place will tear out.

Surgical approach

In the traditional **open operation** the hernia is approached from the outside via an incision in the skin over the swelling, the hernia sac excised or reduced and the abdominal wall repaired and reinforced.

In the **laparoscopic operation** the abdomen is inflated with carbon dioxide, either intra- or extra-peritoneal, the sac reduced into the abdomen, or its neck divided and oversewn, and a mesh is inserted between the peritoneum and the inner surface of the abdominal wall (the pre-peritoneal plane). The actual defect is not repaired.

It is also possible to insert a mesh into the pre-peritoneal plane from outside using an open approach. This is the basis of the *Stoppa* repair, where a mesh is placed in exactly the same place as it would be if placed laparoscopically. This approach has been superseded by the laparoscopic repair because it achieves the same objective without a large external incision.

The choice of approach for each variety of hernia is discussed later.

GENERAL COMPLICATIONS OF HERNIA REPAIR

Mortality

The risk to life following an elective hernia repair in a patient under 60 is negligible, but thereafter it increases with age to approximately 3 per cent in patients over 80.

The risk for operations on large abdominal incisional herniae is greater.

The mortality following surgery for a strangulated hernia is high, approaching 10 per cent. This is because the risk of strangulation rises with age; older patients are more likely to have significant co-morbidity and the risks include the complications that follow operations performed in the presence of damaged bowel.

Thromboembolism

Most hernia repairs carry a very low risk of deep vein thrombosis and pulmonary embolism because the operation and hospital stay is short, often just a few hours. Nevertheless, **prophylactic measures** against thromboembolism should always be applied, particularly in the presence of any specific thrombosis risk factors.

The risk is higher after the repair of major incisional herniae and is similar to that for open abdominal surgery.

Retention of urine

The commonest type of groin hernia is the male inguinal hernia. This hernia is most frequently seen in the older age group. Postoperative retention of urine is therefore quite common as these patients often have a mild degree of symptomless prostatic hypertrophy.

Infection

An elective hernia repair is a clean operation and the chance of infection, usually from skin organisms, is low. However, the consequences of infection when it does occur can be disastrous, as most hernia repairs involve the implantation of a synthetic material which may have to be removed to eradicate the infection, following which the hernia is likely to recur.

For this reason, prophylaxis with a single perioperative dose of a **broad-spectrum antibiotic** is essential and routine.

Haematoma

Repair of a large hernia often requires extensive subcutaneous dissection. If the resulting cavity cannot be closed it may fill with blood that may need evacuating. This risk may be reduced by the use of **closed suction wound drainage**.

Damage to other structures

The testicular vessels and segmental nerves may be injured during the repair or damaged later by postoperative swelling.

Recurrence

The operation may fail to cure the hernia.

INGUINAL HERNIA

At some time in their lives, 9 per cent of males and 1 per cent of females will develop an inguinal hernia. Repair is a routine procedure in developed countries. Places without surgical services sufficient to offer elective repair have an increased incidence of strangulated inguinal hernia, morbidity and death. It can be argued that inguinal hernia repair is perhaps the most important operation in general surgery.

Because of the local pain and discomfort produced by the swelling and the risk of strangulation increasing with time, *surgical repair is the treatment of choice for all reasonably fit patients*. Another significant factor is the cosmetic appearance – patients do not like an obvious swelling.

Techniques of repair of an inguinal hernia

Repair of inguinal hernia became a routine procedure at the end of the eighteenth century as general anaesthesia and antiseptic/aseptic surgery developed. All techniques follow the basic principles of herniotomy and herniorraphy outlined above.

When the hernia is indirect, the peritoneal sac is emptied and then excised.

If the hernia is a sliding hernia, in which a viscus forms part of the wall of the sac, the herniotomy has to be carried out distal to the viscus and the proximal sac reduced into the abdomen.

A direct hernia does not always have a peritoneal sac and may consist solely of extraperitoneal fat which is easy to reduce into the abdomen intact. The anatomy of these varieties of inguinal hernia is discussed in detail in *Symptoms and Signs*.

Open repair

- The **Bassini repair**, described in the nineteenth century, was the first reasonably successful technique to be widely adopted. After the herniotomy, the conjoint tendon is sutured to the inguinal ligament. This results in tension and increases the chance of recurrence. The **Tanner slide**, an incision in the anterior rectus sheath, is a modification that was introduced to reduce the tension and stress at the suture line.
- The **nylon darn** was introduced soon after nylon was invented in the 1940s. The hernia sac is dissected out and excised in the usual way, but instead of suturing the conjoint tendon to the inguinal ligament under tension, the space between these structures is filled with a loose interlocking darn.
- The **Shouldice repair** was devised in Toronto in Canada. It relies upon a meticulous dissection and overlapping repair of the transversalis fascia with stainless steel wire, covered by an overlying loose darn, also with stainless steel wire. Local anaesthesia is used routinely in the Shouldice clinic. This was the first method of repair to be subjected to proper audit and some degree of long-term follow-up and the first to produce good evidence of good long-term results (Table 16.7).

Table 16.7
Results of the open repair of an inguinal hernia

Operation	Long-term chance of recurrence
Bassini with or without a Tanner slide	At least 20 per cent
Nylon Darn	At least 10 per cent
Shouldice repair	1–2 per cent
Lichtenstein repair	1–2 per cent

- The **Lichtenstein repair** was introduced when synthetic mesh of reliable quality became available (Fig 16.2). The herniotomy is carried out in the usual way. The gap between the conjoint tendon and the inguinal ligament is then covered with a mesh that extends from the midline to beyond the internal inguinal ring and spermatic cord. Great stress is placed on achieving a tension-free repair. Its results are comparable to the Shouldice repair but the operation is technically easier.

The Lichtenstein repair is now the standard open procedure for repair of an inguinal hernia. It may be performed as a day case with local or general anaesthetic.

Complications specific to open repair

In addition to the complications listed above for all hernia repairs there are two specific complications that follow open repair of an inguinal hernia.

Testicular infarction This is usually a venous infarction caused by external pressure on the pampiniform plexus at the reconstructed external inguinal ring rather than damage to the testicular artery. It may be immediate with painful postoperative swelling followed by testicular atrophy, or it may be insidious. The incidence is of the order of 1 in 200.

Long-term groin pain Approximately 5 per cent of men have persisting pain in the distribution of the iliohypogastric, ilio-inguinal or genitofemoral nerves after the postoperative pain has resolved. It is not known if this is caused by direct trauma at the time of surgery, nerve ischaemia or late incorporation of the nerve(s) in scar tissue.

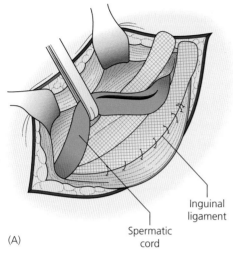

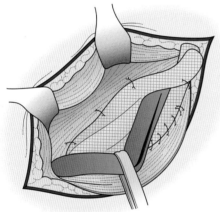

(A)

(B)

Spermatic cord

Inguinal ligament

FIGURE 16.2 Line drawings showing the position of the mesh in a Lichtenstein repair. (A) Mesh covering the posterior wall of the inguinal canal. (B) Tails of the mesh wrapped across the spermatic cord to refashion the internal ring

In about 2 per cent of patients the pain is significant and disabling.

Management is difficult. The pain usually subsides spontaneously but resolution sometimes takes several years.

Laparoscopic repair

Laparoscopic surgery came into general use during the late 1980s and within a few years became the standard method for removing the gall bladder. The advantages gained from avoiding an abdominal incision are a more rapid recovery and a better cosmetic appearance.

Abdominal herniae are clearly seen on laparoscopy as the insufflated carbon dioxide expands the abdominal wall and distends the hernial sac, so it was not surprising that attempts were soon made to repair herniae from the inside of the abdomen.

The benefit in terms of reduced trauma is not so great as with cholecystectomy as the standard open repair of a hernia is not as traumatic as an upper abdominal incision. Laparoscopic repair is also technically more difficult than open repair. A general anaesthetic is always required. Nevertheless, there are real benefits.

There are two laparoscopic approaches, **transabdominal pre-peritoneal repair (TAPP) and transabdominal extraperitoneal repair (TAEP)**.

- In **TAPP**, the peritoneal cavity is entered at the umbilicus and inflated. The peritoneum over the hernia sac is then incised and lifted to allow the mesh to be placed between it and the abdominal wall.
- In **TAEP**, a balloon is inserted and inflated between the abdominal wall and the peritoneum to lift up the peritoneum and expose the inside of the groin on both sides.

Although each has its enthusiastic advocates, there is actually no difference in technical difficulty, results or complications.

The essential steps of a successful laparoscopic repair of an inguinal hernia are:

- reduction (inversion) or excision of the sac
- insertion of a *large* mesh; the standard size is 15 × 10 cm, which will, in most patients, extend from the lateral end of the inguinal ligament to the midline.

If the transperitoneal (TAPP) approach is used it is important to completely cover the mesh with peritoneum to avoid bowel loops adhering to it.

The mesh does not have to be fixed as it is held in place by abdominal pressure once the insufflating carbon dioxide is released, but there are now elegant tacking devices available that are widely used.

Table 16.8   Comparison of open and laparoscopic repair of an inguinal hernia

	Open repair	Laparoscopic repair
Anaesthetic	Local or general	General
Risk	Negligible but increases with age	Negligible, very small risk of major organ damage
Recurrence	1–2 per cent	1–2 per cent
Time to full recovery	4 weeks	2 weeks
Cosmetic appearance	Groin scar	Almost invisible, small scars
Chronic pain	2–5 per cent	Rare
Testicular atrophy	0.5 per cent	Not reported

There is almost unanimous agreement that there are three situations where laparoscopic repair offers a clear advantage over open repair:

- *For recurrent hernia.* The surgeon does not have to dissect out the failed previous repair with increased risk of damage to nerves and vessels. Laparoscopic repair by either approach is carried out in an untouched plane between the peritoneum and the abdominal wall and is usually no more difficult than a first time repair.
- *For bilateral repair.* The trauma from a bilateral open repair is significantly greater than that of a bilateral laparoscopic repair. The trauma of a bilateral laparoscopic repair is the same as that associated with a unilateral repair.
- An additional benefit is that if a clinically occult hernia on the other side is seen during the repair it may be dealt with immediately with no penalty in length of recovery or other morbidity.

Complications specific to laparoscopic repair

Injury to the bowel or other abdominal organs Laparoscopy involves the insertion of a telescope into the abdomen at the umbilicus and so carries a small but not insignificant risk of injury to the gut or other abdominal organs of the order of 1 in 1000. This risk may be reduced by using an open rather than a blind insertion technique.

Hydrocele During a laparoscopic repair, an indirect sac, which often extends into the scrotum, is often divided at the neck rather than excised. The empty sac may fill with fluid and the patient may think the hernia is still there. The swelling may be anywhere along the line of the spermatic cord and around the testis. Resolution is usually spontaneous. If not the fluid may be aspirated percutaneously.

Thromboembolism The risk of thromboembolism after laparoscopic hernia repair is not yet known, so it is mandatory to employ routine prophylaxis.

Infection Infection of the implanted mesh seems to be very rare because it has hardly ever been reported, but this may be because single-dose antibiotic prophylaxis is now used routinely.

Table 16.8 compares the risks and results of open and laparoscopic repair.

RECURRENT INGUINAL HERNIA

Recurrent herniae are more likely to be painful, tend to be direct, are rarely large but more likely to strangulate than a primary hernia. When pain is the main symptom and the hernia small, clinical diagnosis may be difficult. **Herniography** may be helpful or, as a last resort, **laparoscopy**.

The results of open repair of recurrent inguinal herniae are poor, in terms of further recurrence and of morbidity. The evidence for this statement is largely anecdotal as very few studies of the results of the repair of recurrent herniae have been reported, but all surgeons are familiar with unfortunate patients who have had repeated repairs fail.

In the past, orchidectomy was added to the repair as removal of the spermatic cord facilitated the obliteration of the inguinal canal and the internal inguinal ring. For this group of patients the advent of laparoscopic repair, with the advantages detailed above, has been of inestimable value. *There is now little doubt that laparoscopic repair is the procedure of choice for recurrent groin hernia.*

OBSTRUCTED OR STRANGULATED INGUINAL HERNIA

These patients present as an emergency (see Chapter 17). They may be very ill and require intensive resuscitation. **Urgent open exploration** is necessary to identify the constriction point trapping the contents – usually the external inguinal ring. The bowel and any other contents must be inspected to assess their viability. Bowel resection may be necessary. A standard repair is then performed.

The death rate from a strangulated inguinal hernia is high, at least 10 per cent, particularly if the patient is old and frail and the hernia contains dead bowel.

INGUINAL HERNIA IN A CHILD

Groin herniae in children are almost always indirect and inguinal and follow failure of the processus vaginalis to obliterate. If the child has an obvious hernia with reducible bowel contents, operation is indicated as soon as practicable.

When a patent processus vaginalis presents as an infantile hydrocele or an encysted hydrocele of the cord rather than a hernia, resolution may occur in the first year of life but is less likely once the child is walking. *Nevertheless, a definite hernia or persistent hydrocele in a child should be treated surgically.*

It is quite common for a surgeon to be unable to find a swelling even when the child's parents give a good history of seeing a swelling and can indicate the appropriate anatomical area where the swelling appears. They may also have photographic evidence (see *Symptoms and Signs*). In these circumstances an operation may be undertaken on the evidence of the history alone. An indirect sac is invariably found.

Surgical repair

The treatment of a child's hernia need be no more than a simple **herniotomy**.

A general anaesthetic is essential. Some form of local or regional anaesthetic may be added when the child is asleep.

The groin is explored through a small skin crease incision over the internal inguinal ring and the inguinal canal opened. In children the internal oblique muscle extends further medially than in adults and its fibres must be separated to reveal the glistening peritoneal sac which is always in the front of the spermatic cord. If this is dissected and suture ligated above the internal ring, it will retreat back into the abdomen. No formal repair is needed other than to close the anatomical layers of the groin. In females the surgeon should check that the ovary and Fallopian tube are not in the back wall of the sac.

Recovery is immediate and recurrence very rare. Children do not need to be given postoperative instructions about mobility: they will ignore them and do themselves no harm.

FEMORAL HERNIA

This hernia is diagnosed on its physical signs. The femoral canal contains the lymph node of Cloquet. If this is enlarged it may mimic a femoral hernia so accurately that the diagnosis is only made at operation.

All femoral herniae should be repaired, unless the patient has a very short life expectancy, because the risk of strangulation is high.

Surgical repair

The surgical approach to a femoral hernia may be either directly over the swelling (called the *low* approach) or through the inguinal canal (the *high* approach). The latter is nowadays rarely used.

The sac is dissected out, opened, emptied, invaginated or ligated and then divided at the level of the inguinal ligament. The femoral canal is closed by placing a few non-absorbable sutures between the inguinal ligament and the pectineal fascia (Fig 16.3). Care must be taken not to compress the femoral vein. The patient can be fully active within a week and recurrence is very rare. Repair by the low approach is easily performed under local anaesthesia.

A **strangulated femoral hernia** can also be exposed through the low approach. Not uncommonly the sole contents are omentum. Because the femoral canal is narrow a part of the bowel wall may be trapped in the sac – a Richter's hernia. Should bowel resection and an anastomosis be required the femoral canal may be too small to allow the bowel

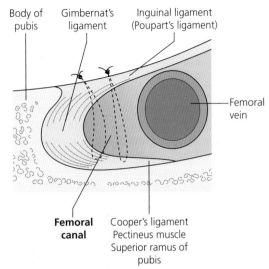

Body of pubis   Gimbernat's ligament   Inguinal ligament (Poupart's ligament)

Femoral vein

Femoral canal   Cooper's ligament
Pectineus muscle
Superior ramus of pubis

FIGURE 16.3   Femoral hernia repair. The femoral canal can be obliterated by placing stitches between the inguinal ligament and the pectineal ligament or blocking the space with a plug or layer of mesh. The dotted line shows the position of the stitches. Care must be taken not to compress the femoral vein

to be returned into the abdomen and the surgeon may have to convert to the high approach or alternatively make a separate laparotomy incision.

A femoral hernia may be repaired laparoscopically, but as recovery is just as rapid after open surgery this approach is rarely indicated.

If a femoral hernia is noticed during the laparoscopic repair of an inguinal hernia it can be dealt with in the same way at the same time. In the unusual event of recurrence of a femoral hernia, or if the hernia is prevascular with the femoral vessels forming the posterior wall of the defect (see *Symptoms and Signs*), laparoscopic repair is ideal.

UMBILICAL HERNIA IN CHILDREN

The vast majority of congenital umbilical herniae disappear spontaneously during the first few years of life. **Management is therefore conservative**, sometimes against the wishes of the parents, particularly when the child is a girl. After the age of 4 years, spontaneous resolution becomes unlikely. This is therefore a convenient time to recommend an operation – before the child starts school.

Surgical repair

The operation is carried out with a general anaesthetic through a curved incision in the lower margin of the umbilical scar, which, when healed, gives an excellent cosmetic result. The peritoneal sac is dissected out, emptied, invaginated or ligated and divided. The defect in the umbilical fascia is closed with simple sutures of a slowly absorbable synthetic material.

Recovery is rapid, with return to normal activity in a day or two. The only complication is the occasional accumulation of a small amount of serous fluid under the redundant umbilical skin. This will absorb without treatment, although anxious parents may have to be placated by aspiration of the collection.

Recurrence following a childhood umbilical hernia repair by simple suture is very rare.

UMBILICAL HERNIA IN ADULTS

In adults, most herniae at the umbilicus are acquired and para-umbilical, but in practice differentiating this variety from a true umbilical hernia is not important.

The defect in the linea alba is often small compared with the size of the sac.

The swelling may consist of extraperitoneal fat only, an empty peritoneal sac with a thick fatty wall or a peritoneal sac filled with omentum or bowel.

The condition is common in middle-aged and elderly people and is associated with obesity. Often the patient has not noticed the swelling. The diagnosis is made clinically.

Management must be tailored to the patient. Strangulation is not rare, but many patients live for many years with an umbilical hernia without problems. An uncomfortable hernia clearly merits repair in a reasonably slim active patient. Morbidly obese patients with a symptomless swelling may be treated conservatively.

The crescent-shaped pit associated with the para-umbilical bulge may contain foul smelling sebaceous secretions because it cannot easily be cleaned. This increases the risk of postoperative wound infection.

Surgical repair

The technique of operative repair in the adult is fundamentally different to that used in children. A number of methods of repair have been tried over the years because simple closure of the defect has a very high failure rate.

The **Mayo repair** mobilizes the fascia at the edges of the defect, overlaps them and then fixes them in place with two layers of non-absorbable sutures.

Because the fundamental principle of hernia repair is to avoid tension, the simple Mayo overlap repair, which involves pulling tissues beyond their normal position, has been replaced by the use of **a mesh** implanted between the deep surface of the abdominal wall and the underlying repaired peritoneum. **Antibiotic prophylaxis is essential**.

With a large hernia, or if there is contaminated skin, excision of the umbilicus simplifies repair and reduces the chance of infection. However, many patients do not want to lose their umbilicus.

No technique for repair of adult umbilical hernia is completely satisfactory and the definite possibility of recurrence must be explained to the patient.

EPIGASTRIC HERNIA

The diagnosis of an epigastric hernia is made on clinical grounds alone. Strangulation and other complications are rare.

Most patients request operation because the swelling is often painful and noticeable.

Surgical repair

Surgical repair is carried out under general anaesthetic via a transverse incision. It is essential to mark the level of the hernia on the skin before the operation as once the patient is anaesthetized the hernia may be impalpable.

The mass is usually found to be mainly extraperitoneal fat, sometimes with a small peritoneal sac, coming through a very small (2–5 mm diameter) defect in the linea alba.

Simple suture suffices. Recurrence is rare.

INCISIONAL HERNIA

An incisional hernia is a hernia through the scar of a previous abdominal operation or stab wound. The incidence is surprisingly high. About 10 per cent of patients who have had an abdominal incision develop a wound hernia, usually within the next 1–2 years but occasionally much later.

Risk factors include increasing age, obesity, diabetes and steroid therapy, but the most important is postoperative wound infection. Postoperative distention and a chronic cough add to the risk.

Investigation

The diagnosis can usually be made with confidence on clinical grounds. If the hernia is irreducible and the incarcerated contents plug the defect there may not be a cough impulse, making a clinical diagnosis less certain. A **CT or MRI scan** may be needed to confirm a clinical suspicion.

Management

The results of surgery for incisional herniae are relatively poor. One reason for this is that many of the factors that led to the breakdown of the initial wound closure will still be present. Second, the technical problems are far from being solved. Countless methods have been described, suggesting that none of them is satisfactory. Recurrence rates of 30–50 per cent are not unusual.

The methods of management that can be employed singly or together are discussed below.

No treatment

Many patients with an incisional hernia may not even have noticed the swelling and are happy to live with it. This is particularly so when the weakness is caused by a diffuse overall thinning of the surrounding tissues rather than a defect with a distinct edge. Complications in this type of hernia are uncommon so doing nothing is safe.

Modification of life style

Many patients know which activities make their hernia painful or larger, e.g. lifting heavy weights. By avoiding them, they can live with their problem.

Diet

If obese patients can be persuaded to lose weight, their hernia will become smaller and less uncomfortable.

Support

A properly fitted support belt will control and alleviate the pain of many abdominal incisional herniae.

Surgical repair

Surgical repair is indicated to relieve symptoms and treat complications, e.g. strangulation. Except in emergency situations the patient should be reasonably fit, aware that the procedure is a major one and that a long-term cure cannot be guaranteed. Prophylaxis against thromboembolism should be routine together with peri-operative antibiotic cover.

Techniques of repair include:

- direct suture closure, if possible
- a 'keel' repair, where the hernia is inverted into the abdomen by successive lines of non-absorbable sutures
- tension-free mesh repair, placing the mesh between the peritoneum and the abdominal wall, or as an onlay
- laparoscopic repair, placing a mesh over the defect from the inside of the abdomen. This may be technically demanding and covering the mesh with peritoneum may be impossible. A special PTFE/rubber mesh may be used to reduce the risk of bowel adhering to the mesh.

RARE HERNIAE

Spigelian herniae occur at the edge of the rectus sheath. They usually present as a diffuse bulge and do not have a narrow neck. The patient may be content to live with the appearance once they know its cause. Repair by an open method can be difficult because there is a general attenuation of the surrounding tissues. Laparoscopic repair, inserting a large mesh beneath the peritoneum from the inside of the abdomen, is the best solution.

Obturator herniae usually present with small bowel obstruction in a slim elderly woman, and are often not diagnosed until the abdomen is explored. The bowel is reduced and the obturator canal closed.

If the mouth of an obturator hernia is noticed during a laparoscopic repair of an inguinal hernia it can be covered by the same mesh used to cover the inguinal defect.

Lumbar herniae sometimes follows trauma to the abdominal wall. They tend to be a diffuse defect and complications are rare. The principles of repair are the same as for Spigelian hernia.

Gluteal herniae are extremely rare and usually develop through a defect in the pelvic floor after an excision of the rectum. Repair is difficult and involves the insertion of a mesh by an open or laparoscopic approach.

DISORDERS OF THE UMBILICUS

EXOMPHALOS

Nowadays this condition is usually diagnosed before birth on routine ultrasound scanning. If not, clinical diagnosis is straightforward. It is a congenital hernia covered by a thin transparent membrane formed from peritoneum and the remnants of the coverings of the yolk sac, which may have virtually no thickness or strength and rupture spontaneously.

The prognosis is poor. Half of the babies born with an exomphalos do not survive, usually because of the presence of other congenital anomalies.

Treatment is surgical and difficult. The principle is to reduce the contents of the sac into the abdomen and cover the defect by any means possible. This may involve using synthetic materials, biologically derived dressings or plastic surgery procedures using whatever skin or muscle is available.

Gastroschisis is another rare neonatal abdominal wall defect, which is not at the umbilicus and does not have a sac. It is easier to repair and the prognosis is better.

UMBILICAL FISTULA

An umbilical fistula that discharges mucus or faeces and presents in early childhood is usually caused by a persistent **patent vitello-intestinal duct**.

Table 16.9
Management of a baby with a discharging umbilicus

Wait. If there is an umbilical granuloma it will resolve

If it does not resolve by 3 months, proceed to contrast X-ray (fistulogram or sinogram):

- Contrast enters small intestine – excise patent vitello-intestinal duct

- No track demonstrated – explore and excise umbilical granuloma

A **patent urachus** that discharges urine may also present in early childhood, but may present in later life if there is associated bladder neck obstruction.

A patent vitello-intestinal duct will usually be suspected on simple clinical grounds, but may be confused with an umbilical granuloma. The instillation of a radio-opaque contrast medium into the orifice of the fistula (a fistulogram) will confirm the diagnosis if the contrast medium enters the small intestine via a Meckel's diverticulum.

Surgical treatment is to explore the fistula through the umbilicus and excise the track and the diverticulum (see Table 16.9).

Patent urachus is discussed in Chapter 19.

UMBILICAL GRANULOMA AND ADENOMA

An umbilical granuloma develops if there is delayed involution of the umbilical cord.

It usually settles in the first month of life. If it does not, the old-fashioned method of applying **silver nitrate** on the end of a wooden stick remains effective.

An umbilical adenoma is an isolated patch of intestinal epithelium without any deep connection. The discharge it produces does not resolve spontaneously. Contrast X-rays should be used to confirm that there is no connection with the gut. Simple **surgical excision** is curative.

OMPHOLITH

An ompholith consists of sebaceous secretions, which dry out and protrude rather like a sebaceous horn. Simple removal and improved personal hygiene are curative.

SECONDARY CARCINOMA (SISTER JOSEPH'S NODULE)

A firm or hard nodule bulging into the umbilicus should be suspected to be a mass of secondary carcinoma from a primary tumour in the abdomen. Almost invariably the patient has many other symptoms and signs, looks unwell and has lost weight.

If there are no specific features to indicate the primary disease, a **core biopsy** and a **CT scan of the abdomen and thorax** will indicate the tissue source and the extent of any intra-abdominal or thoracic disease. Treatment should be that appropriate for whatever disseminated cancer is found.

ENDOMETRIOMA

This exceedingly rare condition should be suspected if there is a history of cyclical pain, swelling and bleeding. Investigations should be conducted by a gynaecologist.

DISCOLORATION OF THE UMBILICUS

A **caput medusa** is a blue tinge around the umbilicus caused by a collection of dilated veins secondary to portal hypertension. Other stigmata of portal hypotension are likely to be present and should be investigated, as described in Chapter 18.

Cullen's sign – umbilical bruising – is discussed in the section on pancreatitis (see Chapter 17). It may also be found in any condition associated with extraperitoneal bleeding. Its associated clinical features will be those associated with its underlying cause, which will indicate the investigations and management necessary.

Abdominal pain

Kevin G. Burnand

This chapter concentrates on patients presenting with abdominal pain. A number of symptoms commonly occur in association with abdominal pain (Table 17.1) and are related to pathology in the alimentary system. Their signs are described in full in *Symptoms and Signs* and their investigation and management is described in Chapter 18.

Pain

Most of the pathological disorders of the upper alimentary system, particularly those of the stomach, duodenum and gall bladder, initially cause a mild epigastric and central abdominal pain that is often related to the ingestion of food and which patients usually call **indigestion** or **dyspepsia**. But not all upper abdominal pain is exacerbated by eating and some conditions such as carcinoma of the stomach may be painless or, in the case of some forms of pancreatic disease, just cause a chronic persistent epigastric discomfort.

The investigation and management of the many conditions which present with abdominal pain as their main symptom are described in this chapter. The common causes of acute pain are listed in Table 17.2.

Dysphagia and regurgitation

Dysphagia and regurgitation (Table 18.1) are most often caused by disease in the oesophagus. It is important to differentiate regurgitation from vomiting.

Anorexia and nausea

Anorexia (a loss of appetite) and nausea (a feeling of sickness or queasiness that makes the patient feel that they are about to vomit) (Chapter 18) are caused by many different diseases, within and without the abdomen. Both symptoms are commonly accompanied by vomiting.

Most patients with gastric, biliary and pancreatic disease experience these symptoms as well as pain. Which symptoms predominate depends on the nature and position of the disease.

The conditions that present with nausea and vomiting are discussed in Chapter 18. Their investigation and management are described later.

Table 17.1

Symptoms occurring in association with abdominal pain

Dysphagia and regurgitation

Anorexia and nausea

Vomiting

Haematemesis

Weight loss

Jaundice

Distention

Colic

Table 17.2

Common causes of acute abdominal pain

Non-specific abdominal pain

Acute appendicitis

Acute cholecystitis and biliary colic

Peptic ulcer disease including perforation

Small bowel obstruction

Gynaecological disorders

Acute pancreatitis

Renal and ureteric colic

Malignant disease

Acute diverticulitis

Vomiting

Vomiting is caused by many different diseases, many outside the abdomen, including disorders of the central nervous system.

Types of vomitus

Vomitus free from bile, in children, is likely to be caused by congenital pyloric stenosis. This vomiting is described as **projectile** in that it spurts effortlessly from the mouth.

Vomiting that does not contain bile, in adults, and often contains undigested food such as tomato skins is usually caused by a fibrotic stenosis of the duodenum or antrum of the stomach that may follow long-standing chronic peptic ulceration. This vomiting is usually effortless and massive.

A similar type of vomitus may occur in patients with a pyloric gastric carcinoma.

Vomitus containing bile implies that an obstruction exists beyond the point in the second part of the duodenum where the bile enters through the ampulla of Vater. Vomiting associated with small bowel obstruction or from a paralytic ileus contains bile but the presence of bile in vomit is not particularly discriminating, apart from ruling out conditions proximal to the ampulla of Vater.

Faeculent vomiting occurs in patients with prolonged small bowel obstruction and rarely in patients with large bowel obstruction (often right-sided bowel cancers). It can also occur with a **gastrocolic fistula** when the vomit, instead of being faeculent, i.e. containing anaerobic organisms with putrifaction, contains actual large bowel contents.

Haematemesis

Haematemesis (Chapter 18, page 463) is vomitus containing blood. The blood may be just a faint 'blood staining' or it may be frank blood. The blood may be dark if it has been in contact with gastric acid for a long period (**coffee grounds colour**).

Patients who have had a haematemesis are usually unreliable witnesses with regard to the volume of blood they have vomited.

A history of dyspepsia or prolonged exposure to steroids or the non-steroidal anti-inflammatory drugs that are known to be associated with acute peptic ulceration may precede a haematemesis from a chronic peptic ulcer but this history is often absent.

A history of considerable weight loss suggests the possibility of a gastric carcinoma.

Patients with alcoholism are more likely to bleed from peptic ulceration than oesophageal varices but both conditions should be considered when excessive alcohol use is discovered. Alcoholics with oesophageal varices have an associated cirrhosis of the liver and so may have the stigmata of liver disease such as spider naevi, palmar flushing and white nails (see Table 18.5).

Bleeding disorders, **antiplatelet drugs** and **anticoagulants** should always be excluded.

Physical examination is often unhelpful apart from looking for signs of liver stigmata. An abdominal mass is rarely palpable. **Rectal examination** may demonstrate dark blood on the glove (**melaena**). The passage of dark blood per rectum is usually associated with gastric haemorrhage, the gastric acid turning haemoglobin to haematin which is responsible for black, tarry and unpleasant smelling stools.

Weight loss

Weight loss (Chapter 18, page 434) is common in patients with upper alimentary system symptoms. A combination of dysphagia and weight loss suggests a malignant tumour of the oesophagus or cardia. A history of a marked weight loss and vague dyspepsia is highly suggestive of a pancreatic carcinoma, especially a tumour arising in the body or tail of the gland. Patients with carcinoma of the head of the pancreas usually become jaundiced as the disease progresses.

Jaundice

Jaundice (Chapter 18, page 437) is a yellow pigmentation of the skin and sclera caused by an increase in the level of the serum bilirubin commonly caused by an obstruction of the biliary system but also by liver disease and increased haemolysis.

Distension

The abdomen may be distended by fluid within the peritoneal cavity or by the enlargement of any of the organs within it. The causes of ascites are listed in Table 18.11.

Colic

Colic is an intermittent griping pain originating from the muscle layers of hollow obstructed conducting viscus such as the small and large bowel and the ureter. Between each severe spasm the pain almost fades away. The pain caused by obstruction of the bile duct is often intermittent in nature and is called biliary colic, even though it does not remit entirely between each spasm and the bile duct has a very weak muscle layer.

ABDOMINAL PAIN AND PERITONITIS

THE 'ACUTE ABDOMEN'

Although the majority of intra-abdominal diseases cause abdominal pain, pain is not always the most prominent or distinguishing feature.

A patient is said to have an '**acute abdomen**' if they have a moderate to severe pain that lasts between a few hours and a few days (1–6 hours and 5–7 days). This type of pain is normally clearly distinguishable from **chronic abdominal pain**, which may last for weeks, months or years, be intermittent and be caused by different pathological conditions.

The principal generic causes of acute abdominal pain are:

- inflammation
- perforation of a viscus
- obstruction of a viscus
- infarction/strangulation
- intraperitoneal/retroperitoneal haemorrhage
- injury
- extra-abdominal and medical causes.

Investigation

Clinical diagnostic indicators

The three most important and significant clinical indicators that must be obtained from the history are the site and the character of the pain and the site of any tenderness.

The site of the pain Acute abdominal pain may be experienced throughout the abdomen or be localized by the patient to their left, centre or right side or be felt mainly in the upper or lower half of the

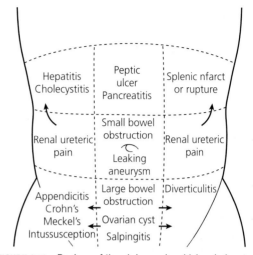

FIGURE 17.1   Regions of the abdomen in which pain is experienced (Reproduced with permission from Burnand *et al.*, The New Aird's Companion in Surgical Studies, 2005, Churchill-Livingstone)

abdomen. The organs and pathologies responsible for pain in the different regions of the abdomen are shown in Fig 17.1.

Some patients cannot localize their pain to any specific part of their abdomen and complain of a 'generalized' abdominal pain. Nevertheless, the principal site of the pain and any accompanying tenderness frequently give a good indication of the underlying problem.

The nature of the pain It is important to try to decide if the pain is 'peritonitic', i.e. constant and accompanied by local tenderness, or 'colicky' and intermittent in nature. There are many causes of peritonitis but fewer causes of colic, which is a pain arising from obstruction of a viscus.

Many patients cannot give a clear description of the character of their pain, and consequently describe it as 'just a pain, doctor' but can usually describe it using adjectives such as mild, discomforting or aching, severe or 'agonizing'.

Localized tenderness, site and severity On examination it is important to decide whether the pain is accompanied by evidence of peritonitis (local persistent tenderness, guarding, rebound, percussion tenderness and rigidity).

Diagnosis is difficult when abdominal pain is poorly localized or felt throughout the whole abdomen and non-specific in character, but most patients are able to differentiate between the constant persistent pain of peritonitis and the intermittent fluctuating pain which is griping in nature and called a 'colic'. When in doubt, a careful clinical re-evaluation and special tests should clarify the diagnosis.

A **differential diagnosis** should be compiled after taking a full history and performing a careful examination followed, if possible, by a single **working diagnosis**.

With knowledge of the severity of the pain and a provisional working diagnosis, the patient can then be assigned to one of the three following management pathways.

1. **An acute abdomen requiring urgent treatment**, e.g. peritonitis with a known or unknown underlying cause.
2. **Abdominal pain** (of known or unknown cause) **requiring pain relief pending further investigation and treatment**.
3. **An abdominal pain** (with no evidence of any clinically detectable intra-abdominal pathology) **that can be observed and investigated later**; i.e. there is time to wait and see.

Put another way:

- I do or not know the diagnosis but the problem needs urgent treatment – possibly an operation.
- I know or do not know the diagnosis but have time to investigate the problem further in order to decide what to do.
- I do not think there is anything wrong and can wait and see whether further investigations are required.

In almost every case, additional investigations are likely to be required to obtain an accurate diagnosis and plan treatment; but when the diagnosis is uncertain *careful monitoring and repeated re-examination are essential to detect any change, progression, or resolution of the problem and ensure the detection of important new physical signs.*

Physical signs often develop over several hours and become obvious, often diagnostic, by the time of a later re-examination.

The diagnostic tests which may be of value in determining the underlying cause of the abdominal pain are described below. The special investigations required for the diagnosis of each specific condition are described later.

The conditions responsible for about 90 per cent of patients presenting with acute abdominal pain are listed in Table 17.2.

Blood tests

Full blood count This may reveal the presence of a low haemoglobin or haematocrit usually indicating a pre-existing anaemia or chronic blood loss. A high haemoglobin and haematocrit is usually caused by dehydration, although polycythaemia should be considered. A leucocytosis is found in many patients with inflammation or peritonitis but is not diagnostic. A very high white cell count supports the diagnosis of severe acute pancreatitis or mesenteric ischaemia.

Blood film This may demonstrate sickle cells or target cells, indicating an underlying haemoglobinopathy (see Chapter 1). **Sickle cell testing** should be carried out preoperatively on all Afro-Caribbean patients.

C-reactive protein and erythrocyte sedimentation rate Raised levels suggest an inflammatory or infective process. A raised C-reactive protein is one of the indicators of severe acute pancreatitis.

Paul Bunnell test A positive test is diagnostic of infectious mononucleosis (glandular fever). The splenic enlargement and lymphadenopathy associated with this condition can cause non-specific abdominal pain.

Urea and electrolytes These should be measured in all patients with severe acute abdominal pain to establish a baseline for future reference. They are **essential** guides to the management of patients who have had severe **diarrhoea**, **vomiting** or appear **dehydrated**.

The **serum potassium, creatinine** and **urea** levels should also be measured because most anaesthetists want to know their baseline level before giving a general anaesthetic and in case there is a hitherto unexpected renal problem which might influence the nature of any fluid replacement. Saline and potassium replacement is indicated if dehydration and hypokalaemia are confirmed (see Chapter 2).

The **serum calcium** is an important prognostic indicator in severe cases of pancreatitis.

Serum amylase/serum lipase These enzymes should be measured routinely in all patients presenting with acute abdominal pain if, after a careful history and examination, the diagnosis remains in doubt. Their levels should always be measured when a diagnosis of acute pancreatitis is suspected **but remember that a raised serum amylase is *not* diagnostic of acute pancreatitis** as the serum amylase can be elevated in patients with a perforated peptic ulcer and mesenteric ischaemia.

Repeated testing, including measuring the amylase/creatinine ratio and the urinary amylase, may provide greater clarity.

Not all of the other enzyme tests that may help are readily available in all hospitals, or outside regular hours.

Blood sugar The blood sugar level must be measured in all diabetic patients presenting with acute abdominal pain, and in all patients found to have glycosuria on routine urine testing. Hypoglycaemia and lactic acidosis can mimic the signs of an ileus or a small bowel obstruction.

Liver function tests, including hepatitis A and B Although these tests may not be readily available out of hours, they should be obtained within 12 hours of admission if the patient appears jaundiced, or if liver failure and ascites are suspected. A markedly **raised serum bilirubin** with evidence of impending renal failure is an indication to intervene urgently in patients suspected of having acute cholecystitis or acute pancreatitis associated with common bile duct stones.

Patients with infectious hepatitis (A or B) can present with upper abdominal pain caused by swelling of the liver capsule. A markedly raised **lactic dehydrogenase** is associated with severe acute hepatitis.

Blood gases and base excess These tests are a prognostic indicator in patients with acute pancreatitis, and should be obtained in all severely ill patients with pancreatitis, mesenteric infarction or a ruptured abdominal aortic aneurysm. They are helpful during resuscitation and may indicate the need for oxygen, ventilation or a bicarbonate infusion.

Pregnancy test (human chorionic gonadotrophin) A pregnancy test should be obtained in all women of child-bearing age whose abdominal pain might be the result of a **ruptured ectopic pregnancy**. A positive pregnancy test strongly suggests this diagnosis in a patient with lower abdominal pain and the signs of hypovolaemic shock.

Urine tests

Blood, protein, sugar, specific gravity All patients with acute abdominal pain should have their urine tested for blood, protein, sugar and specific gravity.

Heavy proteinuria is indicative of chronic renal disease but may also indicate infection. The urinary glucose should be measured to pick up previously undiagnosed diabetes, and should also be tested if the diagnosis is thought to be acute or chronic pancreatitis.

A high specific gravity (dip test or hygrometer) indicates **dehydration**.

Microscopy, culture and sensitivity An aliquot of the urine, preferably a mid-stream specimen, should be examined under a microscope for cells, casts and bacteria. The presence of white cells and bacteria indicates infection. Casts may be found in the urine of patients with chronic viral disease.

Patients presenting with renal colic usually have **microscopic haematuria** but *remember that menstrual blood loss can contaminate urine samples.*

Bilirubin and urobilinogen These should be tested for in any patient with abdominal pain who is thought to be jaundiced. Both may be present in the urine of patients with acute cholecystitis, ascending cholangitis, acute pancreatitis and liver disease. Urobilinogen is not detectable in the urine of patients with obstructive jaundice.

Porphyrins Porphyrins should be measured if a diagnosis of **acute porphyria** is suspected. The urine goes dark on standing (Fig 17.2).

Stool tests

Culture and microscopy Stools should be sent for culture and microscopy in patients suspected of having salmonella, shigella or amoebiasis. Stool culture may also be valuable in diagnosing *Campylobacter,*

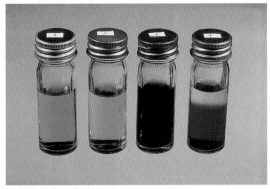

FIGURE 17.2   Porphyrins in urine darkening on standing

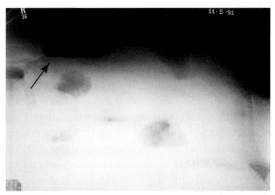

FIGURE 17.4   Free air in abdomen on lateral decubitus film

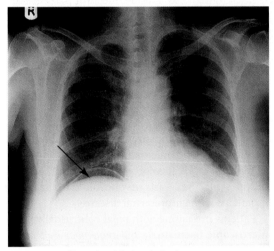

FIGURE 17.3   Air under right hemi-diaphragm

Giardia and *Clostridium difficile* infections. The last one is confirmed by biopsy of the bowel mucosa.

Imaging

Plain abdominal radiograph The presence of free gas, usually indicative of a perforated bowel, is best seen on an erect chest X-ray (Fig 17.3) or a lateral decubitus film (Fig 17.4). Controversy still exists over whether both erect and supine films of the abdomen should be ordered for all patients with undiagnosed abdominal pain in addition to an erect chest X-ray. Some have suggested that the erect abdominal film provides no additional information to the supine film, but it is our experience that it is easy to miss a single dilated gas-filled loop of small bowel on a supine film that is much easier

to see on an erect film because of the fluid levels it usually contains (Fig 17.5).

Dilated bowel visible on the supine film may be a consequence of either large or small bowel obstruction. The presence of a distended caecum separates the two (Fig 17.6). Dilated large bowel is usually situated around the periphery of the abdomen and has a **haustral pattern**, whereas distended small bowel usually lies centrally with a **ladder pattern** (Fig 17.5C) caused by the valvulae conniventes.

Contrast studies may be required to differentiate difficult cases (see below). It must be remembered that paralytic ileus from other intestinal pathology such as acute pancreatitis can produce similar appearances.

The plain abdominal radiograph may also reveal calcification in **lymph nodes, faecoliths, calculi** and the **wall of an abdominal aortic aneurysm** (Figs 17.7A and B).

The haematoma associated with **a ruptured aneurysm** may obliterate one of the psoas shadows or be seen as a soft tissue mass.

Other soft tissue masses that may be seen on a plain abdominal radiograph include a **large bladder**, an **enlarged spleen** or **liver**, a **haematoma**, or an **abscess cavity**, which may contain gas or a fluid level.

Gas in the biliary tree with or without a calcified ring shadow in the right iliac fossa is consistent with a diagnosis of **gall stone ileus** (Fig 17.8).

Occasionally a **gastric volvulus** can cause a fluid level above the diaphragm.

An erect chest radiograph may demonstrate free gas under the diaphragm but this must be

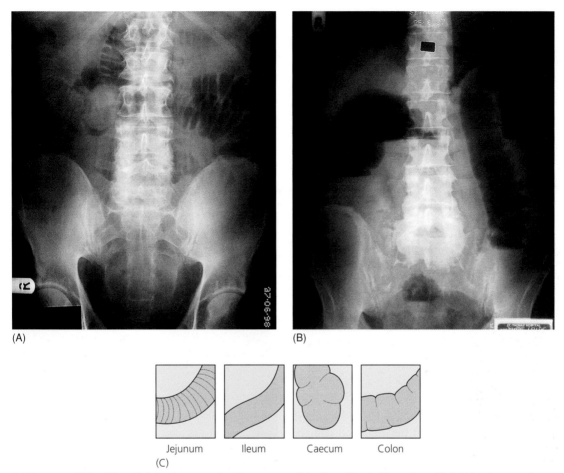

Jejunum   Ileum   Caecum   Colon
(C)

FIGURE 17.5 (A) Small bowel distension on supine X-ray gaseas distention with a ladder pattern; (B) fluid levels on erect plain abdominal X-ray; (C) patterns of bowel when obstructed

differentiated from loops of bowel caught up above the liver (Chilaiditi's sign) (Fig 17.9) or a gastric fluid level.

A chest radiograph can also demonstrate pulmonary consolidation and collapse (conditions which can present with signs similar to those of an acute abdomen) and other extra-abdominal causes of the abdominal pain such as fractured ribs (see Chapter 14).

Contrast radiography

Intravenous pyelography/urography (IVP/IVU) This is helpful when a urinary cause of abdominal pain, especially a **ureteric calculus**, is suspected. Ultrasound and CT scanning are alternative ways of imaging the kidneys and bladder, especially in patients presenting with pain after abdominal trauma (see Chapter 20).

Barium/gastrografin swallow/meal This may be used to confirm **Boerhaave's syndrome** (see page 394). This is used in some centres as a means of diagnosing a perforated peptic ulcer, especially if no free gas can be seen on the plain radiograph. Contrast medium escaping from the perforated viscus is diagnostic.

A small bowel meal/enema This may be helpful in some cases of abdominal pain with subacute obstruction, especially when **Crohn's disease, radiation enteritis**, a small bowel tumour or a lymphoma are suspected. Crohn's disease causes a long

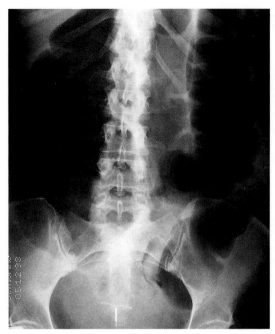

FIGURE 17.6 Distended caecum on plain abdominal X-ray

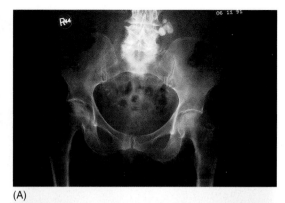

(A)

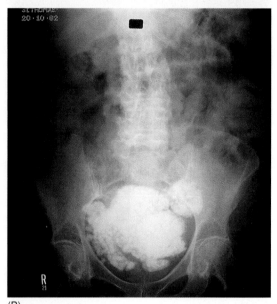

(B)

FIGURE 17.7 Calcification in the abdomen in (A) lymph nodes, (B) fibroids

stricture and the presence of 'skip lesions' is almost diagnostic (see Fig 17.24A) but radiation damage can produce a similar picture. Tumours cause a filling defect.

Barium enema The technique may help separate true large bowel obstruction from pseudo-obstruction. In the latter, the barium passes all the way through the distended bowel whereas in the former its progress is halted at the site of the obstruction (Fig 17.10).

It may sometimes provide useful information on the presence and site of other large bowel pathology. A barium enema can, however, cause perforation of inflamed diverticula of the sigmoid colon. Flexible sigmoidoscopy and colonoscopy (see below) are often more informative.

A barium enema can be therapeutic as well as diagnostic for **childhood intussusception** (Fig 17.11).

Angiography/CT angiography This can provide useful information in patients with chronic mesenteric ischaemia to confirm disease in the mesenteric vessels and may be both diagnostic and therapeutic in patients with severe abdominal haemorrhage when

therapeutic embolization may be used to control bleeding. This is especially valuable in patients with liver or pelvic trauma (see Chapter 6). Angiography is essential if a ruptured intra-abdominal aneurysm is being considered for treatment by the insertion of a stent graft (see Chapter 11).

CT angiography is replacing contrast angiography as a diagnostic test as it avoids the need for an arterial puncture.

Abdominal ultrasound

Abdominal ultrasound is a cheaper test than CT scanning, does not carry the radiation

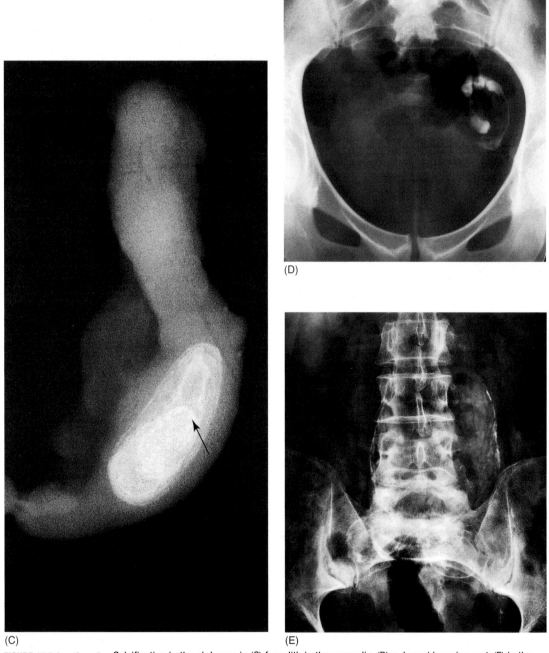

(C)

(D)

(E)

FIGURE 17.7 (continued)   Calcification in the abdomen in (C) faecolith in the appendix, (D) a dermoid ovarian cyst, (E) in the wall an aortic aneurysm

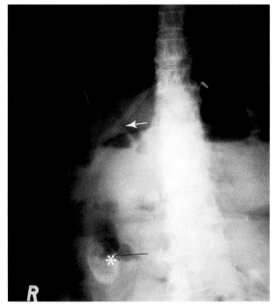

FIGURE 17.8   Gall stone ileus and small bowel obstruction: air in the biliary tree (arrow) and the gall stone (∗)

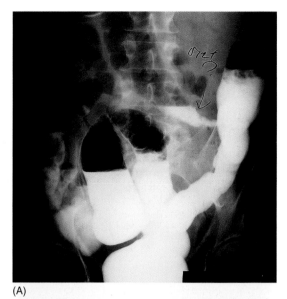

(A)

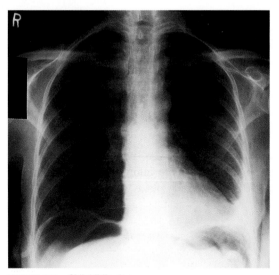

FIGURE 17.9   Chilaiditi's sign

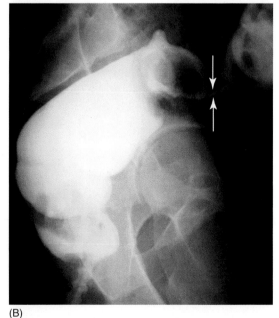

(B)

FIGURE 17.10   Barium enema: (A) obstruction at splenic flexure; (B) obstruction at rectosigmoid junction

hazard and is available in most Accident and Emergency Departments. It is very useful for confirming **gall bladder**, **pancreatic**, **hepatic**, **renal** and **bladder pathology**. Abdominal aortic aneurysms are also easily detected (see Chapter 11), but a CT scan provides more information if rupture is suspected. Ultrasound is good at detecting free intraperitoneal fluid. When free intraperitoneal fluid is seen, it can be accurately sampled using fine needle aspiration and sent for cytological, biochemical or microbiological analysis.

Transabdominal and **transvaginal** ultrasound are both very good at imaging pelvic pathology

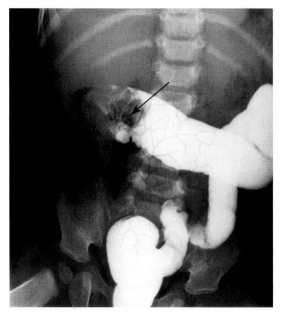

FIGURE 17.11   Barium enema of an intussusception (arrowed)

such as **ovarian cysts**, **twisted fibroids**, **ectopic pregnancies** and **infected fallopian tubes**.

Ultrasound has been used as a diagnostic test of appendicitis but is less accurate than CT scanning (see below) in confirming the diagnosis.

Instant CT imaging of the chest, abdomen and pelvis

There is a growing tendency for all patients presenting with severe unexplained abdominal pain to be 'passed through' the CT scanner. In fact this is now common for all patients who complain of abdominal pain after severe abdominal trauma. This approach has its advantages but is often unnecessary and can delay the commencement of treatment.

CT scanning can detect controlled leaks in patients with palpable abdominal aneurysms who have no signs of hypovolaemia, especially in patients who are very obese.

It can detect small amounts of free gas or trapped gas within the abdomen which is not visible on a plain radiograph.

It scans can display **intra-abdominal abscesses**, **unsuspected secondary deposits in the liver**, **splenic infarcts** and **splenic trauma**.

CT scans may demonstrate colonic and other tumours, especially when combined with a barium enema, and are particularly useful in displaying **pancreatic pathology** such as infarction and pseudo-cysts. Evidence of pancreatic swelling, haemorrhage or infarction will confirm the diagnosis of **acute pancreatitis**.

Although CT scans have been used to confirm the diagnosis of acute appendicitis with some success, the accuracy of CT scanning, like ultrasound, does not approach the 100 per cent accuracy needed for the proper clinical management of this condition.

Cytology

Peritoneal fluid can be collected through an ultrasound or CT-guided needle (see above), and provide useful information. The fluid can be tested for white cells, bacteria, amylase and blood content. This guided approach has largely replaced the blind four-quadrant needle tap and diagnostic peritoneal lavage.

Endoscopy

Proctoscopy and rigid sigmoidoscopy These may be undertaken if rectal pathology is suspected. A **sigmoid volvulus** can be decompressed by passing a flatus tube via a sigmoidoscope through the twist.

Rectal and low sigmoid tumours may be visible through a rigid sigmoidoscope and can be biopsied.

Flexible sigmoidoscopy and colonoscopy These investigations provide more information on large bowel pathology than any other tests and may be valuable in decompressing the bowel of patients with pseudo-obstruction. Colonic tumours and colitis have typical appearances and can be biopsied. Useful information can be obtained about the presence and extent of any colitis, diverticulitis or ischaemic colitis.

The colonoscope can be passed into the distal ileum, which can also be biopsied should Crohn's disease be suspected.

Upper gastrointestinal (GI) endoscopy This investigation provides information on any abnormality in the oesophagus, stomach and duodenum. Boerhaave's syndrome and hiatus hernia may be confirmed and peptic ulceration and carcinoma of the stomach seen and biopsied.

ERCP, cholangiography, percutaneous transhepatic cholangiography and endoscopic ultrasound All these investigations may be used to diagnose and treat bile duct stones, pancreatic duct strictures and pancreatic pseudo cysts in patients with upper abdominal pain associated with jaundice (see Chapter 18).

Laparoscopy

This investigation is now widely used by all general surgeons. It can be both **diagnostic** and **therapeutic**.

When the diagnosis of **acute appendicitis** is in doubt, young women should, if possible, have a diagnostic laparoscopy, before an appendicectomy, to avoid the removal of a normal appendix. Many of these patients will be found to have ovarian pathology (e.g. ruptured mid-cycle cysts).

Laparoscopy may also be used to confirm the diagnosis of a **perforated ulcer** and to close the perforation with sutures, through the laparoscope, at the same time. Laparoscopy is **not** good for examining the structures of the retroperitoneum, i.e. the aorta and pancreas.

Laparoscopy should be avoided when there is bowel obstruction, as the dilated loops of bowel obscure the view and can be perforated during insertion of the canulae especially if the bowel is adherent to the abdominal wall.

Laparotomy

It is debatable if this is an investigation, but it is discussed here as a reminder that this is often **the final diagnostic test** in patients with acute abdominal pain in whom a diagnosis cannot be reached. It must also be considered when there is genuine concern that to delay treatment while complex investigations are undertaken might adversely affect the patient's survival. When a diagnosis cannot be made in an acceptable timeframe a laparotomy for diagnosis and treatment may be essential.

Management

Immediate care

Patients with abdominal pain need immediate care whatever management pathway the clinical indicators and the tests described above indicate.

Patients should be relieved of their pain and resuscitated while the history and examination are being conducted. **Opioid analgesia** can be given before palpating the abdomen without interfering with diagnosis.

Oxygen should be given by a mask to patients who are obviously dyspnoeic or shocked, especially if the pO_2 or saturations reduced.

Intravenous access should be obtained by one or more large-diameter intravenous catheters placed in the antecubital veins in all patients who are in severe pain and shocked. **Crystalloids** should be infused. In most circumstances all patients benefit from a litre of crystalloid, especially if the pain has been present for more the 24 hours, or if they have had repeated vomiting or diarrhoea.

Resuscitation with **intravenous fluids** in patients with a suspected ruptured aneurysm should be administered cautiously as their hypotension is homeostatic and reduces the risk of a fatal rebleed (see Chapter 11).

A **urinary catheter** should be inserted in all shocked or dehydrated patients, as the urine output is an important measurement for assessing the effect of fluid replacement.

A **central venous pressure** (CVP) line should be inserted in patients who appear to be in hypovolaemic shock, especially if they have septicaemia or evidence of cardiac pathology. A CVP line is an excellent method of monitoring the adequacy of fluid replacement and provides a route of rapid access to the circulation.

Antibiotics should be started if infection is suspected. All patients suspected of having acute appendicitis, acute cholecystitis, acute pancreatitis or acute sigmoid diverticulitis should be given broad-spectrum antibiotics active against anaerobic and aerobic organisms, such as a cephalosporin and metronidazole or augmentin. Gentamicin (80 mg bd or tds depending upon blood levels) should be added in cases of severe Gram-negative peritonitis accompanied by septic shock.

Most patients being considered for operation should be aggressively resuscitated in close consultation with the anaesthetist in order to get the patient in the best possible condition for surgery at a specific time. *There is now unequivocal evidence that preoperative resuscitation is beneficial before emergency surgery, but it must be remembered that over or prolonged resuscitation in the presence of continuing sepsis or blood loss is harmful. It is therefore* important to formulate a clear plan of resuscitation and carefully monitor the patient until optimal conditions are obtained. Continuing fluid and blood replacement in the face of patient deterioration must be avoided.

Prophylaxis against deep vein thrombosis and pulmonary embolism should be considered in every case (see page 29).

Management plan

The possible routes for managing acute abdominal pain have been described at the beginning of this section. Although the investigations described above will probably have informed the clinician of the diagnosis and the urgency for treatment, further investigations may be needed before treatment can begin. These will be condition specific and are described later.

CAUSES OF PAIN IN THE UPPER ABDOMEN

The common causes of upper abdominal pain are:

- acute and chronic peptic ulceration
- acute cholecystitis
- perforated peptic ulcer
- acute pancreatitis.

Less common causes of upper abdominal pain are:

- gastric volvulus
- Boerhaave's syndrome
- ruptured abdominal aortic aneurysm
- Curtis–Fitz–Hugh syndrome
- acute hepatitis and liver metastases
- infarction of the spleen
- acute appendicitis
- myocardial infarction
- pneumonia.

The further investigation and management of each of these conditions is described below.

ACUTE PEPTIC ULCERATION/ GASTRITIS

Acute peptic ulcers often develop in response to *Helicobacter pylori*, non-steroidal anti-inflammatory drugs or a noxious stimulus. Systemic inflammatory syndrome (SIRS), severe burns (Curling's ulcer) and a head injury (Cushing's ulcer) are all recognized causes of acute peptic ulceration. Acute ulcers can also develop following a mucosal breach in either the stomach or duodenum. They have very little fibrosis in their bases and can present with haematemesis (see Chapter 18) but rarely perforate or develop into chronic ulceration. *H. pylori*, which are spirochaetal organisms, are often present and can be confirmed by a CLO breath test.

Investigation

Clinical diagnostic indicators

Acute peptic ulceration causes acute upper abdominal pain, usually following eating, which the patient often describes as indigestion. They may have had previous attacks and be taking non-steroidal anti-inflammatory drugs.

Endoscopy

Upper GI endoscopy will confirm the diagnosis.

Management

Prophylaxis in high-risk patients (e.g. those in intensive care) is sensible and usually consists of administering **proton pump inhibitors** (omeprazole, orally or intravenously).

Triple therapy should be used for *H. pylori* eradication as for chronic ulceration (see below).

A clear association has been recognized between acute peptic ulceration, acute gastritis, oesophagitis, duodenitis and multiple gastric erosions. All these conditions are manifestations of hyperacidity, *H. pylori* infection and reduced mucosal resistance. Oesophagitis is covered elsewhere (see Chapter 18). **Acute gastritis** may be related to bile reflux through the duodenum but it is also related to non-steroidal anti-inflammatory drugs, chronic alcoholism and a reduced mucosal blood supply (burns and sepsis). These conditions can present with epigastric discomfort and vomiting but they are often only suspected if a patient has a haematemesis or melaena (see Chapter 18).

All are diagnosed with certainty by endoscopy because they have characteristic appearances (Fig 17.12) and all usually respond to proton pump inhibitors. CLO tests should be carried out and patients started on eradication medication.

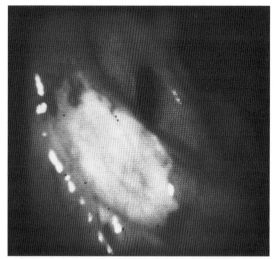

FIGURE 17.12   Chronic duodenal ulcer seen at endoscopy

Table 17.3
Differential diagnosis of chronic peptic ulceration

Chronic cholecystitis

Reflux oesophagitis

Carcinoma of the stomach

Chronic pancreatitis

Carcinoma of the pancreas

Non-ulcer dyspepsia

Irritable bowel syndrome

Sub-acute small bowel obstruction

CHRONIC PEPTIC ULCERATION

Investigation

Clinical diagnostic indicators

Chronic peptic ulceration usually presents with dyspepsia but can present with persistent epigastric pain that may radiate to the back. The pain is characteristically episodic (it has a periodicity with exacerbations lasting days or weeks). The relationship to food is variable, being either made worse by food (suggestive of a gastric ulcer) or made better by food (suggestive of a duodenal ulcer). Patients with duodenal ulcers tend to develop pain at night as the acid levels rise in the absence of food to neutralize the acid. The pain may be associated with water brash. Chronic peptic ulcers may also present with the complications listed in Table 17.4, which are discussed in subsequent sections.

There are often no physical signs associated with uncomplicated peptic ulceration so the main differential diagnoses may be any of the conditions that cause acute and chronic upper abdominal pain. The main other differential diagnoses are chronic cholecystitis and gall stone colic (see Chapter 18) and the other conditions listed in Table 17.3.

Blood tests

Blood tests are not usually helpful. A positive **breath test** or *H. pylori serology* will support the diagnosis of chronic peptic ulceration if positive, but neither is diagnostic.

If endoscopy reveals multiple ulcers extending into the second part of the duodenum or into the oesophagus, the **serum gastrum level** should be measured to exclude the possibility of **Zollinger–Ellison syndrome** (see Chapter 18).

Endoscopy or imaging

A choice has to be made between obtaining **upper GI endoscopy** or an **ultrasound of the gall bladder and pancreas**, because both gall bladder disease and chronic peptic ulceration can co-exist and have similar symptoms.

Unfortunately, many primary care doctors start patients on proton pump inhibitors or even antacids (which many patients have already tried by the time they go to the doctor) without bothering to try to confirm the diagnosis! Although this policy may appear cost-effective, it will fail to detect some patients with an early (treatable) carcinoma of the stomach.

Consequently, it is safer to refer all patients for a CLO test and an upper GI endoscopy, because this will diagnose almost all peptic ulcer pathology, providing it is properly performed by an experienced endoscopist.

Tissue biopsy

Biopsies should be taken from four quadrants of all gastric ulcers to exclude early malignant change.

Patients with dyspepsia and repeated negative tests can be diagnosed as having **non-ulcer**

dyspepsia. Many are probably suffering from irritable bowel syndrome.

Management

Medical management

Almost all patients with a chronic peptic ulcer are treated for 7 days with a **proton pump inhibitor** (**omeprazole** or **lansoprazole**) combined with any two of **amoxicillin**, **erythromycin** or **metronidazole**. Repeated courses of medical treatment can be given without causing harm.

Patients should be advised to avoid non-steroidal anti-inflammatory drugs if possible and be given help to stop smoking. *There is no evidence that changes in the diet or avoidance of 'stress' are of any benefit.*

Gastric protective agents such as bismuth and sucralfate are no longer used as first-line treatment.

Surgical management

There is almost no place for surgical treatment of chronic peptic ulcers today. All gastric surgery has a mortality and morbidity that is now considered unacceptable.

Gastric surgery for peptic ulceration is now reserved for patients with Zollinger–Ellison syndrome, those with complications and those who for some reason will not or cannot take medical treatment.

THE HISTORY OF SURGICAL TREATMENTS

There are many patients who have had surgical treatment in the past and present with the complications of that treatment, so it is important to understand the nature of some now unused operations.

The original Billroth I and Polya partial gastrectomies (Fig 17.13) used to treat gastric and duodenal ulcers were designed to reduce the production of gastric acid by removing the acid-producing part of the stomach. These operations were abandoned because they had a mortality of 1–2 per cent and a considerable morbidity (30 per cent or more, see below) and when it was shown that a similar reduction of gastric acid production could be achieved by vagotomy. Unfortunately, when duodenal ulcers were treated by truncal vagotomy, with pyloroplasty, gastro-enterostomy or antrectomy to avoid gastric hold-up (after dividing the major gastric motor

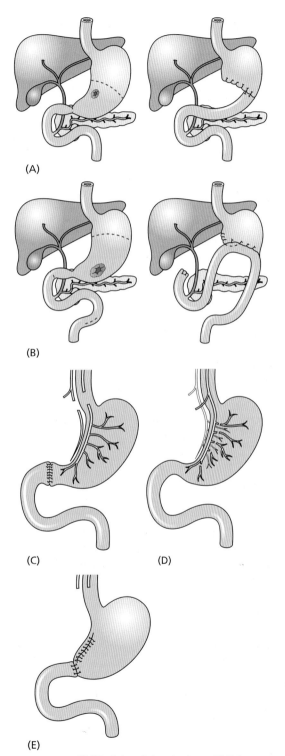

(A)

(B)

(C)   (D)

(E)

FIGURE 17.13 (A) Bilroth I partial gastrectomy. (B) Polya partial gastrectomy. (C) Truncal vagotomy. (D) Highly selective vagotomy. (E) Truncal vagotomy and gastrectomy

nerve), it was found that this caused mild diarrhoea in 10–15 per cent of patients and severe uncontrollable diarrhoea in 2 per cent. The operation of highly selective vagotomy was then developed to conserve the nerve supply of the antrum and abolish the need for a drainage procedure. Although this operation almost stopped the complication of postoperative diarrhoea it has now been replaced by effective antacid compounds (H2 receptor blockers and proton pump inhibitors) and antibiotics effective against *H. pylori*.

COMPLICATIONS OF GASTRIC SURGERY

The mortality from partial gastrectomy was a consequence of anastomotic breakdown, duodenal stump leakage or other complications that follow any major operation. Diarrhoea was the major complication of truncal vagotomy and drainage (see above). Highly selective vagotomy had fewer problems but a higher risk of duodenal ulcer recurrence.

The **post-gastrectomy syndromes** listed below are still seen today:

- small stomach – weight loss
- dumping – early (hyperosmolar load)
- dumping – late (hypoglycaemic swing)
- B12 and folate deficiency – loss of intrinsic factor
- obstruction of proximal or distal loop
- small bowel obstruction
- duodenogastric reflux
- carcinoma developing in the gastric stump
- delayed emptying
- increased risk of infection
- increased risk of gall stones.

Treatment of these complications can be by complex reconstructions, often involving an interposition Roux loop. These operations are only about 50–60 per cent successful.

COMPLICATIONS OF PEPTIC ULCERATION

- Pyloric stenosis (see Chapter 18)
- Perforated peptic ulcer (see below)
- Haematemesis and melaena (see Chapter 18)

- Malignant change – in gastric ulcers (see Chapter 18)
- Gastrointestinal fistula (see Chapter 18)

PERFORATED PEPTIC ULCER

Investigation
Clinical diagnostic indicators

A perforated peptic ulcer usually presents with the sudden onset of severe epigastric pain which then spreads across the abdomen, accompanied by board-like abdominal rigidity, shock and absent bowel sounds.

Patients have often been taking non-steroidal anti-inflammatory drugs and some will give a history of chronic indigestion. The differential diagnoses include all those conditions that can present with acute upper abdominal pain and any that can cause acute peritonitis. **Always consider mesenteric infarction and acute pancreatitis.**

Immediate care

Before proceeding with any diagnostic investigations the patient should be given **opioid analgesia**, **intravenous crystalloids**, **nasogastric aspiration** and **antibiotics**. Continuation of this conservative approach is reasonable when the signs remain localized, the patient's vital signs are stable and there is little leakage of contrast after a gastrograffin meal. A conservative approach may also be preferable if the patient is in a hostile environment (e.g. at sea or in a remote place distant from surgical facilities).

Blood tests

A full blood count and measurement of the blood **urea and electrolytes** are advisable before operation but rarely assist in confirming the diagnosis.

Imaging

An **erect chest radiograph** is likely to confirm the clinical diagnosis because it shows air under the diaphragm in more than 70 per cent of patients with a perforated ulcer. Alternatively, a **lateral decubitus** view may be helpful (see Fig 17.4).

A water-soluble gastrograffin meal may reveal a leak into the peritoneal cavity even when no air is visible on plain radiographs (Fig 17.14). An **ultrasound** examination can demonstrate other pathology, e.g. gall stones.

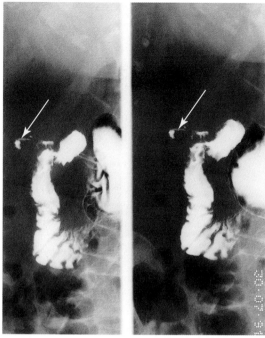

FIGURE 17.14 Leak of gastrograffin through a duodenal perforation

An **abdominal CT scan** can demonstrate small amounts of free gas more efficiently than an erect chest or abdominal X-ray.

Management

The treatment of a perforated peptic ulcer is usually surgical but in some circumstances a conservative non-surgical regimen may be appropriate, especially when the presentation is late and the patient has other serious medical problems.

Surgical closure is performed via a **laparoscope** or a **laparotomy** under general anaesthesia. The perforation is closed with sutures and an omental patch sewn over the suture line (Fig 17.15). There does not appear to be any major advantage to the laparoscopic approach other than the avoidance of a larger scar. If peritoneal lavage is be required it can be more easily and more thoroughly performed through a full-size laparotomy incision.

Whereas perforated duodenal ulcers can be closed by simple suture, the edges of a perforated **gastric ulcer** should be **excised** for biopsy before being closed because some perforated ulcers will be **gastric carcinomata**.

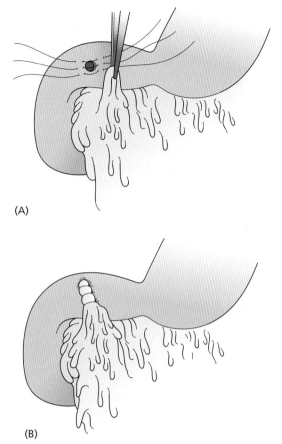

FIGURE 17.15 (A, B) Closure of peptic ulcer perforation with an omental patch

***H. pylori* eradication therapy** should be given once the patient has recovered from the operation, to reduce the risk of reperforation in subsequent years, and the patient should be told to avoid non-steroidal anti-inflammatory drugs.

A conservative regimen may be employed when the presentation is late or the patient has other serious medical problems. It consists of pain relief with **opioid analgesia**, **intravenous crystalloids**, **nasogastric aspiration** and **antibiotics**. Complications such as septic shock and intra-abdominal abscess formation are not uncommon, because the peritoneum is not washed clear of food debris and the natural healing with closure of the perforation by adhesions is slow.

This method of management is now rarely used but should not be forgotten.

Table 17.4
Complications that may follow a perforated peptic ulcer

Abscess
Wound infection
Re-perforation
Lung atelectasis
Pulmonary embolism
Gastric outlet obstruction
Sub-phrenic abscess
Multi-organ failure

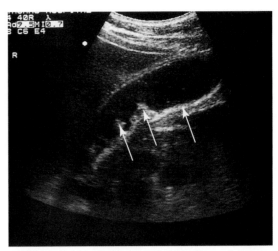

FIGURE 17.16   Ultrasound of gall bladder with a gall stones and thickened wall (arrows)

Complications

The complications that may follow a perforated peptic ulcer are shown in Table 17.4.

The mortality after both open and laparoscopic repair is 5–10 per cent.

ACUTE CHOLECYSTITIS

Investigation

Diagnostic clinical indicators

A history of indigestion coming on several hours after meals may precede the acute attack of pain. The pain is usually severe, central and continuous and often radiates to the tip of the scapula. Associated symptoms include vomiting, which is common. Middle-aged women are most commonly affected.

Tenderness just below the costal margin is almost invariably present. There is a palpable gall bladder mass in 5 per cent. The presence of Murphy's or Boas' sign is highly suggestive of the diagnosis (see *Symptoms and Signs*). Patients are rarely jaundiced but are commonly pyrexial.

Blood and urine tests

A full blood count and **liver function tests** should be obtained within 12 hours, especially if the patient is jaundiced. The urine should be tested for **urobilinogen** and **bilirubin.**

A **serum amylase** may be helpful in excluding a perforated peptic ulcer and pancreatitis.

Imaging

An **upper abdominal ultrasound** is the most important investigation. Diagnostic features are a thickened gall bladder wall and the presence of gall stones seen as filling defects casting acoustic shadows (Fig 17.16). The presence of gall stones is not enough to confirm the diagnosis, but taken with a typical history and a thickened gall bladder wall it is highly suggestive. Upper abdominal ultrasound has about a 95 per cent accuracy for diagnosing acute cholecystitis.

An erect chest radiograph may be helpful in excluding a perforated peptic ulcer and pancreatitis. Rarer differential diagnoses are shown on page 383.

Management

The patient's pain should be relieved by **opioids** before being admitted for bed rest and ultrasound confirmation of the diagnosis.

Oral fluids should be restricted if the patient is nauseated or vomiting. **Intravenous fluids** are administered if the patient has been vomiting or there is evidence of dehydration. (Further tests and investigations are undertaken if the patient is jaundiced, see Chapter 18).

Antibiotics such as a cephalosporin are active against common biliary tract organisms and should be given if the patient is pyrexial or has a marked leucocytosis.

Subcutaneous heparin should be commenced to reduce the risk of deep vein thrombosis.

Once the diagnosis has been confirmed by ultrasound, patients can be treated surgically (cholecystectomy) or conservatively.

Conservative management is selected when the attack has already lasted several days or when the patient is jaundiced. Most patients treated conservatively can be sent home once their pain has subsided and then readmitted for an **elective laparoscopic cholecystectomy** 6–8 weeks later.

An **early operation** (cholecystectomy) has been shown by many studies to be desirable, but only when the duration of the attack is less than 24–48 hours, the patient is fit and the diagnosis has been confirmed by ultrasound.

Most elective cholecystectomies are now performed **laparoscopically** through four ports (Fig 17.17). After the establishment of a pneumoperitoneum, a camera is inserted through a 10-mm port and the fundus of the gall bladder grasped and pulled upwards. The cystic artery and cystic duct are dissected out of Calot's triangle and then clipped, or ligated by endosuture, and divided. The gall bladder with its contained stones is then dissected off the under-surface of the liver and removed through one of the larger ports (Fig 17.18).

Some surgeons believe that this operation should always include **intraoperative cholangiography** but this is not the view of the majority. To obtain an operative cholangiogram, the cystic duct has to be opened and a cannula passed into the common bile duct before the X-ray contrast medium can be injected. An image intensifier is used to take the X-rays. The advantage of this procedure is that it displays the anatomy of the biliary tree and detects any stones in the bile ducts (Fig 17.19).

Patients who develop repeated acute attacks or those who develop **biliary peritonitis**, which is often associated with a **gangrenous** or **perforated gall bladder**, require urgent surgery.

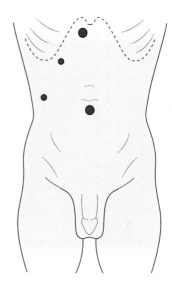

(A)

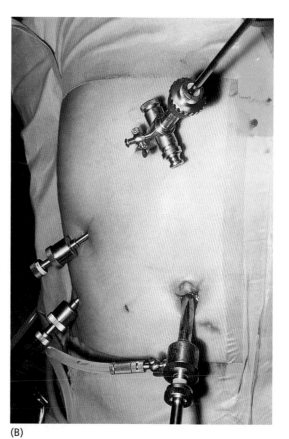

(B)

FIGURE 17.17   (A, B) Ports inserted for laparoscopic cholecystectomy

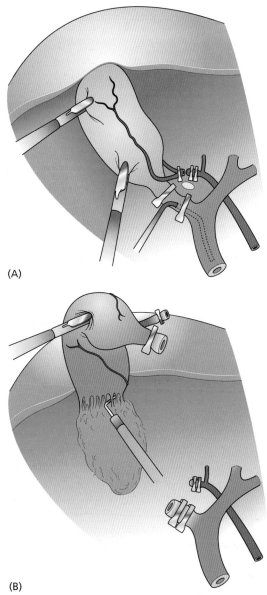

(A)

(B)

FIGURE 17.18   (A, B) Laparoscopic cholecystectomy

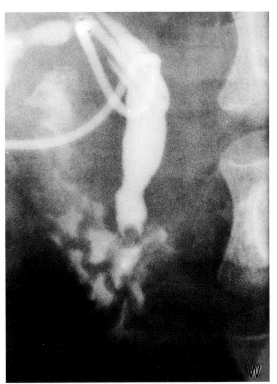

FIGURE 17.19   Stone in common bile duct shown on cholangiogram

Table 17.5
Complications of acute cholecystitis

Obstructive jaundice

Acute pancreatitis

Empyema of gall bladder (pus in the gall bladder)

Mucocele of the gall bladder (mucous distention of the gall bladder)

Mirrizi's syndrome (common bile duct obstructed by stone in Hartman's pouch)

Acute cholangitis

Cholecysto-enteric fistula and gall stone ileus

Complications

The complications of acute cholecystitis are shown in Table 17.5.

Results

The results of laparoscopic cholecystectomy for acute cholecystitis are good. The mortality rate is less than 0.5 per cent provided the bile ducts are not damaged.

There is a 0.2–0.3 per cent risk of **residual stones** being left in the common bile duct (see Chapter 18).

Bile duct damage is rare (>0.5 per cent) but carries a considerable morbidity and increases the mortality rate. Other complications include **leakage of bile** from the cystic duct or **haemorrhage** from the cystic artery if the clips fall off or are incorrectly applied.

CHRONIC CHOLECYSTITIS

Chronic cholecystitis is almost always associated with gall stones. Its investigation and management is therefore similar to that described above for acute cholecystitis.

It commonly causes attacks of pain or discomfort in the right hypochondrium, similar to but milder than the pain of acute cholecystitis and a variety of less diagnostic symptoms such as indigestion and post-prandial flatulence, beginning 30–50 minutes after eating and often associated with eating fatty food.

The investigations required are the same as those described above for acute cholecystitis, the most important being the **ultrasound** detection of gall stones.

The management of chronic cholecystitis is **cholecystectomy** and the removal of any stones in the biliary tree. Many patients may have long symptom-free intervals between each attack so the timing and need for surgical intervention depends upon the frequency and the severity of the attacks.

ACUTE PANCREATITIS

Investigation

Clinical diagnostic indicators

The presentation of acute pancreatitis is often similar to that of acute cholecystitis and perforated peptic ulcer and the many other causes of the acute abdomen.

The pain of pancreatitis is usually experienced in the epigastrium and/or the hypochondrium and often radiates through to the back. **Frequent vomiting is common**.

The patient is often distressed with signs of shock – tachycardia, tachypnoea – and has cool sweaty peripheries. Jaundice and pyrexia are rare.

Upper abdominal tenderness is always present, *but often less marked than the severity of the pain would lead you to expect.* Guarding and rebound tenderness indicates 'peritonism'.

The abdominal signs may be generalized and accompanied by distension, and eventually a loss of bowel sounds. Bruising in the flank (Grey Turner's sign) or around the umbilicus (Cullen's sign) are rare but pathognomonic (see *Symptoms and signs*). An **epigastric mass** indicates a **phlegmon** or a developing pancreatic **pseudocyst** but it rarely presents in the first 24 hours.

There may be the clinical signs of a pleural effusion.

In addition to the causes of acute upper abdominal pain (see Table 17.2), always consider the possibility of **mesenteric infarction** and **small bowel volvulus**, as both these conditions may be associated with a raised serum amylase.

Blood tests

A **serum amylase** three or four times above normal is almost diagnostic. An elevated **serum lipase** may be more accurate but is less readily available. If the patient presents late, the **urinary amylase** may still be raised when the blood amylase level has returned to normal.

Remember, the serum amylase can be mildly elevated in patients with a perforated ulcer, acute obstructive jaundice, a closed loop obstruction of the small bowel and in association with bowel ischaemia.

Haemoglobin, packed cell volume, C-reactive protein and **white cell count** should be measured, as should the **urea and electrolytes**.

The **serum calcium, glucose** and **liver function tests** should be obtained, especially if the patient is jaundiced. These investigations may all be abnormal and indicate the severity of the condition (see later). They should definitely be **measured within 12 hours of the start of the attack**.

Urine tests

The urine should be tested, on admission, for **bilirubin** and **urobilinogen**.

Imaging

Plain abdominal X-rays are useful in excluding a perforated ulcer (free gas), gall stones (10 per cent of which are opaque) and a closed-loop obstruction.

An **erect chest radiograph** may reveal a pleural effusion.

Ultrasound often fails to visualize the pancreas because of associated bowel distension. Nevertheless, an abdominal ultrasound should be

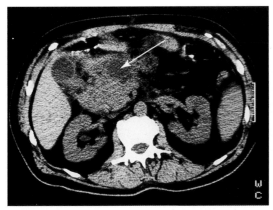

FIGURE 17.20   A swollen pancreas containing liquefaction (arrowed)

Table 17.6
Modified Glasgow criteria

P_aO_2	<60 mmHg (8 kPa)
Albumin	<32 g/L
Calcium	<2.0 mmol/L
White cell count	>15 × 10⁹ cells/L
Aspartate transaminase	>100 units/L
Lactate dehydrogenase	>600 units/L
Glucose	>10 mmol/L*
Urea	>16 mmol/L

*In non-diabetic patients

obtained urgently to determine if there are associated gall stones or biliary tree dilatation.

Any free intraperitoneal fluid seen on ultrasound should be aspirated and sent for amylase or lipase estimation. High levels confirm the diagnosis.

Abdominal CT scanning may show a swollen pancreas.

Dynamic contrast CT scanning is a CT scan performed after the injection of an X-ray contrast medium. If performed between the third and tenth day of the attack it may reveal the extent of any pancreatic necrosis (Fig 17.20) and demonstrate any collections of fluid that may have become infected and require fine needle aspiration and drainage.

Laparotomy

Some patients in whom the diagnosis remains uncertain and in whom there is a real risk of misdiagnosis must be submitted to **laparotomy** to confirm swelling and inflammation of the pancreas. Gall bladder or bile duct pathology, cirrhosis and ascites may also be present.

Evidence of **fat necrosis** (little white plaques occurring most commonly in the omentum and mesentery caused by the release of lipases that digest the fat which then takes up calcium) is diagnostic.

Management

The management is based on the clinical indicators and the tests described above. The decisions are:

- the patient requires an urgent operation
- an urgent operation is definitely not required

- the need for an urgent operation remains uncertain and a management decision cannot be made without further observation and investigation.

In the first set of circumstances the baseline investigations and adequate resuscitation must precede transfer to the operating theatre. In the second and third scenarios the patient should be examined repeatedly and subjected to further investigation after appropriate analgesia and fluid resuscitation.

Calculation of the severity score

Acute pancreatitis needs to be separated into mild and severe disease as the management differs. Table 17.6 shows **a modified Glasgow scoring system.** Unfortunately this system and many others, e.g. C-reactive protein measurement and APACHE 2, are only reliable 48 hours after the beginning of the attack. In future other inflammatory markers or peptides may provide more accurate prognostic information.

The pancreatitis is considered **severe** if three or more of the severity score criteria are exceeded.

Management of mild pancreatitis

Treatment is usually **conservative** unless the pancreas becomes necrotic – a complication that requires surgical intervention.

Monitoring   The temperature, pulse, blood pressure, urine output and blood sugar should be carefully monitored and patients regularly re-examined to detect any change from a mild to a severe condition.

Intravenous fluids should be given especially if nasogastric aspiration is required to relieve repeated vomiting.

Opioid analgesia is usually required to control the pain.

Broad-spectrum antibiotics (augmentin, a cephalosporin or metronidazole) are prescribed by most surgeons.

Deep vein thrombosis prophylaxis must be considered (see Chapter 2).

After care The presence of gall stones and alcohol intake must be assessed before discharge from hospital. It may be necessary to perform a cholecystectomy or endoscopic retrograde cholangiopancreatography (ECRP) and sphincterotomy at a later date. Counselling may be required to prevent recurrence from alcohol abuse if the cause of the attack was alcohol intake.

Management of severe acute pancreatitis

Without expert resuscitation, patients with severe pancreatitis have a mortality rate approaching 50 per cent, so patients with severe acute pancreatitis should be admitted to a high dependency or an intensive care unit.

A central venous catheter, an arterial line and a urinary catheter are essential to assess the state of the circulation and renal function and optimize fluid and blood replacement.

A 7-day course of broad-spectrum antibiotics (cephalosporin or metronidazole) should be given in an attempt to prevent the necrotic pancreatic tissue (the phlegmon) becoming infected. Infection quadruples the mortality rate.

Patients may require **oxygen, inotropes, ventilation** and even **dialysis** to try to prevent the onset of **multi-organ failure**.

ERCP and the removal of bile duct stones

The presence of jaundice, gall stones or a dilated bile duct on an abdominal ultrasound indicates the need for **bile duct sphincterotomy and the removal of bile duct stones**. Early ERCP appears to reduce the mortality of gall stone pancreatitis and must be performed if ascending cholangitis is present.

Surgical drainage

A **pancreatic mass** found on clinical examination or imaging (ultrasound or CT scan) may be observed if it is small, but when its diameter

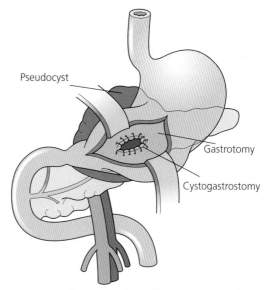

FIGURE 17.21 Cystogastrostomy. Stomach and cyst sutured together through gastrostomy which is then closed

increases above **6 cm** it is likely to contain pancreatic fluid and blood, become infected and **require drainage**. This can be performed **percutaneously or by an endoscopic transgastric route**. A very large cyst may require surgical drainage by open or laparoscopic **cystogastrostomy** (Fig 17.21).

Pancreatic necrosectomy

When a patient is deteriorating despite all the measures described above and there is evidence of massive pancreatic necrosis on a CT scan, or infection in a pancreatic aspirate, the patient should be considered for a **pancreatic necrosectomy**. In this procedure the necrotic pancreas is removed piecemeal at laparotomy and the abdomen washed out. It has a high morbidity and mortality (20–40 per cent).

If it seems likely that the procedure will have to be repeated, the abdomen can be loosely closed with a plastic sheet (a procedure known as a 'laparostomy') so that it can be easily reopened for further necrosectomies and washouts in the subsequent days and weeks.

A necrosectomy can be performed through a flank approach.

Continuing care

The patient should be told to stop drinking alcohol even if the attack was not initiated by an alcoholic 'binge'.

Table 17.7
The complications of pancreatitis

Repeated attacks of acute pancreatitis

Steatorrhoea

Diabetes

Multi-organ failure

Death (haemorrhage)

Table 17.8
Differential diagnoses of gastric volvulus

Perforated ulcer

Boerhaave's syndrome (when the vomiting usually precedes the pain)

Myocardial infarction

Dissecting aneurysm

Cholecystectomy should be recommended if gall stones are demonstrated once the patient has fully recovered.

A search for rarer causes of acute pancreatitis is probably only worthwhile if the condition follows a relapsing course.

Complications

The complications of acute pancreatitis are listed in Table 17.7.

Results

The prognosis following a single episode of mild pancreatitis is excellent with a mortality of less than 1 per cent, provided precipitating factors such as cholelithiasis and alcohol abuse are treated.

By contrast, severe pancreatitis has a mortality rate of around 10 per cent, which rises to 30 per cent if associated with severe necrosis and nearly 40 per cent if necrosectomy is necessary.

BOERHAAVES' SYNDROME

This rare condition occurs when a full thickness longitudinal tear develops at the oesophagogastric junction, usually as a consequence of the patient attempting to suppress a vomit.

Investigation

Clinical diagnostic indicators

This catastrophe commonly follows a suppressed vomit and is followed by the sudden onset of severe epigastric pain which may radiate into the lower chest. Abdominal tenderness, guarding and rigidity are usually present.

The presence of **subcutaneous emphysema** in the cervical region confirms the diagnosis.

The differential diagnoses are included in Table 17.8. **Myocardial infarction** and **dissecting aneurysm** are the most important conditions to exclude.

Imaging

A **chest radiograph** may demonstrate free air in the mediastinum, a pneumothorax or a pleural effusion. Air may also be seen tracking along the cervical muscles in the neck (**cervical subcutaneous emphysema**) (Fig 17.22).

A **barium** or **gastrograffin swallow** will confirm the diagnosis if it shows contrast medium leaking outside the wall of the oesophagus. This investigation should be obtained urgently as delay in treatment is the single most important factor associated with a poor outcome.

Endoscopy may visualize the tear but is rarely required.

Management

There are few indications for conservative management if the diagnosis is made early especially if the rent in the gastro-oesophageal junction is large.

Analgesia, antibiotics, intravenous fluids and the **restriction of all oral intake** are all essential.

It is best to repair the rent by simple **surgical closure** through a high mid-line abdominal incision under general anaesthesia. The repaired area may be covered by a fundoplication, a flap of intercostal muscle or the adjacent diaphragm.

If the diagnosis is delayed or the leak small, a **pleural drain** can be inserted and a conservative approach – fluids, analgesia and antibiotics – continued, but the risks of continuing sepsis and deterioration are high with such management.

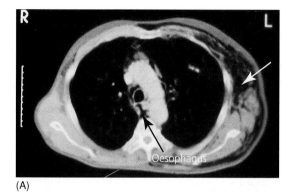

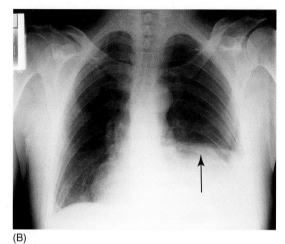

(A)

(B)

FIGURE 17.22 Boerhaaves' syndrome. (A) CT showing surgical emphysema from oesophageal leak; (B) pleural effusion on chest X-ray

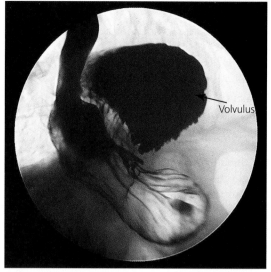

FIGURE 17.23 Gastric volvulus seen on barium swallow (see also page 462)

Imaging

The diagnosis should be suspected if an **erect chest radiograph** shows a fluid level in a section of stomach trapped inside a large hiatus hernia and may be confirmed by a **barium swallow** (Fig 17.23).

Management

The volvulus must be untwisted through an **upper mid-line incision** under general anaesthesia and the stomach reduced into the abdomen. If the stomach is gangrenous it must be resected.

The associated diaphragmatic defect should be repaired and the stomach fixed to the anterior abdominal wall to prevent a recurrence.

Results

The mortality is 10 per cent or less if treated early by surgery, but can rise to 50 per cent if treatment is delayed.

GASTRIC VOLVULUS

This is an extremely rare condition. It is invariably an organo-axial rotation of the stomach within a large paraoesophageal hiatus hernia.

Its **differential diagnoses** are listed in Table 17.8.

Investigation

Clinical diagnostic indicators

Gastric volvulus causes severe epigastric pain which may radiate up behind the sternum. It is usually accompanied by severe vomiting and dysphagia.

INFARCTION OF THE SPLEEN

This rare condition occurs **in pathologically enlarged spleens** and in patients with **sickle cell disease**. It usually causes pain in the left hypochondrium that may radiate to the tip of the left shoulder. Tenderness and guarding is usually present in the left hypochondrium.

The main differential diagnoses are **spontaneous splenic rupture** and **acute pancreatitis** in the tail of the pancreas.

Investigation

Dynamic CT scan with contrast will confirm the diagnosis.

Management

Analgesia and intravenous fluids usually provide sufficient relief until the pain subsides spontaneously, but large spleens with large infarcts may have to be removed by **splenectomy**.

All patients who have had their spleen removed should be given **pneumococcal antitoxin** and **antibiotics**.

CAUSES OF PAIN IN THE CENTRE OF THE ABDOMEN

The conditions that commonly present with central abdominal pain with or without peritonitis are:

- small bowel obstruction
- large bowel obstruction
- intestinal infarction/ischaemia
- small bowel volvulus
- small bowel perforation
- intussusception (usually with colic)
- Crohn's disease (usually with colic)
- leaking abdominal aneurysm.

SMALL BOWEL OBSTRUCTION

Investigation

Clinical diagnostic indicators

The **colicky pain** caused by small bowel obstruction is usually experienced in the central umbilical region of the abdomen. It is severe and gripping in nature. Each attack only lasts a short period. As the pain develops patients feel uncomfortable, and when it is severe they are unable to keep still.

The interval between the pains is short if the obstruction is in the upper jejunum (2–3 minutes) and longer if it is in the lower ileum (15–20 minutes).

There may be a prior history of **previous abdominal operations**, indicating the possibility of adhesions or a known hernia. These two conditions are the most common causes of small bowel obstruction, so the hernial orifices and abdominal scars must always be carefully palpated for irreducible masses.

Vomiting is common but abdominal distension and constipation only develop at a later stage.

On examination the patient may show signs of **dehydration**. Occasionally visible peristalsis may be observed in a thin person. **Abdominal tenderness** may be a sign of **impending infarction**, especially if there is marked **guarding** or **percussion tenderness**.

The **bowel sounds** are infrequent and high pitched. Time must be spent waiting for a peristaltic wave to occur.

Blood and urine tests

The urine will be **concentrated**, the **haematocrit high** and the **urea raised** with a **normal creatinine** if the patient is dehydrated.

Urea and electrolytes should be measured.

Imaging

Plain abdominal radiographs show gaseous distension of the small bowel lumen, which is in the central part of the abdomen and has a **ladder pattern** produced by the valvulae conniventes (see Fig 17.5).

The **erect film** is likely to show fluid levels (see Fig 17.5). A single loop may be all that is visible in a closed loop obstruction, but if this is fluid filled it may not show up until strangulation develops.

Gas in the biliary tree and a large calcified opacity in the right iliac fossa, with signs of small bowel obstruction, suggests obstruction by a gall stone (see Fig 17.8) (known as gall stone ileus).

A **small bowel enema** is only indicated when the obstruction is chronic and the cause obscure. Obstruction caused by **Crohn's disease** and **ascaris lumbricoides** have characteristic appearances (Fig 17.24).

CT scanning may help if the cause remains in doubt, similarly a **colonoscopy** or **barium enema** may help if it is considered that pathology in the large bowel has led to the appearances of small bowel obstruction because of an incompetent ileocaecal valve.

Laparotomy may be the only way to diagnose multiple malignant deposits in the peritoneal cavity and rare small bowel tumours.

Management

For **gastric aspiration**, an 8–10 French nasogastric tube is passed and placed on open drainage to

electrolytes levels, urine output specific gravity or osmolarity, is essential. Gastric aspirate is replaced by normal saline.

Remove the cause of the obstruction. Patients found to have an irreducible tender hernia should have this explored.

Patients who do not have any abdominal tenderness and are thought to have a possible adhesive obstruction may be treated for up to 24 hours with intravenous fluids and nasogastric suction to see if the obstruction will settle. When the cause of the obstruction remains unknown, further **CT scanning** and **small bowel enemas** can be obtained if the symptoms fail to settle or if the obstruction keeps recurring.

Laparotomy is indicated if the pain is worsening, abdominal tenderness is developing, the pulse rising or the nasogastric aspirate increasing in volume. At operation, constricting bands should be divided, bowel untwisted and – if infarcted or diseased – resected.

A primary end-to-end small bowel anastomosis is almost always possible except in patients with an abdomen frozen by adhesions or multiple malignant deposits. In the latter circumstances surgery should be avoided if possible. i.e. **no treatment** or a **side-to-side bypass**.

Enterotomies may be needed to remove foreign bodies. Foreign bodies in the ileum such as a plug of meconium may be milked into the large bowel.

Complications

Other or new adhesions may cause recurrent episodes of obstruction.

Aspiration pneumonia, wound infections, abdominal dehiscence and **incisional hernia** are all recognized complications of surgery for small bowel obstruction.

Results

Operations on otherwise fit patients with small bowel obstruction have a mortality rate of about 1 per cent, but it is much greater in patients who have widespread malignancy or a segment of strangulated bowel (up to 10 per cent).

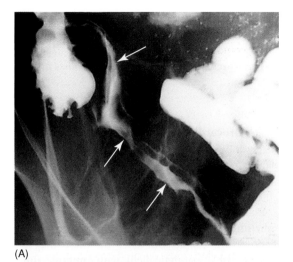

(A)

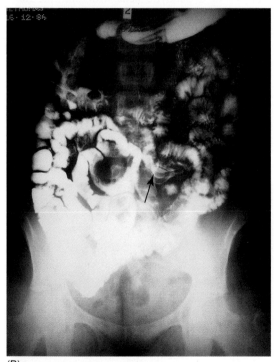

(B)

FIGURE 17.24   Small bowel enema. (A) Features of Crohn's disease (Cantor's string sign). (B) Ascaris lumbricoides, seen as smooth and cylindrical filling defects

reduce distension and prevent aspiration, both of which can compromise ventilation.

Intravenous normal saline and potassium supplements, monitored by measuring the urea and

SMALL BOWEL INFARCTION/ISCHAEMIA

Small bowel infarction can be caused by mesenteric artery thrombosis (50 per cent), arterial embolism (30 per cent), mesenteric vein thrombosis (10 per cent) and, rarely, by an acute aortic dissection.

A low cardiac output in combination with large doses of **inotropes** given for multiple organ failure can cause a patchy ischaemia of both the large and small intestine, as may **vasculitis** and **sickle cell disease**.

Investigation

Clinical diagnostic indicators

Patients may have a history of the prodromal symptoms of bowel ischaemia (intestinal angina and weight loss). Most patients present with central or generalized **constant abdominal pain** of sudden or variable onset. As the pain becomes more severe, patients develop signs of central or general peritonitis (tenderness, guarding, rebound, percussion tenderness and absent bowel sounds).

Some **abdominal distention** is common, as are the signs of **shock**. **Vomiting and diarrhoea** are also quite common.

Evidence of **atherosclerotic disease** at other sites or the presence of **atrial fibrillation** may suggest the possible diagnosis of thrombosis or embolism. Mesenteric ischaemia should be suspected in patients who develop the above symptoms after cardiac or aortic surgery while they are recovering in intensive care, especially if they have required large doses of inotropes or a balloon pump to support their cardiac output.

Mesenteric vein thrombosis is often associated with a thrombophilia and also occurs in women on the contraceptive pill. The patient may know that they have a vasculitis (e.g. Buerger's disease or lupus erythematosis) or they may have sickle cell disease. The patient can become gravely ill by the time the diagnosis becomes obvious, although the symptoms and signs are often mild . A high index of suspicion is required if the diagnosis is to be made at an early stage.

Blood tests

A full blood count often demonstrates a leucocytosis.

The **serum lactate** is commonly raised and a **metabolic acidosis** is often present. The serum amylase and lipase may also be elevated.

The search for a diagnostic blood test has proved elusive.

Imaging

An **electrocardiograph (ECG)** may reveal atrial fibrillation or show evidence of a previous myocardial infarction.

Echocardiography may show thrombus in the left atrium.

Plain radiographs of the abdomen are often unhelpful in the early stages when few bowel shadows are visible, but later on there may be evidence of a paralytic ileus with multiple fluid levels and gas may be seen in a mesenteric vein or in the wall of the bowel. 'Thumb printing' may be present especially in ischaemia of the large bowel (Fig 17.25).

CT angiographic scans may show the absence of contrast medium in the mesenteric arteries or evidence of an aortic dissection. Patients are often too sick to have an arteriogram, but CT arteriography is often diagnostic.

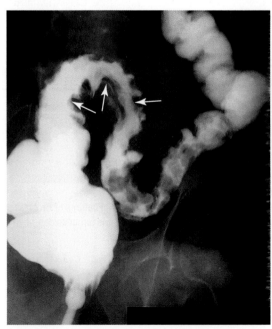

FIGURE 17.25   Barium enema showing thumb printing indicative of large bowel ischaemia

The majority of patients with mesenteric ischaemia require a **laparotomy** to confirm the diagnosis. **Laparoscopy** is usually unhelpful.

Management

There is no place for conservative non-interventional management.

All patients should be given intravenous **fluids**, subcutaneous **heparin** and a **broad-spectrum antibiotic**.

Percutaneous endovascular restoration of mesenteric blood flow by **balloon angioplasty**, **suction embolectomy, thrombolysis** and **stenting** may be successful in the very early stages (before infarction) and avoid the necessity for a laparotomy.

Urgent laparotomy is essential and may reveal pale or gangrenous bowel with poor peristalsis and the absence of pulsating vessels in the mesenteric arteries. There is often an unpleasant smell when the abdomen is open.

Dead bowel must be resected before any attempt is made to restore the blood supply to any bowel with dubious viability. The continuity of the resected bowel can be restored by end-to-end anastomosis or the two ends may be brought out on to the skin surface of the abdomen as stomas. This choice is usually based on the appearances of the remaining bowel, with a stoma being preferable if bowel viability is in doubt.

Embolectomy catheters can be passed up the divided mesenteric vessels to extract emboli. If this fails, the superior mesenteric artery blood supply may be restored by **endarterectomy with a patch graft** or some form of **bypass**.

A 'second-look' laparotomy is usually performed 24 hours after a bowel anastomosis to assess the viability of the bowel and carry out further resections.

Bowel continuity can be restored by **end-to-end anastomosis** at a later stage when the patient has fully recovered.

When the whole of the small intestine is dead or if there is widespread patchy infarction of both small and large bowel and the patient is very sick, old and infirm, it may be necessary to decide that the situation is hopeless, close the abdomen and allow the patient to die with adequate palliation.

Results

Of the patients that develop small bowel infarction 70–80 per cent die. A small number of survivors are left with a short bowel syndrome requiring intravenous nutritional support for weeks, months or the rest of their life. Small bowel transplantation has been attempted in such patients but is of dubious value.

SMALL BOWEL STRANGULATION OR VOLVULUS

Strangulation occurs when the blood vessels that supply a piece of small bowel are compressed by a nearby structure (e.g. the neck of a hernial sac) or the bowel is twisted on its vascular pedicle through 360 degrees (Fig 17.26A and B).

Investigation

Clinical diagnostic indicators

Obstruction and gangrene of the bowel causes severe continuous central abdominal pain often preceded by small bowel colic. Vomiting is common. Patients lie still with the pain, are usually pale and sweaty and have a tachycardia.

Once infarction has occurred the signs of peritonitis soon develop. The bowel sounds which are active or normal at first then disappear. *The hernial orifices must always be palpated to exclude a strangulated hernia*, and a note taken of any previous abdominal surgery. All scars should be examined to exclude a strangulated incisional hernia.

The **differential diagnosis** of small bowel strangulation includes the many conditions listed in Table 17.9.

Blood tests

A full blood count is often normal. The **urea and electrolytes** should be measured if vomiting is a major symptom, dehydration is suspected or the patient scheduled for urgent surgery.

Imaging

Plain abdominal X-rays may not show any abnormality in the early stages. A single dilated fluid-filled loop of bowel may be the only abnormal finding. Signs of small bowel obstruction develop if the condition is left untreated, and eventually, if gangrene and perforation occur, free intraperitoneal gas may be seen on an **erect chest X-ray** or **CT scan**.

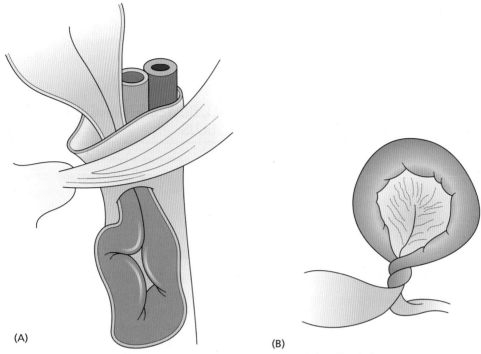

(A)   (B)

FIGURE 17.26   Causes of small bowel obstruction. (A) Hernial neck constriction; (B) volvulus

Table 17.9
Differential diagnosis of small bowel strangulation

Simple small bowel obstruction from a single or multiple adhesions

Intestinal ischaemia/infarction

Acute pancreatitis

Perforated peptic ulcer

Small bowel perforation

Biliary peritonitis

Large bowel volvulus

Gall stone ileus

Malrotation

Intussusception

Perforated appendicitis

Crohn's disease

Management

Small bowel strangulation and volvulus cannot be managed conservatively.

The pain should be relieved with **opioid analgesia** and the patient **swiftly resuscitated** with intravenous crystalloids and antibiotics, before being anaesthetized and treated surgically.

Laparoscopy is **not** an option. **Laparotomy** is usually performed through a central midline incision which can be extended upwards or downwards. *The only exception to this approach is when the strangulated bowel is in a tender hernia.*

The junction between dilated and collapsed small bowel indicates the site at which the bowel and its blood supply are obstructed. The vascular compression may be relieved by dividing a band adhesion; gently pulling the bowel out from the constricting neck of the hernial pouch; or by untwisting a volvulus. Doubtfully viable bowel should be watched for a few minutes, or wrapped in warm moist packs, to see if it recovers its colour, sheen and peristaltic activity. A small area of ischaemic bowel can sometimes be oversewn, but any dubious or frankly dead bowel should be resected and continuity restored by end-to-end anastomosis (Fig 17.27).

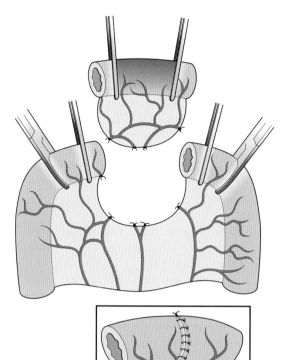

FIGURE 17.27   Resection of ischaemic small bowel with end-to-end anastomosis

Results

The results of the above treatment are usually good unless the diagnosis is missed and treatment is delayed. The mortality rate rises above 5 per cent if the patient is old or infirm and if the resection of dead bowel is delayed beyond 24 hours of its onset.

SMALL BOWEL PERFORATION

The conditions that can cause a small bowel perforation are:

- Crohn's disease
- small bowel infarction/strangulation
- typhoid fever
- foreign bodies, e.g. small bones
- trauma – penetrating sharp or blunt
- potassium tablets
- perforated Meckel's diverticulum
- radiation enteritis
- lymphoma (rare).

Investigation

Clinical diagnostic indicators

The symptoms of a small bowel perforation are similar to those of ischaemia and strangulation of the small bowel, but initially the pain and vomiting are often less severe.

Signs of peritonitis, tenderness, guarding and rebound tenderness develop over a variable period. They may be localized or generalized, depending on how well the perforation is contained by adjacent loops of small bowel, mesentery and omentum. Eventually, if left untreated, the whole abdomen becomes distended, rigid and silent, and the patient develops signs of toxaemia and shock.

The main **differential diagnoses** are conditions with similar clinical features:

- perforated peptic ulcer
- perforated colon (see Chapter 19)
- small bowel ischaemia (see above)
- small bowel volvulus (see above).

Blood tests

A full blood count is likely to show a leucocytosis, and a raised haematocrit. A raised blood urea suggests infection and dehydration.

Imaging

An **erect chest X-ray** or **plain abdominal radiograph** may show free gas under the diaphragm or pocket of air trapped within the abdomen (see Fig 17.3).

A **CT** scan may show small amounts of free gas which may not be visible on a plain radiograph, thickened loops of bowel (Crohn's disease) or the foreign body responsible for the perforation. It is rarely feasible to carry out other diagnostic tests as the patient usually requires urgent resuscitation prior to laparotomy.

Management

Conservative non-interventional management is inappropriate.

Rapid **resuscitation** with intravenous crystal-loids and/or colloids, combined with an intrave-nous broad-spectrum antibiotic (a cephalosporin and metronidazole) is required before proceeding to an **urgent laparotomy.**

Laparotomy is usually performed through a short mid-line incision. The segment of small bowel that is perforated usually requires resection to reduce the risk of reperforation and to obtain tissue for diagnosis. A long segment may require resection with an appropriate segment of mesen-tery if a **malignant process** is suspected, or if there is **evidence of distal obstruction.** End-to-end anas-tomosis restores bowel continuity and the abdomen is carefully washed out with saline or an antibiotic solution before being closed. Peritoneal drainage is usually unnecessary unless there is a localized abscess cavity.

Postoperative care Patients may require **intravenous fluids, intravenous antibiotics** and **nasogastric** aspiration for some days.

Intravenous feeding must be considered if the accompanying paralytic ileus is prolonged (see Chapter 2).

Ventilation, inotropic support and even **haemofiltration** may be required for patients who have signs of septic shock, to avoid **multi-organ failure**, the commonest cause of death.

Complications

Intraperitoneal abscess, wound infection, atelec-tasis and **multi-organ failure** are common. The eventual outcome depends on the underlying cause. For example, foreign body perforation and a per-forated Meckel's diverticulum will be cured by a small bowel resection, while Crohn's disease, a per-forated tumour or a radio necrotic bowel have a high chance of anastomotic leakage and recurrent disease.

Results

The mortality varies between 5 per cent and 10 per cent, depending on the age and fitness of the patient, the cause of the perforation and the period of time that has lapsed between the onset of the perforation and the onset of treatment.

CONGENITAL ANOMALIES OF THE SMALL BOWEL

Congenital abnormalities of the stomach, duo-denum and small intestine usually present with vomiting, abdominal distension and constipation, e.g. signs of small bowel obstruction.

Atresia, **stenosis** and **duplications** are normally treated by resection with end-to-end anastomosis or deroofing of the duplication. Parenteral nutri-tion may be required as feeding is often delayed.

The mortality of surgical correction of these conditions has decreased greatly with the improve-ment of neonatal anaesthesia and should now be less than 10 per cent. Short gut syndrome can occur if an entire volvulus has to be resected and this carries significant morbidity and mortality.

MECONIUM ILEUS

This is almost always a complication of **cystic fibrosis**. Eighty-five per cent of affected children have a two basepair deletion on chromosome 7. The proximal small bowel is distended with multiple meconium pellets and the terminal ileum and colon are narrow and constricted. Children present with symptoms and signs of small bowel obstruction.

Children have a positive sodium sweat test.

Hirschsprung's disease must be considered in the differential diagnosis.

Imaging

The diagnosis is made on a **plain X-ray**. Fluid levels are present in the proximal small bowel. The fat globules in the distended ileum in the right iliac fossa cause translucencies that give a **soap bubble appearance**.

A water-soluble contrast enema will show a 'microcolon' and round filling defects (meconium pellets) in the distal ileum.

Management

The vomiting should be relieved, and the dehydration and electrolyte imbalance corrected with **nasogastric aspiration** and **IV fluids** and **electrolytes**.

Although half of the patients are cured by an **enema** many still require careful fluid replacement over the next few days.

Surgery When surgery has to be performed, an enterostomy is made in the proximal ileum and saline is irrigated distally to wash out the meconium plugs. When this proves impossible, proximal and distal stomas can be brought out onto the abdominal wall. Once the patient has recovered, pancreatic enzyme replacement must be given.

Older children can present with **meconium ileus equivalent**. This causes colicky abdominal pain, tenderness and a mass in the right iliac fossa. Treatment is usually by gastrograffin enemas, but occasionally surgery is required and enterotomies may be necessary to clear out the inspissated masses.

SMALL BOWEL TUMOURS

These are rare and in descending order of frequency include carcinoid tumour (most common in the appendix), lymphoma, gastrointestinal stromal tumours and carcinoma. Other tumours of the small bowel such as adenoma, lipoma, sarcoma and secondary deposits are very rare.

Investigation
Clinical diagnostic indicators
Most small bowel tumours present with subacute obstruction or gastrointestinal haemorrhage.

The **differential diagnosis** is from Crohn's disease, tuberculosis and Meckel's diverticulum.

Imaging
Small bowel enemas, colonoscopy with small bowel intestinal visualization, angiography and nuclear magnetic scans may all be tried, but eventually laparoscopy or laparotomy is required.

Management

Surgical resection of the small bowel and its mesentery to clear the lymph nodes is the only effective treatment. **Chemotherapy** is indicated in patients with a lymphoma or in those who develop the carcinoid syndrome.

Prognosis The prognosis of appendicular carcinoids is very good unless they invade the caecum. Small bowel carcinoids and carcinomas have a far worse prognosis as they often present late: less than 50 per cent at 5 years. Small bowel lymphomas have an intermediate prognosis.

RADIATION ENTERITIS

This occurs when the small bowel is inadvertently injured as part of cancer treatment to tumours in the abdomen or pelvis. The resulting fibrosis, strictures and ulceration often cause subacute obstruction and diarrhoea. A radiotherapist's tattoo is often present!

Collateral damage from radiation most often follows radiotherapy for gynaecological, prostate, bladder and colon cancers.

Investigation
Clinical diagnostic indicators
This diagnosis should be suspected in any patient with diarrhoea, vomiting and colicky pain who has had radiotherapy to the lower abdomen.

Imaging
The diagnosis is by a **small bowel meal (enema)**. **CT scanning** may be helpful.

The main **differential diagnoses** are Crohn's disease and malignancy.

Management

This is conservative unless the diagnosis is in doubt or the symptoms become very severe, when **surgical resection and anastomosis** to healthy bowel may avoid the risk of dehiscence.

Prognosis Many years of poor health often follow this complication. Prevention is better than treatment. Resection carries a 5 per cent risk of anastomotic dehiscence and a 1–2 per cent risk of death.

RUPTURED ABDOMINAL AORTIC ANEURYSM

The investigation and management of the abdominal pain caused by a leaking abdominal aortic aneurysm is described in detail in Chapter 11.

Other conditions that present with abdominal pain and haemorrhagic shock similar to the signs of a ruptured abdominal aortic aneurysm include:

- ruptured spleen
- ruptured liver – see Chapter 6
- torn mesentery
- ruptured ovarian cyst
- ruptured ectopic pregnancy
- large retroperitoneal haematoma.

PAIN IN THE RIGHT ILIAC FOSSA

The many conditions that may present with pain in the right iliac fossa are:

- acute appendicitis
- non-specific abdominal pain
- Meckel's diverticulitis
- mesenteric adenitis
- Crohn's disease in the terminal ileum
- acute gastroenteritis
- intussusception
- carcinoma of the caecum/colon
- solitary caecal diverticulum
- acute sigmoid diverticulitis
- tuberculosis
- actinomycosis
- *Yersinia* pseudotuberculosis
- acute cholecystitis
- perforated peptic ulcer
- ruptured ovarian cyst
- salpingitis
- ectopic pregnancy
- ureteric calculus
- pyelonephritis/cystitis.

All these conditions may be associated with pain elsewhere in the abdomen, and many may present with a colicky pain. They are all important **differential diagnoses of acute appendicitis** and have often been incorrectly diagnosed as acute appendicitis by experienced surgeons. Many, if left untreated, progress to cause generalized abdominal pain and tenderness (peritonitis) and eventually to rupture or infarction.

ACUTE APPENDICITIS

Pain in the right iliac fossa is often assumed to come from the appendix because appendicitis is so common. The other pathological processes that affect the appendix are **mucocele, empyema, carcinoid tumour, adenocarcinoma and lymphoma**.

The condition of 'grumbling' (subacute) appendicitis may not exist, because the pain that gives rise to this diagnosis often persists after removing the appendix, which usually turns out to be normal. The pain may simply be a manifestation of irritable bowel syndrome or gynaecological pathology. Appendicectomy is rarely indicated for chronic right iliac fossa pain.

Adenocarcinoma, lymphoma and malignant carcinoid tumours rarely affect the appendix.

Investigation

Clinical diagnostic indicators

Teenagers and young adults of both sexes are most commonly affected, but appendicitis can occur at any age. The pain, occasionally colicky, usually begins in the mid-line of the **central** or **epigastric region** before moving to the **right iliac fossa** and becoming constant and more severe. The patient may have had similar attacks that have resolved spontaneously. The site of the pain may vary according to the position of the appendix (Fig 17.28). Sometimes the pain is situated in the right loin or upper quadrant (from a retrocaecal or sub-hepatic appendix), or be poorly localized.

Nausea, vomiting, diarrhoea and **dysuria** are common symptoms. The pain becomes generalized and severe if the appendix has perforated.

The most reliable sign is localized tenderness over **McBurney's point**, but foetor oris, a low-grade pyrexia, guarding, percussion tenderness (rebound)

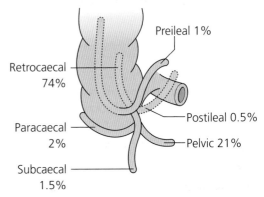

FIGURE 17.28   Positions of the appendix

and the presence of Rovsing's sign all support the diagnosis of appendicitis. Localized hyperparasthesae in Sherren's triangle, positive psoas or obdurator stretch tests and rectal tenderness may all be present, but **rectal tenderness is now rarely sought in children or young adults.**

Repeat examination

No further investigations are required when the clinical diagnosis is not in doubt. When this is not the case, **careful monitoring and repeated evaluation** of the temperature, pulse and abdominal signs in a hospital ward or admission unit are essential.

Clinical scoring

Clinical scoring systems such as the Alvarado system (Table 17.10) have their advocates but do not have a high level of sensitivity or specificity.

Blood tests

A full blood count often reveals a **leucocytosis** but even in cases of severe acute appendicitis the white cell count may be normal.

Urine tests

The **urine** should be dipstick tested for blood and protein and be examined for the presence of cells. The urine may also be dip tested for β-HCG (human chorionic gonadotrophin) in females to exclude pregnancy.

Imaging

Abdominal ultrasound, CT scan and **peritoneal cytology** have been evaluated as potential methods for diagnosing acute appendicitis but none is very accurate – **lower abdominal ultrasound** (80 per cent sensitive), **CT scan** (90 per cent accuracy) – so none has achieved widespread acceptance. At present nothing is better than careful and (when necessary) repeated clinical examination.

Laparoscopy

Laparoscopy is the one investigation that has become accepted as reliable, especially in young women where a pelvic cause of right iliac fossa pain is commonly mistaken for appendicitis. The use of this investigation is discussed below.

Management

Opioid analgesics are indicated if the pain is severe. The patient may benefit from intravenous **crystalloid solutions** if they have been vomiting repeatedly or appear to be dehydrated.

A single dose of a **cephalosporin** and **metronidazole** should be given with the premedication.

DVT prophylaxis should be given to adults, especially elderly patients.

Surgery

Appendicectomy/appendectomy is indicated in all patients with a clear diagnosis of acute appendicitis, especially when there are signs of local peritonitis (Fig 17.29).

Table 17.10
The Alvarado scoring system for acute appendicitis

Indicators	Score
Pain that has moved to the right iliac fossa (RIF)	1
Nausea/vomiting	1
Loss of appetite	1
RIF tenderness	2
RIF rebound tenderness	1
Mild fever	1
Leucocytosis ($>10 \times 10^9$ cells/L)	2
with shift to the left	1
Maximum score	10

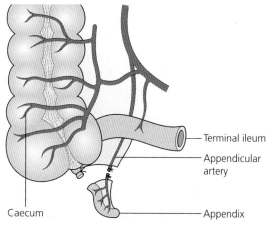

Terminal ileum
Appendicular artery
Caecum
Appendix

FIGURE 17.29 Appendicectomy

Many surgeons now perform a **diagnostic laparoscopy** to confirm the diagnosis before removing the appendix, especially if the patient's pain is non-specific and particularly in females of child-bearing age.

The procedure is performed with the patient in the reverse lithotomy position to encourage the small bowel to move out of the pelvis and into the abdominal cavity. The appendix is inspected via a camera inserted through an umbilical port and, if inflamed, removed using additional ports for dissection and clipping of the meso-appendix. The base of the appendix is closed with staples, or tied off with an endoloop, and the organ removed. The pelvic organs must be carefully inspected if the appendix appears normal.

The patient's abdomen must be explored through an incision in the right iliac fossa if any difficulties are encountered with the laparoscopic approach.

The open surgical approach allows a better inspection of the terminal small bowel for conditions such as an inflamed Meckel's diverticulum, Crohn's disease, intussusception and tumour and is preferable if the base of the appendix and the caecum are friable or involved in the inflammatory process.

The open operation allows the stump of the appendix to be buried, but this is of dubious value.

Complications

Perforation and **general peritonitis** are the important and dangerous complications. Both occur most often when the diagnosis is missed or the patient presents late but they can also follow appendicectomy. The signs of general peritonitis can develop quite quickly and the diagnosis is confirmed if free fluid is seen on an ultrasound or CT scan.

Infected peritoneal fluid and pus should be carefully washed out after an appendicectomy to reduce the risk of a postoperative pelvic or subphrenic abscesses developing. Antibiotics should be given for 5 days.

A pelvic abscess is indicated by a fluctuating temperature and is palpable per rectum. Confirmation by ultrasound is helpful before image-guided drainage.

Results

The mortality of the operation is less than 0.25 per cent, and the incidence of complications 5–10 per cent.

APPENDIX MASS/ABSCESS

Adjacent bowel and the omentum adherent to an inflamed appendix form a mass which may sometimes become an abscess.

Investigation

Clinical diagnostic indicators

The abdomen must be carefully palpated for a right iliac fossa mass in all patients suspected of having acute appendicitis, especially if the history is of pain for several days. It is worthwhile repeating the palpation after a general anaesthetic has been given.

Table 17.11 gives the **differential diagnosis.**

Imaging

An **ultrasound or CT scan** will confirm the diagnosis of a mass and exclude or confirm pus formation.

Management

A mass should be treated expectantly with **antibiotics** and usually resolves. It should be explored if it does not resolve.

Table 17.11
Differential diagnosis of an appendix mass

Carcinoma of the caecum (perforated)
Solitary caecal diverticulum
Crohn's disease
Actinomycosis
Intussusception
Small bowel tumour/lymph nodes
Psoas abscess
Ovarian tumour
Fibroid
Pyo-salpinx
Retroperitoneal mass/tumour
Iliac aneurysm
Spigelian hernia
Ruptured inferior epigastric artery
Transplanted kidney
Malignant change in an undescended testis

An abscess should be **drained** using **ultrasound or CT guidance**.

Resolution of a mass or an abscess after X-ray-guided drainage should be followed by **colono-scopy** to exclude alternative ileocaecal pathology, such as a carcinoma.

Most surgeons advise a laparoscopic appendicectomy a few months later if there are continuing symptoms.

MESENTERIC ADENITIS

Some patients with a generalized non-specific viral infection develop tender, swollen glands within the mesentery. The patient may have had a recent sore throat or upper respiratory tract infection and the cervical lymph nodes may be enlarged, palpable and tender. Placing the patient in different positions (e.g. on one and then the other side) may cause the pain and tenderness to shift position.

Other patients in whom vomiting and diarrhoea predominate may have a **viral gastroenteritis** or some form of **food poisoning**.

INFECTIONS AND OTHER 'NON-SPECIFIC' CAUSES OF RIGHT ILIAC FOSSA PAIN

Some of the problems that lead patients to present with pain in the right iliac fossa, for which no immediate cause can be found after clinical examination and the common routine investigations, are due to the following infections and parasitic helminths (worms).

Tuberculosis

Tuberculosis can present with lower abdominal and right iliac fossa pain, ascites, weight loss and small bowel obstruction. The differential diagnoses are Crohn's disease, starch peritonitis, carcinomatosis and pseudomyxoma peritonei.

A **small bowel meal** may show a stricture. Calcified lymph nodes may be seen on plain abdominal radiographs.

Ultrasound and CT scanning may show free fluid within the peritoneal cavity.

The diagnosis is best assessed by **laparoscopy** with aspiration of any free fluid and biopsy of the omentum or peritoneal tubercles. Occasionally, the tubercle bacillus can be grown from the ascitic fluid.

Treatment is by antituberculous **medication and resection** of any chronically narrowed small bowel.

Actinomycosis

This usually presents with pain, a mass and discharging sinuses in the right line fossa. Microscopy of pus is shown in Fig 17.30.

Typhoid

Typhoid can cause small bowel perforation and present as an **acute abdomen**. Finding air under the diaphragm and on plain radiographs supports

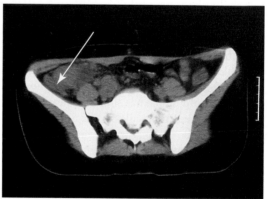

(A)

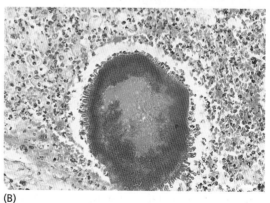

(B)

FIGURE 17.30 Actinomycosis: (A) CT of right iliac fossa mass; (B) *Actinomyces israelii* (a sulphur granule)

the diagnosis. Diarrhoea almost always precedes the pain and *Salmonella* can be cultured from the stools or blood. Perforated bowel should be resected and chloramphenicol given to treat the typhoid.

Yersinia pseudotuberculosis

Yersinia pseudotuberculosis can cause a short-lived terminal ileitis which can be similar to **Crohn's disease** but resolves completely.

Human immunovirus opportunistic infection

Diarrhoea and abdominal pain can result from opportunistic infections with *Mycobacterium avium intracellulari* in patients with human immunovirus. Enlarged mesenteric nodes can sometimes be felt as a mass and there may be signs of small bowel obstruction or peritonitis. The diagnosis is confirmed by finding mycobacteria on small bowel biopsy.

Treatment is with **antibiotics**, either one of the quinalones or amikacin.

Patients with AIDS are more likely to develop small bowel malignancies. Kaposi's sarcoma can cause bleeding or obstruction, as can lymphomas.

The most important **differential diagnosis** is **Crohn's disease**, which has similar appearances on barium meal and tuberculosis. Surgical biopsy or resection may be the only way of making the diagnosis with certainty. The treatment of both conditions is by chemotherapy, supplemented by surgical resection where necessary.

Enterobius vermicularis

Enterobius vermicularis, small threadworms that can live within the appendix, may be responsible for some cases of right iliac fossa pain. They are often found on histological examination of the appendix. The patient, usually a child who may have previously complained of peri-anal irritation, should be treated with an appropriate anti-helminthic agents (e.g. piperazine).

Ascaris lumbricoides

Roundworms can enter the bowel through ingestion, when a tangled mass of worms can cause small bowel obstruction (see Fig 17.24B).

Hookworms

These are an important cause of iron deficiency anaemia.

MECKEL'S DIVERTICULUM

Meckel's diverticulum is the unobliterated end of the vitello-intestinal duct. It occurs in 2 per cent of individuals, approximately 60 cm from the ileocaecal valve, and often lies in the right iliac fossa. Very few of the 2 per cent of individuals who have one develop symptoms.

There is occasionally an associated intraperitoneal band, which can cause small bowel obstruction.

Investigation

Clinical diagnostic indicators

The inflammatory pain and tenderness caused by any ectopic pancreatic tissue that the divericulum may contain are indistinguishable from the symptoms and signs of acute appendicitis.

An ulcer may bleed if the diverticulum contains gastric mucosa and can cause considerable blood loss.

Imaging

Technetium-99m pertechnate scanning can be diagnostic when this radioisotope is taken up by gastric mucosa. It should be considered only after more common conditions have been excluded.

Mesenteric angiography may also confirm the diagnosis and identify the source of bleeding if the bleeding is active. This is usually carried out as a CT angiogram (see Chapter 18).

Management

No action is needed if a Meckel's diverticulum is found incidentally at laparotomy or laparoscopy.

Excision is curative if the diverticulum is causing symptoms. It may be necessary to resect a short length of ileum if the mouth of the diverticulum is wide and the associated ileum inflamed.

SMALL BOWEL CROHN'S DISEASE

Crohn's disease is a chronic full thickness granulomatous inflammation that can affect the wall of the gastrointestinal tract anywhere from the mouth to the anus. The site most commonly affected is the terminal ileum immediately proximal to the ileocaecal valve. Crohn's disease is characterized by multiple 'skip lesions' – short diseased segments separated by lengths of normal bowel. The complications of this chronic inflammatory process are strictures, abscesses and fistulae. Bleeding is usually chronic, not acute and life-threatening.

Crohn's disease is probably multifactorial in origin. Mutations of the NOD2 gene are associated but environmental factors have been implicated. Abnormalities of the immune system, the presence of *Mycobacterium paratuberculosis*, and a refined diet may contribute. Smoking increases the risk of developing Crohn's disease and of recurrence after treatment.

Investigation

Clinical diagnostic indicators

There are two age peaks of presentation, the first in the second and third decades of life, and the second in elderly people.

The principal symptoms are **abdominal pain**, **weight loss** and **intermittent attacks of diarrhoea**. The onset of abdominal pain may be insidious or acute. It is usually colicky in nature but can be continuous when it is most commonly located in the right iliac fossa. Diarrhoea is often associated with the abdominal pain and often precedes its development. Other symptoms include nausea, vomiting, weight loss and lassitude.

The diagnosis may be delayed because these symptoms are similar to the symptoms of the much more common irritable bowel syndrome.

On examination, the thickened inflamed bowel wall can sometimes be felt as a **'sausage-shaped' mass** in the right iliac fossa, or elsewhere in the abdomen.

Such a mass is usually mobile and tender. The **differential diagnoses** are listed in Table 17.12.

Crohn's disease has many serious systemic associations such as **anaemia, erythema nodosum, clubbing, sacro-ileitis, episcleritis and uveitis** (Table 17.13). The presence of these conditions lends support to the diagnosis of Crohn's disease.

Enterocutaneous fistulae and anorectal sepsis are other common associations.

Table 17.12
Differential diagnosis of ileocaecal Crohn's disease

Appendicitis

Lymphoma

Other small bowel tumours

Other causes of stricture such as potassium and ischaemia

Yersinia pseudotuberculosis

Tuberculosis

Human immunovirus

Table 17.13
Systemic effects of Crohn's disease

Anaemia: iron deficiency, B12 and folate

Hypoalbuminaemia

Clubbing of the finger nails

Arthritis

Iritis

Episcleritis

Pyoderma gangrenosum

Sclerosing cholangitis

Sacro-iliitis

Gall stones

Erythema nodosum

Renal stones

Blood tests

Iron deficiency anaemia and a **leucocytosis** are often present and are usually accompanied by an elevated **erythrocyte sedimentation rate** or **C-reactive protein**.

The anaemia can also be normocytic (chronic disease) or macrocytic from associated B12 or folate deficiency.

A raised urea and normal creatinine is indicative of dehydration.

The serum protein/albumin is often low and there may be abnormal liver function tests (raised enzymes).

Stool culture

It is important to remember that exacerbations of the symptoms of Crohn's disease (and ulcerative colitis) may be caused by concomitant infection, so a stool sample should be sent for **culture** and tested for **occult blood**. Bowel infections are also an important differential diagnosis.

Imaging

A **plain abdominal radiograph** may show evidence of small bowel obstruction with fluid levels. An **erect chest X-ray** very occasionally shows free gas, but perforations are unusual.

A **small bowel enema** may show one or more strictures often associated with deep fissuring ulcers. The narrowing may be localized to the terminal ileum (Cantor's string sign) (see Fig 17.24A) or there may be multiple skip areas of luminal narrowing with normal bowel in between. Some of the deep fissuring (rose thorn) ulcers may extend to become fistulae.

MRI is helpful for demonstrating extra-intestinal abnormalities such as abscesses as well as the abnormality of the gut lumen.

CT scanning is often used to detect complications and shows thickened loops of bowel with separation of the loops caused by thickened oedematous bowel.

Biopsy

Biopsies of the small bowel can be taken by a Crosby capsule or through a colonoscope passed through the ileocaecal valve. Rectal biopsies taken through a sigmoidoscope may show evidence of granulomata even when the mucosa appears macroscopically normal.

Management

The management of small bowel Crohn's disease should, if possible, be **conservative** unless there are clear signs of peritonitis or persistent bowel obstruction.

Medical management of acute episode of inflammation

The medical management consists largely of giving **steroids** and **immunosuppressive drugs**, but it must always be remembered that many patients experience a long-term remission with an excellent quality of life after early surgical resection (especially of the terminal ileum).

Severely ill patients with anaemia, a high C-reactive protein, a low albumin and systemic symptoms who need support with **enteral** or **parenteral nutrition**, **antibiotics** and **intravenous fluids** should be admitted to hospital for treatment with either oral or parenteral **steroids**.

Oral prednisolone can produce a remission in up to 70 per cent of patients.

A **proton pump inhibitor or an H2 blocker** should be given with the steroids because of the risk of peptic ulceration,

Calcium supplements should also be prescribed because of the risk of osteoporosis. Careful daily review is mandatory.

Anti-TNF-α drugs such as infliximab and adalimumab may be used if there is failure to respond to the above treatment.

Maintenance of remission

Once the acute inflammation has settled, the remission must be maintained as this is a chronic relapsing condition.

5-Aminosalicylic acid (5-ASA) preparations are effective but the agent must be delivered to the relevant area of bowel. Pure 5-ASA taken orally is absorbed in the stomach and upper small bowel and does not reach the terminal ileum.

Sulfasalazine, the oldest ASA preparation, consists of 5-ASA molecules linked to sulfapyridine, the bond being broken by the bacteria present in the distal ileum and colon where the effect is desired.

Unfortunately, sulfapyridine causes headaches, abnormalities of liver function and indigestion. Modern preparations use resin coating, controlled release spheres and links to inert molecules to prevent the early absorption of the 5-ASA. These drugs have few side-effects, although they have been linked with interstitial nephritis. They produce prolonged remissions in half of the cases treated.

In patients who are judged to be at a high risk of recurrent Crohn's disease, many physicians now use **immunosuppression** with agents such as azathioprine, methotrexate or 6-mercaptopurine. These drugs produce remissions in about half the patients treated but require very careful monitoring. Prolonged use should be avoided.

Infliximab and **adalimumab** (monoclonal anti-bodies to TNF-α) have achieved even more impressive remissions (up to 80 per cent) and some of these drugs seem to maintain remission in low doses.

Polymeric enteral diets, **metronidazole** and **ciprofloxicin** may all help alleviate acute disease and prolong remissions. A high-protein low-residue diet should be supplemented by iron, B12 and folate as required, and diarrhoea may be alleviated by codeine phosphate, imodium and cholestyramine.

Surgical management

Approximately 80 per cent of patients with Crohn's disease of the small bowel will require surgical treatment at some time, usually for the management of complications. Surgery should rarely be performed as an emergency, unless there is a free perforation of the bowel. *The decision to operate should be made on the advice of an enthusiastic physician and a reluctant surgeon.*

Resection of a stricture in the terminal ileum and caecum is often all that is needed, removing as little of the bowel as possible since half the patients who have surgery for Crohn's disease will require further operations over the next 10–15 years.

Limited resections with end-to-end anastomosis is preferable for localized disease in other sites.

Bypass procedures for obstruction are a less satisfactory option.

Stricturoplasty (Fig 17.31) and **balloon dilatation** should be considered for extensive disease causing chronic small bowel obstruction, as these procedures restore the lumen without resection.

Other indications for surgery are perforation with peritonitis, an abscess (which may be managed initially by radiologically guided drainage), fistulae (to other parts of bowel, bladder, vagina or skin), and strictures in other areas of the small bowel.

Complications

The complications following surgery for Crohn's disease are shown in Table 17.14.

Malignancy (adenocarcinoma or lymphoma) is a rare complication of small bowel Crohn's disease and carries a poor prognosis.

Short bowel syndrome can follow massive small bowel resections. Patients with this syndrome present with weight loss and diarrhoea. Similar symptoms can also complicate a fistula or a stoma.

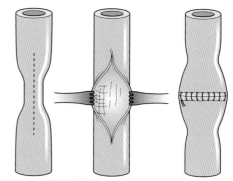

FIGURE 17.31 Stricturoplasty

Table 17.14
Complications following surgery for Crohn's disease

Anastomotic dehiscence

Wound infection

Fistula formation

Abdominal abscess development

Recurrent disease

Perianal Crohn's disease

Both may require **enteral** or **parental** nutrition. Small bowel transplantation may be tried if access sites for parental nutrition become exhausted, but the results of bowel transplantation for this condition are poor.

Results

The mortality of surgery is less than 5 per cent but disease requiring further surgery recurs in 40 per cent within 10 years and in 50 per cent by 15 years.

FISTULAE OF THE SMALL BOWEL

Small bowel fistulae are associated with:

- anastomotic dehiscence
- Crohn's disease
- carcinoma of large bowel
- patent vitello-intestinal duct
- iatrogenic damage, e.g. suture into bowel
- tuberculosis
- bowel ischaemia
- radiation damage

- trauma
- stab wounds.

Patients with small bowel fistulae present with bowel contents leaking out of their wounds or into the bladder (haematuria, faecuria). They can also present with abscesses or peritonitis.

Investigation

Investigation with **barium, gastrograffin** and **CT scanning** will show the extent of the bowel disruption. Contrast medium can also be inserted down the fistula track (a fistulagram).

Management

The sepsis must be controlled by **antibiotics** (e.g. a cephalosporin and metronidazole) and by **drainage**, either radiological or surgical. **Nutrition** must be supplemented to overcome fistula losses. This can be administered either intravenously or orally. The skin must be protected.

Provided there is no distal obstruction, many small bowel fistulae heal spontaneously.

Bowel resection of the fistula with end-to-end anastomosis after a considerable period of conservative management (e.g. up to 6 months) is appropriate. This is usually required if the bowel has completely disintegrated or pathology such as Crohn's disease is associated with the fistula.

Early surgery with defunctioning of the bowel is appropriate in most cases of operative anastomotic failure.

CARCINOMA OF THE CAECUM

Investigation

Clinical diagnostic indicators

Carcinoma of the caecum commonly presents in elderly people with **anaemia, weight loss** and a **right iliac fossa mass.**

Abdominal pain is relatively uncommon, but caecal cancers can ulcerate and if the ulcer extends through the bowel wall it can cause a **paracaecal abscess**. If a caecal cancer or carcinoid tumour occludes the base of the appendix it may present with the symptoms and signs of acute appendicitis and an appendix abscess.

Liver metastases and a mass in the right iliac fossa may be palpable.

Blood tests

A **full blood count** and **blood film** usually show evidence of a **hypochromic microcytic anaemia**. A serum iron will confirm **iron deficiency** with a normal or raised serum ferritin. There will be a **leucocytosis** if there is an associated pericolic abscess or appendicitis.

The **carcino-embryonic antigen** is often raised especially if metastases are present.

Imaging

An **abdominal ultrasound** or **CT scan** may confirm the presence of a mass in the right iliac fossa. A CT scan is often diagnostic and also confirms or excludes large liver metastases.

Colonoscopy is indicated if the diagnosis remains in doubt (see Chapter 19).

Management

The anaemia may require preoperative correction if the haemoglobin level is very low, but usually blood can be transfused at the time of surgery. Metronidazole and a cephalosporin should be given with the premedication to prevent wound infection. DVT prophylaxis should be given as low molecular weight heparin unless contraindicated.

A laparotomy is performed under general anaesthesia, through a transverse, mid-line, paramedian or oblique (Rutherford Morrison) incision. When the diagnosis has been confirmed a **right hemicolectomy** is performed (see Fig 19.13). The right colon, terminal ileum and hepatic flexure are mobilized and resected after the mesenteric vessels have been ligated and divided at their origin. The right ureter and duodenum must be carefully defined as these structures may be damaged during colonic mobilization. The lymph nodes at the base of the mesentery associated with the ligated vessels should be excised with the resected mesentery and bowel. It is important to remove all the local tumour and the lymph nodes to which it drains if good results are to be achieved. Bowel continuity is restored by an end-to-end anastomosis between the terminal ileum and transverse colon.

A **laparoscopic** approach can be used to mobilize the bowel and divide the mesentery and its vessels, but the anastomosis is usually performed extracorporally after the bowel that is to be resected has been brought on to the surface of the abdomen through a short transverse incision. The operation can be carried out completely inside the abdomen using stapling techniques but a small 5- to 10-cm incision is still required to extract the specimen, so little is gained.

Patients should be given intravenous fluids and their oral fluid intake restricted until bowel function returns. More recently, an enhanced recovery programme has supported early feeding to avoid the use of nasogastric aspiration.

Nasogastric aspiration is occasionally required for patients who present with an obstructed bowel, a perforation or a large pericolic abscess.

Complications

Wound infection and **dehiscence of the bowel anastomosis** are the most common postoperative complications.

Metastatic tumour may be found at the time of surgery, or may become apparent in the postoperative period.

Solitary liver metastases may be resected at the time of surgery but this is usually carried out as a separate procedure once the patient has recovered from the bowel resection (see Chapter 19).

Radiotherapy and **chemotherapy**, given after surgery, may reduce the risk of recurrence (see Chapter 19).

Results

The prognosis depends on the pathological staging of the tumour.

- Duke's A stage tumours are rare, but have an excellent prognosis – 95 per cent 5-year survival.
- Duke's B stage tumours have a 40–60 per cent 5-year survival.
- Dukes C stage tumours have a 20–40 per cent 5-year survival.

Other more sophisticated staging systems are available, including a modification of the TNM classification, but they have not been universally adopted (see Chapter 19).

RIGHT-SIDED DIVERTICULAR DISEASE/ SOLITARY CAECAL DIVERTICULUM

Diverticula can develop anywhere in the right colon and caecum. They can cause infection, abscess formation and perforation identical to those seen in the sigmoid colon which are described in full in Chapter 19.

The symptoms and signs in the right iliac fossa of an **inflamed solitary caecal diverticulum** are indistinguishable from those of appendicitis. The mass is often mistaken for a carcinoma of colon. The treatment is resection of the inflamed diverticulum and the bowel from which it has arisen.

PAIN IN THE LEFT ILIAC FOSSA

The causes of pain in the left iliac fossa include:

- diverticulitis/pericolic abscess or perforation
- carcinoma of the colon with pericolic abscess
- ovarian cyst – torted/ruptured
- ectopic pregnancy – bleeding or ruptured
- salpingitis (pelvic inflammatory disease)
- ischaemia or Crohn's colitis
- toxic dilatation/rupture of colitic colon
- ureteric colic/pyelonephritis.

Many of the conditions responsible for pain in the left iliac fossa listed above can cause pain elsewhere in the abdomen (e.g. diverticular disease can present with pain in the centre and lower abdomen and either iliac fossa).

LARGE BOWEL OBSTRUCTION

The two commonest causes of large bowel obstruction are carcinoma of the colon and diverticular disease.

Investigation

Clinical diagnostic indicators

The pain is experienced in the mid-line, usually below the umbilicus and in the suprapubic region. The colic of large bowel obstruction is not usually as severe as small bowel colic and the periods between the pains longer (30–60 minutes). **Abdominal distension and absolute constipation** are indicative of large bowel obstruction. Vomiting is a late symptom.

The distention corresponds to the position of the colon – usually across the epigastrium and in the flanks, in contrast to the central distension of small bowel obstruction.

Occasionally a cancer or diverticular mass is palpable and a large knobbly liver is indicative of liver metastases.

The abdomen is usually not tender. **Obstructive bowel sounds** may be heard.

Rectal examination usually reveals an empty rectum but occasionally a carcinoma or diverticular mass in the rectum or sigmoid colon may be palpable.

Blood tests

Iron deficiency anaemia and evidence of dehydration are often present. Blood should be taken for **haemoglobin**, **packed cell volume**, and **urea and electrolytes**.

Imaging

Sigmoidoscopy whether rigid or flexible may demonstrate the obstructing pathology.

Plain abdominal radiographs may outline the gas-filled distended large bowel.

A **caecal or a sigmoid volvulus** has characteristic features. Plain radiographs cannot separate true obstruction from pseudo-obstruction with complete confidence.

An instant **barium enema** without bowel preparation can be very helpful if sigmoidoscopy does not provide a diagnosis. It is particularly useful for separating **pseudo-obstruction** (Ogilvie's syndrome) from **true obstruction** (see Chapter 19).

A **CT scan** with bowel contrast is often the investigation of first choice.

Colonoscopy can be diagnostic and, by decompressing distended bowel, therapeutic in patients with pseudo-obstruction.

Management

After adequate **rehydration and analgesia** the obstruction must be relieved. A **barium enema** can reduce an **intussusception** in children. **The passage of a flatus tube** via a **sigmoidoscope** can temporarily deflate a **sigmoid volvulus**.

Antibiotics should be given to prevent postoperative wound infection. **DVT prophylaxis** is indicated.

Laparotomy Most causes of large bowel obstruction have to be corrected by open surgery on the next available operating list. It is important to obtain the **patient's consent** for a **temporary defunctioning stoma** before operation and mark its best site.

At operation the obstructing lesion should be **resected** and the ends of the bowel **anastomosed** (usually with a covering proximal colostomy) or **exteriorized.**

Hartman's procedure may also be used (see Chapter 19).

Obstruction of the right side of the colon can usually be treated by a **right hemicolectomy** with immediate anastomosis. This operation can be extended to treat carcinomata as far as the **splenic flexure.**

A **Mickulitz colostomy** is a good treatment for sigmoid volvulus especially if the bowel is of doubtfully viable and requires immediate resection.

Complications Complications are discussed in Chapter 19.

Results Operations on large bowel obstruction have a small but consistent mortality of around 5 per cent. Obstructing carcinomata have a worse prognosis than similarly graded tumours that do not cause obstruction. Presentation with a perforation, either of the tumour or of distended bowel above the tumour, have an even worse prognosis.

ACUTE SIGMOID DIVERTICULITIS, PERICOLIC ABSCESS AND PERFORATION

The investigation and management of these conditions is described in Chapter 19.

COLONIC CROHN'S DISEASE

Although Crohn's disease commonly affects the ileocaecal region it can also develop in any part of the colon. When Crohn's disease affects the descending sigmoid colon it often causes left iliac fossa pain. Colonic Crohn's disease is described in Chapter 19.

OTHER CAUSES OF ILIAC FOSSA PAIN

Mittlesmertz: mid-cycle pain Many women experience mild iliac fossa pain mid-way between menstruation when an **ovarian follicle** ruptures at ovulation.

Some women with chronic long-standing **pelvic sepsis** have recurrent attacks of iliac fossa discomfort.

Iliac fossa pain can arise from **nerve entrapment** in the anterior abdominal wall. The site is usually locally tender and the pain relieved by an injection of local anaesthetic.

Iliac fossa pain may be referred from the back (**musculoskeletal or intervertebral disc pain**). This should be suspected if the pain is exacerbated by spinal movements often in one direction, e.g. lateral flexion.

A number of patients with repeated episodes of iliac fossa pain are eventually diagnosed as having **irritable bowel syndrome** – a diagnosis of exclusion when all other possible causes of pain including **disseminated intraperitoneal malignancy** have been carefully ruled out.

Investigation

The exclusion of more serious conditions may require an **abdominal ultrasound, CT scanning, a small bowel meal, colonoscopy and even laparoscopy**. The patient is usually categorized as having **non-specific abdominal pain** if these tests fail to detect any abnormality, even when the patient is having repeated attacks. Many never present to hospital again.

PELVIC CAUSES OF LOWER ABDOMINAL PAIN

The pelvic causes of lower abdominal pain include:

- pelvic inflammatory disease e.g. salpingitis
- ectopic pregnancy
- ruptured/twisted ovarian cyst
- twisted or degenerating fibroid
- abortion
- cystitis
- acute retention of urine
- pelvic appendicitis.

PELVIC INFLAMMATORY DISEASE, SALPINGITIS, PYOSALPINX AND HYDROSALPINX

Infection in the Fallopian tubes occurs in sexually active women of child-bearing age (15–50). Although it usually develops in the Fallopian tubes (**salpingitis**) it can spread to all the connective tissues of the adjacent pelvic organs (**pelvic inflammatory disease (PID)**).

The Fallopian tubes may become swollen and distended with pus (**pyosalpinx**) or tissue fluid (**hydrosalpinx**).

Investigation
Clinical diagnostic indicators

Pain caused by this infection is experienced in both iliac fossae and the suprapubic region and may be preceded by a low back ache and a vaginal discharge. When the pain is experienced in just one iliac fossa it must be differentiated from acute appendicitis or diverticulitis.

Episodes of sexually transmitted disease often precede pelvic inflammatory disease as the infecting organism is commonly the gonococcus. *Streptococcus*, *Chlamydia* and *Monilia* are also well recognized as causes of pelvic inflammatory disease.

Menstrual irregularities are common.

Pelvic inflammatory disease is a well recognized complication of the puerperium and may follow an abortion. Painful micturition, frequency, rigors and sweating are common and indicate a co-existing urinary tract infection.

On examination the patient appears flushed and often has a **high temperature**. There is tenderness in the suprapubic region which may extend into one or both iliac fossae. A vaginal **speculum examination** may reveal pus exuding through the os cervix. Movement of the cervix usually causes severe pain (**cervical excitation**).

Adenexal tenderness is usually present.

A pyo- or hydrosalpinx can occasionally be felt as a mass on bimanual examination.

Blood tests

A **leucocytosis** is very common.

Microbiology

A **high vaginal swab** confirms the presence of pus cells and may contain organisms. Culture takes

48 hours to obtain. It is also worthwhile culturing a **midstream specimen of urine**.

Imaging

Many patients do not require further investigation before beginning antibiotic therapy. **Abdominal and a transvaginal ultrasound** can be used to determine the presence of a **hydropyosalpinx** and exclude other abnormalities such as a **chronic ectopic pregnancy**, an **ovarian cyst** and **acute appendicitis** – the main differential diagnoses.

Laparoscopy is indicated if the diagnosis remains in doubt.

Management

Patients are usually admitted to hospital until the pain and temperature have settled.

Early and appropriate antibiotic treatment is curative and may prevent future infertility. The antibiotic should be effective against anaerobes and aerobic organisms. **Co-aminoclav** is usually prescribed and can be given intravenously if the temperature is high.

Laparoscopic aspiration of the Fallopian tubes is indicated if the infection has not responded to the antibiotic therapy. The aspirate from the tube should be used to identify the organism and its antibiotic sensitivity.

Salpingoscopy or **tubal fenestration** is occasionally used to treat a massive hydro- or pyosalpinx.

Results

The mortality of this condition is very low (less than 0.5 per cent) but *many patients have repeated attacks which often render them infertile*.

RUPTURED OR TWISTED OVARIAN CYSTS

Investigation

Clinical diagnostic indicators

Ovarian cysts are extremely common in women of child-bearing age and only rarely have any clinical significance.

Mid-cycle (**Mittelschmerz pain**, see above) is extremely common and is the result of a ruptured follicular or luteal cyst. The pain is often relatively mild (similar to dysmenorrhoea), central or in an iliac fossa, usually short-lived and not associated with vomiting, nausea or bowel upset.

Pathological ovarian cysts (e.g. cyst adenomata and dermoid cysts) and ovarian carcinomata can **twist on their pedicles** or **rupture** and **bleed**. When this occurs the pain is severe and persistent.

The pulse may be rapid and hypotension may be present. The patients rarely have a pyrexia. Tenderness is usually maximal suprapubically but may extend into one or both iliac fossae. **Guarding** and **rebound** may be present and the condition must be differentiated from all the differential diagnoses of acute appendicitis. Signs of shock may develop if rupture is accompanied by major bleeding.

Blood tests

The white cell count is usually normal but the **haemoglobin** may eventually fall if there has been significant bleeding.

Imaging

Transabdominal and **transvaginal ultrasound** usually confirm the diagnosis and differentiate ovarian pathology from a ruptured ectopic pregnancy or a twisted fibroid (Fig 17.32).

Management

Small cysts can be treated expectantly until the pain resolves. **Analgesia** may be required.

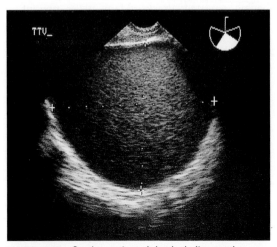

FIGURE 17.32 Ovarian cyst on abdominal ultrasound

Surgical excision Cysts responsible for major **haemorrhage** or those that have **infarcted** should be resected. This can be attempted laparoscopically if the cyst is small. The ovary usually has to be removed completely (**oophorectomy**) if the cyst is large.

The opinion of a gynaecologist should be sought during the operation if the cyst is thought to be malignant, as consideration must be give to performing a combined **bilateral salpingo-oophorectomy and hysterectomy**. When considering performing such an option, the accuracy of the diagnosis and the *exact form of the patient's pre-operation consent are vital factors*.

Results

Success rates are very good unless the cyst is malignant, when the prognosis is extremely poor. An oophorectomy reduces the chance of future fertility.

ECTOPIC PREGNANCY

Investigation

Clinical diagnostic indicators

Severe suprapubic pain of sudden onset in a women of child-bearing age should be considered to be caused by an ectopic pregnancy until proved otherwise because the associated bleeding can be life-threatening.

The diagnosis is strongly supported by a history of **missed or delayed menstruation**, especially if accompanied by **early-morning vomiting** and **swollen and tender breasts**.

Patients often experience a few days of mild intermittent pain before the severe pain (which is frequently associated with faintness and collapse) develops. There may be a history of pelvic inflammatory disease or fertility problems.

On examination the patient is often shocked with a marked **tachycardia**, **pallor**, **sweating** and **hypotension**.

Abdominal tenderness is usually most marked in the **suprapubic** region but may spread over the whole abdomen.

Vaginal examination may cause deterioration even when the patient appears haemodynamically stable and should be carried out by an experienced gynaecologist.

Blood tests

It is always worthwhile obtaining a pregnancy test. Many shocked patients do not require further investigations.

Blood should be sent for **grouping** and **cross-matching**.

Imaging

A transvaginal ultrasound can be used to confirm the diagnosis if the patient is not shocked and the diagnosis in doubt.

Management

Patients should be resuscitated with **intravenous fluids and blood** which, if there are signs of severe shock, can be grouped and given uncross-matched.

Severe unresponsive shock requires **urgent laparotomy**. The control of bleeding usually requires a **salpingectomy**.

Haemodynamically stable patients can have a **laparoscopy** with an attempt at **tubal conservation**.

Results

The mortality from a ruptured ectopic pregnancy is low but patients may be rendered **infertile** by the excision of a Fallopian tube; and even if it is conserved further ectopic pregnancies can occur.

TWISTED OR DEGENERATING FIBROIDS

Investigation

Clinical diagnostic indicators

This abnormality causes suprapubic pain that can extend into either iliac fossa depending on the position of the fibroid. The clinical diagnosis is confirmed by finding, on bimanual examination, a **tender mass attached to the uterus**.

Imaging

An **abdominal** or **transvaginal ultrasound** will confirm the diagnosis.

A calcified fibroid can be seen on a plain **abdominal radiograph** (see Fig 17.7B).

Management

Urgent surgery is rarely required. **Myomectomy** or **hysterectomy** may be considered depending on the patient's history and their child-bearing ambitions.

ABORTION/MISCARRIAGE

Patients who have a spontaneous or therapeutic abortion commonly experience severe labour-like pains as the products of conception are expelled. The diagnosis is usually correctly made by the patient, who notices vaginal bleeding before the cramping pains develop.

Dilatation and curettage (D&C) may be required, if the pain persists or there are accompanying signs of infection, to remove any retained products of conception.

CYSTITIS AND PYLONEPHRITIS (URINARY TRACT INFECTION)

Cystitis and pylonephritis (see Chapter 20) can present with lower abdominal pain but the diagnosis is usually apparent from the accompanying history of **painful micturition** and urinary **frequency**.

Rigors and loin pain suggest the presence of pylonephritis. There may be **tenderness over the bladder or in the loin. Pyrexia** is usually present and the urine looks cloudy.

The causes of loin pain are listed in Table 17.15.

Table 17.15
The causes of loin pain

Ureteric calculus

Pylonephritis

Hydronephrosis

Perinephric abscess

Ruptured renal tumour

Clot colic

Ureteric obstruction

Abdominal aortic aneurysm

Retroperitoneal haematoma/abscess

Psoas abscess

Microbiology

Pus cells and organisms are usually present on **urinary microscopy**. The urine must be cultured to select the most appropriate antibiotic. *Men with cystitis and women with repeated attacks must be fully investigated* to ensure there are no anatomical abnormalities or diseases in the bladder or prostate that are causing the recurrent problems.

ACUTE RETENTION OF URINE

Acute retention of urine causes severe lower abdominal pain associated with a great desire but an inability to pass urine (see Chapter 20).

Patients may have experienced the symptoms of prostatism (poor stream, frequency, hesitancy and dribbling) before the first acute episode. Acute retention may be triggered by an attempt to avoid passing urine during a long journey.

A **large tender palpable bladder** which is dull to percussion confirms the diagnosis.

The passage of a urinary catheter will confirm the diagnosis and relieve the pain. An ultrasound scan of the bladder can be performed if the diagnosis is in doubt.

Further treatment is discussed in Chapter 20.

EXTRA-ABDOMINAL MEDICAL CONDITIONS

The extra-abdominal conditions that may cause abdominal pain include:

- myocardial infarction
- pericarditis
- pneumothorax
- diabetes
- Addison's disease
- uraemia
- porphyria
- haemochromatosis
- spinal disorders
- tabes dorsalis
- sickle-cell anaemia
- Henoch–Schönlein purpura
- leukaemia
- lymphoma

- polycythaemia
- polyarteritis nodosa
- systemic lupus erythematosus
- glandular fever
- herpes zoster.

The majority can be excluded by a careful history and clinical examination.

Most cardiac pulmonary and chest wall causes of pain can be detected by a **chest radiograph**, an **electrocardiogram** and a **troponin T level** assisted if necessary by **echocardiography**, a **chest CT scan** and a **ventilation perfusion scan**.

The urine should be tested for **porphyrins** and the blood and urine tested for **sugar** and **ketones**.

A **sickle cell test** is always worth obtaining in Afro-Caribbean patients.

An **erythrocyte sedimentation rate (ESR)** and an **autoantibody screen** can be helpful in diagnosing **collagen vascular disease**.

When all these tests are negative, many patients end up with a diagnosis of **non-specific abdominal pain** or **irritable bowel syndrome**.

In a few patients it becomes apparent that they are obtaining and dependent on **opioid drugs**.

Patients repeatedly admitted to hospital with symptoms that do not fit a recognized pattern or appear to be self-induced may be associated with the psychiatric disorder called **Munchausen's syndrome**.

Many of the latter conditions that are described in this section are diagnosed by the exclusion of the recognized pathological conditions that can cause acute abdominal pain.

18

Abdominal symptoms, masses, the spleen and obesity surgery

William E.G. Thomas and Kevin G. Burnand

Chapter 17 covers the investigation and management of conditions that present with acute abdominal pain. This chapter complements that by describing the investigation and management of the other major abdominal problems. Inevitably there is some overlap as many conditions are responsible for a variety of problems.

DYSPHAGIA

The term *dysphagia* is defined as an impairment of swallowing and may involve malfunction anywhere from the lips to the oesophagogastric junction. The act of swallowing may be divided into three phases: oral, pharyngeal and oesophageal.

The **oral phase** involves formation of the bolus by means of mastication, tongue movement and the action of saliva. Once a bolus is formed, it is delivered posteriorly by pressure of the tongue on the hard palate, thus delivering it through the pharyngeal fauces into the pharynx.

The **pharyngeal phase** is involuntary and involves delivery of the bolus to the upper oesophageal sphincter while sealing the nasopharynx and protecting the airway. The pharyngeal constrictor muscles propel the bolus through the upper oesophageal sphincter (cricopharyngeus), which serves to prevent aerophagia and reflux reaching the airway.

The **oesophageal phase** is also involuntary. Peristaltic waves propagated in the proximal oesophagus deliver the bolus to the lower oesophageal sphincter, which is under vagal control and provides a barrier to gastro-oesophageal reflux. Any functional abnormality or physical obstruction to any of the three phases of swallowing can result in dysphagia.

Dysphagia may therefore be functional or structural, high or low (see Table 18.1).

High dysphagia, affecting the oral or pharyngeal phase, tends to be functional and caused by a neuromuscular disorder such as a stroke, multiple sclerosis or Parkinson's disease.

Low dysphagia, affecting the oesophageal phase, tends to be structural or obstructive such as a neoplasm or stricture.

Globus hystericus, which is a sensation of having a lump in the throat, must be distinguished from true functional high dysphagia. Its aetiology is not known but it is common and occasionally responds to anxiolytic and antidepressant drugs. **Presbyphagia** is a term used to describe a degree of functional dysphagia resulting from the ageing process, which can prove difficult to manage.

Odynophagia (pain on swallowing) may be caused by infections such as candidiasis but can also occur with neoplasia.

Unfortunately the level at which a patient feels that their food is stuck often correlates poorly with the actual level of the obstructing lesion.

Investigation

Clinical diagnostic indicators

An accurate history is vital and will assist in targeting the investigations. The following features give an indication of the diagnosis.

Speed of onset A sudden onset suggests an obstructed food bolus or foreign body.

Duration of symptoms A short history with associated weight loss suggests malignancy, whereas symptoms that have been present for several years suggest a chronic motility disorder.

Painless progression Progressive dysphagia with a short history suggests malignancy. Long-standing intermittent dysphagia dependent on the nature of the bolus may indicate a stricture from reflux.

Table 18.1
Causes of dysphagia

		High dysphagia	Low dysphagia
Functional		Stroke	Diffuse oesophageal spasm
		Multiple sclerosis	'Nutcracker' oesophagus
		Parkinson's disease	Dysmotility
		Cerebral palsy	■ spasm
		Myasthenia gravis	■ corkscrew oesophagus
		Polymyositis	Scleroderma
		Huntingdon's chorea	Achalasia
		Muscular dystrophy	Chagas disease
		Presbyphagia	Corrosive structure
Structural		Neoplasia	Neoplasia
		Oesophagus/stomach	Oesophagus/stomach
		Pharyngeal pouch	Peptic stricture (reflux)
		Cricopharyngeal web/bar	Post-fundoplication
Rare		Extensive compression	
		Aortic dissection	
		Retrosternal thyroid	
		Mediastinal tumour (e.g. thymoma)	
		Dysphagia lusoria	
		Gastric volvulus	
		Carcinoma of the pharynx	
		Carcinoma of the larynx	
		Carcinoma of the thyroid	
		Carcinoma of the bronchus	
		Gastrointestinal stromal tumour	

Nature and timing Dysphagia to fluids or solids is an indication of the severity of the condition. Regurgitation of undigested food some time after eating suggests a pharyngeal pouch or achalasia.

Recent weight loss This suggests malignancy.

Heartburn or regurgitation soon after eating This suggests gastro-oesophageal reflux and/or stricture development.

Chest symptoms An associated cough may indicate aspiration.

Any history of an associated intercurrent, neurological, medical, rheumatological or psychiatric disease should be sought.

A patient with malignant disease may be **cachectic** (Chapter 4, p59) and have a palpable epigastric mass, liver or cervical lymph nodes.

Any patient with a possible neurological condition should have a full neurological examination.

In high dysphagia, the oropharynx and larynx should be examined.

In many cases the clinical examination is less revealing than the history.

Blood tests

Iron deficiency anaemia may be associated with a pharyngeal web, while patients with long-standing dysphagia or advanced malignancy may be both anaemic and **hypoproteinaemic**.

Imaging

Barium swallow involves giving the supine patient a bolus of barium to swallow and following it from the pharynx to the lower oesophageal sphincter. It is the investigation of choice for patients in whom a pharyngeal pouch is suspected as there is a risk of perforation from endoscopy in these patients.

Single-contrast studies are recommended for detecting strictures, diverticula, hiatus hernia and achalasia ('bird's beaking'), while **double-contrast** studies, giving an effervescent agent prior to swallowing the barium, is superior for visualizing mucosal lesions such as ulcers and nodules.

Gastro-oesophageal reflux can be demonstrated by asking the patient to perform a Valsalva manoeuvre.

Video-fluoroscopy is a modification of the barium swallow in which the act of swallowing the barium in either liquid, solid or semi-solid form is screened and watched by a radiologist and, if available, a speech therapist. This provides information about transit time, function of the oesophageal sphincters, efficacy of peristalsis and the risk of aspiration.

The presence of a speech therapist allows assessment and modification of the swallowing process and can influence treatment.

Chest X-ray and a **computed tomography (CT) scan** of the chest and abdomen are essential for the accurate staging of malignant disease. The role of CT is mainly to provide information about the local and/or distant spread of the disease, rather than confirm the diagnosis.

Endoscopy

Fibreoptic endoscopy is the main method of investigating dysphagia. It provides direct visualization of any mucosal lesion and the ability to biopsy and carry out therapeutic measures. It is the first choice investigation for low dysphagia and is well tolerated and safe, although the perforation rate increases if therapeutic dilatation or stenting is added.

Transnasal endoscopy may allow assessment of the pharyngeal phase of swallowing using liquids or solids with or without dye.

Endoscopic ultrasound can provide an accurate measurement of the depth of penetration of a tumour through the oesophageal wall and detect the presence and size of any adjacent lymphadenopathy.

Further information may be provided by **laparoscopy**, which may demonstrate peritoneal seedings or other metastatic spread not apparent on CT. It also allows peritoneal washings for cytological examination and the use of laparoscopic ultrasound to look for previously undetected secondary deposits in the liver.

Biopsy

All tumours, mucosal abnormalities (e.g. Barrett's oesophagus), or strictures must be biopsied.

Functional investigations

Oesophageal motility disorders require functional assessment. **Manometry** provides an assessment of the function, pressure and relaxation of the lower oesophageal sphincter as well as the peristaltic activity of the body of the oesophagus. All medication that may impact on motility must be stopped before passing a pressure sensor catheter, either solid state or fluid-perfused, via the nose into the stomach. The baseline intragastric pressure is measured and then the catheter is slowly pulled back until the area of maximal pressure, which represents the lower oesophageal sphincter, is reached. The patient then carries out a 'wet swallow' with some water while the ability of the sphincter to relax is assessed.

Oesophageal peristalsis is then assessed by positioning three of the catheter's pressure sensors within the body of the oesophagus and asking the patient to perform further 'wet swallows' at 30 second intervals during which the amplitude, velocity and duration of the peristaltic pressure wave is measured.

Twenty-four-hour pH monitoring is used to assess gastro-oesophageal reflux, which may be responsible for causing dysmotility and ultimately a stricture. This may be done in conjunction with manometry, but any acid-suppressing medication must be stopped for about a week prior to the

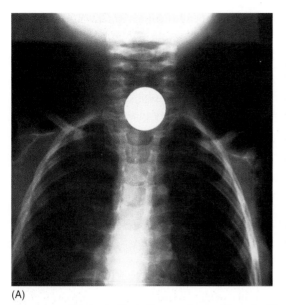
(A)

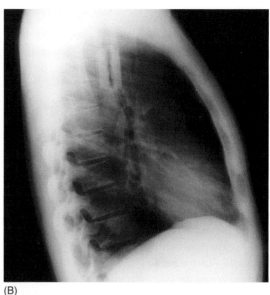
(B)

FIGURE 18.1 Foreign bodies in the oesophagus: (A) a coin; (B) a razor blade

investigation. A transnasal catheter is passed and the pH sensor positioned about 5 cm above the lower oesophageal sphincter as identified by manometry. The patient then undertakes normal activities for the next 24 hours and the pH is recorded using a digital recording device. The data are analysed in relation to the patient's activity, e.g. sitting, lying supine, sleeping, eating, and the patient's symptoms, all of which are recorded by an event marker and by the patient in a diary. By convention, a normal study is accepted as a pH of less than 4 for greater than 4 per cent of the time.

IMPACTED FOREIGN BODIES

Investigation

Clinical diagnostic indicators

This problem usually occurs in a child or an adult when a large food bolus impacts at the back of the throat above the oesophageal sphincter. Sudden onset of dysphagia combined with chest pain and retching indicate the diagnosis.

Imaging

A **plain chest X-ray** may show a foreign body (Fig 18.1) or evidence of surgical emphysema.

Management

First-aid is by **Heimlich's manoeuvre**. This is forcible pressure applied by standing behind the patient and suddenly pressing subdiaphragmmatically to expel the foreign body.

Endoscopy will be required if first-aid fails to visualize any foreign body or bolus and allow its removal by pulling out the endoscope after the obstruction has been caught by grasping forceps. Alternatively it can be pushed onwards into the stomach.

OESOPHAGEAL MOTILITY DISORDERS

The causes of motility disorders are summarized in Table 18.2.

ACHALASIA OF THE OESOPHAGUS

Investigation

Clinical diagnostic indicators

This disorder is most common in females (3:2) aged 30–40 years who present with progressive, often painful dysphagia for both solids and liquids. This may vary from day to day. Patients find it easier to

Table 18.2
Causes of oesophageal motility disorders

Achalasia of the cardia

Diffuse oesophageal spasm

Nutcracker oesophagus

Systemic sclerosis

Chagas disease

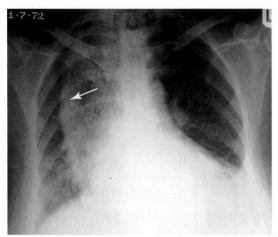

FIGURE 18.2 Large oesophagus containing food residue to the right of the oesophagus

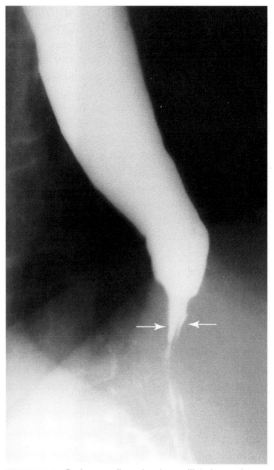

FIGURE 18.3 Barium swallow showing a dilated oesophagus with a smooth stricture (a bird beak) at its lower end

stand when swallowing, which is often accompanied by retrosternal chest pain. Other symptoms can include weight loss and regurgitation, which may cause aspiration pneumonia. Achalasia can predispose to squamous cell carcinoma of the oesophagus.

Blood tests

These are usually unhelpful.

Imaging

A chest X ray may show a widened mediastinum caused by an oesophagus full of food residues (Fig 18.2). Aspiration pneumonia may be present and the gastric air bubble may be absent.

At a late stage, a large flaccid dilated oesophagus containing food residues which smoothly tapers at its lower end can be seen on **barium swallow** (Fig 18.3). At an early stage, lower oesophageal narrowing can be caused by a carcinoma of the oesophagus.

Endoscopy

Flexible oesophagoscopy should be obtained to exclude neoplasia, but cannot diagnose achalasia.

Manometry

This should demonstrate a high-pressure, non-relaxing zone at the lower end of the oesophagus, which is associated with disordered or absent oesophageal peristaltic waves.

Management

This may be expectant at first, but mild to moderate symptoms should be treated by **balloon dilatation**, which disrupts the lower oesophageal sphincter and carries a small risk of causing a perforation. This is successful in relieving symptoms in 80–90 per cent of patients and can be repeated if symptoms recur. H2 receptor blockers or proton pump inhibitors may be required if dilatation is followed by reflux.

Recurrent symptoms with the need for more than one balloon dilatation are indications for **cardiomyotomy (Heller's operation)** (Fig 18.4). This can now be performed laparoscopically or thorascopically. The cardia and lower oesophagus are defined and the longitudinal, circular, smooth muscle of both are divided down to the mucosa. The incision should extend from 3 cm below the cardia to 5 cm above. A **fundoplication** may be carried out to cover the myotomy and prevent reflux (see below).

Early complications

Perforation and bleeding can occur. Late complications include persistent dysphagia, reflux and stricture. Reflux is prevented by fundoplication, which also reduces the risk of perforation and reflux stricture. Balloon dilatation is indicated if symptoms recur.

Prognosis

The mortality of balloon dilatation and Heller's cardiomyotomy is low, less than 1 per cent, and recurrent problems occur in less than 5 per cent of patients after surgery.

DIFFUSE OESOPHAGEAL SPASM

Investigation

Clinical diagnostic indicators

This condition usually presents with intermittent painful dysphagia in a middle-aged or elderly person, usually associated with retrosternal pain that can be mistaken for angina.

Imaging

Barium swallow and **endoscopy** show the appearance of a corkscrew oesophagus, with distorted peristaltic waves (Figs 18.5 and 18.6).

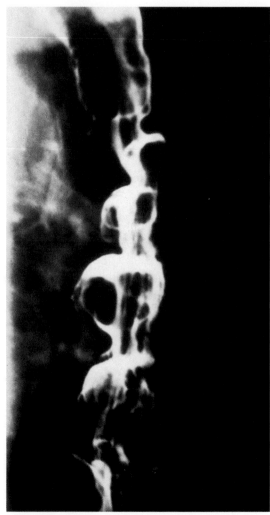

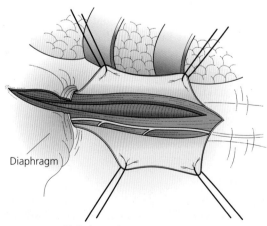

FIGURE 18.4 Heller's myotomy

FIGURE 18.5 Barium swallow of a corkscrew oesophagus with disordered peristaltic waves causing distortion

Manometry

This confirms disordered peristalsis with abnormal relaxation and a raised pressure in the lower oesophagus.

Management

Calcium channel blockers, H2 receptor antagonists, proton pump inhibitors, prokinetic drugs and tricyclic antidepressants can all be tried.

Surgical treatment is by a long **cardiomyotomy** (see Fig 18.4).

NUTCRACKER OESOPHAGUS

This extremely uncommon condition, which can present with chest pain and dysphagia, is a consequence of repeated, forcible peristalsis of unknown cause. The diagnosis can be confirmed by oesophageal manometry. Tricyclic drugs and biofeedback can be tried, but are rarely helpful.

SYSTEMIC SCLEROSIS

This often causes dysphagia, but other stigmata are usually indicative of the diagnosis (see Chapter 11). Oesophageal dilatation may help and proton pump inhibitors are usually prescribed.

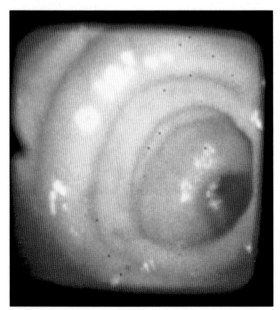

FIGURE 18.6 Endoscopy showing constrictions caused by disordered peristalsis

OESOPHAGEAL NEUROLOGICAL DISORDERS (BULBAR PALSY)

General care is vital for this difficult group of patients. At times seepage of saliva is a problem because of the inability to swallow. A percutaneous endoscopic gastrostomy (PEG) can provide access for enteral nutrition if there are long-term problems with feeding and nutrition (see Fig 1.3).

OESOPHAGEAL STRICTURES

Strictures usually occur as a consequence of acid reflux oesophagitis, but may also occur after ingestion of strong acid or more commonly alkali (attempted suicide). Plummer–Vinson syndrome can cause an oesophageal web. Peptic strictures are usually indicated by a past history of reflux and heartburn.

Investigation

Contrast studies

Barium swallow shows the stricture's length and may show an associated hiatus hernia.

Endoscopy

Oesophagoscopy can be used to confirm the stricture (Fig 18.7) and exclude malignancy by biopsy. Early endoscopy can also assess the extent of the corrosive damage.

Management of corrosive stricture

At an early stage, corrosive injury should be managed by drinking large amounts of water while

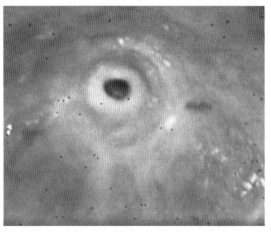

FIGURE 18.7 Endoscopy showing a tight reflux stricture

providing adequate analgesia (e.g. opioids). Early perforation of the oesophagus is usually fatal unless urgent resection is possible.

After the early stages, **oral intake should be avoided** and antibiotics and steroids may be prescribed in an attempt to reduce inflammation and subsequent stricture formation. Nutrition can be provided through total **parenteral nutrition**, a **PEG** or a **feeding jejunostomy** (see Chapter 2). Vomiting should be discouraged by anti-emetics.

Once all the inflammation has settled, symptoms of dysphagia can be treated by **balloon dilatation** or by **oesophageal resection and bypass**, often using jejunum or colon, as the stomach may also have been damaged by the corrosive.

Regular endoscopic surveillance is indicated as malignancy may develop.

Management of reflux stricture

For a benign stricture, Savary–Guillard **bougies** can be used to dilate the narrowing. These are passed over a guide wire. A **balloon** can also be passed over a guide wire, which is inserted under direct endoscopic vision.

H2 receptor blockers and **proton pump inhibitors** are indicated in addition to dilatation in peptic strictures.

An expendable **metal stent** can be inserted if these measures are followed by early restenosis, especially if the patient is unfit for major surgery. Operations include **fundoplication** to prevent reflux (see page 430) or **resection** of the oesophagus with replacement by stomach or oesophagus (see page 434). This may be anastomosed to normal oesophagus in the upper neck.

PHARYNGEAL POUCH

Investigation

Clinical diagnostic indicators

Elderly men present with regurgitation of recognizable food, halitosis, gurgling in the neck, a visible lump and symptoms of dysphagia.

Imaging

Barium swallow demonstrates a pouch (Fig 18.8). **Endoscopy** will confirm the presence of the pouch and reveal its contents.

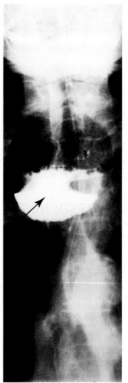

FIGURE 18.8 X-ray showing a pharyngeal pouch with barium hold-up

Management

Endoscopic stapling has largely replaced open surgical resection of the pouch with myotomy of the oesophagus.

Prognosis

This is very good for either technique with a low mortality of less than 1 per cent and a low risk of recurrence. Aspiration pneumonia can occasionally be disastrous if the condition passes unrecognized.

REFLUX OESOPHAGITIS

Reflux oesophagitis is caused by the reflux of gastric acid into the oesophagus. A certain minor degree of retrograde movement occurs as a normal physiological event during eating and drinking, but reflux of gastric contents into the oesophagus can result in unpleasant symptoms, including reflux oesophagitis, Barrett's oesophagus, peptic structuring of the oesophagus and carcinoma.

Gastro-oesophageal reflux (GOR) is usually caused by an inadequacy of the lower oesophageal sphincter with low basal sphincter pressures. This may be exacerbated by a hiatus hernia, which can cause sequestering of gastric contents in the herniated stomach. The hernia itself is usually but not always the sole cause of GOR. Other exacerbating factors include obesity, smoking, excessive alcohol, caffeine or fat ingestion, scleroderma and delayed gastric emptying.

Investigation

Clinical diagnostic indicators

The most common presentation of GOR is **heartburn, indigestion and regurgitation**. These symptoms are often worse at night when the patient is lying down, and can sometimes be confused with ischaemic heart pain. Regurgitation can be associated with aspiration, chest infection and chronic cough, especially if it is marked and occurs at night when the patient is lying down. It is essential to investigate patients to confirm the diagnosis and exclude other pathology, especially when there are atypical or **alarm symptoms** such as dysphagia, odynophagia (painful swallowing), haematemesis, choking sensations and weight loss.

Endoscopy

Oesophagoscopy may reveal oesophagitis (Fig 18.9), which is graded as:

- A: non-confluent mucosal breaks no longer than 5 mm
- B: non-confluent mucosal breaks >5 mm long
- C: confluent mucosal breaks between mucosal folds but <75 per cent of the oesophageal circumference
- D: mucosal breaks that involve >75 per cent of the oesophageal circumference.

Endoscopy may also show up mucosal lesions such as Barrett's oesophagus, peptic ulceration, infective oesophagitis from *Candida* or even a carcinoma.

It also provides the opportunity to treat strictures with dilatation and stents.

Imaging

Barium swallow studies can display a hiatus hernia, and the stress of a head-down position or a Valsalva

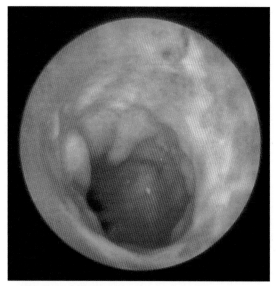

FIGURE 18.9 Endoscopy showing oesophagitis

manoeuvre may stimulate barium reflux into the oesophagus. Any associated strictures will also be seen.

Physiological function tests

Twenty-four-hour pH monitoring and **oesophageal manometry** (see page 423) detects the amount of acid reflux in the course of a day; the latter picks up any associated sphincter disturbance or motility disorder.

Management

A significant number of patients with mild or moderate symptoms have these effectively controlled by general measures and medical management. These measures include:

- **Lifestyle changes** such as:
  - weight reduction (sometimes bariatric surgery should be considered in the morbidly obese patient) (see page 469).
  - avoiding spicy, acidic, fatty foods
  - elevating the head of the bed – sleeping upright with additional pillows
  - reduction in smoking and alcohol intake
  - avoiding large meals late at night.
- **Medical management** is with:
  - antacids
  - H2 receptor blockers

- □ proton pump inhibitors (first line treatment usually)
- □ prokinetic therapy to assist with gastric emptying (metoclopramide).

Anti-reflux surgery

This is advised for patients who do not respond to the above measures or those with severe oesophagitis or recurrent strictures and symptomatic Barrett's oesophagus. Also, patients who develop side-effects from medical therapy or those who do not want to be on long-term medication may wish for anti-reflux surgery. Management of other conditions or complications such as stricture or carcinoma are dealt with elsewhere.

Laparoscopic fundoplication is now the established surgical treatment for GOR. The partial Nissen fundoplication (Fig 18.10) controls the majority of reflux episodes and reduces the risk of gas bloat and dysphagia. The long-term efficacy of reflux control may however be less than a 360-degree wrap.

A laparoscopic fundoplication involves mobilization of the cardia and lower oesophagus, with reduction of the hiatal hernia. The posterior crura are approximated over an intra-oesophageal bougie and the mobilized fundus is wrapped around the back of the oesophagus using non-absorbable sutures. *The crural sutures and the 'wrap' should not be too tight as this will result in dysphagia and gas bloat.*

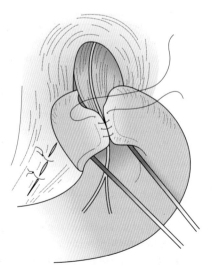

FIGURE 18.10   Nissen fundoplication

Complications

Intraoperative These include gastric perforation and bleeding.

Postoperative The patient may complain of vomiting, dysphagia or gas bloat. These symptoms may also be caused by a repair that is too tight and may require re-operation if they do not settle once postoperative oedema has settled.

Patients may develop **recurrent GOR**, which needs to be investigated as before and treated either medically or by re-operation, depending on the outcome of the investigations.

GOR is an important cause of vomiting in neonates. Thickening feeds, alginates and H2 receptor blockers are usually effective, but some infants who fail to thrive or who develop complications require fundoplication.

Newer innovative techniques are being explored within clinical trials, such as endoscopic plication of the cardia mucosa, intrasphinteric injections of polymers, and induction of scarring of the cardia tissues by radioablation. None of these techniques is established in clinical practice.

Prognosis

The majority of patients, 90 per cent, have their symptoms relieved by medical management. Ninety per cent have reflux cured by laparoscopic Nissen fundoplication. The mortality is less than 1 per cent.

HIATUS HERNIA

Investigation

Clinical diagnostic indicators

Patients with a sliding type of hiatus hernia usually present with reflux oesophagitis, but those with a large para-oesophageal hernia may present with shortness of breath, palpitations, arrhythmias, hiccupping and vomiting (Fig 18.11A and B).

A large para-oesophageal hernia may be found by chance on a chest X-ray or CT scan.

Imaging

Chest X-ray may show a widened mediastinum with a large fluid level sitting behind the heart.

Barium swallow confirms the presence of the stomach in the chest and reflux of barium can be seen on tipping the patient.

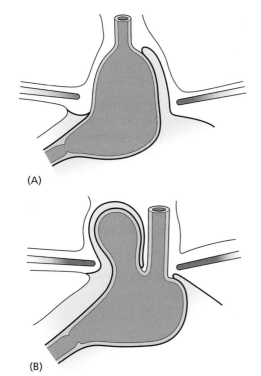

(A)

(B)

FIGURE 18.11 (A) Sliding and (B) rolling hiatus hernias

Endoscopy may show the presence of a hiatus hernia and evidence of reflux oesophagitis see (Fig 18.7).

Twenty-four-hour pH monitoring confirms low pH in the oesophagus.

Management

This is usually conservative if the patient has no symptoms. Medical treatment is the same as for reflux oesophagitis. Surgical treatment is also the same as for reflux oesophagitis if the patient has a sliding hiatus hernia and symptoms of reflux. Para-oesophageal hernias require the stomach to be repositioned in the abdomen before the diaphragm is repaired either directly or with a mesh.

Prognosis

This is very good unless a gastric volvulus occurs.

BARRET'S OESOPHAGUS

A Barret's oesophagus is an oesophagus lined, mainly in the lower part, with gastric epithelium. It

develops as a result of repeated reflux. It is usually found during an endoscopy when investigating the symptoms of reflux or stricture.

Investigation

Endoscopy and biopsy confirms the presence of gastric mucosa in the oesophagus with evidence of dysplasia.

Management

This should be with **proton pump inhibitors** and **repeated biopsy**. *There is no evidence that anti-reflux surgery is beneficial in preventing the development of malignancy.* A case can be made for oesophagectomy when severe dysplasia is present or if the patient has *in situ* carcinoma.

BENIGN OESOPHAGEAL TUMOURS

These tumours are rare, most being gastrointerstitial stromal tumours (GIST) previously called leiomyomas. They usually present with bleeding or dysphagia.

Barium swallow shows a filling defect and **CT** may demonstate a mass in the wall of the oesophagus.

Endoscopy may visualize the tumour and allow biopsy, although this may fail as the tumour is submucosal.

Treatment is by **enucleation**, which has very good results, a low morbidity and low mortality.

MALIGNANT OESOPHAGEAL TUMOURS

A multidisciplinary team approach is required to determine the optimum management for each oesophageal neoplasm. Unfortunately, the majority of patients with oesophageal carcinomas are unsuitable for radical surgical excision by the time they present because of advanced locoregional disease or distant metastases. Many are unfit for radical surgery.

Investigation

Clinical diagnostic indicators

Painless dysphagia that progresses from solids to liquids is the most common presentation. Odynophagia and aspiration pneumonia can also occur. Weight loss, anorexia and cachexia are common, and hoarseness may indicate invasion of the recurrent laryngeal nerve. It is worthwhile examining for enlarged cervical lymph nodes and the presence of hepatomegaly.

Blood tests

A **full blood count** should be carried out as the patient may be anaemic. **Liver function tests** may show signs of poor nutrition with hypoalbuminaemia.

Imaging

Barium swallow usually shows an irregular stricture in the oesophagous, often in its lower third with some proximal dilatation (Fig 18.12). The **differential diagnosis** is from a benign stricture or achalasia.

CT scans help with staging the disease. The presence of liver or lung metastases indicates inoperability.

Endoscopy

Oesophagoscopy is usually diagnostic and a biopsy should be taken to discover whether the tumour is an adenocarcinoma or a squamous cell carcinoma (Fig 18.13). **Bronchoscopy** may confirm spread to the lungs.

Biopsy

The presence of malignancy in distant nodes may be confirmed by fine needle aspiration cytology.

Laparoscopy

This confirms or excludes peritoneal spread.

Management

Palliation

Palliative treatments include:

- **intubation** using expandable metal mesh stents (Fig 18.14)
- **ablation** using argon beam coagulation
- **radiotherapy**, administered intraluminally or with an external beam, to reduce pain and improve the quality of life. This can be curative in some squamous cell carcinomas
- **chemotherapy** can be associated with a modest survival benefit

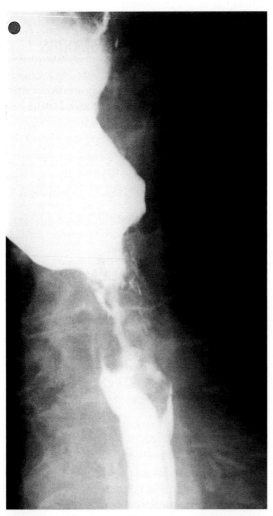

FIGURE 18.12   Carcinoma of the oesophagus with proximal oesophageal dilatation

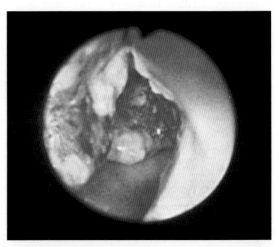

FIGURE 18.13   Endoscopy showing cancer of the oesophagus

psychological and social support given by palliative care teams working in the hospital and in primary care should provide analgesia and terminal care.

Surgery

Attempted curative surgery, with or without preoperative neoadjuvant **chemoradiotherapy**, performed in a tertiary referral specialist centre gives the best results. Neoadjuvant therapy aims to improve operability by downstaging the tumour prior to surgery.

The surgical aim is to remove all macroscopic and microscopic disease (R0 resection) and remove any involved abdominal and mediastinal lymph nodes.

The surgical methods for resection (Fig 18.15) include the following.

- A standard **two-stage (Ivor Lewis) oesophagectomy** uses abdominal and right thoracic incisions to mobilize the lower oesophagus and stomach on its vascular pedicles. The oesophagus is then resected through the right chest and the stomach brought up through the hiatus and anastomosed to the proximal oesophagus.
- A **McEwan three-stage oesophagectomy**. In this operation the oesophagus and stomach are mobilized in the neck, chest and abdomen. The stomach is brought up on its vascular pedicle into the neck. The oesophagus is resected and continuity is restored by end-to-end anastomosis of the oesophagus to the stomach in the neck.
- **Transhiatal subtotal oesophagectomy**. The stomach is again mobilized on its vascular pedicle, but the hiatus is widened and the lower oesophagus is mobilized into the lower chest by the abdominal surgeon while the cervical surgeon mobilizes the upper oesophagus into the chest. The mobilized oesophagus and stomach are pulled up into the neck and the fundus of the stomach is anastomosed to the divided cervical oesophagus. *This avoids a thoracotomy.*
- Total **gastrectomy and Roux-en-Y jejunal reconstruction** is carried out for tumours at the cardia. This is usually done through a thoraco-laparotomy incision, which carries a high risk of chest complications.
- Minimally invasive **transhiatal laparoscopic or thorascopic approaches** are also being used to mobilize the stomach or the oesophagus in the abdomen or chest, but there is concern over the adequacy of cancer clearance and the risk of vascular damage to the pedicles leading to gastric ischaemia.

Small bowel or colon are alternative means of reconstruction if the stomach cannot be used because of previous resections or infiltration with tumour (see Fig 18.15E).

Complications

Postoperative care should be in a high dependency unit. Cardiac arrhythmias and lung atelectesis are common. Nutrients may be provided through a **feeding jejunostomy** (which itself can cause complications) or intravenous feeding.

Anastomotic leakage occurs in 5–10 per cent and persistent chyle leakage can occur in a few patients when the thoracic duct is damaged.

Prognosis

The early mortality is usually related to anastomotic leakage (5–10 per cent). Of the 30 per cent of tumours that are resectable, about 30 per cent survive 5 years. The prognosis is better for early-stage lower oesophageal tumours without lymph node spread. It is also good for patients with severe dysplasia associated with Barrett's oesophagus, and transhiatal surgery is probably indicated for these patients.

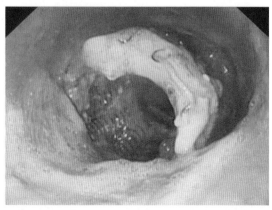

FIGURE 18.14 Endoscopy showing cancer of the oesophagus with a stent

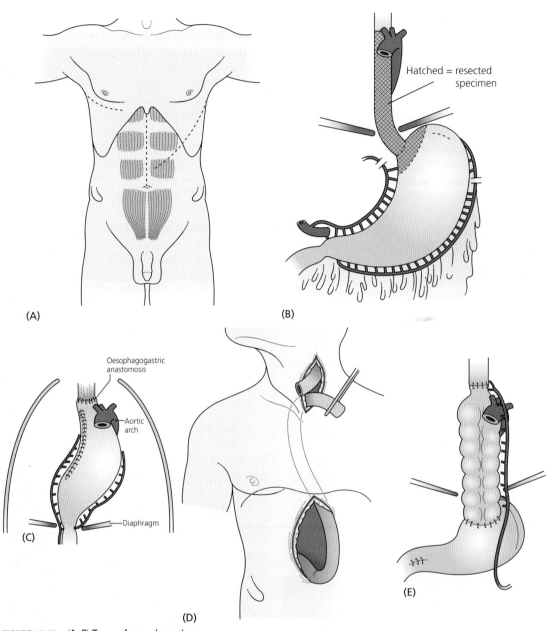

FIGURE 18.15 (A–E) Types of oesophagectomy

ANOREXIA AND WEIGHT LOSS

These symptoms are usually associated with gastric neoplasms and pancreatic carcinoma. Other intra-abdominal malignancy, generalized sepsis, AIDS, diabetes and renal failure are alternative causes that must be excluded.

GASTRIC NEOPLASMS

Benign tumours are very rare. Occasionally, gastric adenomas are found but must be assessed for their malignant potential. They can be treated by endoscopic snare resection or local excision with a cuff of normal gastric mucosa. Leiomyomata, now known as gastrointestinal stromal tumours (GST), are discussed under upper GI haemorrhage. Carcinoid tumours, ectopic pancreas and vascular malformations can occasionally arise in the stomach.

Malignant tumours are usually adenocarcinomata, although leiomyosarcomata (gastrointestinal stromal tumours), lymphomata (non-Hodgkin's) and malignant carcinoid tumours can also occur. Very rarely, the stomach can contain metastatic tumours from a malignant melanoma or other primary carcinoma.

ADENOCARCINOMA OF STOMACH

Investigation

Clinical diagnostic indicators

Adenocarcinoma of the stomach normally presents with the following symptoms and signs.

Symptoms

- anorexia
- weight loss
- epigastric pain
- nausea
- vomiting
- dysphagia
- evidence of distant spread.

Signs

- anaemia
- jaundice
- lymphadenopathy in the neck
- abdominal masses, including stomach, omentum and liver
- ascites
- abdominal distension
- pelvic mass
- cachexia
- visible peristalsis (pyloric obstruction)
- distant metastases (liver, lung, bone).

Blood tests

These should include a **full blood count**, a blood **film** and measurement of the **serum B12 and folate**. Pernicious anaemia is a predisposing factor.

Endoscopy for screening

In Japan where carcinoma of the stomach is very common, **endoscopic screening** is utilized. The cure rate is dramatically improved as the cancer is detected early with more than 75 per cent of patients having a chance of cure.

Endoscopy for diagnosis

Upper GI endoscopy has replaced barium studies in the diagnosis of carcinoma of the stomach (Fig 18.16). It can miss linitis plastica (leather bottle stomach), where the tumour extends beneath the mucosa (Fig 18.17), but the thick-walled stomach will usually be seen on abdominal CT scans.

Tissue biopsy

Multiple deep biopsies and repeated examination are very important if the diagnosis remains in doubt. All '**benign gastric ulcers**' must be considered to be potentially malignant and biopsies should be taken from four quadrants.

Staging

Once there is histological confirmation of the diagnosis, the tumour should be staged and evidence of metastatic spread sought.

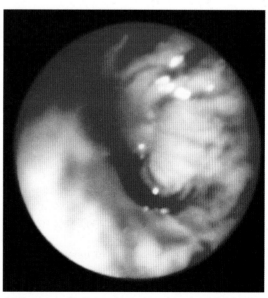

FIGURE 18.16 Gastroscopic appearances of cancer of the stomach

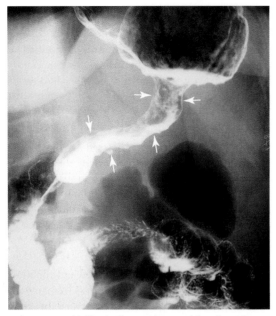

FIGURE 18.17   Linitis plastica carcinoma of the stomach

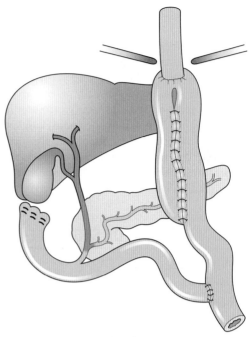

FIGURE 18.18   Reconstruction after total gastrectomy

Whole body CT scanning, endoscopic ultra-sound (to assess the depth of invasion), positron emission tomography (**PET**) **scanning** and **laparoscopy** can all be utilized. Not all investigations should be used on every occasion *but multislice rapid CT scanning is now considered almost essential before surgery is undertaken.*

Management

Treatment should be determined in specialist centres after a discussion by multidisciplinary teams, when further diagnostic investigations can be ordered and treatment plans formulated.

Palliative treatment is appropriate for patients with distant metastases and few symptoms, and also for patients with very advanced tumours that are irresectable. **Self-expanding stents** placed through the cardia or the pylorus via an endoscope may relieve the symptoms of patients who are vomiting and unable to eat.

Surgical bypasses by **gastro-enterostomy** or **local resections** (partial gastrectomies) can be considered if stenting fails.

Anaemia and dehydration should be corrected.

A decision may have to be made to withhold surgery and just give opiates and anti-emetics.

There is little or no place for palliative chemotherapy or radiotherapy.

Curative surgical resection. (Fig 18.18) There has been considerable controversy over the merits of radical total gastrectomy with resection of all R2 nodes and more localized surgical resections with only the local lymph nodes (e.g. omental nodes) being removed. The Japanese literature suggests that although radical R2 resections carry a higher mortality, they give better cure rates, but this has not been confirmed by randomized trials carried out in the West. *At present, the case for R2 total gastrectomy remains 'unproven'.*

Preoperative and postoperative chemotherapy with **epirubicin cisplatin** and **5-fluorouracil** has demonstrated a small but significant improvement in overall survival when combined with radical surgical resection.

Adjuvant radiotherapy may also improve survival.

Prognosis

The incidence of this tumour appears to be declining in Western nations (20 per 100 000 of the population) but remains high in Japan (125 per 100 000 of the population) where surgery and early diagnosis appear to improve survival. In early tumours, i.e. those confined to the mucosa and submucosa, the 5-year survival rate is around 80–90 per cent, but for invasive cancers with nodal spread this drops to 30–20 per cent. Patients with distant metastases rarely survive for prolonged periods of time.

LYMPHOMA

Lymphoma accounts for between 5 per cent and 10 per cent of all gastric malignancies. They are always **non-Hodgkin's lymphomas** and may be related to previous *Helicobacter pylori* infection. They diffusely infiltrate the stomach and often have to be differentiated from a linitis plastica adenocarcinoma of the stomach (see Fig 18.17).

Deep biopsies at endoscopy are required to confirm the diagnosis. **CT scanning and laparoscopy** may allow more accurate staging.

Surgical resection, radiotherapy, chemotherapy and even *H. pylori* eradication have been used with some success.

Provided there is no distant spread, the prognosis is usually reasonable with about 50 per cent of patients surviving for 5 years.

CARCINOID TUMOURS

Carcinoid tumours can occur in the stomach. Other rare tumours of the stomach include the schwannoma, chorion-epithelioma and carcino-sarcoma. All are treated by **gastrectomy** if feasible.

BENIGN DUODENAL TUMOURS

Duodenal adenoma and villous adenoma, lipoma and leiomyoma (gastrointestinal stromal tumours) all occur in the stomach. **Snare excision** is the treatment of choice if possible but otherwise they must be resected.

MALIGNANT DUODENAL TUMOURS

These include adenocarcinoma, lymphoma and carcinoid tumours. Periampullary tumours often cause jaundice. Resection is the treatment of choice.

JAUNDICE

Jaundice may be defined as an increase in the serum bilirubin, leading to the clinical manifestation of **yellow pigmentation of the skin and sclera**. It may result from hepatocyte failure, i.e. primary liver disease such as hepatitis and cirrhosis, or from obstruction within the biliary tree. **Jaundice is a physical sign and not a diagnosis**.

Obstruction to the flow of bile (cholestasis) may occur within the intrahepatic ductules (hepatic cholestasis) or in the extrahepatic biliary system (extrahepatic cholestasis). This latter group is usually referred to as cases of '**obstructive jaundice**'.

The early diagnosis and timely treatment of obstructive jaundice is important because pathological changes such as secondary biliary cirrhosis and hepatorenal failure can develop in the liver if the obstruction is not relieved. The investigation and management of 'jaundice' should be supervised by multidisciplinary teams, preferably in specialized centres.

CLASSIFICATION AND FEATURES OF JAUNDICE

Pre-hepatic jaundice is caused by an increased load of unconjugated bilirubin being presented to the hepatocytes, which is usually the sequel of **excessive haemolysis**. The liver itself may be normal, although in some cases, such as in haemolytic disease of the newborn, the hepatocytes may be immature and therefore less able to conjugate the increased load of bilirubin. The serum levels of the transaminases and alkaline phosphatase do not change.

Hepatic jaundice is caused by a failure of the hepatocytes to excrete conjugated bilirubin. This may be caused by **hepatitis or primary liver disease**. The serum transaminases are usually raised, reflecting hepatocyte damage; and, although there may be a raised level of conjugated bilirubin in the blood, there is often a mixed picture depending on the underlying disease process.

Post-hepatic jaundice has traditionally been used to describe obstructive jaundice but it is more accurate to refer to it as **cholestatic jaundice**; as n can occur within as well as outside the liver. Cholestasis, which can occur at any point between the hepatocytes and the ampulla of Vater, is accompanied by a raised serum conjugated bilirubin and alkaline phosphatase.

Preliminary investigation of jaundice

Blood tests

These should be performed on all jaundiced patients on presentation before beginning any special investigations.

Full blood count and film may show evidence of a haemolytic anaemia with sickle cells, elliptocytes or spherocytes present on the blood film (see Chapter 4).

Clotting screen international normalized ratio (INR) or prothrombin ratio and activated partial thromboplastin time (APTT) are often abnormal in liver disease because of malabsorbtion of vitamin K.

The serum urea, which will become elevated if hepatorenal failure is developing, **creatinine and electrolytes** should also be measured.

Liver function tests consist of:

- ▥ **bilirubin:** the conjugated/unconjugated ratio is now rarely used
- ▥ **alkaline phosphatase:** high levels are typical of obstructive jaundice
- ▥ **aminotransferases** (transaminases: AST/ALT) may be raised in the presence of active infection (cholangitis) but are typically not as high as the levels seen when major hepatocyte damage occurs as for example severe viral hepatitis
- ▥ **albumin:** usually normal but may fall in the presence of long-standing malignant bile duct obstruction or persisting infection
- ▥ **blood cultures** should be taken if the patient is septic or febrile. Cholangitis (inflammation in the bile ducts) is usual caused by organisms from the gut including *Escherichia coli*, *Streptococcus faecalis* and *Klebesiella*. Anaerobic organisms are more frequently present in patients who have had previous biliary surgery.

Urine tests

Urinary bilirubin and urobilinogen levels can sometimes be helpful.

In *prehepatic jaundice* the excess bilirubin is unconjugated and fat soluble and therefore not excreted in the urine (acholuric jaundice).

In *obstructive jaundice* the bilirubin is conjugated and water soluble allowing it to be excreted in the urine, when it produces a very dark (yellow/brown) colour. The urine does not contain urobilinogen, as no bilirubin is reaching the gut for conversion into urobilinogen before being reabsorbed and excreted in the urine.

Immunology

The following immunological studies should be requested immediately if primary liver disease is suspected, as they take some time to perform.

Test for plasma auto-antibodies, particularly **smooth muscle** antibodies (chronic active hepatitis) and **mitrochondrial** antibodies (primary biliary cirrhosis).

Hepatitis status (especially **hepatitis B** and **C**) should be known before performing any endoscopic or invasive investigations.

In immunocompromised patients, it is important to exclude cytomegalovirus and Epstein–Barr (EB) virus infections. An obstructive liver function test pattern may be seen in certain stages of hepatitis.

Preliminary management of jaundice

As many jaundiced patients are seriously ill, it is important to consider whether the following general measures are required before undertaking special investigations and treatment.

- ▥ **Correction of dehydration** with intravenous fluids including plasma expanders in patients with endotoxic shock.
- ▥ **Monitoring of urine output.** Jaundiced patients are at risk of developing acute renal failure (tubular necrosis). Assessing **osmolarity, urea concentration** and **sodium and potassium levels in a 24-hour urine specimen** are useful base line measurements.
- ▥ **Restoration of fluid balance** with mannitol or frusemide and appropriate intravenous fluids and inotropic support (e.g. dopamine 3 μg/kg/minute) may be needed on occasions.
- ▥ **Correction of clotting disorders** with intravenous vitamin K (10 μg daily) until the international normalized ratio (INR) or prothrombin time returns to normal.

■ **Control of sepsis** with an intravenous broad-spectrum cephalosporin (second or third generation) with gentamicin or Tazocin (a combination of piperacillin and tazobactam). The use of anti-anaerobic agents (e.g. metronidazole) must be considered in 'complex' situations particularly for those who have had previous biliary surgery or interventional procedures for benign strictures.

Further Investigation of jaundice

Imaging

It is vital to know whether the bile ducts are dilated, a finding diagnostic of biliary obstruction. The first imaging investigation should be an **abdominal ultrasound**. There is no reason to begin with a plain abdominal X-ray, as only 10 per cent of gall stones are radio-opaque, and pneumobilia and pancreatic calcification, which are uncommon, should be picked up by the ultrasound scan.

A **chest X-ray** should however be performed if malignant disease is suspected to look for lung metastases, which, if present, may exclude the need for other complex investigations and alter management.

Abdominal ultrasound

An abdominal ultrasound will detect dilatation of the **upstream bile ducts** and show the site of the obstruction and its cause if the jaundice is caused by an obstruction in the extrahepatic biliary tree. The ultrasound findings may be all that is required to direct subsequent management. The combination of the definition of the anatomical level of the obstruction revealed by the biliary dilatation and the relevant clinical details may help decide the likely cause or guide further appropriate investigations when the cause of the obstruction is not apparent on the initial ultrasound examination.

Interpretation of ultrasound findings

The vast majority of patients presenting with **distal common bile duct (CBD) obstruction** will have a **bile duct stone** or a **carcinoma of the head of pancreas**. In both conditions there is dilatation of both the intra- and extrahepatic bile ducts down to the level of the pancreas/distal

CBD. The cause of the obstruction (cancer or stones) may be apparent on ultrasound.

The appropriate management is obvious if a stone is detected in the bile duct; but if a mass is detected in the pancreas, attention must be focused on deciding whether or not it is a potentially operable tumour. If not (e.g. in the presence of liver metastases), then a **biopsy** can be arranged **under ultrasound guidance** for histological confirmation of the diagnosis once the biliary obstruction has been relieved. A **liver biopsy** should *not* be performed prior to decompression of the biliary tree as this may result in a bile leak and biliary peritonitis.

Patients with potentially resectable tumours should have further staging with **CT** or **magnetic resonance imaging** (MRI) *prior* to any endoscopic intervention, as the presence of a stent may cause difficulty in interpreting these scans.

Distal obstruction may also be caused by a tumour at the ampulla or in the duodenum. Both can be biopsied, if visible at **endoscopy**.

Proximal obstruction is obstruction in the region of the porta hepatis. It causes dilation of the intrahepatic ducts, without dilatation of the CBD. It is relatively unusual but is the classical presentation of a **hilar cholangiocarcinoma** (Klatskin tumour).

A similar appearance can, however, be caused by local infiltration from gall bladder pathology (e.g. a primary carcinoma or an inflammatory mass, Mirizzi syndrome), or from metastatic lymphadenopathy from a known or unknown primary tumour.

These cases can be difficult to assess, and further imaging with CT, MRI or both may be required. Doppler ultrasound can delineate the relationship of a hilar tumour to the adjacent vascular structures. This is important when assessing resectability.

Dilated common bile duct only. The 'normal' CBD diameter is often quoted as being <6 mm, but a 'baggy' CBD (>6 mm) is not an uncommon finding during routine ultrasound examination, particularly in patients who have had a cholecystectomy. It is rarely significant if the liver function tests are normal. Obstructive dilatation of the CBD in the jaundiced patient is usually associated with concomitant dilatation of the intrahepatic ducts, but there are some exceptions.

Spontaneously resolving or fluctuating levels of jaundice strongly suggest the presence of a CBD stone. A stone may have passed or disimpacted from the ampulla by the time of the ultrasound examination, so that the intrahepatic ducts are no longer dilated. If, in this situation, a CBD stone is not seen on ultrasound examination, **magnetic resonance cholangiopancreatography (MRCP)** (Fig 18.19) should be used to discover if the stone is still present.

In cases of distal obstruction with co-existing cirrhosis, the intrahepatic ducts may be prevented from dilating by the underlying parenchymal liver disease, leaving the dilatation confined to the extrahepatic ducts. This may cause confusion over whether the derangement in liver function is related to the underlying liver disease or an element of extrahepatic obstruction. An MRCP may help resolve this conundrum.

When the **bile ducts are not dilated**, the cause of the jaundice is assumed to be 'medical', i.e. primary hepatic in nature. Liver metastases are often included in this category. **Only very large multiple metastatic deposits cause clinical jaundice.** A more likely cause of jaundice in a patient with metastatic disease and jaundice is biliary tree obstruction caused by infiltrated lymph nodes at the porta

hepatis or a centrally placed liver deposit. In these patients the ducts will be dilated *but beware of paying attention just to the cause and missing the opportunity of providing symptom relief with palliative stenting.*

Other abnormalities A micro- or macronodular heterogeneous liver, splenomegaly, ascites and oesophageal varices can be detected on ultrasound and usually indicate chronic liver disease as the underlying aetiology.

In many cases of 'medical' jaundice, biliary dilatation is absent, and no other abnormality is detected. Further imaging is seldom of any help, other than to guide a percutaneous liver biopsy for histological assessment.

Occasionally ultrasound assessment may be suboptimal, e.g. in an obese patient, or when the head of the pancreas is obscured by bowel gas. In cases where the ultrasound findings are inconclusive, alternate imaging with a CT or MRI scan is appropriate.

CT or MRI scans

These investigations are used when further information is needed following the initial ultrasound assessment. Either can be used for tumour staging, but CT is the more commonly used investigation. An MRI examination is usually limited to one area (upper abdomen), whereas CT can assess the whole body (chest, abdomen and pelvis). CT is poor at detecting gall stones, unless they are calcified, so MRCP is preferred if CBD stones are suspected (see Fig 18.19). MRCP provides exquisite detail of both the pancreatic and bile ducts and has effectively replaced the diagnostic applications of endoscopic retrograde cholangiopancreatography (ERCP).

Percutaneous transhepatic cholangiography

Percutaneous transhepatic cholangiography (PTC) is a highly invasive investigation that was used as an alternative to ERCP, particularly for imaging the proximal biliary tree. It has now been largely superseded by MRCP. Currently PTC is only used to guide the stenting of a proximal bile duct tumour when the endoscopic route is not possible or appropriate.

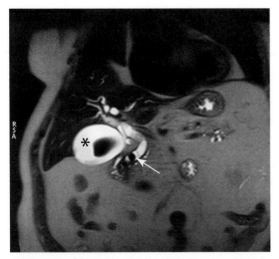

FIGURE 18.19   Magnetic resonance cholangiopancreatography showing stone in the common bile duct (arrow) as well as a stone in the gall bladder (*)

Radionuclide scanning

Radionuclide scanning may be used in several ways. A scan of the liver after an intravenous injection of ^{99}Tc sulphur colloid, which is taken up by the Kupffer cells of the liver, may demonstrate focal liver disease, but has largely been supplanted by the improving quality of ultrasound and CT.

Gallium scanning using ^{67}gallium citrate may be useful in the detection of a hepatomata.

Liver abscesses may be demonstrated using Tc-labelled white cell scanning.

Another form of scanning examines the biliary tree after the intravenous administration of a ^{99m}Tc-labelled iminodiacetic acid compound (^{99m}Tc-HIDA). This is secreted in the bile and gives a degree of functional information but has been largely supplanted by the greater accuracy of other investigations.

Endoscopic retrograde cholangiopancreatography

When distal obstruction is present on ultrasound examination and CBD stones suspected, but not confirmed, the traditional next step is to carry out endoscopic retrograde cholangiopancreatography (ERCP). This is still appropriate, but if there is any possibility that the obstruction could be caused by a tumour, staging investigations should be performed first.

Furthermore, obstruction by stone disease may resolve spontaneously. *Therefore in a well patient whose jaundice is improving, it may be worth performing a non-invasive MRCP to check that a stone is still present.*

Tumour staging

Pancreatic cancer has a dismal prognosis even after resection (see page 450), and yet surgery remains the only known cure. The purpose of imaging is therefore to identify patients with a potentially curable tumour while avoiding a futile attempt at surgery in a patient with an already limited life expectancy.

Staging should be undertaken before any attempt at endoscopic intervention is made as any subsequent pancreatitis or the presence of a stent may make the interpretation of further scans difficult.

Although the incidence of clinical pancreatitis following ERCP is low, 'radiological' pancreatitis is common. In fact, some inflammatory changes are detected on CT in the majority of patients even after an uncomplicated ERCP. This makes accurate staging very difficult. An episode of pancreatitis following ERCP may also make surgery very difficult if not impossible. Consequently, patients with **potentially resectable tumours** shown by the initial staging investigations *should not routinely undergo ERCP or endoscopic stenting preoperatively.*

When preoperative decompression is thought necessary it should be done percutaneously with an external biliary drain using ultrasound guidance, fluoroscopy or both. **Endoscopic stenting is best reserved for inoperable disease.**

Both CT and MRI tend to underestimate the extent of malignant disease. Most studies show that a significant minority (up to one-third) of patients thought to have operable tumours turn out to have unresectable disease at surgery. Unfortunately, disease thought to be inoperable on preoperative imaging is rarely found to be resectable. Staging laparoscopy has been used to try to improve staging accuracy.

Laparoscopic ultrasound can be used to display the relationship of the tumour to the superior mesenteric artery, the superior mesenteric vein and the portal vein, information which increases the sensitivity for unresectability.

Endoscopic ultrasound can also evaluate the relationship of a tumour to the vascular structures and can be used therapeutically to aspirate cysts and biopsy lesions but is very operator dependent.

A **hilar cholangiocarcinoma** (Klatskin tumour) is notoriously difficult to detect, although the biliary dilatation that results is relatively easy to image. A cholangiogram during an ERCP may demonstrate the anatomy well, but the proximal extent is not always clearly demonstrated. MRCP is particularly useful at showing the proximal extent of involvement – information used in the assessment of resectability.

Because metastatic carcinoma with disease at the porta hepatis can present a similar picture, a whole-body CT scan (chest, abdomen and pelvis) should be performed to look for an alternative primary tumour or other evidence of metastatic disease.

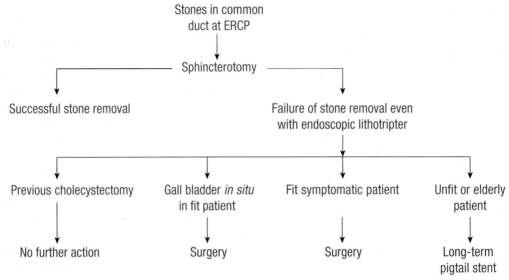

ERCP, endoscopic retrograde cholangiopancreatography.

FIGURE 18.20 Therapeutic options for choledocholithiasis

BILE DUCT STONES

Once jaundice has been confirmed as being caused by bile duct stones, there are several management choices (Fig 18.20). These include:

- ERCP and endoscopic sphincterotomy – either as definitive treatment or preceding cholecystectomy
- laparoscopic cholecystectomy and exploration of the common bile duct
- open cholecystectomy and exploration of the common bile duct.

The patient's clinical condition, their age and intercurrent disease, whether or not the patient has previously undergone cholecystectomy, and the clinical expertise available determines which of these options is chosen.

Endoscopic retrograde cholangiopancreatography and endoscopic sphincterotomy

This treatment has a success rate of around 90 per cent, with a low complication rate in the hands of an experienced endoscopist. Complications such as bleeding from damage to a branch of the superior pancreaticoduodenal artery, bowel perforation and acute pancreatitis can occur, as well as failure to cannulate the ampulla or an inability to perform an adequate sphincterotomy.

Once an adequate endoscopic sphincterotomy has been performed, stones may be allowed to fall out, but preferably the duct should be cleared at the same time. This can usually be performed with a balloon catheter or Dormia basket (Fig 18.21), although the balloon may occasionally burst and the stone can impact at the lower end of the duct or in the ampulla itself while still in the Dormia basket. In the majority of cases, however, the duct can be cleared and this should be confirmed by a post-clearance X-ray of the duct.

A stone that is too large to pass may be crushed *in situ* using a mechanical lithotripter. This is a difficult instrument to use and can cause damage to the lining of the duct.

Specialized units have other ways of reducing the size of the stone including:

- perfusion with monoctanoin through a nasobiliary tube
- external shockwave lithotripsy

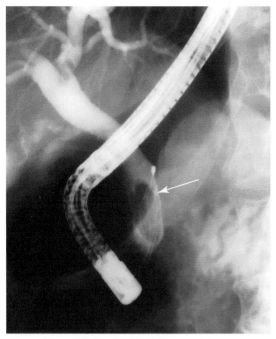

FIGURE 18.21   Stone removal with Dormia basket from the lower end of the common bile duct

■ endoscopically guided ultrasound or laser contact lithotripsy using a 'mother and baby' scope to view the stone.

These techniques are not in routine use. When there is a single large stone or multiple irretrievable stones, a stent or pigtail catheter can be placed endoscopically to improve the passage of bile into the duodenum, relieve the jaundice and prevent the residual stones impacting at the ampulla. This technique is especially useful in elderly patients who are not suitable for open surgery. **Such stents can remain *in situ* indefinitely and if they become blocked can be removed and replaced.**

Laparoscopic exploration of the common bile duct during laparoscopic cholecystectomy

Intraoperative cholangiography will occasionally demonstrate the unexpected presence of common duct stones. Cholangiography is therefore strongly indicated in all patients having a laparoscopic cholecystectomy who have been jaundiced, have abnormal liver function tests, a dilated common bile duct

on ultrasound (>7–8 mm), and in patients with a history of acute pancreatitis.

In direct **laparoscopic choledochotomy**, an incision made in the common bile duct enables the surgeon to extract common bile duct calculi and insert a T tube. Alternatively, when the stone is small and the cystic duct lumen negotiable, a Fogarty catheter or stone basket may be passed into the bile duct to extract a calculis or push it through the ampulla. The stones must be in the bile duct distal to the entry of the cystic duct for this method to be used.

This technique is time consuming and requires considerable laparoscopic expertise, and is rarely the procedure of choice in patients presenting with obstructive jaundice.

Most of the patients with common duct stones who request and are suitable for a laparoscopic cholecystectomy are advised to have an **ERCP** and an **endoscopic sphicterotomy** *preoperatively* to clear the duct prior to surgery.

Open exploration of the common bile duct

Many surgeons advise fit patients who are jaundiced and still have their gall bladder *in situ* to have an open cholecystectomy with a standard supraduodenal choledochotomy and duct exploration through a medially placed transverse subcostal incision. This approach allows all relevant pathology to be dealt with at the same time, saving the patient from multiple procedures and hospital admissions.

Other drainage procedures are indicated when the bile duct is very dilated, contains multiple stones, drains poorly or has a stone impacted at its lower end that has resisted all efforts at removal. In these situations **choledochoduodenostomy** or **transduodenal sphincteroplasty** (Fig 18.22) are safe and effective especially in elderly people. The former procedure, which involves anastomosing the duodenum to the opened duct, is simple and safe as long as the duct is dilated (>1 cm). A transduodenal sphincteroplasty is more appropriate if the duct is small or a stone is impacted at its lower end. The duodenum is opened opposite the ampulla, before the ampulla is cannulated and cut in the line of the duct. This opens the duct and allows the removal of any impacted stones, before the mucosa of the duct and the duodenum are sutured together to hold the lower end of the common bile duct widely open. The duodenotomy is then closed.

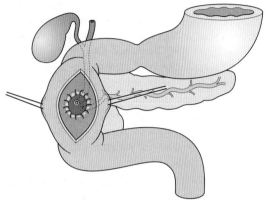

FIGURE 18.22   Transduodenal sphincteroplasty

MALIGNANT STRICTURES

In those patients who have a malignant cause for their jaundice, *it is first necessary to decide whether the tumour is resectable.* This will depend on the nature, site, extent or spread of the tumour as well as the age and co-morbidity of the patient. Radiological evidence of unresectability includes **liver or peritoneal metastases, ascites, enlarged lymph nodes, or a tumour that involves adjacent blood vessels,** especially the superior mesenteric vein and portal vein.

The multidisciplinary team should decide a management strategy based on the radiological staging and the age and co-morbidity of the patient (Fig 18.23).

Preoperative histological confirmation of malignancy may not be possible if there is concern that

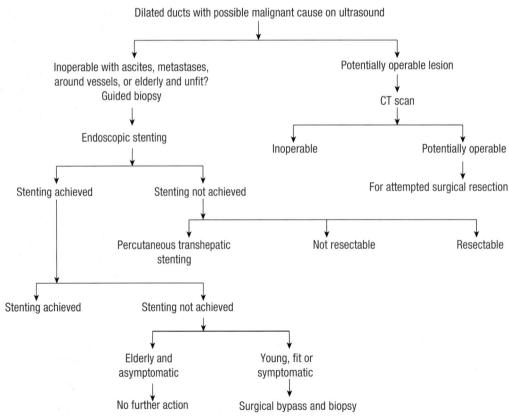

FIGURE 18.23   Therapeutic options for malignant disease

a tissue biopsy might cause cellular spread, but it should be sought whenever possible, even in patients who are not having definitive excisional surgery. This allows the prognosis to be given to the patient. Chemotherapy can be considered as treatment.

If a patient is considered to have a potentially resectable tumour, treatment depends on the site of the lesion. Tumours may be broadly considered as either **distal** or **proximal**.

Distal malignant obstruction

Tumours obstructing the distal common bile duct are usually cholangiocarcinomata, ampullary carcinomata or carcinomata in the head of the pancreas or adjacent duodenum. The treatment of choice is a **standard pancreaticoduodenectomy (Whipple's procedure)** (Fig 18.24). In certain situations a pylorus-preserving procedure may be appropriate, e.g. for distal cholangiocarcinoma of the bile duct or certain ampullary carcinomata. Most surgeons feel this approach is inappropriate for carcinoma of the duodenum or pancreatic head, where greater clearance is required.

The patient may benefit from a palliative **choledochojejunostomy** and **gastrojejunostomy** (Fig 18.25A) (often referred to as a triple bypass if an entero-enterostomy is added) if at operation the neoplasm is unexpectedly found to be unresectable for any reason.

Cholecystojejunostomy is less favoured because of the potential future obstruction of the cystic duct by the expanding neoplasm, especially if the cystic duct insertion is low in the common bile duct. The requirement for open palliative biliary bypass operations is much less since the development of precise investigation and less invasive methods of palliation.

Proximal malignant obstruction

Surgery for operable lesions situated proximally in the duct system (including the Klatskin tumour involving the confluence of the hepatic ducts) should be undertaken in specialized units where liver surgery is regularly performed. Multidisciplinary support and the special equipment such as ultrasonic dissectors, argon coagulators and lasers required for liver resection must be available.

Central **liver split procedures** may be required with subsequent **hepatodochojejunostomy**. This can now be performed with minimal blood loss and morbidity.

In cases where resection is impossible, a bypass procedure may be carried out, utilizing a **hepatodochojejunostomy** with a Roux-en-Y loop of

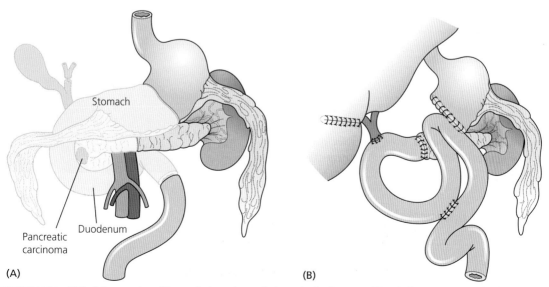

FIGURE 18.24 Whipple's procedure (A) resected specimen of stomach, duodenum and head of pancreas (faded), (B) reconstruction

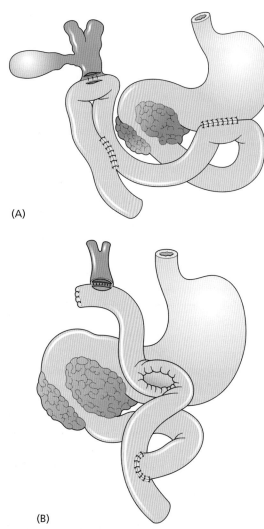

(A)

(B)

FIGURE 18.25 (A) Choledochojejunostomy.
(B) Hepatodochojejunostomy with a Roux en Y anastomosis

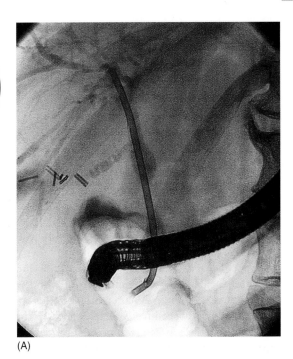

(A)

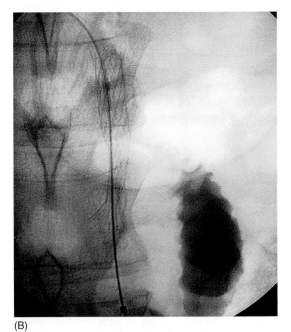

(B)

FIGURE 18.26 Stents in the common bile duct: (A) plastic;
(B) metal

jejunum being anastomosed to the left hepatic duct once it has been lowered from the liver plate, or anastomosis of a Roux loop to the segment III duct of the liver.

Stenting of unresectable obstruction

One of the commonest clinical presentations is that of an elderly frail patient with extensive co-morbidity and an unresectable neoplasm. Most of these patients will at some time require the insertion of a biliary stent. There are different forms of stent in current use and different approaches for their insertion (Fig 18.26).

Route of insertion

Endoscopic stenting is preferred to percutaneous transhepatic stenting, especially for lower bile duct or pancreatic lesions. Angulation at the site of the tumour may, however, prevent this approach. A percutaneous transhepatic approach is required in these cases and for proximal lesions.

Type of stent

Following negotiation of the malignant stricture with a guide wire, a biliary stent is passed over the guide wire. **A plastic stent is preferable** if there is any possibility that future surgery may be possible. An expandable metal or wall stent is better if resection is not an option.

When it is not possible to insert a stent because of oedema or other technical reasons, it is vital to leave an external proximal percutaneous catheter *in situ*. Otherwise the patient will be left with an obstructed system, a perforation in the biliary system upstream to the obstruction, and be at risk of developing a biliary peritonitis and/or an infected biliary tree.

The bile draining externally should be cultured at regular intervals to ensure the early detection of any infection.

Complications of stenting

The immediate complications of stenting are:

- sepsis
- haemorrhage
- acute pancreatitis
- perforation and bile leak (peritonitis).

The late complications are:

- recurrent jaundice caused by:
  - □ stent displacement
  - □ sludge in the stent
  - □ overgrowth of the stent by neoplasm
- erosion of the stent into an adjacent viscus.

BENIGN STRICTURES

The commonest avoidable cause of a benign biliary stricture is damage to the common duct or its blood supply at the time of gall bladder surgery.

Provided the damage is identified when it occurs, the best treatment is immediate reconstruction by an experienced biliary surgeon.

The treatment of delayed strictures includes endoscopic balloon dilatation, stenting and surgical reconstruction.

Dilatation, although of value, often fails to provide good long-term results even if repeated on multiple occasions.

Stenting is frequently complicated by sludging and cholangitis, which require multiple admissions for antibiotic control and stent replacement.

In cases where a metal Wall stent has been used, a plastic stent may be inserted through the blocked lumen of the metal stent but the results are not entirely satisfactory (Fig 18.26).

Surgical bypass (hepatodochojejunostomy) in the hands of an experienced hepatobiliary surgeon is therefore the preferred definitive treatment. For this reason it is wise not to insert a metal stent if reconstruction at a later date is to be considered as these stents cannot be removed.

GALL BLADDER DISEASE

Acute and chronic cholecystitis are covered in Chapter 17 as they usually present with pain. There are, however, a number of other conditions of the gall bladder which will be briefly discussed.

Acalculus choleycystitis

This is common in patients admitted to the intensive care unit with major trauma, sepsis and splanchnic shutdown. Gangrene and perforation of the bladder may develop and this is fatal if left untreated.

The diagnosis is difficult as the patients are often unconscious on a ventilator. It requires a high index of suspicion and may only be diagnosed by a speculative ultrasound in an otherwise extremely sick patient.

In very sick patients, the management is by **percutaneous drainage**. Early cholecystectomy is curative if the patients' general condition allows.

Cholesterosis (strawberry gall bladder)

This is a pathological entity caused by cholesterol deposition and is only relevant if associated with gall stones or cholecystitis.

Adenomyomatosis

This is mucosal diverticulitis in a thickened gall bladder wall. It can be seen as a filling defect on ultrasound and is only diagnosed by investigation of the gall bladder, e.g. ultrasound. The differential diagnosis is from carcinoma of the gall bladder.

Mucocoele of the gall bladder

This occurs when Hartman's pouch or the cystic duct is obstructed by a stone and the gall bladder does not become infected. It often causes some discomfort and a gall bladder mass may be detected. Treatment is by cholecystectomy.

Empyema of the gall bladder

This is the same as a mucocoele but the gall bladder contents have become infected. Fever, pain and a mass situated beneath the liver that is tender and moves on palpation indicates the diagnosis. Confirmation is by ultrasound and treatment is by cholecystectomy.

Emphysema of the gall bladder

This occurs in diabetics when anaerobic bacteria proliferate in the gall bladder, which then contains gas. Plain X-rays show the gas, which can also be seen on CT or ultrasound.

Treatment is cholecystectomy with metronidazole cover.

Gangrene of the gall bladder

Gangrene of the gall bladder (Fig 18.27) often develops as a complication of acalculus cholecystitis, acute cholecystitis or empyema of the gall bladder. The patient becomes extremely sick with signs of generalized peritonitis (see 'Acute abdomen'). Free bile can be imaged in the peritoneal cavity. Management is **urgent cholecystectomy**.

This condition has an appreciable mortality – greater than 10 per cent.

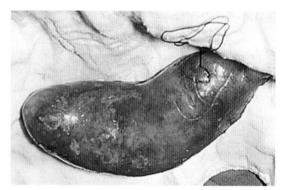

FIGURE 18.27   A gangrenous gall bladder that has been removed by cholecystectomy

Carcinoma of the gall bladder

This rare condition is invariably related to gall stones. Patients often present with symptoms or signs of acute or chronic choleycystitis. Progressive jaundice is common and a result of bile duct invasion.

It is rarely diagnosed with certainty preoperatively, but ultrasound will demonstrate gall stones and sometimes a filling defect or mass around Hartman's pouch. This can be confirmed by CT, and an MRCP may show a high bile duct obstruction.

It may be treated conservatively by **cholecystectomy and stenting** or aggressively by **central liver resection** followed by **chemotherapy**.

The prognosis is poor whatever the treatment. Less than 5 per cent of patients survive 5 years.

ASIATIC CHOLANGIOHEPATITIS

This is common in China and Japan. Patients present with pyrexia, rigors and jaundice.

Ultrasound shows dilated bile ducts. MRCP confirms dilated ducts containing multiple filling defects and stones.

Antibiotics and stone removal may be followed by **choledocoduodenostomy** or **hepaticojejunostomy** to allow residual stones to pass spontaneously. Radical hepatic resection is indicated for localized liver destruction with abscesses.

PRIMARY SCLEROSING CHOLANGITIS

The cause of this condition, which presents with thickening and inflammation of the bile ducts, is not known. It is associated with ulcerative colitis (75 per cent) and other autoimmune conditions.

Intermittent attacks of obstructive jaundice become permanent and progressive.

The **liver function tests** show an obstructive picture with a raised bilirubin and alkaline phosphatase.

Ultrasound shows dilated intrahepatic ducts and an MRCP shows a beaded appearance.

ERCP and stenting with **biopsy** confirms the diagnosis and excludes a primary bile duct carcinoma (see below). Eventually, **liver transplantation** may be required for patients developing liver failure.

CHRONIC PANCREATITIS

Investigation

Clinical diagnostic indicators

This condition presents with chronic epigastric pain, often radiating through to the back. Weight loss, steatorrhoea and diabetes can occur. Occasionally duodenal obstruction (vomiting) and splenic vein thrombosis (portal hypertension and haematemesis) and obstructive jaundice can be presenting symptoms.

Blood tests

The **amylase and lipases** are occasionally elevated but these are not diagnostic. The **bilirubin and alkaline phosphatase** can be raised if there is obstructive jaundice. Random blood sugars and a glucose tolerance test may confirm the presence of associated diabetes.

Faecal fat

Levels above 5 g per day on a normal diet are indicative of **steatorrhoea**. Fat absorption and excretion can also be measured by an isotope test.

Imaging

Plain abdominal X-rays may show calcification, which can be confirmed to be in the pancreas by CT (Fig 18.28).

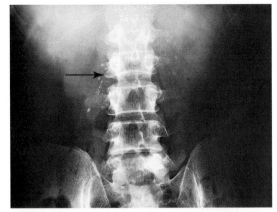

(A)

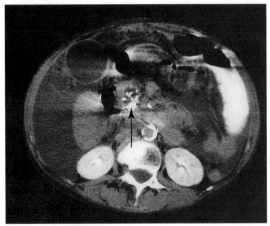

(B)

FIGURE 18.28 Calcification in the pancreas: (A) plain X-ray and (B) CT

Ultrasound or **CT** shows an enlargement of pancreatic gland, often containing cystic collections and calcification.

ERCP may confirm biliary obstruction and an abnormal pancreatic duct system.

Endoscopic ultrasound should *not show* a localized mass in the head as this is suggestive of a neoplasm. Pancreatic juice can be sent for cytology to exclude a carcinoma.

Management

Pain relief and abstinence from alcohol will improve the patient's condition, even if they are jaundiced. Pancreatic extracts (creon) can help diarrhoea, and

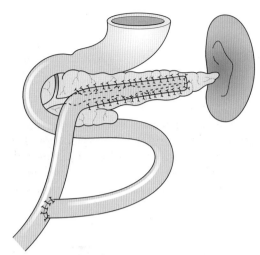

FIGURE 18.29   Pancreaticojejunostomy for chronic pancreatitis

if the patient is diabetic they may require hypoglycaemic tablets or insulin. A coeliac plexus block may provide short-term pain relief. Jaundice can be treated by inserting a stent (see above).

Surgical options

Pancreaticojejunostomy (Fig 18.29) may provide drainage of an obstructed duct system and relieve symptoms in 60–70 per cent of those treated.

Pancreaticoduodenectomy is a more radical option but can preserve the tail of the pancreas, and as a consequence preserve endocrine function.

Total pancreatectomy is a last resort, resulting in severe diabetes and loss of exocrine function with steatorrhoea and frequent stools.

Prognosis

This is often poor, with many patients being constantly readmitted to hospital over many years, and only 60–70 per cent remaining free of severe pain even after radical surgical treatment. Results are better in patients who give up alcohol. Sadly, many become drug addicts and Munchausen's syndrome is always a possibility.

NEOPLASMS OF THE PANCREAS

These can be divided into **exocrine** and **endocrine** tumours.

There are a **few benign neoplasms of the pancreas**, usually cyst adenomas, which are only detected by chance when abdominal scans are obtained for other reasons. They can be symptomatic when they become very large and have to be differentiated from pseudocysts and cyst adenocarcinomas.

Malignant pancreatic neoplasms are usually ductal adenocarcinoma (see below), but cyst adenocarcinomata and acinar cell carcinomata are also reported.

Adenocarcinoma of the pancreas

Investigation

Clinical diagnostic indicators

Two-thirds of these tumours arise in the head of the pancreas, where they usually present with obstructive jaundice (see above). This is painless and progressive. Dark urine, pale stools, pruritis, weight loss and epigastric pain radiating through to the back are common associated symptoms. Pain and weight loss are the main symptoms when the tumour arises in the body or tail of the gland, and diabetes and steatorrhoea may develop in any pancreatic carcinoma.

A palpable gall bladder in the presence of jaundice (**Courvoisier's law**) is suggestive of a carcinoma of the head of pancreas. Liver metastases may cause an enlarged, knobbly mass in the right hypochondrium, but a pancreatic mass is rarely palpable. Thrombophlebitis migrans (**Trousseau's sign**) is a rare late complication.

The **differential diagnosis** is shown in Table 18.3.

Blood tests

Anaemia is common when jaundice is present. Tumour markers may be raised. Liver function tests show an obstructive picture. A random or fasting blood sugar may be raised.

Stools

There may be evidence of steatorrhoea with raised faecal fats as in chronic pancreatitis (greater than 5 g per day). Occult blood in the stool may indicate an ampullary tumour.

Table 18.3
Differential diagnosis of carcinoma of the pancreas

Chronic pancreatitis

Cystadenocarcinoma of pancreas

Lymphoma of the pancreas

Cholangiocarcinoma of bile ducts

Vipoma

Gluconoma

Insulinoma

Sclerosing cholangitis

Gastric carcinoma

Duodenal carcinoma with secondary deposits in the portahepatis

Urine tests

Bilirubin is present and urobilinogen is absent when there is total obstruction of the common bile duct.

Imaging

Ultrasonography and **CT scans** can detect bile duct dilatation and tumours in the pancreatic gland, but cannot differentiate tumours from chronic pancreatitis with certainty.

An **MRCP** can usually differentiate between gall stone obstruction and cholangiocarcinoma of the bile duct, although ampullary tumours may be difficult to diagnose without endoscopic biopsy.

Endoscopy

Duodenoscopy and biopsy can confirm the diagnosis of an ampullary cancer and can be combined with **ultrasound and biopsy** to positively diagnose carcinomata of the pancreatic head.

Endoscopic retrograde cholangiopancreotography is mainly used to pass stents for treatment rather than as a diagnostic test, as it can cause severe pancreatitis.

Cytology

The pancreatic juice can be collected for cytology at the same time as a stent is passed to relieve biliary obstruction.

Laparoscopy

This may be used to try to detect spread to the liver or peritoneum, but it is dubious if this adds a lot to the CT scan.

Laparotomy

It may still not be possible to differentiate chronic pancreatitis from carcinoma at laparotomy. **It is important to try to obtain a correct preoperative diagnosis if possible** to avoid radical and dangerous surgery being offered to patients with chronic pancreatitis.

Management

The management of jaundice is discussed above. Curative treatment for pancreatic neoplasms requires pancreatic resection, but *only 10 per cent of all patients with malignant tumours are suitable for surgery.*

Curative treatment

Whipple's procedure of radical pancreaticoduodenectomy is the best treatment for resectable carcinomas of the head of the pancreas (see Fig 18.24). In this operation the head of the pancreas is resected with the duodenum, gall bladder and lower half of the common bile duct. The continuity of the pancreatic bile duct and intestine is restored by anastomosing a Roux loop to the stomach, pancreas and bile ducts. The mortality of this procedure is now less than 5 per cent but the survival is only 10–20 per cent at 5 years in these highly selected patients.

Pylorus preserving operations and **radical total pancreatectomies** (the only procedure for extensive tumours of the body of the pancreas) have similar survival rates with few discernable benefits.

Distal pancreatectomy may be possible for tumours in the tail of the gland. Adjuvant radiotherapy and chemotherapy may marginally improve survival at the cost of increased side-effects.

Palliative treatment

The palliation of jaundice is discussed above. **Endoscopic stents** are now used more commonly than **triple bypass**. Within 1 year 90 per cent of patients are dead.

Radiotherapy and chemotherapy are not indicated for palliation and pain relief by analgesics, coeliac plexus block and splanicectomy may all be required.

Insulinoma

Clinical diagnostic indicators

Patients often present with **palpitations, sweating and tremors** following a lack of food (fasting). They may also develop **neuropsychiatric problems** with personality changes. Hypoglycaemic coma can occur if the symptoms are left untreated. Attacks are relieved by taking glucose. The major **differential diagnosis** is from psychosis, epilepsy and space-occupying lesions of the brain.

Blood tests

The blood sugar falls after fasting while the blood insulin levels remain high even when the blood sugar is low.

Imaging

Abdominal ultrasound rarely picks up small tumours and **multislice CT is more accurate** but still only detects 40–50 per cent of insulinomata.

Angiography or CT angiography does not improve this accuracy greatly, but **intraoperative and endoscopic ultrasound** may pick up smaller tumours.

Management

Surgical resection of the tumour, or rarely tumours in patients with MEN1, is the treatment of choice. The whole of the pancreatic gland is exposed at laparotomy by 'Kocherizing' the duodenum, taking down the right colon and dividing the gastrocolic ligament. Careful palpation of the gland is supplemented by intraoperative ultrasound. Once the tumour has been located it can be locally excised (shelled out). Tumours are usually solitary and are 2 cm or less in diameter.

When no tumour can be found, it is probably better to withdraw than perform a blind distal pancreatectomy, which may achieve nothing.

Diazoxide can be used to control the blood sugar postoperatively and an attempt can be made to locate the tumour by selective venous sampling for insulin levels in the splenic vein. Ten per cent of insulinomata are malignant and should be radically resected if possible. **Streptozotocin** should be tried for inoperable tumours or metastases and diazoxide can be used to control hypoglycaemia.

Gastrinoma

Clinical diagnostic indicators

These tumours cause the Zollinger–Ellison syndrome (MEN1) where the high gastric acid levels cause multiple **recurrent peptic ulceration** at atypical sites. They can also cause **severe diarrhoea** and steatorrhoea.

Blood tests

Serum gastrin levels and gastric acid secretion are both elevated.

Imaging

CT scans, **MRI** and **selective angiography** may detect multiple tumours.

Management

The tumour should be **resected** where possible, although it is sometimes multifocal and can undergo malignant change. Control of acid secretion is then important and **proton pump inhibitors** can be used to achieve this.

Glucagonomas and Vipomas

Clinical diagnostic indicators

Glucagonomas cause glossitis, stomatitis, necrotizing dermatitis, bowel upset, weight loss, diabetes and anaemia.

Vipomas cause watery diarrhoea with secondary hypokalaemia and achorhydria causing metabolic alkalosis.

Blood tests

The finding of increased **glucagon or vaso-inhibitory polypeptide** in the serum is indicative of the diagnosis.

Imaging

This is again by **CT, MRI and angiography** of the pancreas.

Management

Resection either locally or by subtotal pancreotectomy is ideal. Symptom control may be by streptozotocin and octreotide if this cannot be performed.

JAUNDICE IN CHILDREN

Most jaundice in neonates is caused by rhesus incompatibility, prematurity and neonatal sepsis. Prolonged progressive jaundice in an infant is usually the result of **biliary atresia**, which is an uncommon condition.

BILLIARY ATRESIA

Clinical diagnostic indicators

Beside jaundice, the liver and spleen may be palpably enlarged.

Blood tests

Liver function tests show an obstructive picture with a raised bilirubin and alkaline phosphatase.

Imaging

Ultrasound usually shows intrahepatic biliary dilatation. An **MRCP** may show the site of obstruction to be either intra- or extrahepatic.

Management

Surgery using a '**Kasai' bypass** (a Roux-en-Y loop anastomosed to the intrahepatic bile ducts in the liver), or a **liver transplant**, may give reasonable long-term results.

Prognosis

Liver transplantation may give better results than the Kasai bypass.

CHOLEDOCHAL CYSTS

This is a rare cyst usually arising at the lower end of the biliary tree, compressing both the common bile duct and the pancreatic duct.

Clinical diagnostic indicators

Jaundice can develop in neonates, although it is unusual, and more commonly cysts remain symptomless until later in life. Intermittent pain and jaundice is a common presentation in the adult, and patients may also present with recurrent attacks of acute pancreatitis.

Blood tests

Liver function tests show an obstructive jaundice picture with a raised alkaline phosphatase and the serum amylase may be raised if pain persists.

Imaging

Ultrasound shows bile duct dilatation and may demonstrate the cystic swelling. **MRCP** confirms the diagnosis by showing a cystic swelling sometimes causing a long stenosis of the bowel and pancreatic ducts.

Management

Choledochal cysts should be excised as they can become malignant. Prolonged biliary and pancreatic obstruction can also lead to permanent liver damage.

LIVER DISEASE

CIRRHOSIS OF THE LIVER (PORTAL HYPERTENSION)

This is the result of damage to hepatocytes with fibrosis and nodular regeneration. The fibrosis damages hepatic function and also obstructs the portal vein radicals leading to portal hypertension.

The causes of portal hypertension are listed in Table 18.4.

Investigation

Clinical diagnostic indicators

Symptoms of liver failure include anorexia, weight loss, jaundice and eventually encephalopathic coma. Abdominal distension from ascites and bleeding problems can also cause patients to seek medical advice.

The symptoms of portal hypertension may predominate with haematemesis and melaena being the clinical presentation in about 40 per cent of patients from either oesophageal varices or peptic ulceration.

The stigmata of liver disease including jaundice are often present (Table 18.5), and splenomegaly

Table 18.4
Causes of portal hypertension

Presinuoidal

Extrahepatic

Portal vein thrombosis or atresia

Splenic vein thrombosis

Portal arteriovenous fistula

Pancreatitis

Hypersplenism

Intrahepatic

Schistosomiasis

Cirrhosis

Postsinusoidal

Budd–Chiari syndrome

Congestive heart failure/pericarditis

Veno-occlusive disease

Table 18.5
Stigmata of liver disease

White nails

Dupuytren's contractures

Liver palms

Liver flap

Spider naevi

Gynaecomastia

Loss of axillary and pubic hair

Foetor hepaticus

Ascites

Caput medusa

and hepatomegaly may be detected in addition to the presence of ascites.

Blood tests

Iron deficiency and megaloblastic anaemias are common, the latter from B12 and folate deficiency. **Liver function tests** often show a mixed picture of liver failure (raised bilirubin, low albumin and raised transaminases) and intrahepatic cholestasis (raised alkaline phosphatase).

Imaging

Ultrasound shows a small, shrunken, fibrotic liver without any filling defects. In the early stages, hepatomegaly with fatty infiltration and fibrosis may be detected (fibroscan). Ascites can usually be seen.

An **MRCP** is normal and a **CT scan** excludes liver metastases or a hepatocellular carcinoma (see page 457).

CT angiography may demonstrate portal vein occlusion and the presence of varices with evidence of other sites of portosystemic shunts.

Endoscopy

Upper GI endoscopy may show oesophageal varices (Fig 18.30) or the presence of peptic ulceration.

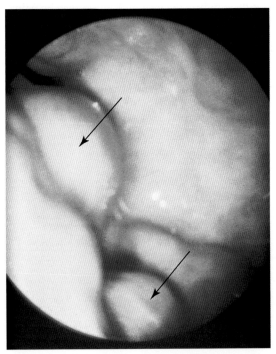

FIGURE 18.30   Endoscopy demonstrating Oesophageal varices

Proctoscopy or **flexible sigmoidoscopy** may show severe haemorrhoids.

Liver biopsy

This confirms the presence of cirrhosis by finding the features of **fibrosis and nodular regeneration**. Bleeding can be a problem after the biopsy, which

Table 18.6
Child–Pugh grading system for liver disease

Variable	Number of points		
	1	2	3
Bilirubin (μmol/L)	<34	34–51	>51
Albumin (g/L)	>35	28–35	<28
Prothrombin time	<3	3–10	>10
Ascites	None	Mild	Moderate to severe
Encephalopathy	None	Mild	Moderate to severe

Grade A, 5 or 6 points; grade B, 7–9 points; grade C, 10–15 points.

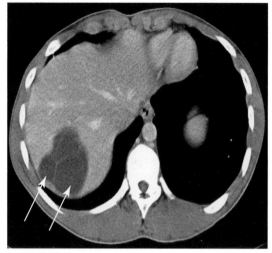

FIGURE 18.31   Hydatid cyst in liver

can be taken through the internal jugular vein via the hepatic veins.

Management

The severity of liver disease can be staged using the Child–Pugh grading system (Table 18.6) and treatment based on the grading.

Alcohol must be avoided. Schistosomiasis should be treated and steroids may be tried for patients with primary biliary cirrhosis.

Prophylactic oesophageal variceal banding or **transjugular intrahepatic portosystemic shunt (TIPS)** procedures are probably not indicated. They are, however, valuable when patients start to bleed from their varices (see page 465).

Liver transplantation is indicated if liver failure progresses. The management of gastrointestinal bleeding is dealt with elsewhere.

A few patients may benefit from splenectomy when hypersplenism is present, and patients with the Budd–Chiari syndrome can also be treated by a TIPS procedure.

Portocaval shunt procedures have now become a rarity.

Prognosis

This is very poor once patients have reached Child's B or C grade, with only 10 per cent surviving 5 years.

HYDATID DISEASE OF THE LIVER

Clinical diagnostic indicators

Right upper quadrant pain, dyspepsia, vomiting and acute anaphylactic reactions are more common than jaundice as presenting symptoms.

Jaundice sometimes develops when a hydatid cyst ruptures into the biliary tree and is associated with secondary infection. Cysts may also cause hepatomegaly and chest symptoms from diaphragmatic perforation. They can be quiescent and are then only found on imaging studies being carried out for other reasons.

Intraperitoneal rupture of a cyst can lead to generalized abdominal swelling with ascites.

Blood tests

Eosinophilia is found on blood films and a **hydatid compliment fixation test** may be positive, indicating that infestation has occurred at some stage.

Imaging

X-rays may show an elevated diaphragm with a pleural effusion and occasionally ring calcification may be seen over the liver on chest X-ray or plain abdominal X-rays.

Ultrasound or **CT scan** shows the characteristic appearances of a thick-walled cystic space containing multiple daughter cysts (Fig 18.31).

Management

This may be 'expectant' for burnt out small cysts, but a strongly positive compliment fixation test or eosinophilia usually indicates the need for treatment. This is by an **albendazole**, which should be given for several months.

Large symptomatic cysts can be **excised** taking special precautions to avoid spillage into the peritoneal cavity. Normally the cysts are killed by injecting normal saline into them before resection, and spillage of daughter cysts is avoided by attaching specialized devices to the surface of the liver.

Prognosis

This is good, unless there is widespread biliary or peritoneal spillage. Anaphylaxis can be lethal.

PYOGENIC LIVER ABSCESS

Clinical diagnostic indicators

Pyrexia, rigors and pain in the right hypochondrium are more common than jaundice as a presentation. There is usually a preceding history of appendicitis, diverticulitis, cholecystitis or some other type of infection in the structures drained by the portal vein. On examination pyrexia, hepatomegaly and tenderness should be sought.

Blood tests

The **white cell count** is usually raised and **liver function tests** may be abnormal.

Imaging

A **chest radiograph** may show basal lung collapse, a right pleural effusion and a raised right hemidiaphragm.

Ultrasound and CT show a circular, fluid-filled mass in the liver with an enhancing capsule. An abscess can be confirmed by technicium-labelled **white cell scanning**.

Management

Percutaneous drainage under ultrasound guidance with installation of **antibiotics** should be combined with a prolonged course of systemic broad-spectrum antibiotics. This is usually coamoxyclav, 1 g tds. The abscess is monitored by ultrasound and can be re-aspirated with further antibiotics being instilled.

Prognosis

This is usually good, provided the diagnosis is made and treatment instituted.

AMOEBIC LIVER ABSCESS

This follows a bout of amoebic dysentery. Presenting symptoms are usually **pyrexia, rigors, night sweats and pain** in the right hypochondrium. Jaundice is unusual, but nausea and anorexia can occur. On examination, tender hepatomegaly may be present.

Blood tests

Serology for **amoebae** may be positive and they may be present in the stools.

Imaging

Chest radiographs may demonstrate basal collapse with a pleural effusion and a raised hemidiaphragm. **Ultrasound and CT scans** again show a spherical enhancing mass in the liver.

Management

Metronidazole should be given systemically and the abscess aspirated. The prognosis is good.

Benign tumours of the liver

These tumours are usually found by chance at laparotomy or laparoscopy, or on imaging. They can occasionally produce **upper right-sided abdominal pain** from bleeding. Adenomas usually occur in women on the contraceptive pill.

Focal nodular hypoplasia and primary and secondary liver malignancies are the main **differential diagnoses**. Abscesses rarely cause problems.

Blood tests

The **alpha-fetoprotein** tumour marker is negative.

Imaging

CT scans with contrast and **MRI scans** all demonstrate filling defects in the liver. Biopsies of angiomata and adenomata can cause dangerous bleeding.

Management

Most benign tumours (haemangiomata and haematomata) can be left alone unless they are symptomatic. Adenomata often have to be excised as they may be mistaken for a small hepatocellular carcinoma and they can bleed spectacularly.

PRIMARY MALIGNANT TUMOURS OF THE LIVER

Hepatocellular carcinoma (hepatoma)

Clinical diagnostic indicators

Many patients who develop this tumour have cirrhotic livers and may be jaundiced. Others have ascites or present with a gastrointestinal bleed. **When a tumour develops there is often a rapid deterioration in liver function associated with upper abdominal pain, weight loss, fever and a mass.** These are late signs in patients where the tumour develops in a normal liver. A single large mass in the liver is highly suggestive, but generalized hepatomegaly is more commonly present.

Blood tests

The **liver enzymes and bilirubin** may be raised, as may the alkaline phosphatase, although this is not usually very high. **The alpha-fetoprotein** may be elevated in up to a third of patients with a hepatocellular malignancy.

Imaging

A **dynamic CT scan** of the abdomen and chest allows resectability and secondary spread to be assessed (Fig 18.32).

Angiography is not considered essential any longer, but **gallium citrate scanning** can be diagnostic.

Tissue biopsy

Ultrasound-guided biopsy should provide the diagnosis.

Management

Surgical resection is the only definitive treatment but may be impossible in patients with severe cirrhosis who have a poor liver reserve. Tumours are often multifocal in cirrhotic patients and are too extensive for resection.

Combination chemotherapy can be tried, but responses are limited. **Chemoembolization**

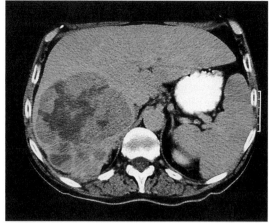
(A)

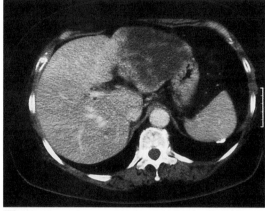
(B)

FIGURE 18.32   CT scans of hepatocellular carcinoma of the liver: (A) posterior part of right lobe; (B) most of left lobe

through the hepatic artery may be more successful. Normally a **partial left or right hepatectomy** is satisfactory, but occasionally a **hepatectomy and liver transplant** offers the only prospect of success.

Prognosis

The 5-year survival for partial hepatectomy for hepatoma is around 10 per cent, unless it is a fibrolamellar tumour when the results are somewhat better.

Cholangiocarcinoma

Clinical diagnostic indicators

This is far less common than a hepatocellular carcinoma in most Western countries, but is much more common in the Far East, where it is associated with 'helmintic' infection of the biliary tree. It normally presents with **jaundice** and **right upper quadrant pain**. Hepatomegaly is commonly present.

Blood tests

Liver function tests show an obstructed picture. The **alkaline phosphatase** is usually very elevated.

Imaging

Ultrasound and CT may demonstrate a liver tumour.

Management

Liver resection is required for a cure. This may be impossible and a **total hepatectomy with transplant** may be the only other option. Bile duct tumour management is described earlier under jaundice.

Rare primary malignant tumours of the liver

These include angiosarcomata, haemangiomta endotheliomata and hepatoblastomata. Their clinical indicators, investigation and management are similar to other primary tumours of the liver, but cytotoxics and radiation may provide better palliation.

Metastic tumours in the liver

Clinical diagnostic indicators

Metastases are 20 times more common than primary liver tumours. The most common primary site is from carcinoma in the abdomen (colon, stomach, oesophagus, pancreas, ovaries and kidneys). Malignancies such as carcinoid tumours, melanomata, bronchial carcinomata, breast carcinomata and sarcomata may all occasionally spread to the liver.

Jaundice, weight loss, pyrexia and right upper quadrant pain are common presenting symptoms, and jaundice, ascites and hepatomegaly may be found on examination.

Blood tests

Liver function tests are often abnormal. The bilirubin, aspartate transaminase and alkaline phosphatase may all be raised. There may be evidence of anaemia and the C-reactive protein (CRP) and erythrocyte sedimentation rate (ESR) can be elevated. The alpha-fetoprotein is not elevated.

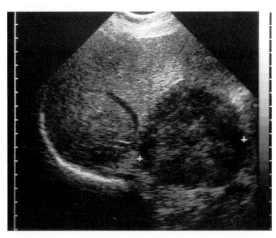

FIGURE 18.33   CT scan of metastatic tumour of the liver

Imaging

Ultrasound and **CT scans** with contrast can both detect metastases, but the resolution of CT scan with contrast is better. These imaging techniques can be used to take a guided fine needle aspiration to confirm the diagnosis.

Management

Most tumours are inoperable because metastases are present throughout both liver lobes. Treatment is then **palliative** with radiotherapy, chemotherapy and hepatic artery embolization. More recently, **laser destruction of individual metastases** has been used. In the terminal stages analgesia is indicated.

Solitary tumours or those confined to a single lobe can be treated by **partial hepatectomy**, with some gratifying long-term survivors, although level-1 evidence for the benefit of liver resection for metastases does not exist.

Prognosis

Thirty per cent of carefully selected patients having resections have survived for 5 years.

VOMITING AND COLIC

Vomiting frequently accompanies colic, especially when caused by intestinal obstruction, so here they are considered together. The many causes of both problems include:

- upper, small and large bowel obstruction
- gall bladder and bile duct calculi/choleycystitis
- gastroenteritis
- paralytic ileus
- systemic disorders (e.g. typhoid)
- diabetic ketoacidosis
- uraemia
- drugs (e.g. morphia)
- raised intracranial pressure
- viral infections
- ureteric and renal calculi
- uterus (labour)
- Fallopian tube ectopic pregnancy/salpingitis
- bladder outlet obstruction.

Almost all these conditions are associated with anorexia and nausea.

SMALL AND LARGE BOWEL OBSTRUCTION

See Chapter 17 for investigation and management of these conditions.

MECONIUM ILEUS

This is almost always a complication of **cystic fibrosis**. Eighty-five per cent of affected children have a two basepair deletion on chromosome 7. The proximal small bowel is distended with multiple meconium pellets and the terminal ileum and colon narrow and constricted.

Affected children have a **positive sodium sweat test**.

Hirschsprung's disease must be considered in the differential diagnosis.

Imaging

The diagnosis is made on a **plain abdominal X-ray**. Fluid levels are present in the proximal small bowel. The fat globules in the distended ileum in the right iliac fossa cause translucencies that give a **soap bubble appearance**.

A water-soluble contrast enema will show a 'microcolon' and round filling defects (meconium pellets) in the distal ileum.

Management

The vomiting should be relieved and the dehydration and any electrolyte imbalance corrected with **nasogastric aspiration** and **iv electrolytes**.

Although half of patients are cured by the contrast enema many still require careful fluid replacement over the next few days.

When **surgery** has to be performed, an **enterostomy** is made in the proximal ileum and saline is irrigated distally to wash out the meconium plugs. Proximal and distal stomas can be brought out onto the abdominal wall if this proves impossible. Once children have recovered, **pancreatic enzyme replacement** must be given.

Older children can present with **meconium ileus equivalent**. This causes colicky abdominal pain, tenderness and a mass in the right iliac fossa. Treatment is usually by gastrograffin enemas but occasionally surgery is required when enterotomies may be necessary to clear out the inspissated masses.

CONGENITAL HYPERTROPHIC PYLORIC STENOSIS

Investigation

Clinical diagnostic indicators

Congenital hypertrophic pyloric stenosis presents in the first 2 months of life with projectile, non-bile-stained vomiting with signs of dehydration and weight loss usually 2–3 weeks after birth.

Successful palpation of the tumour after nasogastric intubation and feeding with an electrolyte solution is diagnostic.

The **differential diagnosis** is shown in Table 18.7.

Table 18.7
Differential diagnoses of congenital hypertrophic pyloric stenosis

Duodenal atresia	Gastro-oesophageal reflux
Malrotation	Gastroenteritis
Small bowel atresia	Systemic infections
Meconium ileus	Raised intracranial pressure
Duplication cysts	Feeding difficulties/food allergies

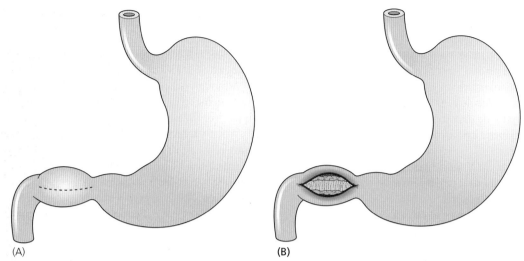

(A)   (B)

FIGURE 18.34   Ramstedt's pyloromyotomy. The mucosa should not be incised.

Imaging

An abdominal ultrasound reveals the hypertrophied pylorus if the tumour is impalpable.

Management

For successful **fluid replacement**, the fluid and electrolyte balance (usually a hypochloraemic acidosis) must be corrected by providing **intravenous normal saline with potassium**.

Emptying the stomach should be accomplished by nasogastric aspiration and washouts to stop the vomiting.

If **conservative regimen** is applied, very occasionally the muscle hypertrophy will regress, but waiting for this to occur increases the risks of dehydration and weight loss, so immediate operation is always advisable.

Ramstedt's pyloromyotomy (Fig 18.34) should be carried out through a transverse right upper quadrant incision or through a laparoscope under either local or general anaesthesia. Oral feeding can be resumed as soon as the infant is awake. The child can be discharged 24–48 hours later.

Complications

Complications include continued obstruction and vomiting, if the myotomy is inadequate, and peritonitis, if the duodenal mucosa is perforated during the myotomy. Wound infection can also occur.

Results

With modern paediatric anaesthesia and fluid balance control, the once very high mortality rate of this condition is now less than 1 per cent.

ADULT PYLORIC STENOSIS

Investigation

Clinical diagnostic indicators

Pyloric stenosis presents with **projectile vomiting** containing undigested food (e.g. tomato skins). The vomitus does not contain bile and is often foul smelling. There may be a history of the symptoms of peptic ulceration but this is often lacking. **Visible peristalsis** and a **succussion splash** are diagnostic physical signs. There are usually accompanying signs of dehydration and weight loss.

The **differential diagnoses** of adult pyloric stenosis are listed in Table 18.8.

Blood tests

The **haematocrit, potassium, urea** and **electrolytes** and the **specific gravity of the urine** all help assess the degree of dehydration. A hypochloraemic alkalosis is usually present.

A CLO test should be performed.

Table 18.8
Differential diagnoses of adult pyloric stenosis

Antral gastric carcinoma

Duodenal carcinoma (very rare)

Pancreatic or bile duct carcinoma

Small bowel obstruction

Carcinoma of the pancreas

Chronic pancreatitis

Imaging

A **plain abdominal radiograph** will often show a large stomach containing a fluid level. This can be confirmed by a barium or gastrograffin meal (Fig 18.35).

Endoscopy

Endoscopy and **biopsy** should be performed after washing out the stomach with a large-bore **nasogastric tube**.

Management

Most patients require **rehydration** with intravenous normal saline, usually with added potassium, depending on the serum potassium level.

A **stomach washout** will relieve the vomiting.

Endoscopy, biopsy and **the passage of a guidewire through the stenosis** is followed by balloon dilation of the pylorus or duodenum. This can often produce immediate and long-term relief of the symptoms.

H2 receptor antagonists or **proton pump inhibitors** are then prescribed and *H. pylori* eradication therapy carried out if there is a positive CLO test (see Chapter 17).

Pyloroplasty or **gastro-enterostomy without vagotomy** may be needed if recurrence occurs in spite of long-term medical treatment.

Prognosis

Recurrent pyloric stenosis can occur after balloon dilatation and may require redilatation. Surgical treatment is very successful but has the morbidity and mortality risk of 1–2 per cent.

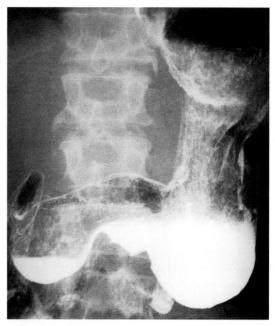

FIGURE 18.35   Acute pyloric obstruction: note the huge stomach with food residues floating on the barium

GASTRIC VOLVULUS

This is an extremely rare condition. It is invariably an organo-axial rotation of stomach within a large para-oesophageal hiatus hernia.

Investigation

Clinical diagnostic indicators

Gastric volvulus causes severe **epigastric pain** that may radiate up behind the sternum. It is invariably accompanied by **severe vomiting**.

Imaging

The diagnosis should be suspected if an **erect chest radiograph** shows a fluid level in a section of stomach trapped inside a large hiatus hernia and may be confirmed by a **gastrograffin swallow** (Fig 18.36).

Management

The stomach must be **untwisted** through an upper abdominal incision and the hiatus hernia repaired. The stomach needs to be fixed to the abdominal wall or partially resected. A gastrectomy is required if the volvulus has become gangrenous.

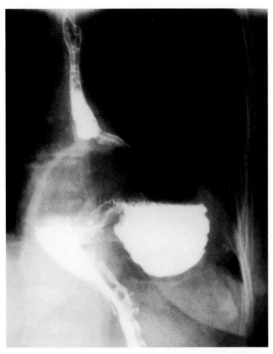

FIGURE 18.36   Gastric volvulus: a rotated stomach is seen within a large para-oesophageal hiatus hernia in the chest

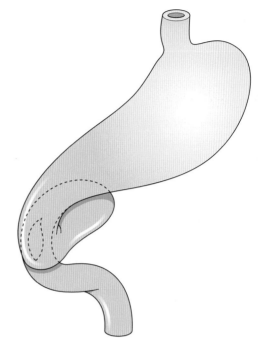

FIGURE 18.37   Duodenoduodenostomy

ACUTE GASTRIC DILATATION

This complication can occur after any abdominal operation and can lead to death if it causes an aspiration pneumonia. The patient is usually **nauseated** and there are signs of upper abdominal distension with **hiccupping and belching**. It is not uncommon in patients taking psychotrophic drugs and quite common in very sick patients in intensive care units. It is often missed or misdiagnosed.

A **plain radiograph** will show gastric dilatation with a large gastric fluid level.

It is treated by continuous gastric aspiration until normal peristalsis resumes. Sympatheticomimetic drugs and metoclopramide may help prevent recurrence.

DUODENAL ATRESIA

Investigation

Clinical diagnostic indicators

Duodenal atresia should be suspected if a routine pre-natal ultrasound detects **hydramnios** when the child is born. **Bilious vomiting** begins soon after

birth. The stomach is distended and there are signs of dehydration.

There may be other **associated congenital abnormalities**, including Down's syndrome, cardiac anomalies, anorectal anomalies and oesophageal atresia.

The **differential diagnosis** is similar to that of congenital pyloric stenosis (Table 18.7).

Imaging

A **plain radiograph** will show the **double-bubble sign**. The installation of a liquid contrast medium will reveal the site of the obstruction.

Management

Resuscitation is identical to that described above for congenital pyloric stenosis. The tension and height of the fontanelle can be used to monitor the adequacy of fluid replacement.

The atretic section of the duodenum must be bypassed by performing a **duodenoduodenostomy** (see Fig 18.37).

Postoperatively, nasojejunal feeding may be required for a few days.

Prognosis

Survival is now greater than 95 per cent but is affected by any other associated anomalies.

MEGADUODENUM

High intestinal obstruction can be caused by compression of the duodenum by the superior mesenteric vessels. It is diagnosed on **barium meal** and **CT scanning with contrast**.

It is treated by **duodenoduodenostomy** (see Fig 18.37) or gastro-enterostomy. No attempt should be made to elevate or move the superior mesenteric artery.

BILIARY COLIC

The symptoms of biliary colic are very similar to those of acute cholecystitis (see page 388) except that the pain is more acute and gets worse with each episode. The treatment is the same as for acute cholecystitis.

URETERIC COLIC

This is discussed in Chapter 20. Haematuria is usually present. The pain is experienced in the right or left loins. It is usually very severe, making the patient roll around and sweat. The pain rarely remits completely between each attack.

OTHER CAUSES OF COLIC

Colicky pain can also come from the uterus, Fallopian tube and an obstructed bladder.

HAEMATEMESIS AND MELAENA

Bleeding from any part of the gastrointestinal tract may cause haematemesis or melaena. Severe bleeding from the oesophagus, stomach, duodenum and bleeding from the upper small bowel which enters the stomach is likely to be expelled by vomiting (haematemesis). Less severe bleeding, even from these sites, may continue down the gastrointestinal tract and appear as melaena.

Bleeding from the upper colon is usually occult, but severe bleeding from any part of the colon may appear as frank, unaltered blood (see page 472).

Table 18.9
The causes of gastrointestinal haemorrhage

Common	
Acute peptic ulceration	
Gastric erosions	80 per cent
Chronic peptic ulceration (gastric or duodenal)	
Oesophageal varices	5 per cent

Less common

Oesophagitis
Leiomyomas of stomach (GIST tumours)
Gastric adenocarcinoma
Mallory Weiss tears
Aorto enteric fistula
Haemobilia
Dieulafoy syndrome
Bleeding disorders
Meckel's diverticula
Jejunal diverticula
Intussusception
Angiodysplasia
Peutz-Jegher's syndrome
Leiomyoma/leiomyosarcoma of small bowel (GIST tumours)
Lymphoma
Haemangioma (Osler Rendu Weber)
Henoch–Schönlein purpura

The causes of haematemesis and melaena are shown in Table 18.9.

Initial management

Patients presenting with massive haemorrhage require prompt and adequate resuscitation.

A rapid assessment should be made of the circulation by measuring the **pulse** (>100 = marked hypovolaemia) and the **blood pressure** (a systolic of <100 mmHg = serious blood loss).

Table 18.10
Risk assessment following a haematemesis

Low risk	Moderate risk	High risk
Age >60	Age >60	Age <60
Pulse >80	Pulse < 90	Pulse <100
BP <120 systolic	BP 105 systolic or above	BP under 100 systolic
Hb 12–15	Hb 10–12	Hb >10
ASA Grade 1	ASA 2–4	ASA 5

ASA, American Society of Anesthesiology; BP, blood pressure; Hb, haemoglobin.

Two large-bore **intravenous catheters** should be inserted, one into each antecubital fossa. Blood should be sent for **cross-matching** as the intravenous cannulae are inserted and **4 units should be requested**.

Intravenous saline or **a plasma expander** can be given while grouped or cross-matched blood is awaited.

Although the majority of patients are in a relatively stable state when they are admitted to hospital they should still be treated as potentially unstable. Intravenous lines should still be inserted to provide rapid access to the circulation if required. Blood should be sent to the laboratory for cross-matching, although this need not be urgently requested. An **electrocardiogram** (ECG) and **chest radiograph** should be obtained in elderly or unfit patients and those with known cardiovascular disease. Haemoglobin, urea and electrolytes, liver function tests, platelets and a coagulation screen (if thought necessary) can also be requested. The patient should remain starved and fluid restricted so that they are ready for theatre should they deteriorate. **Patients should be jointly managed by a team of gastrointestinal surgeons and physicians**.

At their initial assessment, patients can be placed into a low-, moderate- or high-risk category (Table 18.10). The first two categories of patients can be admitted to a general ward, preferably with a high-dependency bay and an endoscopy organized for the next convenient opportunity.

Management of high-risk patients

These patients should be admitted from the emergency department to a high dependency or intensive care ward where they can be fully resuscitated (see below) and monitored, preferably with a central venous pressure line.

They should be endoscoped as soon as possible (see below).

Patients who have suffered a *major haemorrhage* may have to be given uncross-matched group O negative blood while the correct grouped cross-matched blood is awaited.

The great majority of patients will stabilize after correction of their hypovolaemia with blood transfusion. It should be remembered that only 1 L of plasma expander should be given if coagulation and oxygen carriage are to be maintained.

Oesophagogastroduodenoscopy (OGD) (upper GI endoscopy) should be carried out as soon as possible once the patient has been stabilized. This policy should be adhered to even when the patient has had a small bleed without accompanying hypovolaemia, although the endoscopy may wait for a convenient time in daylight hours.

Endoscopy is the essential investigation. In experienced hands, it will provide a diagnosis and determine the site of bleeding in more than 80 per cent of patients. Continued massive blood loss and a failure to wash out adherent clot can hinder diagnosis.

Endoscopy may reveal a chronic peptic ulcer, oesophageal varices, a Mallory–Weiss tear, an acute ulcer, Dieulafoy syndrome and haemorrhagic erosions. It can sometimes avoid an abdominal operation if it reveals a condition best treated endoscopically or medically.

CT angiography can be considered as a first line investigation if OGD does not determine the cause of bleeding.

Selective mesenteric angiography should be considered when CT angiography shows an abnormality. It may confirm the CT angiographic findings and therapeutic embolization can be utilized to arrest haemorrhage.

Radioisotope scanning can be used to localize the bleeding, especially if a Meckel's diverticulum is considered to be the likely source, but it is rarely diagnostic.

Angiography has the advantage that it can be both diagnostic and therapeutic. The bleeding vessel can be selectively embolized using microspheres. The risks are of causing bowel or organ ischaemia and there is also a risk of rebleeding.

Patients with massive haemorrhage should be endoscoped under general anaesthetic in theatre. A Sengstaken tube can be passed and a vasopressin infusion started if there is evidence of bleeding oesophageal varices.

Emergency laparotomy is indicated for massive bleeding from a peptic ulcer. A gastrostomy or duodenotomy is made and the bleeding ulcer underrun with a strong Vicril suture. A duodenotomy should be closed as a pyloroplasty.

There is now rarely, if ever, an indication for more radical surgery such as a partial gastrectomy or vagotomy and antrectomy.

These patients should receive a course of proton pump inhibition and *Helicobacter* eradication in the postoperative period followed by repeat endoscopy 6 weeks later to ensure the ulceration has healed.

The bleeding of low or moderate-to-high risk patients usually stops spontaneously and can be treated by restoring the diet with acid suppression therapy. A CLO test should be performed before eradication treatment is carried out.

Patients can usually be discharged after 3–4 days if no further bleeding is experienced. A follow-up endoscopy at 6 weeks is sensible to ensure that all ulceration has healed.

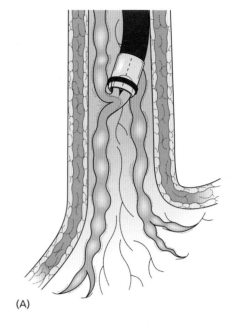

(A)

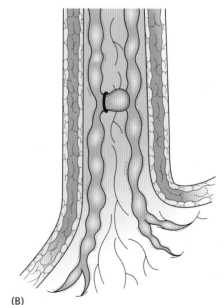

(B)

FIGURE 18.38 Banding of bleeding oesophageal varices

Disease-specific management

After control of bleeding oesophageal varices by a Sengstaken tube and a vasopressin infusion, the varices should be injected with a sclerosant. Alternatively, an elastic band should be placed around the base of each varix (see Fig 18.38). Recurrent bleeding is an indication for a TIPS procedure. A needle and catheter are forced through the liver substance to develop a channel between the portal and systemic venous systems. The channel can be held open by a stent.

Oesophageal transaction and surgical portosystemic shunts are now rarely required.

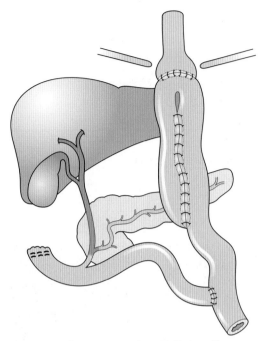

FIGURE 18.39   Total gastrectomies with Roux en Y

Gastric erosions can usually be satisfactorily treated with proton pump inhibitors.

Acute and chronic peptic ulcers are usually treated by injecting adrenaline in saline (1:1000) around the ulcer base in an attempt to occlude the bleeding vessels.

Laser or photocoagulation may also be used to try to close an open a vessel in the base of an ulcer but this is an ominous finding that often presages rebleeding.

Rarely, CT angiography to try to discover a source of unexplained bleeding (see below) can be followed by therapeutic embolization.

A **Dieulafoy lesion**, in which an atherosclerotic vessel protrudes through a small acute ulcer, should be treated by **surgical under-running** if it continues to bleed after attempts at conservative measures (laser, photocoagulation or clipping) fail.

Carcinoma of stomach is a rare cause of upper gastrointestinal bleeding and is usually apparent at endoscopy (see page 434). Whenever possible the diagnosis should be confirmed by tissue biopsy. Usually the bleeding stops spontaneously but continued bleeding can be treated by **total gastrectomy** (see Fig 18.39). Radiotherapy may occasionally be used to stop the bleeding.

Gastrointestinal stromal tumours (leiomyomas and leiomyosarcomas) of stomach can bleed rapidly and repeatedly from a central ulcer where the tumour necroses. Treatment is by local excision with a cuff of normal surrounding stomach. A more radical resection can be undertaken for malignant tumours.

Aorto-enteric and **aorto-graft-enteric fistula** are discussed in Chapter 11. They are rare but should be considered in any patient who has had an aortic graft inserted or a palpable or previously diagnosed abdominal aortic aneurysm. The graft has to be removed with an alternative route used as reconstruction (axillo-femoral graft), or the deep femoral vein used as an autograft.

Haemobilia is very rare but can occur after hepatic trauma or interference with the bile duct. Surgery and endoscopy, together with sphincterotomy and cholelithotomy, may be required.

Bleeding disorders require correction.

Angiodysplasia is more common in the large intestine but vascular malformations can cause repeated small bowel haemorrhage.

An **ulcerated Meckel's diverticulum** can bleed into the small intestine and the blood may then pass upwards and downwards towards the stomach and the rectum. A combination of haematemesis and frank rectal bleeding occurring simultaneously suggest the possibility of a bleeding Meckel's diverticulum. The treatment is surgical excision (see Chapter 17).

Unexplained recurrent bleeding

CT angiography is now the investigation of choice for unexplained gastrointestinal bleeding. The suggested source of the bleeding can then be confirmed by selective angiography and treated by embolization.

Prognosis

The prognosis for patients with haematemesis has improved since the introduction of combined management by specialist gastroenterologists and surgeons. A 10 per cent mortality has been reduced to 2 per cent in specialist units. Bleeding oesophageal varices have a much higher mortality (30 per cent), although this depends upon the severity of the liver disease.

ABDOMINAL DISTENSION

The common causes of abdominal distension are best remembered as the six Fs:

- fat
- fluid: ascites
- faeces: faecal impaction
- flatus: obstruction
- foetus
- fibroids.

In practice the common gastrointestinal causes are bowel obstruction, ascites and paralytic ileus.

Investigation

Clinical diagnostic indicators

Bowel obstruction classically presents with acute **abdominal distension** with **colicky pain, vomiting** and **constipation**. The symptoms depend on the level of obstruction, with vomiting and pain being more prominent in upper small bowel obstruction while large bowel obstruction presents more gradually, usually starting with constipation and then distension (see Chapter 17).

Irritable bowel syndrome is a frequent cause of **intermittent abdominal bloating**.

Distension caused by malignant and benign ascites (Table 18.11) is gradual in onset. A significant degree of ascites may cause shifting dullness.

Paralytic ileus is a postoperative phenomenon.

Blood tests

Routine standard blood tests may give some clues. **Anaemia** suggests **right colon cancer**. Abnormal coagulation with a **low albumin** suggests **ascites** secondary to chronic liver disease.

Imaging

A **plain abdominal X-ray** may reveal distended loops of bowel. Ascites causes a ground-glass appearance.

Table 18.11
Differential diagnosis of abdominal distension caused by ascites

Liver failure (portal hypertension)

Hyperproteinaemia

Carcinomatosis

Tuberculosis

Pseudomyxomatous peritonii

Chylous ascites

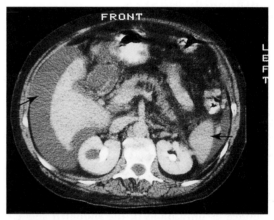

FIGURE 18.40 Ascites seen as ground glass homogeneous fluid surrounding the liver and spleen

Distended large bowel is typically seen around the periphery of the abdomen, with unevenly spaced haustrations, whereas **distended small bowel** lies more centrally with valvulae conniventes visible across the loops. A clear cut-off point may be visible and if the obstruction is complete no gas should be seen in the distal bowel.

In **irritable bowel syndrome** there may be non-specific gaseous distension or faecal loading.

In **paralytic ileus** distension of both small and large bowel is usual.

An **abdominal ultrasound** confirms the diagnosis of ascites but a **CT scan of abdomen and pelvis**, preferably with oral and intravenous contrast, is the key investigation. Ascites can be easily seen (Fig 18.40).

Colonoscopy may be needed if the diagnosis remains in doubt, especially in patients with the irritable bowel syndrome, which often presents with troublesome symptoms but a paucity of clinical signs. **A warning – patients with irritable bowel syndrome may not be able to tolerate the passage of the instrument.**

Management

Management will depend upon the underlying cause but the symptoms caused by ascites may be temporarily relieved by **paracentesis**.

ABDOMINAL MASSES

Masses in the abdomen can arise from the liver, gall bladder, spleen, kidneys, omentum, stomach, pancreas, small and large bowel, aorta, bladder uterus, ovaries and Fallopian tubes. The retroperitoneal tissues can also give rise to masses. The physical signs will often distinguish the organ from which the mass arises (see *Symptoms and Signs*).

Investigation

An intravenous pyelogram, barium meal, barium enema, laparoscopy or laparotomy are now rarely required as **ultrasound of the abdomen** and **CT scanning** can almost always confirm the diagnosis of a mass.

Fine needle aspiration cytology can be obtained from solid masses not involving the bowel.

Further investigations are usually guided by the findings on ultrasound and CT. These include upper GI endoscopy, ERCP, colonoscopy and transvaginal ultrasound.

A large mass of lymph nodes in the retroperitoneum may require an open biopsy if a lymphoma is suspected.

Management

The management of the mass depends upon the organ involved and the underlying pathology.

THE SPLEEN

This organ was originally thought to serve little function after foetal life, although it is a major

Table 18.12
Causes of an enlarged spleen

Rheumatoid arthritis (Felty's)

Amyloid and sarcoidosis

Malaria

Sub-acute bacterial endocarditis

Tuberculosis

Sepsis

Infectious mononucleosis

Brucellosis

Leishmaniasis

Schistosomiasis

Hydatid disease

Myelofibrosis

Portal hypertension

Cirrhosis

Chronic cardiac failure

Budd–Chiari disease

Lymphomas

Leukaemia

Polycythaemia rubra vera

Other tumours (secondaries) are very rare

Cysts and abscesses

reservoir of reticulo-endothelial cells, which destroy effete red blood cells. It is now recognized to have an important immunological function (both T and B cells), which may be seriously impaired by splenectomy. The causes of a large spleen are shown in Table 18.12.

Investigation

Ultrasound or **CT** of the abdomen confirms that the spleen is enlarged and separates splenic masses from renal, colonic and gastric masses. Filling defects may be seen within the spleen, although these are rare.

Indications for splenectomy

The spleen is removed when it is severely damaged (see Chapter 6), when it is very enlarged or when red cells or platelets are being removed or broken down excessively. This last indication is usually for **haemolytic anaemia** (spherocytosis, elliptocytosis or autoimmune disease), **idiopathic thrombocytopenic purpura** and **pancytopenia**. Medical measures such as haematinics, transfusions and steroids should be tried initially, but splenectomy is indicated if these do not cause a prolonged improvement.

Splenectomy

Splenectomy may be carried out through a vertical or transverse laparotomy incision and more recently a laparoscopic approach with morcellation of the spleen in a bag has been introduced.

Preoperatively, blood should be cross-matched and platelets may be required if the patient has idiopathic thrombocytopenic purpura. These should be given once the splenic vessels are controlled and about to be clamped.

Postoperative complications include **wound infection, chest infection** and **bleeding**, which may indicate the need for re-exploration.

There is an increased risk of **deep vein thrombosis** and low-dose heparin prophylaxis is usually indicated.

Pancreatitis can occur in the tail of the spleen from inadvertent damage to the organ during removal of the spleen. **Pancreatic fistulae** are very rare.

The risk of **overwhelming post-splenectomy infection (OPSI)** is real in 1–2 per cent of those undergoing splenectomy. It is most common in the 3 years after surgery. Any intercurrent illness may lead to septicaemia and disseminated intravascular coagulation. Vaccinations should be carried out as prophylaxis against pneumococcus, *Haemophilus influenzae* B and the meningococcus. All febrile illnesses should be treated with antibiotics and some would recommend prophylactic lifelong penicillin 250 mg bd. Dental work should probably be covered. The condition has a very high mortality.

CONDITIONS CAUSING CHRONIC ABDOMINAL PAIN

All the conditions that have been described as causes of acute abdominal may also be the cause of chronic

Table 18.13
Causes of chronic abdominal pain

Hiatus hernia/reflux oesophagitis/oesophageal spasm

Chronic peptic ulcer

Carcinoma of the stomach/lymphoma/leiomyoma

Coeliac artery compression

Chronic pancreatitis

Chronic cholecystitis (acalculus)

Carcinoma of the gall bladder

Carcinoma of the pancreas

Chronic liver disease/liver metastases

Chronic mesenteric ischaemia

Abdominal dissection (dissecting aneurysms)

Metastatic peritoneal tumours

Inflammatory aneurysms/retroperitoneal fibrosis

Ovarian carcinoma

Tuberculosis

Small bowel tumours/lymphomas

Diverticular disease/irritable bowel syndrome

Adhesions with recurrent obstruction

Cancer phobia anxiety state

Chronic lumber disc disease

Endometriosis

Other gynaecological causes

abdominal pain (see Chapter 17). All those listed in Table 18.13 may cause pain for weeks, months or years.

GASTRIC SURGERY FOR MORBID OBESITY

Obesity is defined as a body weight 100 per cent greater than ideal. The aim of surgery is to reduce the morbidity (osteoarthritis, sleep apnoea and diabetes) and the mortality caused by the obesity. **Type II diabetes can be cured by gastric bypass.**

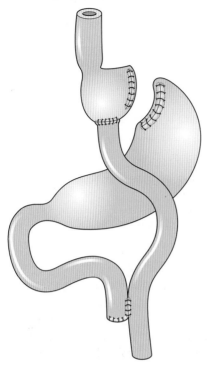

FIGURE 18.41   Gastric bypass for obesity

Management

Patients should be assessed by a multidisciplinary team, including a physician, a nutritionist, a psychiatrist and a surgeon.

Treatments include jaw wiring, jejuno-ileal bypass, gastric bypass and gastric banding. Gastric bypass can be performed laparoscopically and is currently in favour because it cures Type II diabetes (see Fig 18.41).

Postoperatively, deep vein thrombosis prophylaxis, physiotherapy and monitoring of the haemoglobin, proteins and vitamins are essential.

Prognosis

Patients may lose up to 10 per cent of their initial weight. The mortality of gastric banding and bypass is less than 1 per cent.

19

The colon, rectum and anus

Ruth McKee

Diseases of the colon, rectum and anus include cancers and inflammatory bowel disease, as well as perianal disorders. A careful history and clinical examination aided by simple sigmoidoscopy and proctoscopy, as described in detail in *Signs and Symptoms*, will often reveal the diagnosis.

PROBLEMS CAUSED BY DISEASES OF THE COLON

- Abdominal distension (see Chapters 17 and 18)
- Colicky pain
- Change in bowel habit
- Rectal bleeding
- Weight loss
- Bowel dysfunction
- Screen-detected abnormalities

ABDOMINAL PAIN AND COLIC

The various types of abdominal pain caused by disease of the colon are described in detail in *Symptoms and Signs*, and their treatment is covered in Chapter 17.

The common causes of colicky pain that appear to arise from the colon are bowel obstruction, obstructions of other hollow organs, e.g. gall stones, or ureteric colic and irritable bowel syndrome.

Investigation

Clinical diagnostic indicators

Inflammatory conditions in the colon mainly affect its left and sigmoid part and so the **pain** they cause is usually experienced on the **left iliac fossa**. There may be a **palpable mass** in the left iliac fossa.

There may be an intermittent or hectic fever if a pericolic abscess develops.

Blood tests

A raised **white blood cell count** suggests the presence of an inflammatory process and infection. Colic may come from the obstruction caused by the inflammation.

Imaging

A **plain abdominal X-ray** often distinguishes bowel obstruction from the other causes of acute severe colic such as biliary and renal colic.

An **ultrasound scan**, which may reveal an inflammatory mass, is the best investigation to demonstrate colic arising from gallstones or calculus obstructing the renal tract.

CHANGE IN BOWEL HABIT

The common causes of a change in bowel habit are:

- gastroenteritis
- inflammatory bowel disease
- colorectal cancer
- diverticular disease
- radiation enteritis
- irritable bowel syndrome
- coeliac disease.

Investigation

Clinical diagnostic indicators

Infective gastroenteritis should be considered when a patient presents with the **sudden onset of diarrhoea**, **vomiting** and **abdominal pain** and a stool culture should be arranged. In the absence of infection, and if symptoms continue, investigation will be needed.

An alteration towards looser stools is generally more concerning than constipation with hard stool. Remember to be clear what patients mean by the terms 'diarrhoea' and 'constipation' (*Symptoms and Signs*, page 448).

Faecal blood test for screening

Blood mixed in the stool in the younger patient suggests inflammatory bowel disease, whereas in the older patient colorectal cancer must be excluded. Inspection of the stool may reveal blood on its surface, mixed within it or a red to black discoloration, suggestive of altered blood. Bedside tests and laboratory tests are available for the detection of occult blood.

Stool culture

Each laboratory issues its own instructions concerning the timing (hot or cold stools), storage and delivery of specimens of faeces. A series of specimens may have to be collected.

Serology

The possibility of coeliac disease is initially investigated by testing the serum for either tissue transglutaminase antibody or anti-endomysial antibody.

Imaging

Rigid sigmoidoscopy visualizes the rectum. **Flexible sigmoidoscopy** visualizes the rectum and sigmoid colon. In most older patients it is necessary to proceed to either **colonoscopy**, **barium enema** or computed tomography (**CT**) **colonography** to assess the remaining colon.

RECTAL BLEEDING

The common causes of rectal bleeding are

- anal disease (see page 489)
- colorectal cancer
- colorectal polyps
- inflammatory bowel disease
- radiation enteritis
- diverticular disease
- angiodysplasia.

The most common cause of massive colonic bleeding is probably **angiodysplasia of the colon**, although it is often attributed to diverticular disease because that condition is often found on elective investigation in that age group. True major bleeding from an artery eroded in the neck of a colonic diverticulum does occur but is rare.

A few patients have recurrent colonic bleeding with no cause found.

Severe bleeding from the colon that requires emergency surgery is fortunately rare. It may not be possible to localize the source of bleeding beforehand.

Investigation

Clinical diagnostic indicators

The loss of **small amounts of blood on defaecation** is the common way rectal bleeding presents. It is usually caused by anal disease such as **haemorrhoids**. However, unless the diagnosis of anal bleeding is entirely clear from the history, examination and an **outpatient sigmoidoscopy**, endoscopy or imaging of the lower gastrointestinal (GI) tract is essential.

A few patients, usually middle-aged or elderly, are admitted to hospital with **major blood loss** from the rectum. Fortunately this type of bleeding is uncommon and usually settles spontaneously. The first step is resuscitation, and then an attempt is made to identify the site of the bleeding.

Vigorous bleeding from **oesophageal varices** or an **artery in the base of a peptic ulcer** can cause apparently fresh bleeding from the rectum, as can the rare **aortoenteric fistula** (see Chapter 18).

Blood tests

Routine blood tests are required to help indicate the severity and duration of the bleeding and, if the blood loss is massive, for grouping and cross-matching. If there is any doubt, endoscopy of the stomach and duodenum is mandatory.

Imaging

If the standard outpatient procedures fail to reveal the source of the bleeding, **colonoscopy** and **barium contrast studies** may be needed.

If no upper GI source is found by **endoscopy of the stomach and duodenum** in patients presenting with significant bleeding, and the bleeding continues, **colonoscopy** and **selective mesenteric angiography** may be required. Neither is ideal.

Colonoscopy may be very difficult as bowel preparation is impossible and blood and clots will almost certainly obscure the view. However. if the bleeding point is seen, it may be possible to achieve haemostasis with argon beam or laser coagulation.

Selective mesenteric angiography requires the immediate availability of an expert radiologist and angiography must be carried out while bleeding is continuing. **Embolization of the bleeding point may be possible**.

If no source is found and the bleeding has ceased without specific treatment, a further elective colonoscopy should be performed to exclude serious pathology such as colorectal cancer, although a cancer is much more likely to cause small amounts of blood loss than life-threatening bleeding.

IRON DEFICIENCY ANAEMIA

See Chapter 4.

WEIGHT LOSS

See Chapter 18.

BOWEL DYSFUNCTION

There is a group of patients with long-standing bowel symptoms who do not have any demonstrable disease of the colon or rectum but who nevertheless find their lives made miserable by their condition. They complain sometimes of difficulty in defaecation or incontinence. They are sometimes described as having '**functional bowel disorder**'. There is an overlap between this vague diagnosis and the common irritable bowel syndrome.

Investigation
Clinical diagnostic indicators
Patients with very chronic bowel dysfunction symptoms are less likely to have either colorectal cancer or inflammatory bowel disease than patients with recent-onset symptoms. Nevertheless, these dangerous conditions should be excluded by special investigations.

Faecal incontinence is much more common in women, and related to obstetric trauma.

Function studies
Chronic constipation can be investigated with X-ray or radionucleotide **transit studies**, X-ray or MR **proctography**, and **pressure studies** of the colon, rectum and anal canal.

Faecal incontinence is investigated by combining **ultrasound scanning** and **pressure studies (manometry) of the muscles of the anal canal**.

ABNORMALITIES DETECTED DURING SCREENING OR COINCIDENTAL INVESTIGATIONS

Common coincidental findings include:

- colorectal polyps
- colorectal cancer
- rare tumours such as carcinoids.

Investigation
Clinical diagnostic indicators
It is important to review the patient's history.

Colorectal polyps or small cancers may bleed very slowly without producing any obvious change in the stools or any other symptoms. Faecal occult blood testing is very sensitive and will pick this up. Although routine testing gives many false-positive results caused by minor perianal disorders, and even eating meat that has been cooked rare, a significant number of patients with positive occult blood tests do have polyps or early cancer, and a survival benefit has been demonstrated from screening.

Screening for colorectal cancer using faecal occult blood testing is being rolled out in the UK.

Imaging
Screened patients with positive findings should be referred for **colonoscopy**, which must reach as far as the caecum, because occult lesions are more common in the right side of the colon.

Inevitably screening will often produce incidental findings such as lipomata of the bowel and small carcinoid tumours.

CONDITIONS OF THE COLON

DIVERTICULAR DISEASE

Colonic diverticular disease is common. It is found in at least 50 per cent of the population over 50 years of age who eat the so-called 'western diet'.

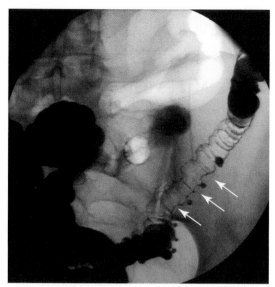

FIGURE 19.1   Barium enema showing diverticular disease

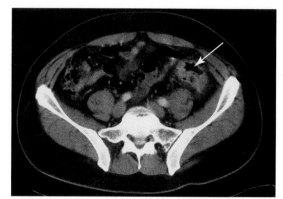

FIGURE 19.2   Computed tomography scan showing inflammatory mass of the sigmoid colon due to diverticulitis

The likely cause is increased intraluminal pressure associated with a diet low in fibre residue.

The colonic mucosa herniates through the muscularis mucosa and inner circular muscle layer, between the taeniae coli, at the point of entry of the small arteries.

The process starts distally at the rectosigmoid junction. The sigmoid colon is the most commonly affected site.

Diverticula do not develop in the rectum because the taeniae join at the rectosigmoid junction to form a complete outer longitudinal muscle layer.

The clinical problems caused by colonic diverticula are abdominal pain, inflammation, (diverticulitis), perforation, bleeding and fistula formation.

The expression *diverticulitis* should be reserved for the acute inflammatory condition.

Investigation

The orifices of diverticula can be seen at **colonoscopy** and **fibreoptic sigmoidoscopy**, but not at rigid sigmoidoscopy, because this instrument rarely passes beyond the rectosigmoid junction.

Colonic diverticula show clearly on **barium enema** (Fig 19.1) and **CT colonography**.

A **CT scan** will also demonstrate diverticulitis or a diverticular abscess (Fig 19.2).

SYMPTOMLESS DIVERTICULAR DISEASE

Symptomless diverticular disease does not require treatment. Patients are usually advised to increase their fibre and fluid intake.

ACUTE SIGMOID DIVERTICULITIS

Acute inflammation around the sigmoid colon, with pain, tenderness and often a fever and leucocytosis, is called acute diverticulitis.

Clinical diagnostic indicators

Acute sigmoid diverticulitis accounts for about 5 per cent of all admissions to hospital with abdominal pain. Patients are usually middle-aged or elderly people and present with **left iliac fossa pain**. The pain may be colicky in nature if large bowel obstruction (caused by inflammation or stricture) predominates (see Chapter 17).

Patients are usually constipated but a few develop diarrhoea. There is often accompanying nausea.

The pain may spread across the whole abdomen if either a diverticulum or a pericolic abscess ruptures causing generalized peritonitis.

Urinary symptoms can occur if the inflamed colon lies against the bladder. Diverticulitis can cause *right* iliac fossa pain if the sigmoid loop flops over to the right.

Patients usually have a pyrexia and mild tachycardia.

Tenderness, guarding and percussion tenderness are usually present in the left iliac fossa, and a **'sausage-shaped' mass** may be palpable.

Centralized abdominal tenderness and guarding suggest the presence of a perforation causing generalized peritonitis.

Rectal examination excludes a low carcinoma of the colon or rectum and must be carefully performed as it can cause severe pain.

Blood tests

Polymorphonuclear leucocytosis is common.

Urine tests

The urine should be tested for **blood, protein cells and bacteria**, and a mid-stream urinary specimen (MSU) sent for **culture**, if the patient has any urinary symptoms.

Imaging

Plain abdominal radiographs and an **erect chest X-ray** should be obtained if the patient has symptoms of obstruction or generalized peritonitis, to exclude a perforation.

CT scanning is very useful in confirming the diagnosis as clinical diagnosis is unreliable. A CT scan will demonstrate diverticulitis and a diverticula abscess.

Management

Conservative treatment

Patients without abscess or perforation should be managed conservatively with **intravenous fluids and antibiotics** (a **cephalosporin and metronidazole**) for 5–7 days, unless the condition deteriorates. Most patients settle with conservative treatment and can then be investigated later.

If there is a clear deterioration, indicated by a fever that does not settle, continuing pain and tenderness, a tachycardia, or **widespread guarding and percussion** tenderness, the patient should be rapidly resuscitated and taken to theatre.

DVT prophylaxis should be started on admission and a urinary catheter inserted.

DIVERTICULAR ABSCESS

If investigation demonstrates a unilocular collection of pus of reasonable size, a diverticular abscess, it may be susceptible to **radiological drainage**. This treatment is less effective for multilocular abscesses.

PERFORATED DIVERTICULAR DISEASE

Perforated diverticular disease presents in two ways, not always easy to distinguish preoperatively.

- If diverticulitis proceeds to the formation of a pericolic abscess that bursts into the peritoneal cavity but does not communicate with the bowel, the patient will develop a *purulent peritonitis*. This is often described as 'perforated diverticular disease' but it is in fact the pericolic abscess which has perforated, not the colon.
- If the orifice of the diverticulum is patent there will be a true connection between the bowel and the peritoneal cavity through which faeces may enter the peritoneal cavity causing *faecal peritonitis*. This condition carries a **mortality of at least 50 per cent** and is characterized by septic shock (see page 47).

Management

Resuscitation is with appropriate fluids and monitoring (Table 19.1). Infection control is with **broad-spectrum and anti-anaerobe antibiotics**. There

---

Table 19.1
Management of perforated diverticular disease

Resuscitation with appropriate monitoring

Broad-spectrum antibiotics

Review after resuscitation: If improved continue with conservative treatment. Purulent peritonitis may resolve

If not improving, laparotomy

If septic shock is caused by faecal peritonitis, there may be no response to resuscitation; but if patient has prospect of survival, laparotomy is indicated

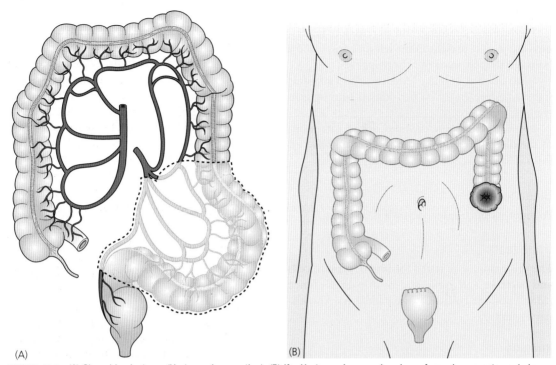

(A)   (B)

FIGURE 19.3   (A) Sigmoid colectomy (Hartmann's operation). (B) If a Hartmann's procedure is performed no anastomosis is made. The proximal end of the bowel is brought out as an end-colostomy, and the rectal stump is stapled or oversewn and left in the peritoneal cavity

should be **continuous observation and monitoring** so that if the patient's general condition does not improve emergency surgical intervention can be instigated. Hartmann's operation (Fig 19.3) is the safest option in a debilitated acutely ill elderly patient with complicated diverticular disease, because it does not involve leaving an anastomosis that might leak.

When patients have recovered from the acute episode they can be discharged to regain their strength and readmitted several months later for closure of their stomas or re-anastomosis of the Hartman's procedure. This delay ensures that they are fully recovered and allows the adhesions and stomas to mature. Patients must be taught to manage their stoma until it is closed, and a number of elderly unfit patients never have their stoma closed as the risks of reoperation will be considered too great.

Resection with primary anastomosis of the bowel is the ideal but is often not attempted because of the perceived risks in patients in poor condition.

Postoperative care Antibiotics should be continued. Patients with severe sepsis (**faecal peritonitis**) should be nursed on an intensive care unit.

Careful fluid management, **inotropic support, ventilation and haemofiltration** may be required to prevent or treat **multi-organ failure**.

Repeated ultrasound or CT scans may show an **intra-abdominal collection** that requires **radiological drainage**.

Complications

Complications are not uncommon after either conservative or operative treatment of complicated sigmoid diverticular disease (Table 19.2). These complications must be recognized immediately and appropriately treated.

Results

The prognosis of mild diverticulitis is very good, though patients may develop further attacks. The

Table 19.2
Complications of treatments for complicated diverticular disease

Peritonitis

Anastomotic leak

Paralytic ileus

Multi-organ failure secondary to sepsis

Left ureter and bladder damage during dissection

mortality rises to more than 5 per cent if sigmoid resection is required, and rises again to between 20 and 50 per cent if faecal peritonitis develops from a diverticular perforation in a frail, elderly patient.

VESICOCOLIC FISTULA

A pericolic abscess arising from an infected diverticulum may adhere to another organ and burst into its lumen. If the luminal orifice of the diverticulum is patent, a fistula may develop between the colon and the organ to which it has become adherent. A vesicocolic fistula is the most common fistula to develop after an episode of diverticulitis because the sigmoid colon often lies in the pelvis against the dome of the bladder.

Investigation

Clinical diagnostic indicators

The cardinal symptom is **pneumaturia**, described by the patient as the passage of bubbles. For obvious reasons, males notice this more readily.

The urine may be discolored or contain obvious **faecal material**. This may block the internal urinary meatus and cause **urinary retention**.

Curiously, ascending infection is rare, presumable because the ureteric junctions are competent.

Endoscopy

Cystoscopy (fibre or rigid) may show a reddened area in the dome of the bladder, occasionally emitting bubbles. A normal examination must **not** be considered to exclude the condition.

A **barium enema** will demonstrate diverticular disease and may show barium in the fistula entering the bladder. Conversely a **cystogram** may show the contrast medium entering the colon.

Management

Sigmoid colectomy is needed. At operation there is often an inflammatory mass. When the colon is separated from the bladder it may not be possible to demonstrate the hole in the bladder. The diseased colon must be removed and bowel continuity restored with an end-to-end anastomosis. The bladder is kept empty for 7–10 days.

A vesicocolic fistula caused by an infiltrating cancer of the colon or bladder is usually a complication of advanced disease and difficult to manage.

COLOVAGINAL FISTULA

This may develop when there has been a previous hysterectomy and an inflamed sigmoid colon adheres to the peritoneal closure at the vaginal vault. (The intact uterus and vagina in the pouch of Douglas are thick muscular organs and are not susceptible to fistula formation.) **Gas and faeces are passed through the vagina.**

Speculum vaginal examination reveals faecal contamination. Occasionally the orifice of the fistula is visible.

Barium enema will show diverticular disease and sometimes fill the fistula and upper vagina with barium.

Management is the same as for vesicocolic fistula.

CROHN'S DISEASE

Crohn's disease is a chronic full thickness granulomatous inflammation which can affect the GI tract anywhere from mouth to anus. The site most commonly affected is the terminal ileum immediately proximal to the ileocaecal valve, but the large bowel may also be affected. *The investigation and management of small bowel Crohn's disease are discussed extensively in Chapter 17.*

Colonic Crohn's disease is becoming more frequent. Crohn's disease is characterized by multiple 'skip lesions' – short diseased segments separated by lengths of normal bowel. The complications of this chronic inflammatory process are strictures, abscesses and fistulae of the bowel. Bleeding is usually chronic rather than life-threatening.

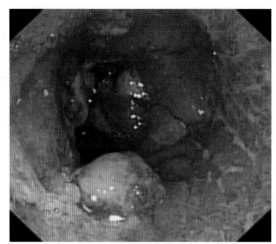

FIGURE 19.4   Colonoscopy of inflammatory bowel disease

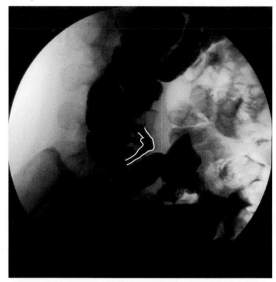

FIGURE 19.5   Small bowel barium follow-through showing a terminal ileal stricture due to Crohn's disease

Investigation

Clinical diagnostic indicators

There are two age peaks of presentation: in the second and third decades of life, and in older people.

▦ Colonic Crohn's disease affecting a continuous length of distal colon usually causes **diarrhoea** and **bleeding** so may be difficult to distinguish from ulcerative colitis.

▦ Crohn's disease of the **anus** may present with **abscesses, fistula-in-ano, fissure** and rarely **excavating ulcers**.

▦ Many patients have extra-intestinal manifestations such as **uveitis, iritis, spondyloarthropathy, pyoderma gangrenosum** and **erythema nodosum**.

Blood tests

It is important to assess the degree of any **anaemia** and measure the **CRP and plasma albumen**.

Stool culture

It is important to remember that exacerbation of inflammatory bowel disease, both Crohn's disease and ulcerative colitis, may be due to concomitant infection, and to send stool samples for **culture**. The stools should be tested for **occult blood**.

Imaging

Diagnosis is made by **endoscopy** (Fig 19.4) and **biopsy. Contrast X-rays** of the small bowel are standard (Fig 19.5), but **MRI** is better at demonstrating extra-intestinal problems such as abscess as well as the abnormality of the gut lumen. **CT scanning** is often used to detect complications.

Management

Medical management of an acute episode of inflammation follows the principles described in Chapter 17 for small bowel cancer. Indications for surgery are also described.

The most common procedure is resection of the terminal ileum and caecum for terminal ileal stricture.

Patients with Crohn's disease throughout the colon may require **panproctocolectomy and permanent ileostomy** (Fig 19.6). Unfortunately this operation cannot be guaranteed to provide a lifetime cure as the disease may reappear in the small bowel.

Complications

The complications specific to large bowel resections for Crohn's disease are

▦ anastomotic leakage in up to 10 per cent of cases, which may require the formation of a stoma
▦ intra-abdominal abscess, usually drained by radiological guidance
▦ the chance of recurrence, an ever-present long-term problem.

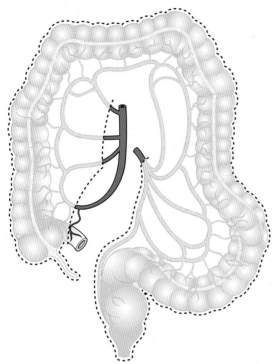

FIGURE 19.6 Panproctocolectomy, removing all of colon, rectum and anus and bringing out the terminal ileum as an ileostomy

ULCERATIVE COLITIS

Ulcerative colitis is a chronic inflammatory process that affects and destroys the colonic mucosa. The inflammation extends from the rectum proximally and may affect any length from a few centimetres to the entire colon. Its acute complications include toxic megacolon (acute colonic dilatation), perforation and bleeding. Patients with long-standing, severe and extensive ulcerative colitis have a higher incidence of colorectal cancer which increases with duration of the disease.

Investigation

Clinical diagnostic indicators

Ulcerative colitis presents in the second or third decade of life. The main diagnostic clinical feature is incessant **diarrhoea**, which may contain **blood.**

Extra-intestinal manifestations can affect the skin, eye and joints.

Table 19.3
Indications for surgery for ulcerative colitis

Emergency indications

Acute life-threatening fulminating colitis not responding to medical treatment

Toxic dilatation of the colon

Elective indications

Chronic ill health

Severe extra-colic complications

To prevent cancer in long-standing active colitis

Blood tests

Anaemia and hypo-albuminaemia are common.

Stool culture

The first and essential step in all suspected cases is to exclude an infective cause by **stool culture**, repeated if necessary.

Imaging and tissue biopsy

Colonoscopy and a **mucosal biopsy** will give the diagnosis.

In acute severe colitis a **plain abdominal X-ray** must be taken as it is important to look for any dilatation that indicates the **presence of a toxic megacolon**.

Management

The medical management of ulcerative colitis is similar to that of colonic Crohn's disease, namely **steroids** for acute inflammation and **5-ASA compounds** to maintain remission. The indications for surgical management are given in Table 19.3.

Ulcerative colitis affects only the large bowel and is cured by **total removal of the colon and rectum**, known as **panproctocolectomy** (Fig 19.6).

This is major surgery and leaves the patient with a permanent stoma – an **ileostomy**. The terminal ileum is brought out through the abdominal wall at an appropriate point. Digestion of the skin by the effluent from the ileum is prevented by fashioning the terminal ileum into a spout that protrudes above the level of the skin – the **Brooke ileostomy**.

Ileostomies act continuously. The effluent is never formed, but does not smell. Very little gas is produced. An ileostomy does not prevent a patient returning to normal life. Panproctocolectomy has been performed safely for over 50 years and usually rapidly restores the patient to general good health.

In the emergency situation or if the diagnosis is in doubt a subtotal **colectomy with ileostomy** is the operation of choice. This allows a more accurate histological assessment and reduces immediate postoperative complications. Should the patient be found to have Crohn's colitis the continuity of the bowel can be restored later by an anastomosis of the ileum to the rectum.

If ulcerative colitis is confirmed, it leaves the option of fashioning an ileo-anal pouch (see below).

A stoma may be avoided for those who wish by means of a **restorative proctocolectomy**, in which an artificial pouch is constructed from ileal loops and joined to the anal canal (Fig 19.7). This operation is possible in 80–90 per cent of those who want it done.

Bowel function after pouch surgery is not normal. The patient has three to six actions each day.

This surgery is complex and if there is leakage into the pelvis from the various anastomoses the subsequent pelvic sepsis is difficult to eradicate. To avoid this dreaded complication many surgeons fashion a proximal temporary loop **ileostomy** after constructing the pouch.

It is vital to be sure that the colitis is not caused by Crohn's disease, which may recur in the terminal small bowel and ileostomy after removal of the colon.

Patients who have had pouch surgery or panproctocolectomy are liable to suffer small bowel obstruction from adhesions.

ACUTE SEVERE COLITIS AND TOXIC MEGACOLON

Patients with extensive ulcerative colitis and occasionally Crohn's disease can develop a fulminating condition in which the whole colon rapidly dilates and if left untreated may perforate. Persistent pain accompanying severe diarrhoea suggests the likely diagnosis. Pyrexia, dehydration, abdominal distention and localized tenderness

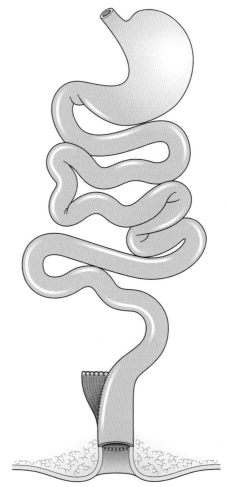

FIGURE 19.7 Restorative proctocolectomy (ileoanal pouch) where the rectum is divided at the anorectal junction and a neo-rectum formed from the distal ileum

usually precede perforation and the signs of generalized peritonitis.

Investigation

Blood tests

Anaemia and **leucocytosis** are common in all these conditions.

Imaging

Plain chest and **abdominal radiographs** may show evidence of **dilatation** of the colon or of **free perforation**. An instant barium enema is *inadvisable* as it may rupture the colon. A carefully performed **flexible sigmoidoscopy** is preferable.

Management

Patients should be given **intravenous fluids** and **broad-spectrum antibiotics**. They should be carefully re-examined to see if abdominal signs of peritonitis are developing.

Plain radiographs should be repeated daily to discover if the dilatation is developing or subsiding.

Systemic steroids in large doses should be given to patients suspected of having early acute toxic dilatation.

Laparotomy is indicated if the patient's condition deteriorates, especially if a perforation or a full thickness bowel infarct is suspected.

Total colectomy with an **ileostomy** will be needed. The abdomen should be carefully washed out if there is evidence of faecal contamination.

Results

Emergency colonic surgery carries a high mortality (5–10 per cent) when performed for complications in patients who are often malnourished, toxic and immunosuppressed.

INFECTIONS

This topic is mentioned briefly because it is a possible diagnosis in any patient presenting with diarrhoea.

GI infections spread by the faeco-oral route are a major cause of child mortality in developing countries. Presentation is with diarrhoea. The mainstay of treatment is oral or parenteral **rehydration** therapy.

In the UK the most common cause of infectious diarrhoea are the rotaviruses. *Campylobacter* is the most common bacterial cause followed by *Salmonella*. *Giardiasis* is a common protozoal infection.

IRRADIATION DAMAGE

The most common site of bowel radiation injury is the ileum and rectum following pelvic radiation for cervical or prostatic carcinoma.

Soon after undergoing pelvic radiotherapy patients may suffer from diarrhoea because of the mucosal inflammation and damage caused by the radiation. The diarrhoea may be severe and distressing but generally settles spontaneously.

Late disease may occur after many years. Small vessel thrombosis caused by the radiation can lead to ischaemia, fibrosis and fistula formation. These complications present in many ways and may be difficult to distinguish from cancer recurrence.

Investigation

Radiation damage should be considered in any patient who has had abdominal radiotherapy. The investigations should be appropriate to the presenting symptoms. **Tissue biopsy** by some means may be necessary.

In making the diagnosis and planning treatment it is important to exclude metastatic disease and recurrence of the original cancer that initiated the radiotherapy. A **CT scan** may be required.

Management

Early radiation enteritis is treated symptomatically. Late disease symptoms tend to wax and wane, and surgery can usually be avoided. Surgery for strictures and fistulae can be difficult and require stoma formation.

Irradiation damage to the small bowel is covered in Chapter 17.

ISCHAEMIA OF THE COLON

Investigation

Full thickness colonic infarction is rare. It occurs at the splenic flexure and left colon, where the arterial supply is tenuous.

Clinical diagnostic indicators

Symptoms are of **bloody diarrhoea with pain**.

Imaging

The appearance on a **barium enema** is of a long smooth narrowed area in the descending colon, sometimes with a *'thumb printing'* appearance in the mucosa (see Fig 17.25).

Endoscopy

The diagnosis is made by **colonoscopy and biopsy**.

Management

Colonic ischaemia without signs of peritonitis is treated expectantly and usually resolves, presumably because the ischaemia is mucosal rather than full thickness. It is unexpected that an ischaemic condition can cause bleeding, but this is the case. Many elderly patients who have a colonic bleed which settles without treatment and have subsequent normal investigation probably have had transient colonic ischaemia.

A few patients develop colonic strictures which need resection and a few require urgent resection for full thickness infarction.

MEGACOLON

The **toxic megacolon** associated with ulcerative colitis and occasionally Crohn's disease is discussed above.

Hirschsprung's disease

This is caused by a lack or shortage of ganglia in the myenteric plexuses in the wall of the colon or rectum. It usually presents in neonates with intestinal obstruction or in infants with constipation and failure to thrive. The colon proximal to the contracted aganglionic segment becomes grossly distended.

A small number of patients with Hirschsprung's disease confined to a short segment do not present until adulthood.

Idiopathic megacolon

This is another cause of chronic colonic distension in young people. It is associated with faecal impaction and overflow diarrhoea with incontinence. In most cases there are no obvious abnormalities on histology of the bowel and the cause is unknown.

Chagas' disease

Chagas' disease, South American trypanosomiasis, is the most common worldwide cause of megacolon.

Pseudo-obstruction of the colon

Pseudo-obstruction of the colon, sometimes known as Ogilvie's syndrome, is dilatation of the colon in the absence of mechanical obstruction. It occurs in older patients, often with systemic illness, who have been immobilized. Its importance is that it mimics large bowel obstruction caused by carcinoma.

Investigation of megacolon

An abdominal X-ray gives the diagnosis of megacolon.

Patient's with Hirschsprung's disease have an absent anorectal inhibitory reflex and a **full thickness rectal biopsy** is needed to confirm the diagnosis.

There is no single diagnostic test for idiopathic megacolon.

Chagasic megacolon is associated with mega-oesophagus and cardiomyopathy. **Antibodies to** *Treponema cruzi* can be identified.

Pseudo-obstruction syndrome can be distinguished from sigmoid volvulus or large bowel obstruction by **water-soluble contrast enema**.

Management

Hirschsprung's disease is treated by **resection of the affected segment** of bowel with very low anastomosis, often achieved by bringing normal colon down to the anal canal. Attempts are usually made to treat idiopathic megacolon and rectum by conservative means with regular laxatives, but some patients require bowel resection.

Chagasic megacolon may also require resection.

Surgery should be avoided in elderly infirm patients who suffer from pseudo-obstruction. Colonoscopy with decompression may help. Neostygmine may help in the acute situation if there are no cardiac contraindications.

CAECAL AND SIGMOID VOLVULUS

Long, mobile lengths of the caecum or sigmoid colon may twist on their mesentery and form a volvulus. In the UK volvulus is most common in older people, but in Africa sigmoid volvulus is common in young males, undoubtedly related to their high-residue diet. If the torsion does not resolve spontaneously the colon beyond the twist may become ischaemic, then necrotic.

Investigation
Clinical diagnostic indicators

Distention, localized **pain** or the colic of obstruction should all raise the suspicion of volvulus.

Imaging

An **abdominal X-ray** shows dilated large bowel with a 'kidney bean' configuration originating in either the left or right iliac fossa. The diagnosis is confirmed by **water-soluble contrast enema** (Figs 19.8 and 19.9).

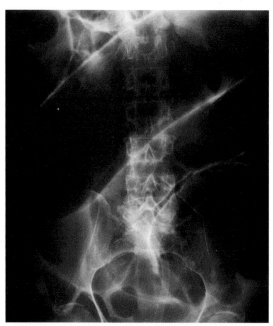

FIGURE 19.8 Plain abdominal X-ray showing sigmoid volvulus

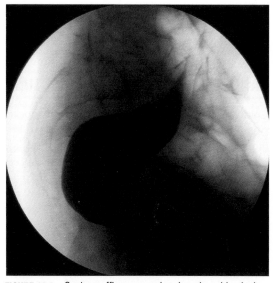

FIGURE 19.9 Gastrograffin enema showing sigmoid volvulus

Management

A sigmoid volvulus can often be **decompressed** by passing either a rigid or a flexible sigmoidoscope through the twist into the dilated bowel. Decompression of the bowel by this manoeuvre confirms the diagnosis.

Caecal volvulus always requires **resection**, as does a sigmoid volvulus if it shows any signs suggestive of bowel ischaemia.

INTESTINAL POLYPS

Polyps of small bowel and colon may be

- hamartomatous: malformations of normal mucosal tissue
- hyperplastic: polyps with normal individual cells but distortion of the crypt architecture
- adenomatous: dysplastic polyps with abnormal cell mitoses, implicated in the adenoma-to-carcinoma sequence during the development of colorectal cancer.

Adenomata may be tubular or villous, but are mostly mixed. Increasing polyp size, villous architecture and more severe dysplastic change carry a higher risk of invasive carcinoma. *It is vital to know the histology of any polyp in the colon or rectum. All adenomatous polyps have the potential to become cancers.*

Polyps may have a long stalk (pedunculated) or be flat with no stalk like a cauliflower (sessile) (Fig 19.10). The pathological process is the same. Sessile polyps tend to occur in areas where the bowel is wide (caecum and rectum), while pedunculated polyps are seen in narrow areas and presumably have been pulled out on a stalk by peristalsis and colonic movements.

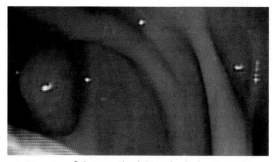

FIGURE 19.10 Colonoscopic picture of colonic adenoma

Patients with **familial adenomatous polyposis** (FAP) have hundreds of adenomata and develop colorectal cancer because the tumour-suppressor APC gene on the long arm of chromosome 5 is not functioning. New mutations without any family history are common in this autosomal dominant disease.

Investigation

Clinical diagnostic indicators

Small polyps are often **symptomless** but larger polyps may cause **bleeding**, particularly in the distal colon.

Imaging and biopsy

Colonoscopy and **biopsy** confirm the diagnosis and may also allow destruction of small polyps by diathermy or their excision using a snare. Regular colonoscopy may be required.

Patients with FAP have a higher risk of upper GI cancer and should have endoscopic surveillance of stomach and duodenum.

Genetic screening

In FAP it may be possible to identify the mutation in the APC gene and thus provide a blood test to screen all family members. If the mutation cannot be identified, regular endoscopic examination is needed from the mid-teens.

Management

All polyps seen at colonoscopy should be removed and sent for **histological examination**. Follow-up colonoscopy is recommended for patients with multiple or large polyps. Rectal polyps may be removed by various procedures through the anus. More proximal large polyps may require **bowel resection**.

Patients with FAP should be considered for prophylactic colectomy. The safest option is to remove all the mucosa at risk in the colon and rectum by **panproctocolectomy**, with or without a restorative pouch. An alternative is to leave the rectum with an ileorectal anastomosis, but in this event regular sigmoidoscopy must be carried out thereafter.

VILLOUS ADENOMA OF RECTUM

This is a variety of rectal adenomatous polyp with a broad base and a frondular surface that exudes large quantities of mucus. It is slow growing and may present with hypokalaemia as intestinal mucus contains a lot of potassium (see *Symptoms and Signs*).

Investigation

Clinical diagnostic indicators

The repeated passage of liquid, grey, mucous-like stool is almost a diagnostic symptom.

Blood tests

The **blood potassium** level must be measured if the polyp is very large.

Imaging

The lesion or lesions are usually easy to see with a rigid **sigmoidoscopy**. If there is malignant change the induration may be palpable on digital examination and the mucus visible on the examining glove. It is important to perform a **colonoscopy** as there may be polyps elsewhere.

Management

There are a variety of ways in which the lesion may be **excised or ablated** through the anus. If there is malignant change, it is treated as for any other rectal cancer. Occasionally a villous adenoma without malignant change covers the entire rectum. The only way to extirpate it is with an **abdominoperineal resection** (see below).

CANCER OF THE COLON AND RECTUM

Colorectal cancers are almost invariably adenocarcinomata, and together are the second most common cause of cancer death in the UK. The peak age is between 55 and 70 years. Most colorectal cancers are thought to arise from adenomata. Their most common site is the rectosigmoid, followed by the caecum. Spread is through the bowel wall, then to local lymph nodes, with the liver the most common site of distant metastases.

Dukes' classification (1932), which was the first time that a correlation between the pathological stage of a cancer and the prognosis was ever demonstrated, is highly relevant to management and remains in general use, sometimes with modification. The TNM classification is more detailed. Definitive staging can only be done on the resected bowel specimen (Tables 19.4 and 19.5).

Investigation

Clinical diagnostic indicators

Colorectal cancer must be considered as a likely diagnosis in all patients who present with a **change in bowel habit**, **rectal bleeding** and/or **iron deficiency anaemia**.

A quarter of all cases of colorectal cancer present as **emergencies** with **bowel obstruction** or **perforation.** Their prognosis is much worse than those presenting electively, not just because staging and management may be less than ideal but because more quickly growing aggressive tumours are more likely to present in this way.

Blood tests

Check the patient's haemoglobin level.

Imaging and biopsy

Initial outpatient rigid **sigmoidoscopy** will detect rectal cancer. **Colonoscopy** (or flexible sigmoidoscopy combined with either **barium enema or CT colonography**) (Figs 19.11 and 19.12) is then required. Complete examination of the colon is needed in all cases to exclude synchronous cancers, found elsewhere in the colon in 5 per cent of patients.

An **abdominal X-ray** generally suggests the diagnosis of large bowel obstruction.

A **CT scan** may show a mass at the site of obstruction and may show metastatic disease.

A **double-contrast water-soluble enema** gives a better assessment of the colon and confirms an obstruction lesion, but affords no opportunity to assess distant disease.

Preoperative staging is essential in addition to an assessment of the patient's fitness for surgery. Up to 30 per cent of patients present with metastatic disease.

Table 19.4
Dukes' classification of colorectal cancers

Stage	Extent	Approximate 5-year survival (%)
A	Confined to the bowel wall	90
B	Penetrating full thickness of bowel wall	70
	No lymph node involvement	
C	Involvement of regional lymph nodes	30
D	Presence of distant metastases	<5

In Dukes' classification the tumour in Stage A is confined to the bowel wall, not to the mucosa as in the TNM classification). D was not part of the original classification.

Table 19.5
Tumour, nodes, metastases classification of colorectal cancers

T		N		M	
1	Confined to the mucosa	0	No lymph node involvement	0	No distant metastases
2	Invading the muscularis propria but not penetrating through	1	<4 nodes involved Apical node not involved		
3	Penetrating the entire muscularis propria	2	≥4 nodes involved and/or apical node involved	1	Metastases
4	Penetrating through the serosa into adjacent structures				

The T, N and M scores are independent.

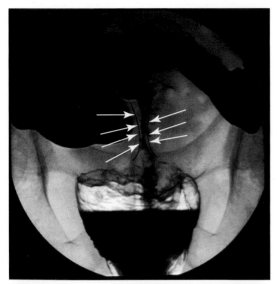

FIGURE 19.11   Barium enema of carcinoma of the rectum

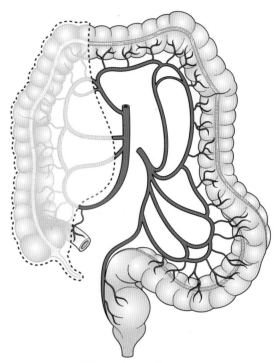

FIGURE 19.13   Right colonic resections for cancer

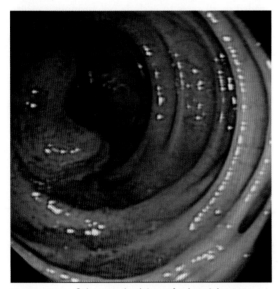

FIGURE 19.12   Colonoscopic picture of colorectal cancer

Staging

With colon cancer, the main purpose of staging is to detect distant metastases, since it is rare that local resection of the tumour with clear margins is impossible. **CT scanning**, with particular attention to the liver, is usual but **chest X-ray and ultrasound** scan may have to suffice if it is not readily available.

In rectal cancer, the aim of staging investigation is to determine if the tumour can be resected completely, as this is by no means always possible in the confines of the true pelvis.

Thin slice MRI is the preferred method of assessing the potential circumferential margins of a rectal cancer.

In small cancers, **endoluminal ultrasound** is useful to assess the penetration of the tumour through the bowel wall. Either **CT or MRI** is used to exclude distant metastases.

Examination under anaesthetic is helpful in assessing the precise site of the tumour, its mobility and the potential for re-anastomosis of the bowel.

All elective cases of colorectal cancer should be discussed at a multidisciplinary team (MDT) meeting attended by surgeons, radiologists, pathologists and oncologists. This is particularly important in preoperative decision-making for rectal cancers.

Management of colon cancer

Surgical resection is the only treatment that can achieve cure. The aim is to remove the tumour with its field of lymphatic drainage in the mesocolon, i.e. **right or left hemicolectomy** (Fig 19.13).

Wide resection is carried out not just to make sure there is wide clearance of bowel, but to remove as many lymph nodes as possible. However, a good blood supply to resected bowel margins must be retained if the anastomosis is to heal.

Patients that present with large bowel obstruction require either colonic or an emergency laparotomy. Wherever possible the primary tumour should be resected at the first operation. Anastomosis is usually possible on the right side of the colon, but when the cancer is in the sigmoid colon proximal distention may be massive and anastomosis difficult and hazardous. Hartmann's operation, as described for diverticular disease, is then appropriate.

Presentation with perforation, either of the tumour or of distended bowel above it, carries a very poor prognosis.

Colonic resection is major surgery in a middle-aged and elderly population and carries all the complications discussed in Chapter 2.

Hospital stay is 7–10 days for traditional open surgery. However, as in all other areas there is increasing use of the minimally invasive approach. The introduction of **laparoscopic colorectal resection** for cancer was cautious because of fears that it might not be possible to achieve the same clearance. However, developing techniques supported by large clinical trials have shown that the results in pure oncological terms are at least equivalent to those obtained from open surgery. All the usual advantages of laparoscopy apply.

Complications

The principal complication specific to colonic resection is **anastomotic leakage**, which occurs in up to 5 per cent of cases. This generally requires re-laparotomy and stoma formation.

MANAGEMENT OF RECTAL CANCER

Preoperative radiation and chemotherapy

If preoperative staging indicates a tumour of such size that complete excision by surgery may not be possible, preoperative neoadjunctive chemotherapy and radiotherapy should be considered. The aim is

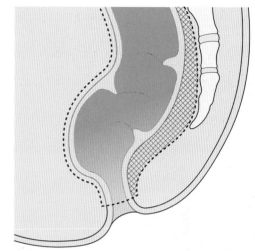

FIGURE 19.14   Total mesorectal excision for rectal cancer, ensuring that all of the circumferential margins of the mesorectum are dissected cleanly and removed down to the anorectal junction

to decrease the size of the tumour and allow removal with margins of normal tissue free of tumour.

Traditional long-course radiotherapy consists of a 6-week course delivering around 60 gray by external beam radiotherapy.

Newer techniques include **conformal radiotherapy**, which delivers treatment more precisely, and **multifractionated** (multiple small doses), which may improve efficacy.

Chemotherapy given in combination with radiotherapy is usually based on 5-fluorouracil and increases radiosensitivity. Surgical resection is delayed for a 6-week interval to allow the tumour to shrink as much as it is going to.

Several studies have shown a reduction in local recurrence (but not in survival) by giving short-course radiotherapy for all rectal cancers: 25 gray of external beam radiotherapy is given over a week with surgery a week later.

Anterior resection

Good surgical technique is important in the resection of rectal cancers. The aim is to make local recurrence unlikely by excising the rectum as widely as possible including the mesorectum. This is known as **total mesorectal excision** (TME) (Fig 19.14).

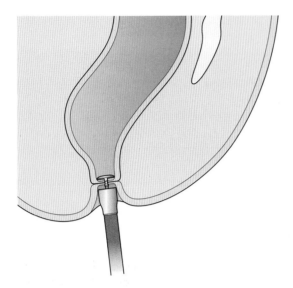

FIGURE 19.15   The circular stapling gun is placed via the anal canal to simplify distal anastomosis

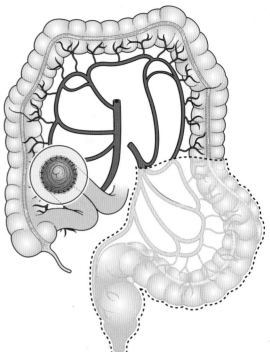

FIGURE 19.16   Low anterior resection of the rectum to be followed by a stapled colo-anal anastomosis and a temporary loop ileostomy

If after removing the tumour with adequate margins it is possible to join the two ends of the bowel, the operation is termed an **anterior resection**. This is now achieved in many more patients than in the past: first because it is now realized that clearance of rectum below the tumour need not be more than 2 cm (lateral clearance is the critical factor); and second because of technical advances such as the use of circular stapling devices (Fig 19.15), which can be inserted into a very short anal stump. It is usual to protect a low pelvic anastomosis with a temporary loop colostomy which is closed in a relatively minor operation several months later after complete healing of the anastomosis has been demonstrated by a contrast enema (Fig 19.16).

Abdominoperineal resection

If the cancer is less than 5 cm from the dentate line, or if it is large or poorly differentiated, an anastomosis may not be possible. The anal canal is then removed together with the rectum: an abdominoperineal resection (Fig 19.17). This is usually carried out synchronously by two surgeons, one working in the abdomen and the other in the perineum. A permanent end colostomy must be performed.

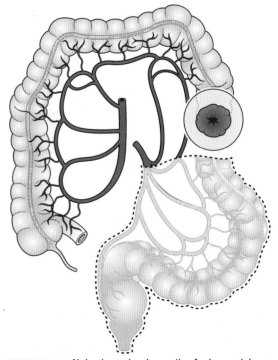

FIGURE 19.17   Abdominoperineal resection for low rectal cancer, with end colostomy

ADJUVANT TREATMENT FOR COLON AND RECTAL CANCER

Some patients benefit from postoperative chemotherapy, particularly those with lymph node involvement. Agents used include oxaliplatinum, irinotecan, 5-fluorouracil and its oral equivalent capecetibane, given for between 6 months and 1 year. The benefit is not huge, improving 5-year survival by 3–5 per cent.

When histology shows that the margins of the rectal resection margins are involved with cancer, postoperative radiotherapy is indicated, provided it has not been employed before surgery.

Liver resection for metastases

Patients who have either a single or several liver metastases may be offered liver resection if this is technically possible and there is no other metastatic disease. Five-year survival of up to 25 per cent has been reported in individual series. If the liver metastasis is found at presentation, liver resection can be performed at the same time as resection of the primary tumour (see Chapter 18).

Palliative treatment

Regrettably, many patients present with multiple and extensive metastases. Palliative resection should be avoided if possible as complications are common and survival poor but may be required if there is painful obstruction. **Endoscopic insertion of a stent** is an option. **Palliative radiotherapy and chemotherapy** are used to relieve specific symptoms.

Follow-up

It is traditional to see patients for 5 years after surgery to search for resectable and even curable liver metastases with ultrasound or CT scanning.

Because patients who have had a colorectal cancer are more likely than the general population to get another, it has become customary to undertake life-long surveillance with regular colonoscopy to look for metachronous cancers.

OTHER NEOPLASMS OF COLON AND RECTUM

Lipomata of the colon are occasionally found and do not usually require treatment. They lie deep to the mucosa and appear as a smooth bulge on endoscopy or contrast X-rays.

Carcinoid tumours are an occasional incidental histological finding in an inflamed appendix. If the lesion is large or showing any signs of malignant change, right hemi-colectomy is indicated.

Gastrointestinal stromal tumours (GISTs) originate from the connective tissue of the bowel. They are very rare except in the stomach. Treatment is resection.

Melanomas of the rectum are rare but can be resected.

RECTUM AND ANUS

Many of the problems related to diseases of the rectum and anus may be produced by colonic disorders and have been considered above, but there are a number of other problems specific to the anus:

- anal pain
- pruritus
- anal swelling
- anal discharge
- faecal incontinence
- tenesmus.

ANAL PAIN

The causes of anal pain include

- abscess
- anal fissure
- prolapsed haemorrhoids
- anal or low rectal cancer.

Diagnostic investigations

Examination under anaesthetic (EUA) is necessary if pain is severe and a diagnosis cannot be made otherwise. Endo-anal ultrasound scanning or perineal MRI are used to assess complex sepsis or malignancy.

PRURITUS

Itching in the perianal region is a common symptom. Pruritis may be caused by:

- diet
- local manifestation of a generalized skin disease, such as psoriasis

- virtually any perianal condition, typically a fistula, fissure, or haemorrhoids
- worm infestation, particularly in children
- no demonstrable cause.

Diagnostic investigations

Routine clinical rigid sigmoidoscopy and proctoscopy will detect any perianal conditions. Skin biopsy may be necessary if carcinoma *in situ* is suspected.

ANAL SWELLINGS

Anal swellings may be caused by:

- haemorrhoids
- anal skin tags
- perianal haematoma
- anal cancer
- rectal prolapse
- anal warts.

Diagnostic investigations

Digital rectal examination, rigid sigmoidoscopy and proctoscopy and/or EUA with biopsy should reveal the diagnosis.

ANAL DISCHARGE

Anal discharge is caused by

- haemorrhoids
- fistula-in-ano
- villous adenoma of rectum.

Diagnostic investigations

Digital rectal examination, rigid sigmoidoscopy and/or EUA with biopsy should be diagnostic.

FAECAL INCONTINENCE

Faecal incontinence usually follows:

- anal sphincter injury or neurological damage at childbirth
- anal surgery
- neurological disease
- rectal prolapse.

Diagnostic investigations

Inflammatory or malignant bowel disease should be excluded by endoscopy and/or contrast X-rays. Endo-anal ultrasound scanning will detect sphincter defects and anorectal manometry will assess sphincter function.

TENESMUS

Tenesmus is usually associated with:

- rectal cancer
- villous adenoma of rectum
- inflammatory bowel disease.

Diagnostic investigations

Digital rectal examination and rigid sigmoidoscopy are mandatory. If there is any suspicion of disease proximal to the rectum it is essential that endoscopy or radiological imaging of the whole colon be performed.

HAEMORRHOIDS

Haemorrhoids are prolapsed anal cushions (see *Symptoms and Signs*). Presentation is usually with prolapse and bleeding on defaecation, but may be as an emergency with acute prolapse.

Investigation
Clinical diagnostic indicators

Haemorrhoids have a typical pattern of bleeding which is described in *Symptoms and Signs*.

Imaging

Haemorrhoids cannot be felt but can be seen during **proctoscopy** or may be visible protruding from the anus.

If rectal bleeding is a major symptom, then colorectal cancer or inflammatory bowel disease should be excluded by **colonoscopy**.

Management

Patients with minor symptoms such as minor streaks of blood on the stools and who are not anaemic do not require specific treatment provided you are certain that the haemorrhoids are the source of

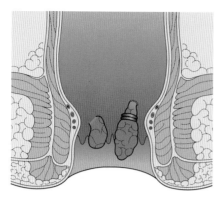

FIGURE 19.18   Banding of piles

the bleeding. Recurrent symptoms of itching, prolapse and bleeding may be treated by:

- **injection** of submucosal sclerosants just above the pile
- **rubber banding**, to strangulate the pile (Fig 19.18). Care must be taken to apply the bands above Hilton's white line or the procedure will be very painful for the patient
- surgery, in the form of **haemorrhoidectomy.** This is used for patients who have large skin tags as well as internal haemorrhoids, and have significant symptoms. The piles are excised, taking care to preserve a bridge of skin and mucosa between each area excised.

Some patients have troublesome postoperative pain and haemorrhoidectomy not be undertaken lightly. It does however give excellent long-term results.

Acutely prolapsed piles are usually treated conservatively. After resolution, they can be treated electively as above. Occasionally they are so painful that an emergency haemorrhoidectomy is necessary.

PERIANAL HAEMATOMA

This is a thrombosed vein in the subcutaneous plexus and presents as a painful swelling. Diagnosis is clinical, and the condition must be differentiated from an acutely prolapsed pile.

Resolution of the pain and the lump is invariable. In the first 48 hours when the clot has not become adherent to surrounding structures it is possible to evacuate it through a small skin incision made with local anaesthetic. This should only be done if the diagnosis is certain. Incision of a prolapsed pile is not recommended.

ANAL FISSURE

Midline posterior and anterior fissures are common and usually self-limiting. The tear is caused by straining at stool, the pain by the resulting sphincter spasm.

Investigation
Clinical diagnostic indicators

An anal fissure can be diagnosed from the history of the relationship of the pain to defaecation and in most cases by careful digital examination but an EUA is sometimes needed.

Management

The fissure will heal if the sphincter spasm resolves. This is achieved in three ways.

- **Natural dilatation** of the anus by formed stools. This requires an adequate intake of fluid and fibre, with **stool softeners** if the motions are hard. **Topical local anaesthetic gel** helps some patients.
- **Pharmacological relaxation**. Nitric oxide is a neurotransmitter in the internal anal sphincter and can be blocked by **glyceryl trinitrate** and the calcium antagonists **nifedipine and diltiazem**. They are administered as creams applied to the perianal skin. Headache due to vasodilatation is a possible side-effect, least likely with diltiazem, the current agent of choice.
- The anus may be **dilated under anaesthesia** or the internal sphincter may be divided laterally by a fine blade inserted through a small skin puncture – **sphincterotomy**. Both carry a risk of incontinence, particularly anal dilatation. They should be reserved for intractable cases.

Anal fissure in children is best treated by application of local anaesthetic gel to the fissure by the parents. The tubes and nozzles supplied for use in the urethra for catheterization serve well.

ANAL FISTULA

A fistula-in-ano connects the lumen of the rectum or anal canal with the perianal or ischiorectal skin. The key distinction is between low level, which does not involve a significant amount of sphincter muscle, and high-level, which does.

Investigation

Clinical diagnostic indicators

Diagnosis is usually clinical based on seeing the external openings of the fistulae. It is confirmed by examination under anaesthetic and demonstration of the presence of a track by the passage of a probe.

Complex high level fistulae can be elegantly demonstrated by **MRI scanning**.

Management

An anal fistula will never heal spontaneously, although there may be quiescent periods. This is because in the process of defaecation, mucus is forced along the track preventing closure.

If an EUA reveals a simple low-level fistula, a probe is passed along it, taking extreme care not to damage the sphincter muscle and the track **laid open**. This converts the fistula into an open ulcer, which is then allowed to heal by granulation. The excised tissue should always be sent for histology in case there is underlying Crohn's disease.

If there is a significant amount of muscle around or below the tract, i.e. the fistula is high, management is debatable. Many different operative procedures have been described, a testament that no method is ideal.

The principles are to drain any sepsis, establish the anatomy of the fistula at EUA or with MRI and then operate with minimal sphincter damage.

Staged surgery, using a progressively tightened suture (known as a Seton) passed through the fistula, which cuts slowly through the involved muscle, is one approach. An alternative, which will not cure the fistula, is to leave the suture in place to provide permanent drainage and prevent abscess formation.

A reasonably successful operation is to excise the internal and external openings of the track without laying the whole length of it open. The external incision can be closed by suture and the internal closed by an advancement flap of mucosa.

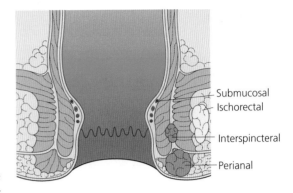

FIGURE 19.19   Perianal and ischiorectal abscess formation

ANORECTAL ABSCESS

Abscesses arise in the anal intersphincteric glands and may be perianal or ischiorectal (Fig 19.19). An abscess in the natal cleft is pilonidal and has no connection with the anal canal.

Investigation

The diagnosis rests on the classical signs of an abscess: calor, dolor and tumour.

An **MRI scan** is helpful in delineating a complex abscess.

Management

Acute abscesses are **incised under anaesthetic**. It is important that all loculi of pus are broken down and the incision is large enough to allow continued drainage. Approximately half will heal without further treatment. If the orifice of the intersphincteric gland in which the abscess arose remains patent, a fistula-in-ano develops. It is rare for the internal opening to be obvious at initial abscess drainage, and it should not be sought as there is a risk of sphincter damage.

PILONIDAL SINUS

A pilonidal sinus is a midline pit commonly containing hair, occurring in the natal cleft, most commonly in young men. Presentation may be as an acute abscess but most patients complain of chronic discharge and irritation.

Investigation

Clinical diagnostic indicators

The position of the sinus and the presence of hair protruding from it is diagnostic.

Sinogram

If necessary, the track can be demonstrated by the injection of a radio-opaque contrast material, a **sinogram.**

Management

A pilonidal abscess requires **incision and drainage.** Approximately half the patients will require a further procedure to deal with recurrent symptoms.

Chronic pilonidal sinus is treated traditionally by **wide excision** of the sinus and any secondary tracts, leaving the wound open to heal by secondary intention.

Since some patients have extensive branching sinuses, this can lead to prolonged recovery with a large, uncomfortable, slow-healing wound.

Local hair must be regularly removed until healing is complete.

Less extensive day case procedures to excise the pits and curette any abscess have become popular recently.

An intractable sinus may require a more extensive procedure, excising the sinus and closing the defect with a **skin flap.** The aim is to obliterate the natal cleft and have a wound away from the midline. This removes a probable cause and gives a greater chance of primary healing.

ANAL WARTS

Anal warts are diagnosed on clinical grounds and treated in the same way as warts anywhere else in the body. If they are sexually transmitted, contacts must be traced and treated in the usual way.

ANAL SKIN TAGS AND POLYPS

Diagnosis is clinical. If skin tags cause difficulty with personal hygiene or anal polyps are painful they can be **excised** under anaesthetic.

CARCINOMA OF THE ANAL CANAL

Carcinoma of the anus is associated with papilloma virus infection and may be preceded by dysplastic changes similar to those seen in cervical cancer. This process is termed anal **intraepithelial neoplasia** or AIN. The cancer arises in the anal skin and is therefore a **squamous carcinoma.** It spreads to the inguinal lymph nodes, not the intra-abdominal nodes.

Investigation

Biopsy of any suspicious anal lesion is essential, particularly in immunosuppressed patients. If carcinoma is confirmed, **staging by CT scan** is usual.

Management

Anal carcinoma is sensitive to **radiotherapy and chemotherapy.** Ninety per cent of patients do not require surgery. If the tumour does not respond to chemoradiation, **abdominoperineal excision** is necessary.

RECTAL PROLAPSE

Rectal prolapse may be either a prolapse of the mucosa or a prolapse of the full thickness of the rectum.

Mucosal prolapse is associated with straining during defaecation. Full thickness prolapse is usually associated with a weak pelvic floor caused by a childbirth injury or neurological disease, but may, rarely, also occur in nulliparous women and in men.

Investigation

The prolapse should be visible or appear with straining. An **EUA** may be needed to confirm that a full thickness prolapse is indeed present.

Assessment of the anal sphincter and colonic function may influence the type of surgical treatment.

Management

Mucosal prolapse can be treated by **banding** or **by stapling** (stapled prolapsectomy).

In children the condition is self-limiting, provided the parents can be persuaded to be **patient.**

Perineal excision and abdominal rectopexy. Full thickness prolapse is difficult to treat, as evidenced by the many operations described.

In the frail and elderly patient, a common situation, a perineal procedure is preferred to an abdominal operation. This may involve plication of the prolapsed rectal muscle (Delorme's procedure) or perineal excision of the prolapse. The recurrence rate for a perineal procedure is between 20 and 33 per cent, but it can be repeated if necessary.

Abdominal rectopexy (-pexy means fixing) attaches the rectum to the pre-sacral fascia The recurrence rate is less than 5 per cent. However, even after these operations the patient may have continuing symptoms of bowel dysfunction, particularly if they are present before surgery.

PERIANAL INFLAMMATORY BOWEL DISEASE

More than a quarter of patients with Crohn's disease have perianal manifestations – fissures, fistulae, ulcers and abscesses with characteristic purplish skin discoloration. This is the presenting feature in 5 per cent of patients.

Investigation

Diagnosis is made histologically by **biopsy**. The rest of the gut should be assessed by **radiological contrast studies** and **endoscopy**.

Management

Management depends on the manifestation of Crohn's disease elsewhere. In general, surgery for inflammatory anal problems should be cautious.

Once sepsis has been controlled, **medical treatment**, often with **immunosuppressants**, is indicated. Crohn's disease is chronic and relapses of its anal manifestations are common.

20

The urinary tract

Hari L. Ratan and Christopher P. Chilton

Diseases of the urinary tract encompass some of the most common benign and malignant conditions encountered in surgical practice. They present with a number of common symptoms and signs. A thorough history and examination followed by a logical approach to diagnostic imaging and other investigations will usually reveal the underlying pathology.

RENAL AND URETERIC PAIN

The causes of renal and ureteric pain are summarized in Table 20.1. The most important conditions are upper tract infection, stone disease, upper tract obstruction, and renal malignancy. Although the most common cause of ureteric colic is passage of a renal calculus, other diagnoses such as a sloughed renal papilla in diabetics and passage of clot in the presence of an upper tract urothelial tumour should be borne in mind.

Investigation

Clinical diagnostic indicators

Renal **pain** is felt **in the flank**, and when asked to localize it the patient will place his or her hands over an area spanning the lower border of the twelfth rib

---

Table 20.1
Common causes of renal and ureteric pain

Renal trauma

Renal calculus

Renal cell cancer

Infection (pyelonephritis)

Passage of ureteric calculus, clot or sloughed renal papilla

Pelviureteric junction obstruction

Urothelial malignancy

---

and the posterior superior iliac spine, lateral to the erector spinae muscle mass. The pain is visceral in nature and therefore often poorly localized. The severity can range from an occasional dull ache to a severe persistent pain. Pain may **radiate** round the loin into the groin; in men it may even be felt in the testis or in women the labia.

Patients suffering from **ureteric colic** characteristically experience agonizing pain in the loin, radiating to the groin. The pain is not characteristically colicky in the same way as pain arising from small bowel obstruction for, although the pain waxes and wanes, it is rarely described as griping and rarely eases off completely (see Chapter 17).

Patients in severe pain with ureteric colic require fluids to correct dehydration and must receive adequate analgesia *before embarking upon diagnostic tests*. Non-steroidal anti-inflammatory drugs (NSAIDs) such as diclofenac are effective, but the patient often requires opiate analgesia and anti-emetics.

Urine analysis

Urine **dipstick testing** may reveal the presence of **blood**, or there may be evidence of **leucocytes** and **nitrites**, which taken together are strongly indicative of **urinary tract infection**. Approximately 85 per cent of patients with ureteric colic caused by stone disease will have **microscopic haematuria**. Urine microscopy and culture will provide a more accurate measure of haematuria and the presence of infection. If there is any suspicion of tuberculosis, **three early-morning urine specimens** should be submitted for culture using Lowenstein–Jensen medium if there is any suspicion of tuberculosis.

Blood tests

A standard **full blood count** should be performed and the **serum urea and electrolytes** measured to check renal function.

Imaging

A **plain abdominal X-ray** with a field that includes kidneys, ureters and bladder (**KUB**) must be obtained. This may reveal the presence of renal tract calculi, although differentiating urinary tract calcification from other abdominal and pelvic calcification can be difficult.

Renal tract ultrasound scanning (**USS**) is effective at providing images of the kidneys themselves and differentiates between cystic and solid masses. Renal stones are usually seen clearly.

Intravenous urography (**IVU**) employs an intravenous radio-opaque contrast medium which is excreted rapidly through the kidneys. After an initial plain X-ray, KUB films are taken at intervals following contrast injection. This test delineates the pelvi-calyceal systems, the ureters and the bladder. The IVU is of particular value in detecting upper tract obstruction and the anatomy of the kidney and ureter and gives some idea of the relative function of the two kidneys.

Computed tomography (**CT**) scans provide detailed images of cross-sectional anatomy, and are valuable in the diagnosis of urological pathology. In many institutions, **non-contrast-enhanced CT scan** has replaced IVU as the investigation of choice in ureteric colic, as it has a higher sensitivity for the detection of stones (approaching 98 per cent), does not need intravenous contrast, and is quick. Its radiation dose is similar to a full series IVU.

HAEMATURIA

The common causes of haematuria are listed in Table 20.2.

Investigation

Clinical diagnostic indicators

Haematuria is defined on urine microscopy as the presence of more than three red blood cells per high-powered microscope field. Clinically, haematuria may turn the urine **pink** or **deep red with clots of blood** or be invisible. It may therefore be characterized as painful or painless, microscopic or frank.

Painful haematuria implies an inflammatory or infective process such as urinary tract infection or the passage of a calculus, although malignancies

Table 20.2
Common causes of haematuria

Kidney
Trauma
Infection
Calculus
Malignancy (either renal cell cancer or urothelial cancer of the pelvi-calyceal system)
Glomerulonephritis
Interstitial nephritis

Ureter
Trauma
Calculus
Urothelial cancer

Bladder
Trauma
Infective cystitis
Chemical cystitis, e.g. following cyclophosphamide chemotherapy
Radiation cystitis
Bladder cancer
Bladder calculus

Prostate/urethra
Urethral trauma
Benign prostatic hyperplasia
Prostatitis

such as *carcinoma in situ* of the bladder may also give rise to painful haematuria. Approximately 85 per cent of patients with renal or ureteric colic will have microscopic haematuria. **Painless haematuria** strongly suggests the presence of a tumour somewhere in the urinary tract.

Urinalysis

Microscopy is essential to confirm the diagnosis. In addition, it may detect excreted malignant cells.

Imaging

A **renal ultrasound scan** will show the anatomy of the kidney.

A **plain X-ray** (KUB) and **intravenous urography** (IVU) will reveal the anatomy of the renal tract and any calculi.

Endoscopy

Cystoscopy, usually flexible, is used to evaluate the bladder and urethra.

It is important to evaluate completely both the upper and lower urinary tract of any patient presenting with haematuria. In the **one-stop haematuria clinic** all investigations can be completed in one visit. This involves two investigations:

- a renal ultrasound scan and KUB X-ray to visualize the upper urinary tract
- cystoscopy, usually flexible, to evaluate the bladder and urethra.

In the case of microscopic haematuria, if the KUB, renal ultrasound and flexible cystoscope examinations are normal, no further diagnostic imaging is required unless there is particular suspicion of malignancy, as with a heavy smoker.

If the haematuria is macroscopic but investigation normal, an IVU should be done to provide further information about the pelvicalyceal anatomy and demonstrate the rare ureteric tumour.

PROBLEMS WITH MICTURITION

The functional activity of the bladder has two phases, storage and voiding. The normal bladder spends most of the time in the storage phase. It is a highly compliant organ and can accommodate increasing volumes of urine without large increases in intravesical pressure. During the voiding phase, the detrusor contracts while the urethral sphincter relaxes in a coordinated fashion, resulting in a normal voiding pattern. 'Lower urinary tract symptoms' (**LUTS**) is an umbrella term for symptoms arising from derangement of either the storage or voiding phase.

Investigation

Clinical diagnostic indicators

- *Storage phase symptoms*
  - **Urgency**: a sudden compelling desire to void which is difficult to defer.
  - **Increased daytime frequency**: the complaint by the patient who considers that he or she voids too often during the day.
  - **Nocturia**: the individual has to wake one or more times at night to void.
  - **Incontinence**: any involuntary leakage of urine.
- *Voiding phase symptoms*
  - **Slow stream**
  - **Hesitancy**: difficulty initiating micturition
  - **Intermittency**: a urinary stream which stops and starts
  - **Straining**: use of muscular effort from the abdominal wall to initiate or maintain flow
  - **Terminal dribble**: prolonged conclusion of micturition when the flow slows to a dribble.

The investigation of lower urinary tract symptoms depends upon the age and sex of the patient and the pattern of the presenting symptoms. For example young women with diurnal storage symptoms in whom urinary infection has been excluded are usually diagnosed as having an **idiopathic overactive bladder**. No special tests are required in the first instance to confirm this.

Elderly men with voiding symptoms and prostate enlargement on digital rectal examination are likely to have **bladder outflow obstruction** secondary to **benign prostatic hyperplasia**.

An important concept in the management of LUTS is estimation of how bothersome the symptoms are to each individual. Urinary symptoms are perceived very differently. Getting up to void once at night might be seen as normal by some individuals but unacceptable by others. The impact of urinary symptoms on quality of life has been quantified by a number of validated instruments including the International Prostatic Symptom Score questionnaire.

Frequency voiding charts

A diary of fluid input and output is very useful in most cases of LUTS. The patient is asked to record his or her daily fluid consumption, frequency of micturition and voided volume on a pre-printed chart, ideally for 1 week. This yields a wealth of information about bladder function, including maximum functional capacity, and the relationship of nocturia to fluid intake.

Urinalysis

A urine dipstick test or urine culture is vital to exclude infection.

Blood tests

Serum creatinine and electrolytes should be measured to exclude the presence of upper urinary tract deterioration secondary to lower tract dysfunction.

Serum prostate-specific antigen (PSA) measurement may be appropriate if benign prostatic hypertrophy or prostate cancer is suspected.

Uroflowmetry

Uroflowmetry is a useful outpatient test. The patient is asked to void into a funnel-shaped receptacle which is linked to a measurement device. The patient's urinary flow rate is calculated and a plot of flow rate against time produced.

Normal males void with a maximum flow rate (Qmax) above 15 mL/second – in young men much higher. In men there is a gradual decline in flow rate with increasing age, and characteristic flow rates in men with bladder outflow obstruction are likely to be below 10 mL/second.

Flow rates in women tend to be higher and do not change with age.

Uroflowmetry does not diagnose outflow obstruction. A poor flow may be caused by either obstruction or poor contractility of the detrusor. Conversely, *a normal flow rate does not exclude obstruction*, as the initial response to bladder outflow obstruction may be the detrusor generating higher pressures to maintain flow rate. However, as a quick, non-invasive and cheap test of voiding function, uroflowmetry is useful, especially when combined with a **post-micturition ultrasound scan of residual bladder volume**. This simple ultrasound scan estimates the **post-void residual urine volume**, which should normally be less than 50 mL. A large post-void residual volume may indicate the presence of chronic retention.

Cystoscopy

Cystoscopy may be valuable in patients in whom storage symptoms predominate in order to rule out an intravesical lesion. It is mandatory in those with concurrent haematuria.

Urodynamic studies

Urodynamics is the study of detrusor pressure during bladder filling (cystometrogram) and voiding phases. It is an invasive test requiring placement of a small urethral filling catheter and pressure transducer into the bladder. Intravesical pressure is a composite of detrusor pressure and the intra-abdominal pressure measured by means of a monitoring device inserted into the rectum. The true detrusor pressure is obtained by subtracting the intra-abdominal pressure from the total intravesical pressure.

During the filling phase, warm saline is instilled into the bladder at a constant rate. In a normal bladder, the detrusor pressure should change very little as the bladder fills until the maximal capacity is reached, when the pressure rises slightly. **Unstable contractions** may be observed in an overactive bladder and may be associated with urinary leakage. The patient is asked to report the first sensation of filling and then when discomfort is felt. **Provocative manoeuvres**, e.g. asking the patient to cough or perform the Valsalva manoeuvre, are used to demonstrate **stress incontinence** or **detrusor overactivity** associated with raised intra-abdominal pressure.

Once maximal bladder capacity has been reached, the patient is asked to void and pressure flow plots are obtained. These data allow differentiation between poor flow resulting from obstruction, when the detrusor pressure is usually high, and poor flow caused by a hypocontractile detrusor.

HYDRONEPHROSIS

Hydronephrosis is dilatation of the pelvicalyceal system of the kidney and is often secondary to upper-tract obstruction. However, it is an anatomical as opposed to a functional diagnosis, so it is entirely possible to have a hydronephrotic kidney which is not obstructed. For example, during pregnancy there is a so-called **physiological hydronephrosis**.

Antenatal and infantile hydronephrosis constitute an important and extensive topic and will not be discussed further in this text. Causes of obstructive hydronephrosis in adults are summarized in Table 20.3.

Investigation

Clinical diagnostic indicators

The main and often only symptom is renal pain but this can occur with many other conditions.

Table 20.3
Common causes of obstructive hydronephrosis

Intrinsic or luminal

Stones

Ureteric tumour

Blood clot

Papillary necrosis

Ureteropelvic junction obstruction

Ureteric stricture

Tuberculosis

Ureterocele

Extrinsic, from external pressure

Retroperitoneal malignancy

Retroperitoneal lymph node enlargement

Aortic aneurysm

Retroperitoneal fibrosis

Arising from the bladder

Bladder cancer

Neuropathic bladder

Arising from the urethra

Benign prostatic hyperplasia

Urethral stricture disease

Imaging

An **ultrasound examination of the kidney** will detect hydronephrosis but cannot usually differentiate the obstructive from the non-obstructive varieties. Long-standing hydronephrosis may result in loss of renal parenchymal tissue and this can be seen clearly on ultrasound images. Loss of cortical thickness is associated with obstructive pathology.

Intravenous urography (IVU) can also demonstrate hydronephrosis, but the quality of the image is dependent on there being sufficient residual renal function to excrete the contrast. In cases of severe obstruction, pelvicalyceal anatomy may only be demonstrated on delayed films obtained many hours after contrast injection.

Retrograde ureteropyelography involves direct retrograde instillation of contrast through a ureteric catheter placed inside the ureteric orifice via a cystoscope. This technique gives very clear anatomical information and is not dependent on renal function.

Dynamic radioisotope renography (Fig 20.1) is the most accurate radiological method of assessing upper tract obstruction. A technetium-99-labelled compound (either mercaptoacetyltriglycine (MAG3) or diethylenetriaminepentaacetic acid (DTPA)) is injected intravenously, and images of the kidneys are acquired dynamically by a gamma camera.

Furosemide is usually administered with the radioisotope to stimulate a brisk diuresis. MAG3 is filtered as well as actively excreted by the renal tubule so tends to give clearer images than DTPA, which is filtered only, and thus is more dependent on the glomerular filtration rate (GFR).

A normal renogram has a triphasic curve: an initial rapid uptake followed by a short plateau and then rapid elimination as the pelvicalyceal system empties of radioisotope. In the presence of obstruction, the second and third phases of the curve continue to rise as **the radioisotope accumulates within the dilated renal pelvis**. This is illustrated in Fig 20.1.

As well as giving an indication of the presence of obstruction, renography allows an estimate of the relative contribution of each kidney to the overall renal function. In cases of long-standing obstructive hydronephrosis, there may be very little residual renal function.

CT scanning may detect extrinsic causes of upper tract obstruction and demonstrate pathology such as retroperitoneal fibrosis or retroperitoneal lymph node enlargement.

Management

The management of hydronephrosis resulting from upper tract obstruction is dependent on the severity of obstruction, clinical symptoms and signs, renal function, and the underlying cause of the obstruction.

Emergency drainage (Table 20.4) of the kidney is indicated when there is:

- sepsis in an obstructed system
- obstruction of a single kidney
- intractable pain
- derangement of renal function (obstructive renal failure).

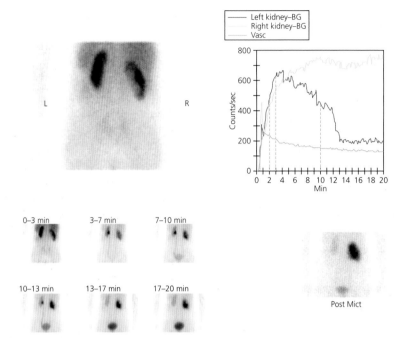

FIGURE 20.1   A DTPA (diethylenetriaminepentaacetic acid) renogram with furosemide given at 10 minutes. The left (purple line) kidney displays the normal triphasic pattern of uptake and rapid excretion, especially following furosemide administration at 10 minutes. The right (yellow line) kidney shows uptake but no excretion, signifying obstruction. This can be clearly seen on the scintigraphy images. Note that despite the presence of obstruction, the right kidney is still functioning well, contributing 47 per cent of total renal function

Table 20.4
Indications for surgical drainage of an obstructed kidney

Sepsis

Intractable pain

There is only one functioning kidney

If there is no indication for emergency drainage, the first step is to identify the underlying cause.

Effective non-emergency **drainage** of the hydronephrotic kidney may be accomplished either by **radiologically guided percutaneous passage of a nephrostomy tube**, or retrograde passage of a **ureteric stent** via a cystoscope. The former may be safer in patients with severe sepsis or septic shock as it can be accomplished under local anaesthetic coupled with light sedation rather than requiring general or regional anaesthesia.

Nephrectomy In cases of long-standing obstructive hydronephrosis in which renal function has been lost, nothing need be done if the patient is symptomless or too frail. However, if there is recurrent pain, infection or stones in the hydronephrotic kidney, **nephrectomy** is indicated, nowadays probably by the laparoscopic route.

The management of stone disease is detailed below.

URETEROPELVIC JUNCTION OBSTRUCTION

This is an important cause of hydronephrosis. It is a congenital condition resulting in impaired drainage of the renal pelvis, most likely due to an aperistaltic segment of proximal ureter. It often presents with episodes of acute loin pain in a young adult, often after imbibing large quantities of fluid. The diagnosis is confirmed by **IVU or retrograde pyelography**, and renal function in the affected kidney is assessed by **isotope renography**. If there is a useful degree of renal function, more than say 15–20 per cent of total function, the patient should be offered surgery.

Pyeloplasty involves excision of the obstructing segment of the UPJ or upper ureter and reconnection of the ureter to the renal pelvis, making sure that there is a wide anastomosis. This is a major abdominal operation which can be done by open or laparoscopic means and is usually curative.

RENAL INFECTIONS

Acute bacterial pyelonephritis is the commonest renal infection, and is most frequently caused by virulent coliform bacilli that have arisen in the lower urinary tract. Haematogenous spread may also occur.

Pyonephrosis is an obstructed kidney laden with pus. This is a very dangerous condition which can result in irreversible renal damage followed by death of the patient.

Occasionally renal infections, particularly those occurring in obstructed kidneys, can perforate with development of a **perirenal abscess**. These collections may be confined by Gerota's fascia to the flank although pus may track down along the ureteric sheath.

These patients are often dehydrated, nauseated and pyrexial and require urgent intravenous fluid replacement.

Investigation
Clinical diagnostic indicators
Acute bacterial pyelonephritis is characterized by an acutely ill patient with loin pain, high fever, rigors and lower urinary tract symptoms.

Blood tests
A **full blood count** should be obtained and the serum **electrolytes** estimated. **Blood cultures** should be requested.

Urinalysis
The urine should be examined by microscopy and **cultured**.

Imaging
Diagnostic imaging allows differentiation of acute bacterial pyelonephritis from pyonephrosis. Initial **ultrasound scan** of the kidneys will demonstrate any obstruction as well as a perirenal collection. **IVU** is useful to show drainage. In complex cases or where there may be a perinephric abscess, a **CT scan** of the abdomen is helpful.

Management
Patients with a suspected renal infection should be admitted to hospital and given immediate parenteral broad-spectrum antibiotics, prior to investigation.

Acute bacterial pyelonephritis is treated with a course of parenteral preferably bactericidal antibiotics, including **gentamicin** and a **cephalosporin**, changing to oral administration after the fever has subsided.

Pyonephrosis is a life-threatening condition and requires **emergency drainage** of the obstructed kidney usually by placement of a **percutaneous nephrostomy** tube under local anaesthesia with ultrasound or X-ray guidance.

Once the acute infection has subsided, the cause of the obstruction, usually stone disease, must be attended to before the nephrostomy tube is removed.

RENAL TRACT TUBERCULOSIS

Infection with *Mycobacterium tuberculosis* has become resurgent in the UK in recent years and urinary tract manifestations of tuberculosis must be considered in the assessment of patients with urinary symptoms. Urinary tract tuberculosis is one of the long-term consequences of haematogenous dissemination of the bacillus at the time of initial infection. The kidney is usually the first organ of the urinary tract to become infected. Typically, caseating granulomas develop bilaterally in the renal cortices. Other parts of the urinary tract become involved by direct extension.

Investigation
Clinical diagnostic indicators
Urinary tract symptoms apart from frequency are uncommon. The diagnosis may be suspected by the patient's general symptoms of **malaise** and **weight loss**.

Urine analysis
Urine **microscopy** demonstrates, in most cases, the classical finding of a persistent **sterile pyuria** – the

presence of leucocytes without any bacterial growth. Microscopic haematuria may also be present. Urine samples are best collected first thing in the morning, which is the time when the numbers of bacilli are highest. As *M. tuberculosis* is a fastidious organism, three separate specimens must be sent. A slide can be examined with **Ziehl–Neelsen staining** looking for the characteristic acid- and alkali-fast bacilli (AAFB), but more often the diagnosis can only be made by culturing the urine for 6–8 weeks on **Lowenstein–Jensen medium**. Newer molecule-based assays are becoming available and may allow more rapid confirmation of tuberculous infection.

Imaging

Plain X-rays of the kidneys, ureters and bladder may show renal calcification of typical distribution.

An **IVU** series may demonstrate multiple abnormalities, including:

- distortion of calyceal anatomy
- blunting or loss of calyces
- parenchymal loss, leading in advanced cases to so-called 'autonephrectomy'
- a dilated segment of ureter above a vesico-ureteric junction stricture.

Cystoscopy

The bladder mucosa should be inspected directly and bladder capacity measured. The bladder may be scarred and non-compliant. Biopsies are rarely indicated for diagnosis, which is made by urine culture.

Management

The definitive management of urinary tract tuberculosis is by multiple agent **chemotherapy**, usually a combination of **rifampicin, isoniazid, pyrazinamide and ethambutol**. Various regimens are used, usually under the care of a specialist physician. Treatment is for at least 6 months.

If **retrograde pyelography** reveals a significant hydronephrosis secondary to a stricture of the vesico-ureteric junction, **a stent** may be inserted.

The indications for **surgery** are few. Even heavily calcified non-functioning kidneys may be managed conservatively if the patient becomes asymptomatic following completion of chemotherapy.

A non-functioning kidney producing persistent symptoms, or one in which malignancy cannot be excluded because of the distortion found on imaging, requires **nephrectomy**.

Ureteric strictures often resolve with chemotherapy alone, but, if persistent, the **ureter may be reimplanted** into the bladder.

A small-capacity bladder can be enlarged surgically by **augmentation cystoplasty** in which the bladder capacity is increased by the incorporation of a pouch of intestine.

RENAL TRAUMA

The kidneys are injured relatively infrequently in blunt trauma, being protected by the rib cage and their mobility. They may be injured by penetrating wounds of the flank.

The American Society of Trauma Surgeons has classified renal trauma by the degree of injury (Table 20.5).

Table 20.5
Classification of renal trauma

Grade 1	Subcapsular haematoma
Grade 2	Parenchymal laceration usually not extending more than 1 cm
	Non-expanding perirenal haematoma confined to the retroperitoneum
Grade 3	Parenchymal laceration more than 1 cm with no involvement of the collecting system
Grade 4	Parenchymal laceration extending through renal cortex, medulla, and collecting system
	OR
	Main vessel injury with contained haemorrhage
Grade 5	Shattered kidney
	OR
	Avulsion of renal pedicle resulting in devascularized kidney

Investigation

Clinical diagnostic indicators

The usual presentation is with **flank pain** and tenderness, a loin mass or extensive flank bruising and **haematuria**. There may be **hypovolaemic shock** from massive retroperitoneal haemorrhage. A thorough general examination is important.

Urinalysis

Microscopy will reveal any haematuria.

Imaging

Patients who are haemodynamically stable and have isolated flank trauma with microscopic haematuria do not require any specific diagnostic imaging unless the mechanism of injury (such as deceleration) suggests that other organs may be damaged.

Contrast-enhanced CT scan is the modality of choice, if imaging is required, because it can accurately stage a renal injury and confirm the presence of a normal contralateral kidney (Fig 20.2).

Intraoperative renal imaging can be rapidly obtained by performing a single-film IVU after injection of double-dose contrast medium.

Laparotomy may have to be the investigation of last resort if there is no response to resuscitation and a CT scan not possible.

Management

As these patients often have other major injuries, management should be based on advanced trauma and life support (ATLS) principles, with initial focus on airway, breathing and circulation. **Resuscitation** with fluids, colloids and blood may be required to stabilize a shocked patient.

Most renal injuries of low grade can be managed conservatively with **bed rest, analgesia** and careful **monitoring**. In most cases, the haematoma is held stable by tamponade in the retroperitoneal space. Even if the injury results in urinary extravasation, conservative treatment will result in spontaneous resolution in the vast majority of cases.

A **repeat CT scan** a few days after the original injury is useful to re-stage the injury and ensure that resolution is occurring.

The indications for immediate operative management are a **grade 5 renal injury** or a haemodynamically unstable patient. If the patient is already undergoing laparotomy for concurrent intra-abdominal injury, an expanding retroperitoneal haematoma is the main indication to explore the retroperitoneal space.

Nephrectomy may be required if a major renal injury is found. In these circumstances it is reassuring to have an intraoperative IVU to confirm the presence of a kidney on the other side.

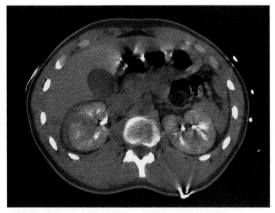

FIGURE 20.2 A contrast-enhanced CT showing renal trauma. This CT demonstrates the effects of blunt trauma to the right kidney with a renal parenchymal laceration and accompanying perirenal haematoma. Note the presence of the normal left kidney and the fact that both kidneys are well vascularized

CANCER OF THE KIDNEY

Renal cell carcinoma is the most lethal of all urological malignancies. It represents around 3 per cent of all solid tumours and occurs predominantly in older people. Smoking is the only known environmental risk factor. Most are clear cell carcinomata. Other subtypes include papillary tumours, which are more likely to be multifocal, and chromophobe carcinoma.

Investigation

Clinical diagnostic indicators

The classic triad of **pain, haematuria and flank mass** is seen in fewer than 30 per cent of cases. Most renal cell carcinomata are detected incidentally on US or CT scans performed for other purposes.

The tumours characteristically **metastasize** via the circulation to **bone, lung and brain**. A number of paraneoplastic syndromes may occur, including **hypercalcaemia**, **polycythaemia** and **hepatic dysfunction**. These are listed in detail in *Symptoms and Signs*.

Urinalysis

Urine dipstick or microscopy usually reveals haematuria.

Blood tests

Routine tests of renal and liver function are essential to exclude renal failure or metastatic disease (see Chapter 18).

Imaging

Ultrasound scan allows differentiation between solid and cystic masses. If a solid mass is found, **a contrast-enhanced CT scan** (Fig 20.3) will demonstrate malignant masses and stage the disease. An X-ray **skeletal survey** may reveal skeletal metastases and a **chest X-ray** any lung metastases.

Management

Radical nephrectomy performed either open or laparoscopically is the only treatment that offers a prospect of cure. The surgical principle is early control of the renal vessels followed by excision of the kidney within Gerota's fascia. Tumour thrombus in the inferior vena cava (IVC) may be excised by opening the vein. Even patients with supradiaphragmatic IVC involvement may be amenable to curative surgery, sometimes with cardiopulmonary bypass.

Laparoscopic radical nephrectomy is superseding the open approach. It appears to offer equivalent oncological clearance, with smaller scars and a shorter postoperative recovery period.

Patients with multifocal bilateral tumours or those with a tumour in a solitary kidney, as well as those at risk of future renal failure such as patients with diabetic nephropathy, may be suitable for **nephron-sparing surgery**, in which the principle is to preserve as much normal kidney tissue as possible. This is a technically demanding operation, and the kidney may have to be cooled with saline slush and the vasculature clamped during the excision.

Cure rates for tumours confined to the kidney are excellent and 5-year survival exceeds 80 per cent.

Immunotherapy and chemotherapy. Metastatic RCC has a poor prognosis with 5-year survival rarely exceeding 30 per cent. Most patients are dead within a year of diagnosis. These tumours are chemo- and radio-resistant. In fit patients immunotherapy with either **interferon-α** or **interleukin-2** has been shown to have some effect especially following a cytoreductive nephrectomy, an operation designed to remove as much tumour as possible.

Highly targeted **anti-angiogenic tyrosine kinase inhibitors** have been introduced recently and early results from trials are encouraging.

RENAL AND URETERIC STONE DISEASE (UROLITHIASIS)

Renal calculi (stones) are common. The lifetime risk of stone formation in Western countries is as high as 15 per cent, depending on gender, race and geographical location. Caucasian men with sedentary lifestyles living in arid environments constitute the group with the highest risk. In a few cases, underlying metabolic disorders such as cystinuria or renal tubular acidosis are found.

Most stones are calcium salts, with calcium oxalate being the most common. Other stones consist of calcium urate and struvite (magnesium ammonium phosphate). Struvite stones arise in alkaline urine, such as may occur during urinary tract infection with urease-producing microorganisms such as *Proteus mirabilis*.

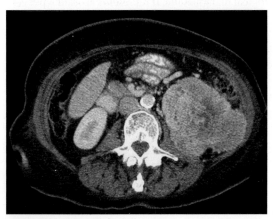

FIGURE 20.3 A large left renal cancer

Investigation

Clinical diagnostic indicators

The emergency investigation of patients presenting with **ureteric colic** caused by stones is described above (see page 495). Other patients may have no symptoms or can present with **haematuria, urinary tract infection** or **chronic flank pain**.

Blood and urine analysis

Serum calcium and **urate** levels should be measured, the urine cultured to look for infection and the urinary **pH** tested.

Imaging

Plain KUB X-ray will demonstrate approximately 70 per cent of stones, predominantly those containing calcium salts, and is thus a valuable initial investigation (Fig 20.4).

Renal ultrasound will often demonstrate stones in the renal pelvicalyceal system but is much less sensitive for ureteric calculi.

Intravenous urography is used to detect urinary tract obstruction secondary to urolithiasis.

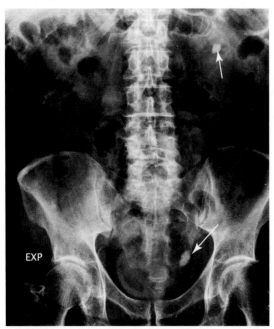

FIGURE 20.4   Kidney, ureter and bladder (KUB) X-ray showing large lower left ureteric and renal calculi

Non-contrast-enhanced CT has now become the investigation of choice for suspected ureteric calculi as it detects over 90 per cent of stones and can be performed quickly and without the risks of intravenous contrast injection.

Metabolic screening of blood and urine

Most patients presenting with urolithiasis have no underlying metabolic abnormality, so a full metabolic screen is not required for first-time stone formers.

Patients who present with recurrent urolithiasis should be evaluated by a **24-hour urine collection** to detect **hypercalciuria** and rare metabolic disorders such as **cystinuria**.

Management of renal calculi

Regular observation

Small symptomless stones within the renal calyces may be managed conservatively. There is some evidence that these stones can gradually increase in size and subsequently become symptomatic, so **annual follow-up** with a KUB X-ray to monitor any enlargement is indicated.

Fragmentation

Extracorporeal shockwave lithotripsy (ESWL) is the mainstay of management of small to medium-sized (5–20 mm) renal stones. This relies on the generation of an acoustic shock wave which can be focused on the renal stone, thus shattering it into smaller fragments which can be passed in the urine. Modern machines are compact and use piezo-electric or electromagnetic shock-wave generators. The shock waves are focused by acoustic lenses or parabolic reflectors. In most cases ESWL can be accomplished as an outpatient procedure under opiate analgesia or light sedation.

Success rates are as high as 80–90 per cent for smaller renal stones but fall as stone burden increases. Multiple treatments may be required to treat larger stones.

For bigger stones, ESWL is less effective and more invasive techniques may be required.

Ureteroscopy and laser fragmentation involves the passage of a narrow-gauge instrument up the ureter from the bladder, giving access to the pelvicalyceal system. A **holmium laser fibre** can be passed through the ureteroscope and used to fragment the stone. This technique is particularly useful for smaller stones in the lower pole of the kidney, or for hard stones which fail to fragment with lithotripsy.

Surgical excision

Large stones are best treated by **percutaneous nephrolithotomy** (PCNL). This technique involves a percutaneous radiologically guided antegrade puncture into a renal calyx. The patient lies prone. Using the Seldinger technique, the tract is dilated to allow passage of a nephroscope. Instruments may then be passed via the nephroscope to directly fragment and remove the stone.

Despite technological advances and increasing expertise, there are a few stones which may resist minimally invasive management, and there is still a place for **open pyelolithotomy** (removal of a stone from the renal pelvis) or **nephrolithotomy** (removal of a stone from the renal substance).

Management of ureteric calculi

The management of ureteric calculi is influenced by:

- the size of the stone
- the site of the stone
- the degree of obstruction
- whether there is sepsis.

If the ureteric calculus is causing high-grade obstruction, characterized by a delayed dense nephrogram phase on the IVU series, or if there is any sign of sepsis, *the obstructed kidney should be drained prior to definitive management of the stone* (see Table 20.5).

Drainage may be accomplished by cystoscopy and retrograde passage of a **'double-J' stent** up the obstructed ureters, past the calculus.

Alternatively, an **external nephrostomy** tube may be placed by radiologically guided percutaneous puncture of the hydronephrotic collecting system.

Stones less than 5 mm in diameter are likely to pass spontaneously and **expectant management** can be adopted. The patient is provided with adequate analgesia and once comfortable can be discharged home safely. A follow-up KUB X-ray or limited IVU can be performed 1 or 2 weeks later to confirm passage of the stone. Surprisingly large stones may disappear from the X-ray without the patient noticing that they have passed them, but on other occasions the final passage is extremely painful. *Indications for abandoning expectant management include signs of sepsis, intractable pain or a failure to pass the stone after a few weeks.*

Stones larger than 5 mm in diameter less commonly pass spontaneously. Those larger than 1 cm rarely do. Some form of intervention is required in these patients and there are various options available. ESWL (see above) is widely used and modern lithotripters allow targeting of stones in all parts of the ureter. **Visualization of stones masked by bony prominences can still prove difficult.**

Most ureteric stones are accessible to either a flexible or rigid ureteroscope passed in a retrograde direction from the bladder. The calculus is fragmented with holmium laser or pneumatic lithotrite.

Open or laparoscopic ureterolithotomy is rarely used in the modern age of endo-urology.

INFECTIVE CYSTITIS

Inflammation of the bladder is usually caused by bacterial infection with perineal and faecal organisms. Cystitis is common in women because of the easy retrograde migration of organisms up the short female urethra. The most common pathogen found in community-acquired urinary tract infection (UTI) is *Escherischia coli*. It is responsible for more than 60 per cent of cases. Different pathogens such as methicillin-resistant *Staphylococcus aureus* (MRSA) may be encountered in nosocomial infections. A greater degree of antibiotic resistance is usually found in hospitals.

Investigation

Clinical diagnostic indicators

Women with cystitis typically present with **dysuria, frequency, urgency and foul-smelling urine**.

It is important to differentiate those patients with *recurrent* UTI caused by different strains of bacteria on each presentation from those with *relapsing* UTI in whom the same organism is cultured repeatedly. Recurrence is caused by genuine reinfection, whereas relapse is usually related to a persistent infection caused by an underlying abnormality such as stone disease or urinary tract obstruction.

UTI in young men is uncommon and is likely to be associated with a urinary tract abnormality.

UTI in older men is usually the result of bladder outflow obstruction, and is discussed below.

UTI in children is an important topic and full discussion is beyond the scope of this book. Functional and anatomical abnormalities of the urinary tract are the common causes of UTI in children and must be thoroughly investigated.

Urinalysis

Use the urine dipstick test for **nitrites** and **leucocyte esterase**.

In cases of recurrent UTI, it is helpful to perform urine **microscopy, culture and sensitivity** to determine the infecting organism and guide appropriate antibiotic therapy.

Imaging

Recurrent urinary tract infections in women and most infections in men should be investigated with an **ultrasound scan** and **KUB X-ray**.

Management

Most cases of uncomplicated urinary tract infection may be treated empirically with a short oral course of agents such as **trimethoprim, nitrofurantoin, a penicillin or a cephalosporin**. If the symptoms do not resolve a further urine culture is required.

Recurrent UTI may become intractable. Once underlying abnormalities have been excluded, it may be necessary to prescribe **long-term antibiotic prophylaxis** with a once-daily low dose of trimethoprim, nitrofurantoin or cefalexin. These agents may be rotated monthly to reduce the risk of drug resistance developing.

TRAUMA TO THE BLADDER

The bladder is usually damaged only when it is full. Blunt abdominal trauma can result in rupture and urinary extravasation. The bladder may also be injured by a penetrating injury or from a fracture of the pelvis.

Iatrogenic perforation may occur from technical error during endoscopic resection of bladder tumours.

Bladder injury may be *extraperitoneal* or *intraperitoneal*.

Investigation

Clinical diagnostic indicators

Bladder injury is usually suspected on the basis of the history – **pain, an absence of micturition and haematuria**.

Urinalysis

Haematuria, overt or microscopic, is always present with bladder trauma.

Imaging

The diagnosis can be confirmed by a **retrograde cystogram**. Water-soluble contrast medium is instilled via the urethra to distend the bladder and obtain radiographic proof of the extravasation and establish whether it is intraperitoneal or extraperitoneal.

Management

Extraperitoneal rupture following blunt abdominal trauma may be managed conservatively by keeping the bladder empty with a **urethral catheter**. This is because urinary extravasation is confined to the retroperitoneal space, which is not a cavity. The cystogram is repeated after 2 weeks to confirm healing of the perforation. The catheter may then be removed.

Intraperitoneal rupture requires **laparotomy and repair** of the bladder to prevent the otherwise inevitable development of urinary peritonitis.

Penetrating abdominal injuries that damage the bladder are rare but if found during laparotomy should repaired.

BLADDER CANCER

The bladder is the site of the commonest urological cancer. Men are more commonly affected. The peak ages of incidence are the sixth or seventh decades. The most important cause of bladder cancer is exposure to environmental carcinogens excreted in the urine. Cigarette smoking is the usual source, although exposure to carcinogens in the dye and rubber industries was once responsible for a large number of cases.

Histologically most bladder cancers arise from the urothelium and are thus **transitional cell carcinomata**. If there is chronic bladder irritation

Table 20.6
Staging of bladder tumours

No muscle invasion	Muscle invasion
Ta: non-invasive papillary	T3: invasive beyond the muscle and into fat outside bladder
T1: invasive but not into detrusor muscle	T4: invasive into surrounding structures such as prostate
Tcis: carcinoma *in situ* with malignant cells but no invasion	

(long-term catheterization, schistosomial infection, bladder stone), squamous metaplasia of the urothelium occurs with subsequent development of squamous cell carcinoma. In the UK, the transitional cell type accounts for over 90 per cent of bladder cancers, but in parts of the world where schistosomiasis is endemic the squamous cell type are more common.

Bladder cancers are *graded* histologically from 1 to 3 (low–high grade) and *staged* using the TNM system (Table 20.6).

The behaviour of these two types of tumours is markedly different.

- Low-grade tumours that do not invade muscle rarely metastasize or progress to higher grade or stage lesions, but do tend to recur after treatment (in over 70 per cent of cases). High-grade non muscle-invasive G3 T1 and Tcis lesions tend to progress to become invasive and are thus termed high-risk disease.
- Muscle-invasive tumours if not properly treated invariably metastasize and have a poor prognosis.

Investigation

Clinical diagnostic indicators

Bladder cancer usually presents with frank, **painless haematuria**.

Urinalysis

Urine cytology is rarely useful in cases of low-grade cancer but it may be positive in high-grade lesions and Tcis.

Cystoscopy and imaging

The investigation must always include **cystoscopy**. The typical lesion seen on cystoscopy is illustrated in Fig 20.5.

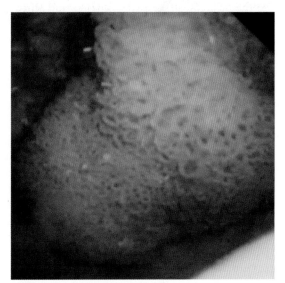

FIGURE 20.5 Cystoscopic appearance of superficial transitional cell carcinoma of the bladder

Upper tract imaging by means of an **IVU** is essential to see if there is also upper tract urothelial tumour, a finding in 2–4 per cent of cases.

Patients found to have muscle-invasive bladder cancer require staging by means of **chest X-ray and CT scan of the abdomen and pelvis** (Fig 20.6).

Management

Transurethral resection of the visible lesion with an electrocautery loop is the initial management of bladder cancer.

Specimens of detrusor muscle deep to the tumour must be obtained to assess whether muscle invasion has occurred. The management then depends on the stage and grade of the cancer.

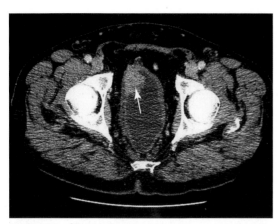

FIGURE 20.6 CT scan showing right anterior muscle invasive transitional cell cancer of the bladder (arrow)

For most low-grade Ta and T1 tumours, the initial transurethral resection is often curative. Nevertheless, because of the high risk of recurrence subsequent regular cystoscopic inspections are essential, their frequency depending on the histology of the tumours. Recurrences can be cauterized or resected.

Intravesical instillation of a chemotherapeutic agent such as **mitomycin C** has been shown to reduce the risk of recurrence.

Immunotherapy. High-grade T1 tumours or Tcis are dangerous because of their propensity to progress to muscle-invasive disease. Initial treatment is with weekly intravesical instillation of bacille Calmette–Guérin (**BCG**), a live attenuated vaccine, over a 6-week period. This stimulates an antitumour immunological response in over 60 per cent of cases. Subsequent maintenance courses of BCG may be given every 6 months and the response monitored cystoscopically.

Patients who fail BCG treatment or with non-metastatic muscle-invasive disease should be offered radical treatment in the form of either **radical cystectomy** or **radical radiotherapy**:

- **Cystectomy** is an operation with high morbidity and 2–4 per cent mortality. The bladder, prostate and seminal vesicles are removed en bloc. Urinary tract reconstruction is by diversion of the ureters into an **ileal conduit** or construction of an **orthotopic neobladder from an ileal segment**.

- **Radical radiotherapy** to the bladder is given in fractions over a 5- to 6-week period. Although the bladder is preserved, the side-effects include early haemorrhagic cystitis and later bladder fibrosis, as well as radiation proctitis and damage to small bowel. Even with radical therapy, the 5-year survival of patients with invasive bladder cancer is only 50 per cent. Metastatic bladder cancer has a poor prognosis.

- **Systemic chemotherapy** has a very limited response rate.

A transitional cell carcinoma may also occur in the ureter and renal pelvis, usually presenting with haematuria, and often associated with bladder tumours. It is rarely if ever amenable to endoscopic removal and requires excisional surgery, usually **nephro-ureterectomy**, an operation ideally suited to the laparoscopic approach.

BENIGN PROSTATIC HYPERPLASIA

Benign prostatic hyperplasia is a progressive pathological process in which there is hyperplasia of stromal and glandular elements of the prostate gland concentrated in its peri-urethral and transitional zones. The stromal proliferation usually predominates.

As the prostatic hypertrophy progresses, bladder outflow obstruction may occur giving rise to voiding symptoms. The detrusor's response to obstruction is to hypertrophy and increase voiding pressure so that, initially, the flow rate may be maintained. A consequence of detrusor hypertrophy is detrusor overactivity, giving rise to urgency, daytime frequency and nocturia. As obstruction progresses, however, the detrusor fails to compensate, leading to acute or chronic retention. Other complications include urinary tract infection, bladder stone and prostatic bleeding.

Investigation

Clinical diagnostic indicators

The common symptoms are **urgency, daytime frequency and nocturia** sometimes leading on to acute or chronic retention.

Digital rectal examination will usually indicate the presence of **prostatic enlargement** and may detect features suspicious of malignancy. It is important to note that benign prostatic hyperplasia is a histological diagnosis, which cannot be made on clinical evidence alone.

The International Prostatic Symptom Score (IPSS) questionnaire is calculated from a series of questions assessing the impact of urinary symptoms on quality of life and is scored up to 35. Patients can be graded as having mild, moderate or severe symptoms.

Urinalysis

The urine should be **cultured** to exclude infection.

Blood tests

The **electrolytes, urea and creatinine** should be measured to determine whether there is any renal damage.

Prostate-specific antigen is a glycoprotein detectable in the serum produced by prostate cells. An elevated PSA is associated with prostate cancer, but is neither sensitive nor specific enough to be used for the definitive diagnosis of this malignancy; but a high level is an indication for a biopsy of the prostate (see page 513). It is known that PSA level is directly related to the size of the gland, and so patients with advanced benign hypertrophy may have elevated PSA levels.

A high PSA is an important prognostic indicator for disease progression, including subsequent development of retention.

Uroflowmetry

Results may be normal, or there may be a typically 'obstructed pattern'. As discussed above it is impossible to differentiate this pattern from that observed in cases of detrusor failure. **Post-void residual volume** may be absent in early benign prostatic hyperplasia, but may build up and progress eventually to chronic retention.

Urodynamics

Filling and voiding urodynamic studies may be of value in the investigation of patients with symptoms suggesting predominantly problems with storage (urgency, frequency, urge incontinence) and in young patients with LUTS. During the filling phase idiopathic detrusor instability may be demonstrated, although this may be secondary to bladder outflow obstruction. Measurement of **detrusor pressure** during the voiding phase helps to clarify whether a poor urinary stream is caused by bladder outflow obstruction (in which case the detrusor pressure is usually high) or detrusor failure (when it is low).

Cystoscopy

The size of the prostate as observed during cysto-urethroscopy correlates poorly with the degree of urodynamic obstruction or severity of symptoms, but it must be done to exclude intravesical pathology in patients with predominantly storage symptoms.

Prostate biopsy

Refer to page 514.

Management

The management of bladder outflow obstruction secondary to benign prostatic hyperplasia depends on how much the patient is bothered by the symptoms and whether there are complications such as UTI or urinary retention.

Patients with mild symptoms and no complications need no treatment until symptoms deteriorate or complications develop. There is then a choice of pharmacotherapy or surgery.

Pharmacotherapy

Two varieties of pharmacotherapeutic agents are employed in the treatment, first **alpha-blockers** (prazosin, doxazosin, terazosin, alfuzosin and tamsulosin), and second **5-α-reductase inhibitors** (finasteride and dutasteride).

Alpha-blockers act upon the α-adrenergic receptors in the prostatic stroma which are responsible for contraction of the myofibroblasts. By reducing the resting tone of these cells, the degree of bladder outlet obstruction may be eased. Treatment with α-blockade is usually first-line medical therapy.

Finasteride and dutasteride inhibit the 5-α-reductase enzyme responsible for converting testosterone into its more active metabolite dihydrotestosterone (DHT). 5-α-reductase inhibitor therapy makes the glandular elements of the prostate shrink with consequent improvement of symptoms in men with large glands. Combinations of a drug from each class have been shown to act synergistically.

Surgery

Prostatectomy has been the surgical management for many years. The classic procedure was **open enucleation** of the enlarged prostatic tissue from within the compressed outer layers of the gland.

Development of endo-urological technology led to **transurethral resection** of the prostate by means of monopolar electrocautery. This is now the current 'gold-standard' surgical treatment. Initially only small glands could be dealt with endoscopically, but with improved techniques large glands can be treated in this way so that the use of and expertise in open surgery is now rare.

New developments include the use of lasers to either ablate or enucleate the prostate.

The indications for surgery include:

- failed pharmacotherapy
- acute urinary retention
- persistent haematuria
- bladder stones
- recurrent UTI
- rising post-void residual urine volume
- high-pressure chronic retention.

Surgical treatment usually results in the best available symptom improvement with measurable increase in flow rate and sustained long-term results.

Early complications such as **bleeding and infection** can be serious.

Late complications include **retrograde ejaculation, impotence** and rarely **incontinence**.

Hospital stay is short, but patients must 'take it easy' for several weeks afterwards until the prostatic bed has re-epithelialized and there is no risk of secondary haemorrhage.

ACUTE RETENTION OF URINE

Acute urinary retention is a complete inability to void accompanied by severe suprapubic discomfort, which then progresses to the visceral pain of bladder distension. There may be preceding lower urinary tract symptoms, particularly progressive voiding symptoms such as hesitancy and dwindling stream. Occasionally retention may be provoked by putting off passing urine during a long journey, or drinking a large quantity of fluid.

In men, acute urinary retention is commonly the end result of bladder outflow obstruction secondary to **benign prostatic hyperplasia**, with an acutely decompensated (failing) detrusor muscle. Other important causes include **infection** and **constipation**, particularly in elderly patients. In younger males **urethral stricture disease** may be responsible. Acute retention in women is uncommon and raises the possibility of an obstructing **pelvic mass** such as an ovarian tumour or a retroverted gravid uterus.

In either sex, neurological disease such as spinal injury, cord compression, cauda equina syndrome and multiple sclerosis can all give rise to retention. A thorough neurological examination must therefore be performed in cases of retention if there is any doubt about the cause.

Investigation

Investigation is usually deferred until the patient's discomfort is relieved by passage of a **urethral catheter**, a simple manoeuvre with gratifying results! If it is not possible to pass a urethral catheter, a catheter may be inserted percutaneously in the suprapubic area, but only if there is an easily palpable bladder. The residual volume drained is typically between 600 and 1000 mL.

Clinical diagnostic indicators

The diagnosis is usually obvious but it is important to elucidate, by a thorough clinical examination, the cause of the retention.

Digital rectal examination will allow a relatively inaccurate assessment of the degree of prostatic hypertrophy and may reveal the presence of a palpable prostatic malignancy.

Urinalysis

Urine dipstick or microscopy and culture must be performed to exclude an infection.

Blood tests

Serum **creatinine** and **electrolytes** should be measured to check renal function. It must be noted that measurement of **PSA can be misleading** after acute retention as it may be raised by benign hypertrophy as well as further elevated by urethral catheterization.

Management

Relieve the patient's pain by passing a **urethral catheter**. Any underlying cause of the retention such as UTI or constipation must be treated before removing the catheter.

Pharmacotherapy. Alpha-adrenergic antagonists such as **alfuzosin** have been shown to increase the likelihood of successful removal of the catheter after the first episode of a retention secondary to prostatic hypertrophy. The alpha-blocker should be started immediately following catheterization and at least two doses taken prior to trial without catheter.

If this fails, the options are either to replace the catheter and try again 2 weeks later, or advise an early transurethral resection. While awaiting operation, the patient can be safely discharged from hospital with an indwelling catheter fitted to an inconspicuous and easily concealed leg bag.

Permanent catheterization. A few patients are unwilling to undergo resection or are unfit for surgery. They can be shown how to pass a disposable urethral catheter on themselves to empty the bladder several times a day (**intermittent self-catheterization**, ISC). This requires motivation and manual dexterity and is not appropriate for all patients. It is particularly valuable, however, for the management of women with acute retention as well as those with neurological injury awaiting return of detrusor function. Simple plastic guides are available to assist women to find the urethral meatus.

CHRONIC RETENTION OF URINE

Chronic retention occurs in older patients and has an insidious course. Often, the patient will still be voiding but the residual volume will be high.

Investigation

Clinical diagnostic indicators

One of the commonest presenting features is **overflow urinary incontinence**. Pain is usually absent. Abdominal examination will usually reveal the presence of a **grossly distended bladder**.

Blood tests

Measurement of **serum creatinine** is vital as patients with chronic retention are at risk of renal failure secondary to obstructive uropathy, which occurs if the bladder is able to maintain high voiding pressures. It is known as *high-pressure chronic retention*. If there is total detrusor failure, *low-pressure chronic retention*, the upper tracts usually remain well preserved as there is no back pressure.

Urinalysis

Urine culture is important as these patients often harbour infection.

Imaging

A plain X-ray may reveal the presence of a bladder stone. Upper tract imaging by means of an **ultrasound scan** may demonstrate bilateral hydronephrosis, especially if there is renal failure.

Management

Catheterization of the bladder is the first step. The residual urine volume is high, often several litres. It is important to **monitor urine output** carefully as patients with obstructive uropathy may experience a post-obstructive diuresis once the obstruction is relieved, producing large volumes of dilute urine. This inability of the kidneys to concentrate urine is usually self-limiting and recovers, but the patient may require support with **intravenous fluid and electrolytes**.

If there is impaired renal function recovery may never be complete. Once a steady state has been reached the patient's condition should be reassessed. Chronic retention often occurs in very frail and elderly patients in whom an indwelling urethral catheter may be the only practical option.

In fit younger patients with high-pressure chronic retention, **transurethral resection** is effective. In patients with low-pressure chronic retention the chance of voiding following the operation is much lower because the bladder wall is weak. *The patient must be warned of this possibility.*

Pharmacotherapy with α-blockers or 5-α-reductase inhibitors is generally of no benefit in chronic retention.

BLADDER DIVERTICULUM

Congenital diverticula of the bladder usually arise in children and are more common in boys. They are rare.

Acquired diverticula of the bladder are a consequence of bladder outflow obstruction in elderly men. Years of chronically raised voiding detrusor pressure causes hypertrophy and trabeculation (massive bars) of the detrusor muscle so that a pouch of mucosa is forced out between bundles of muscle fibres.

Diverticula may be clinically significant if they are large or empty poorly. Under such circumstances they can harbour a large volume of residual urine, which is stagnant and becomes infected. Long-term consequences include recurrent symptomatic infections, bladder stone formation, incontinence (due to leakage of residual urine) or even development of malignancy within the diverticulum.

Investigation
Clinical diagnostic indicators
Most of these patients have a history of having had to strain to micturate for many years and have a palpable bladder.

Imaging
Diverticula may be seen on the **post-contrast IVU films** as out-pouchings of the bladder mucosa. The post-micturition film may demonstrate incomplete emptying of the diverticulum. A more detailed examination of the diverticula may be obtained by a **voiding cysto-urethrogram**. This involves intravesical instillation of contrast medium after which the patient is asked to void while being screened by fluoroscopy. This investigation provides accurate visualization of the lesion.

Endoscopy
Cystoscopy allows determination of the size, site, and careful inspection of the interior of the bladder and any diverticula.

Management
Most acquired diverticula are small and associated with bladder outflow obstruction. Treatment is thus directed at relieving this obstruction, usually by a **transurethral resection** or a **long-term catheter** in unfit patients. After the obstruction is relieved, most diverticula will empty satisfactorily. Diverticula that remain symptomatic following relief of the outflow obstruction may have to be excised.

Malignancy within a diverticulum is thankfully rare. It is difficult to manage as endoscopic measures are impossible because of the thin wall consisting of mucosa only. It is a dangerous situation as there is no barrier to the spread of the malignant change. Surgery is needed, usually **total cystectomy**.

CANCER OF THE PROSTATE

Prostate cancer is the most common malignancy in men in the UK, with approximately 20 000 new cases and 9000 cancer deaths each year. It is a disease of the older population and results in an important socioeconomic burden. Age is the most important risk factor but the incidence is much higher in Western countries, suggesting an environmental contribution to carcinogenesis.

Carcinoma of the prostate is an adenocarcinoma arising from the peripheral zone of the gland in 85 per cent of cases. It is graded by the Gleason system on a scale of 1 to 5 according to the degree of disruption of the glandular architecture. The grading is done twice, once on the majority pattern and again on a minority pattern that must represent at least 5 per cent of the tumour. The scores are added together, so the minimum is 2 and the highest 10.

The Gleason sum score correlates well with prognosis:

- 2–5 low-grade and best prognosis
- 6–7 intermediate-grade
- 8–10 high-grade and worst prognosis.

Prostate cancer is also staged by the TNM system with T1 and T2 tumours being confined to the prostate and T3 and T4 tumours becoming progressively locally advanced.

Investigation
Clinical diagnostic indicators
Early prostate cancer is symptomless but diagnosed more often nowadays because of PSA testing. Advanced prostate cancer produces symptoms of **urinary obstruction** caused by malignant enlargement of the gland, and **back pain** following pathological **spinal collapse** in the most common site for metastases – the vertebrae.

Digital rectal examination is neither sensitive nor specific enough for reliable detection of prostate cancer, and there is a great deal of observer variability. Characteristically, a malignant prostate feels hard and nodular with obliteration of the midline sulcus.

Blood tests

A **raised PSA** suggests malignancy, but there are other conditions that cause it to rise. It is not raised by digital examination but may be by ejaculation. Its lack of sensitivity and specificity means that **an elevated PSA must be followed with a biopsy** to confirm the malignancy. Many men now arrange unofficial PSA screening tests and this is now the commonest means of presentation of prostate cancer.

Imaging and tissue biopsy

Transrectal ultrasound-guided biopsy is performed by inserting a biopsy needle into the prostate via the rectum under the guidance of an ultrasound probe.

Under anaesthetic, multiple guided biopsies, at least six and often more, may be obtained by an expert radiologist from any suspicious hypoechogenic areas. Although there is a chance of sampling error, this technique is the most reliable method of diagnosing prostate cancer.

Staging investigations

Magnetic resonance imaging of the pelvis helps determine whether the disease is confined within the prostate or has spread beyond the capsule. Enlarged pelvic lymph nodes are also demonstrated clearly by MRI.

Bone scintigraphy using an intravenous radioisotope labelled compound (usually methylenediphosphonate) demonstrates bony metastases as 'hot spots' on the gamma camera images.

A plain X-ray may show bony metastases with a sclerotic appearance, although this appearance is not invariable.

Management

The management of prostate cancer is complex, evolving and gives rise to heated debate. Only the general principles are outlined here.

The main distinction to be made is between early, organ-confined prostate cancer and advanced metastatic disease. With the former cure is possible, whereas treatment of the latter is essentially palliative.

Early prostate cancer in fit and healthy men may be managed in a number of ways – active monitoring, radical prostatectomy and radical radiotherapy.

Active monitoring. Serial PSA measurement may be most appropriate for older men with low-grade tumours because these patients are usually symptomless and their chance of a prostate cancer-related death is low.

Radical surgery. Younger men or those with more aggressive tumours may opt for radical surgery to remove the prostate gland, or radiotherapy to the gland. **Radical prostatectomy** is a major procedure, performed abdominally by open or laparoscopic surgery. It results in excellent cure rates in early prostate cancer, but is associated with serious complications such as **impotence** and **incontinence**.

Radiotherapy. Radiation may be delivered by external-beam therapy or implantation of radioactive seeds (brachytherapy, see Chapter 2). Both give excellent rates of control of the disease.

Hormone therapy. Patients with locally advanced disease, or those with metastatic disease (N1+ or M1),cannot be cured. Treatment is by **suppression of endogenous testosterone**. Prostate cancer cells are exquisitely sensitive to the mitogenic effects of androgens and withdrawal of androgenic stimulation often leads to disease remission, with symptomatic improvement. Hormone ablation may be achieved by **surgical castration**, or alternatively by pharmacological means. Drugs which act on the hypothalamo-pituitary axis, such as **goserelin** and **leuprolide**, have become the mainstay of treatment for metastatic prostate cancer, and can be administered in convenient depot injections lasting for months at a time. Eventually, however, most prostate cancers relapse despite hormone ablation. This is referred to as androgen-independent or hormone-escape disease and invariably leads to death within a year. There is very limited effective intervention available at this stage, although **chemotherapy with docetaxel** has shown a modest survival benefit.

URETHRAL STRICTURE

The male urethra consists of the anterior penile and bulbar urethra along with the posterior membranous and prostatic urethra. Strictures may occur at any site, depending on the underlying disease process. The common causes of urethral strictures are:

- iatrogenic – e.g. urethral instrumentation
- traumatic – e.g. falling astride an object or from a pelvic fracture
- inflammatory – e.g. after gonococcal infection
- lichen sclerosus et atrophicus at the meatus.

Investigation

Clinical diagnostic indicators

The patient typically presents with a slow urinary stream and incomplete bladder emptying, occasionally with recurrent infections.

Urinalysis

Recurrent infection must be excluded.

Uroflowmetry

Uroflowmetry will usually reveal a slow flow with a characteristic 'plateau' due to the fixed obstruction created by the narrow urethra.

Retrograde micturating urethrocystography

Urethrography demonstrates the site and length of a suspected stricture. A Foley balloon catheter is placed just inside the tip of the penis and the balloon inflated with a small volume of water to occlude the distal urethra. Water-soluble contrast material is then injected through the catheter during X-ray imaging. Once the contrast has reached the bladder, the patient is asked to pass urine and further images are obtained of the posterior urethra and bladder neck area.

Management

Management depends on the site and length of the stricture. Traditionally, short strictures of the bulbar urethra are first managed by either urethral dilatation or optical urethrotomy.

Urethral dilatation involves the passage of a series of curved metal sounds of increasing calibre into the bladder. (They are called 'sounds' because they were used for centuries before X-rays were available to diagnose bladder stones. As the metal instrument struck a stone a clinking sound could be heard.) Adequate dilatation should be confirmed by subsequent **urethrocystoscopy**.

Optical urethrotomy is the use an endoscopically directed knife to cut open the area of fibrosis under direct vision.

These procedures are reasonably effective, resulting in a 50 per cent cure rate. The other half recur despite repeated procedures. The recurrence rate may be reduced by asking the patient to pass a catheter on themselves at set intervals to dilate the urethra (**intermittent self-dilatation**).

Anastomotic urethroplasty. In younger patients, the best chance of affecting a cure even for a short bulbar stricture is by open surgery. In **anastomotic urethroplasty** the strictured segment of urethra is excised and the two healthy cut ends anastomosed. Long-term cure rates of 85 per cent have been reported.

On-lay urethroplasty. Longer strictures and particularly strictures of the penile urethra unsuitable for excision and anastomosis are best managed by a primary surgical flap or graft procedure. The scarred narrow area is cut open along its long axis and a skin flap or free graft is sutured into the gap to provide a wide lumen. Buccal mucosa is one possible source of donor material. Such on-lay urethroplasties have a higher rate of failure than anastomotic procedures and may need revision many years after the primary procedure.

TRAUMA TO THE URETHRA

The urethra may be injured in various ways. Sexual intercourse may injure the penile urethra. Falling astride an object may injure the bulbar urethra if it is compressed against the inferior pubic arch. Pelvic fracture may result in rupture of the membranous urethra if the prostatic urethra, which is held against the pubic rami by the strong pubo-prostatic ligaments, is pulled away from the urogenital diaphragm.

Investigation

Clinical diagnostic indicators

Urethral injury presents with **inability to void**, **blood at the urethral meatus** and either or both **perineal and penile bruising**.

Haematoma and extravasated urine in bulbar urethral injuries is confined by the attachment of Colles' fascia, leading to perineal bruising in the 'butterfly pattern'. Rupture of the membranous urethra leads to an extraperitoneal collection of urine and blood which appears in the lower abdomen deep to Scarpa's fascia and does not extend into the thigh.

Rupture of the membranous urethra is supposed to be demonstrated on rectal examination by a boggy swelling and high-riding prostate. This is a difficult clinical sign to detect in a patient with multiple injuries.

The mechanism of injury and the clinical signs suggest the possibility of urethral injury.

Imaging

Diagnosis is made by an **ascending urethrogram**, as described above for urethral stricture (see page 515). With the patient in an oblique position, contrast is instilled into the urethra and images are taken of its whole length. A urethral injury is revealed by the extravasation of contrast. The disruption of the urethra may be complete or partial.

Management

The immediate management of urethral trauma is to **drain the bladder and bypass the injury**. With partial rupture, one gentle attempt may be made to pass a **urethral catheter**.

In all cases of total rupture, and in cases of partial rupture when urethral catheterization is found to be impossible, drainage should be accomplished by means of a **percutaneous suprapubic catheter**. This procedure may be difficult if there is a large pelvic haematoma and if the bladder is not distended. It is best performed under ultrasound guidance and may have to be done by open surgery.

There are differing views on the best subsequent management of urethral injury. Many advocate a repeat urethrogram 6 or 8 weeks after the injury to delineate the injury accurately, followed by elective surgical repair 3 months after the initial episode.

Injuries of the bulbar and membranous urethra are normally amenable to repair by **excision and anastomosis** of the scarred disrupted segment. Injuries of the penile urethra or any long segment are challenging and may require **reconstructive flaps or grafts** as described above for urethral stricture (see page 515).

21

The external genitalia

Benedict T. Sherwood and Christopher P. Chilton

Diseases of the external genitalia are frequently encountered by physicians working in almost all areas of clinical practice. The key to an accurate diagnosis of the cause of the presenting problem is a careful, systematic clinical examination, but a good understanding of the underlying pathological processes is also essential to guide correct investigation and treatment.

PROBLEMS CAUSED BY DISEASES AND ABNORMALITIES OF THE EXTERNAL GENITALIA

The common presenting problems caused by diseases and abnormalities of the external genitalia are:

- a non-retractable foreskin
- abnormal micturition
- erectile dysfunction
- ulcers and lumps on the penis
- swellings in the scrotal skin and within the scrotum
- pain in the scrotum
- an absent testicle.

A non-retractable foreskin

An inability to pull the prepuce back over the underlying glans penis is most often caused by a congenitally narrow opening at its end, a **phimosis**. This may be a congenital abnormality or be caused by inflammation (balanitis xerotica obliterans, BXO), recurrent balanoposthitis or malignant disease (carcinoma of the penis). Rarely it is caused by adhesions between the foreskin and the glans penis.

The history and examination usually reveal the cause of the problem.

If a congenital phimosis is very tight, the patient or their parents will complain of ballooning of the foreskin or spraying of the urinary stream during micturition.

Patients with a recurrent balanoposthitis will have a history of episodes of pain and discharge from beneath the foreskin.

Sexual function may be affected because of pain or splitting of the foreskin during an erection.

The severity of the phimosis can be detected on examination by attempting to retract the foreskin as far as possible. This also allows inspection of the glans penis and may reveal whitish areas of thickened, depigmented skin on the prepuce or glans penis – BXO (Fig 21.1).

When severe phimosis or adhesions prevent retraction, the glans penis should be carefully palpated through the prepuce for any swelling suggestive of a **carcinoma**. Enlarged or tender inguinal lymph nodes suggest the presence of cancer or infection.

A tight foreskin once retracted may present acutely as a **paraphimosis** (see below).

Abnormal micturition

The urethra usually ends on the tip of the glans penis but it may, if there is a defect in its intrauterine development, open anywhere on the ventral surface

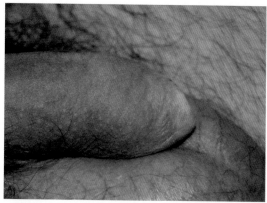

FIGURE 21.1 Balanitis xerotica obliterans (BXO) causing phimosis

of the penis – **hypospadias** – or sometimes on the dorsal surface of the glans penis – **epispadias**.

The patient is usually a neonate and the appearance of urine from an unusual site noticed by the infant's mother. The site is easy to see.

Erectile dysfunction

Patients may complain of an inability to obtain an erection – a form of **impotence** – curvature and pain in their penis when erect – **Peyronie's disease** – and of a persistent erection in the absence of sexual stimulation – **priapism**.

Ulcers or lumps on or in the penis

Possible causes of ulcers and lumps on the penis are:

- intraepithelial neoplasia
- carcinoma
- balanitis xerotica obliterans
- syphilitic chancre
- genital warts
- herpes simplex
- Peyronie's disease.

Most of these conditions can be identified from their history and physical signs.

It is vitally important to distinguish between benign and malignant or pre-malignant conditions. The duration of symptoms is an important clinical feature, together with the presence or absence of pain or urethral discharge. In cases of malignancy, weight loss and anorexia may indicate disseminated disease.

Patients should be asked about associated phimosis or problems with erection.

Some infective lesions will be acquired sexually, for example syphilis and herpes simplex, so a detailed sexual history must be taken.

Pre-malignant conditions, e.g. intraepithelial neoplasia, typically show a well-circumscribed erythematous patch on the glans or prepuce, often with a scaly or crusted surface.

Penile cancer which is unusual in younger men may present as a small papillary or ulcerated lesion, or a fungating mass. Both may be painless. The inguinal lymph nodes may be palpable.

A syphilitic chancre begins as an erythematous, papular lesion and then becomes a painless, infectious (and sometimes infected) non-bleeding ulcer.

The dorsal hard plaque in the corpus cavernosum of Peyronie's disease may be palpable.

Swellings in the scrotal skin and within the scrotum

The common causes of swellings in the scrotal skin and within the scrotum are:

- sebaceous cysts
- scrotal carcinoma
- hydrocele
- varicocele
- epididymal cysts
- tumours of the testis.

All the above can usually be diagnosed by a careful clinical examination. Few are accompanied by pain.

The skin of the scrotum is so mobile that it is usually obvious when a swelling is actually in the scrotal skin or deep to it.

Sebaceous cysts in the scrotal skin become painful when infected or are complicated by abscess formation.

Varicoceles may give rise to an aching discomfort, particularly after long periods of standing.

Epididymal cysts, uncomplicated hydroceles and most testicular tumours present as painless swellings but some testicular cancers are associated with acute pain and swelling.

Varicoceles and epididymal cysts may be palpably separate from the testes, whereas testicular cancers and hydroceles cannot be felt separately. Cystic swellings (hydroceles, large epididymal cysts) will transilluminate.

The ability to 'get above' the swelling, i.e. feel the spermatic cord above it, differentiates it from an inguinal hernia. (These clinical signs are covered in detail in *Symptoms and Signs*.)

Any skin changes should be noted.

An acutely painful, swollen, erythematous scrotum indicates a different underlying problem (see below).

Pain in the scrotum

The common causes of pain in the scrotum are:

- epididymo-orchitis
- torsion of the testis or a testicular appendix

- scrotal abscess
- Fournier's gangrene
- testicular tumour
- referred pain from renal colic.

Patients with acute scrotal pain must be assessed urgently. Where testicular torsion cannot be excluded on clinical assessment, the patient should be taken immediately to the operating theatre for exploration.

Pain caused by **torsion** is usually rapid in onset, whereas the pain from **infection** tends to build up slowly. It should be remembered that some testicular **cancers** can present with acute pain and swelling.

On examination, there may be obvious swelling and erythema of the scrotal skin.

The presence of crepitus or necrotic skin will alert the clinician to the possibility of **Fournier's gangrene.**

In testicular torsion the testis is classically riding high, lying transversely and exquisitely tender.

Torsion and epididymo-orchitis often need to be separated by urinalysis, culture of the urine, blood tests and ultrasound imaging to distinguish between torsion and infection.

Abscesses may be fluctuant with visible 'pointing'.

If the pain is referred from the renal tract there will be no scrotal signs.

An absent testicle

The diagnosis is obvious and invariably made by the patient. In the adult patient, a careful history must be taken to distinguish between a retractile testis, in which an active cremasteric reflex causes the testis to sometimes retract up into the inguinal canal, a true undescended testis (**cryptorchidism**) and an atrophic testis.

Although a testis may become impalpable if it atrophies following trauma or ischaemia (Table 21.1) its spermatic cord should still be palpable.

Examination will confirm the absence of the testicle from the scrotum and any associated under development of the scrotal sac. The inguinal canal, the base of the penis and the perineum should be examined carefully to look for an **ectopic testis**. General examination will detect any associated congenital defects.

Table 21.1
Classification of undescended testes

Retractile

Ectopic

Truly undescended

Absent/atrophic

DISEASES AND ABNORMALITIES AFFECTING THE MALE EXTERNAL GENITALIA

PHIMOSIS

Investigation
Clinical diagnostic indicators
The common causes of phimosis are described on page 517. The small opening in the prepuce is usually obvious on clinical examination. There may be a purulent discharge from it.

Microbiology
Swabs should be taken of any discharge for microbiological examination.

Tissue biopsy
Any suspicious lesion on the underlying glans penis should be biopsied. If a circumcision is performed a histological examination of the excised foreskin is essential to identify any inflammatory changes or any evidence of dysplasia or malignancy.

In adulthood, phimosis is often the result of poor penile hygiene leading to recurrent subpreputial infection and inflammation. **Balanitis xerotica obliterans** may be the underlying pathology (Fig 21.1).

Phimosis may occasionally conceal the presence of a squamous cell carcinoma of the penis.

Management
Any active infection should be treated with the appropriate antibiotics.

Circumcision (removal of the foreskin) should be recommended for adults. In children, circumcision should be reserved for those with recurrent

Table 21.2
Indications for adult circumcision

Phimosis

Recurrent paraphimosis

Malignancy

Uncertain pathology

(Cultural or religious demand)

Table 21.3
Types of hypospadias

Glandular: opening on proximal glans

Coronal: at the coronal sulcus

Penile shaft

Penoscrotal

Perineal

balanitis. The indications for adult circumcision are given in Table 21.2.

Preoperatively, patients should be warned of the risks of bleeding, wound infection and altered penile sensation. Fitness for anaesthesia should be considered carefully when there is significant co-morbidity. If necessary, the procedure may be carried out under local or regional anaesthesia. Once the foreskin is retracted or removed, the glans must be inspected carefully. Any areas on the penis suspicious of malignant or *in situ* disease should be biopsied and the foreskin sent for histological examination.

PARAPHIMOSIS

In this condition the foreskin becomes held in the retracted position, behind the corona, where it becomes a constricting band and causes considerable pain and swelling. Untreated paraphimosis can lead to ischaemia of the glans penis and the skin beneath the constricting ring and ultimately cause tissue necrosis. The condition usually occurs when the foreskin is not replaced by the patient after intercourse or a careless clinician after performing a urethral catheterization.

There will often have been some degree of pre-existing phimosis, but the patient may not have been aware of this and consider his foreskin to be normal.

Management

Prompt recognition and **reduction** is vital to prevent complications. Topical anaesthetic jelly should be applied or a penile nerve or ring block employed. The glans penis and retracted foreskin should be compressed manually by the surgeon for a number of minutes, to reduce the oedematous swelling. Time and patience are required before attempting the reduction, which is usually successfully achieved, to the great relief of the patient.

Very rarely, it is necessary to divide the constricting ring of the prepuce. This is done on its dorsal aspect (**a dorsal slit**).

The patient may be offered an **interval circumcision** after a manual reduction to prevent recurrence of this unpleasant condition.

HYPOSPADIAS

Hypospadias is a congenital anomaly in which the urethral meatus opens on the ventral surface of the penis as a result of incomplete closure of the urethral folds during foetal development. It is found in approximately 3 in 1000 live births. The severity of the condition depends on the distance of the urethral meatus from the tip of the glans. The different forms of hypospadias are classified in Table 21.3. More extreme cases of hypospadias may represent abnormal sexual differentiation.

Investigation
Clinical diagnostic indicators

In the younger patient and in cases where the meatus is close to the anatomically correct position, the condition may not be noticed.

There may be spraying or dribbling of the urinary stream. Patients with **penoscrotal** or **perineal hypospadias** have to micturate in the sitting position.

Where there is significant **chordee** there may be difficulty with sexual intercourse and these patients sometimes present complaining of infertility.

The diagnosis is made by a careful clinical examination.

Chromosome karyotyping

A **buccal smear** for chromosome karyotyping is mandatory in severe cases to confirm the sex of the child.

Imaging

Further investigation with **cystourethroscopy**, **excretory urography** (**IVU**) and **cross-sectional imaging** (**CT** or **MRI**) may be required if associated urinary tract abnormalities are suspected.

Management

Mild cases of glandular hypospadias require no treatment.

Surgical repair is indicated where there is severe deformity, voiding difficulty or predicted impairment of sexual function. To minimize psychological morbidity, surgery is best performed at between 6 and 12 months of age, when the patient will not remember it.

A variety of corrective procedures have been described for each form of hypospadias. Extra urethral length may be created by mobilizing skin flaps from adjacent tissues such as the penile shaft or foreskin, or by using free on-lay grafts, for example of buccal mucosa. The new urethral tissue is then made into a tube and the meatus thereby restored to the correct anatomical position. Such repairs are sometimes complicated by fistula formation requiring revision surgery.

Patients with hypospadias should never be circumcised as the foreskin may provide useful grafting material.

CHORDEE

Chordee (a ventral curvature of the penis) can occur with or without associated hypospadias. It is thought to result from the shortened urethra and fibrosis in the tissues surrounding the corpus spongiosum. A redundant foreskin is found on examination, with deficient skin ventrally.

Management

Correction of a chordee (**orthoplasty**) may be part of surgery for hypospadias. In minor cases, simple degloving and reattachment of the penile skin is effective. Otherwise, plication sutures on the dorsal surface of the penis or excision and grafting of the fibrosed urethra may be required.

EPISPADIAS

Epispadias is very rare, 1 in 12 000 live births. The ectopic urethral opening is on the dorsal aspect of the penis. It may lie as far back as the junction of the penis with the pubic bone (complete epispadias), when it can be associated with **bladder extrophy** (failure of closure of the infra-umbilical midline structures, with exteriorization of the open bladder).

Less severe cases (**penile or glandular epispadias**) are less common than the complete variety. If the defect is proximal to the sphincters, there will be urinary incontinence.

Investigation

The diagnosis is apparent on careful clinical examination and should be made at the first neonatal examination.

The diagnosis may be suspected *in utero* during a routine ultrasound scan if there is bladder extrophy.

Management

Complex **reconstructive surgery** is the only effective treatment. The aim is to produce a functional, cosmetically acceptable penis with continence of urine. Many techniques are described.

When the extrophy is too extensive for reconstruction of the bladder, patients may be best served by urinary diversion, usually into an ileal conduit (see Chapter 20).

BALANITIS

Balanitis is inflammation of the prepuce. Where the glans penis is also inflamed the term **balanoposthitis** should be used. Poor local hygiene is the major cause of this condition. Where inflammation is recurrent or chronic the foreskin may adhere to the glans, or phimosis may develop. There may even be stenosis of the urethral meatus with urinary obstruction.

Balanitis xerotica obliterans is the penile manifestation of *lichen sclerosis* and is a specific form of chronic, probably autoimmune, inflammation. It is characterized by whitish plaques and does not present as acute inflammation.

Investigation

Clinical diagnostic indicators

Pain, discharge and preputial oedema are the dominant physical signs. There may be evidence of inadequate body care and poor hygiene.

Microbiology

Swabs should be taken for microbiological examination, culture and antibiotic sensitivity.

Tissue biopsy

If the presence of a malignant process is suspected a tissue biopsy must be obtained.

Management

Antibiotic therapy should be commenced if there is active infection. Advise the patient to retract the foreskin daily and to wash the glans penis and the preputial cavity thoroughly.

Circumcision is required to prevent relapse if there is phimosis.

SYPHILIS

Syphilis is an infection caused by the microaerophilic spirochaete *Treponema pallidum*. Transmission is usually by sexual intercourse with an infected partner. In the primary phase of the disease (usually within 3 weeks of contact with an infected individual), a **syphilitic chancre** develops on either the penis or scrotum.

Investigation

Clinical diagnostic indicators

A **chancre** appears as an erythematous, papular lesion that becomes a painless, infectious, non-bleeding ulcer. It may develop anywhere on the penis or scrotum, usually within 3 weeks of sexual contact with an infected partner. Spontaneous healing usually occurs after a few weeks. The systemic symptoms of secondary syphilis develop later.

The syphilitic chancre can easily be confused with the multiple, painful vesicular lesions on the glans, prepuce or shaft of the penis caused by the **herpes simplex virus**, which typically appear 3–14 days after exposure.

Serology

The diagnosis is confirmed by serological assay with the *Treponema pallidum* inhibition test or the VDRL test.

Tissue biopsy

A biopsy of the ulcer may be needed to differentiate the lesion from a squamous cell carcinoma.

Management

Penicillin remains the mainstay of antimicrobial chemotherapy.

Instruct the patient to avoid contaminating others.

CANCER OF THE PENIS

Penile cancer is an uncommon squamous cell carcinoma accounting for less than 1 per cent of all male cancers and arising most commonly in the sixth decade of life. **Poor local hygiene** with retention of smegma is the most important aetiological factor. The disease is extremely rare in men who have been circumcised in early childhood.

Infection with human papilloma virus is also implicated.

Sometimes, invasive cancer is preceded by a premalignant lesion such as **erythroplasia of Queyrat** or **Bowen's disease**, known collectively as **penile intraepithelial neoplasia**.

Premalignant lesions typically appear as a well-circumscribed erythematous patch on the glans penis or prepuce, often with a scaly or crusted surface.

Investigation

Clinical diagnostic indicators

Penile cancer is unusual in younger men. Most patients are in their sixth decade or older. Cancer of the penis usually affects the glans penis or prepuce and there is often an associated phimosis.

It may present as a small **papillary or ulcerated lesion or a fungating mass** (see *Symptoms and Signs*). It is usually painless. The lack of pain and fear of the diagnosis often delay patients from presenting to the doctor until the tumour has ulcerated, become fungating and spread. The inguinal lymph nodes must be palpated to look for evidence of metastatic spread.

Microbiology

Swabs should be taken for microscopy and culture if an associated bacterial infection is suspected.

Similarly if syphilis is suspected, the diagnosis should be made or excluded by serological assay (see page 522).

Blood tests

In advanced malignancy, **anaemia** may be present if the disease has metastasized. Liver or bone metastases may cause biochemical abnormalities.

Imaging

Once the diagnosis is made, **staging investigations** are required, usually **chest X-ray, CT scan and bone scintigraphy**. MRI is of value in defining the extent of local invasion prior to surgery.

Tissue biopsy

A biopsy is diagnostic. Circumcision may be needed to expose the tumour. If the prepuce is the primary site, a circumcision may give both the diagnosis and provide definitive primary treatment.

Cytology

Palpable enlargement of the inguinal lymph nodes may be caused by infection rather than metastatic spread. **Fine needle aspiration cytology** will usually give the diagnosis. If clinically suspicious nodes persist despite cytology, suggesting reactive changes only, and treatment of infection, **sentinel node biopsy** may help to diagnose nodal involvement and subsequent block dissection of the nodes. The principles of this technique are discussed in Chapter 15.

Management

Treatment depends on the stage of the disease.

Surgical excision is the most effective treatment of the primary tumour. The aim is to excise the primary carcinoma with an adequate margin of normal tissue. If there are palpable inguinal lymph nodes with cytologically confirmed metastatic tumour, an **inguinal node block dissection** should be carried out at the same time.

Excision with preservation of the penis may be possible when the primary tumour is at an early stage (Tis, Ta, possibly T1) using techniques such as:

- **micrographic surgery** (progressive slicing of the area around the lesion with immediate histological examination until clearance is achieved)
- **laser obliteration**
- **excision of the glans alone**.

For more advanced disease more major procedures are required.

- **Partial excision of the penis**. The distal corpora are excised and a penile stump is preserved.
- **Radical penectomy** is amputation of the entire penis with the creation of a **perineal urethrostomy**.

External beam **radiotherapy** is used selectively in diseases of lower stage and is able to preserve penile function in many cases.

In cases of inoperable disease, **chemotherapy** and/or **radiotherapy** may provide some degree of palliation.

PRIAPISM

Priapism is a persistent painful erection of the penis in the absence of sexual stimulation. The condition affects only the corpora cavernosa, so the glans penis remains soft.

Low-flow priapism is more likely to result in thrombosis of the corpora cavernosa and subsequent ischaemia, scarring and permanent loss of function. The causes are listed in Table 21.4, although a third of cases are idiopathic.

Table 21.4
Types and causes of priapism

Low-flow priapism	High-flow priapism
Sickle cell disease	Traumatic arteriovenous fistula
Drug therapy: antipsychotics, sildenafil, papaverine injections	
Leukaemia	
Malignant infiltration of corpora by bladder or other cancer	
Neurogenic: spinal cord injury or autonomic neuropathy	

High-flow priapism is caused by an arterio-venous fistula that develops after a perineal injury.

Investigation

Clinical examination will reveal the problem; the investigations are directed towards identifying the cause.

Blood tests

Blood tests will detect the presence of **sickle-cell disease** or **leukaemia**.

Blood gas analysis of a sample of blood taken from the corpora cavernosa may help to differentiate between low- and high-flow priapism.

Imaging

Colour Doppler ultrasound scanning may also help differentiate between the low- and high-flow varieties.

Arteriography may be needed to identify the site of an arteriovenous fistula.

Management

Although many cases of priapism resolve spontaneously, the condition must be treated as an emergency.

Low-flow priapism is managed initially by **aspiration of blood from the corpora** using a butterfly needle. If this is unsuccessful, **phenylephrine**, a sympathetic alpha-blocker, may be **injected into the cavernosa** until the priapism resolves. Careful monitoring is required as phenylephrine has significant cardiovascular side-effects.

If simple measures fail, the distended corpora cavernosa must be decompressed permanently, generally into the corpus spongiosum or glans (which are not affected) by:

- **Percutaneous puncture of the fibrous capsule** using a core biopsy needle to establish a connection between the glans penis and one or both corpora cavernosa.
- Open perineal surgery to fashion an anastomosis between the corpus spongiosum and the corpus cavernosa (**spongiocavernostomy**).
- Open anastomosis of the corpora cavernosa to the divided long saphenous vein (**saphenocavernostomy**). This approach is rarely used.

Any underlying haematological cause should be treated appropriately.

High-flow priapism requires arteriography to locate the site of the fistula, followed by definitive treatment, i.e. embolization of the internal pudendal artery or the branch that is supplying the fistula.

PEYRONIE'S DISEASE

Peyronie's disease consists of a fibrous plaque in the tunica albuginea of unknown origin, which makes erections painful and deforms the erect penis.

It is occasionally associated with Dupuytren's contracture in the hands.

In the early stage of the disease patients complain of painful erection, and biopsy shows vasculitis. As the inflammation resolves pain ceases but the plaque contracts and produces deviation of the erect penis towards the affected side. Plaques are most common anteriorly. Sexual intercourse may be awkward or painful.

Investigation

Clinical diagnostic indicators

The diagnosis is largely clinical. The skin moves freely over the hard dorsal plaque palpable in the corpus cavernosum. A digital photograph taken by the patient can provide objective evidence of the deformity of the erect penis.

Tissue biopsy

Biopsy is occasionally required to exclude other causes of a lump in the body of the penis.

The plaque of Peyronie's disease shows vasculitis and fibrosis.

No other special investigations are necessary.

Management

When the deformity is minimal most cases improve spontaneously, so **conservative management** is appropriate. Medical therapies such as vitamin E or tamoxifen have no proven benefit.

Surgery Those few patients with significant persistent deformity may be offered surgical correction, deferred until the disease enters the stable phase with no pain or progression of the deformity. This usually takes a year or more.

Several procedures have been described; **Nesbit's operation** is the most commonly performed. The skin of the penis is incised in a circle and retracted (degloving) to expose the plaque. An ellipse of tunica albuginea is excised on the side of the penis opposite to the plaque. The resulting elliptical defect is then closed to correct the deformity, in effect shortening the normal side. Erection is then induced using a tourniquet around the base of the penis and saline injections, to confirm adequate correction, before replacing the penile skin and completing the operation.

There may be some minor shortening of the erect penis, the likelihood of which should be explained to the patient before the procedure.

Patients with concomitant erectile dysfunction that is refractory to medical therapy may need to be treated with the insertion of malleable **penile rods** or an **inflatable prosthesis** when the deformity is corrected.

SCROTAL SEBACEOUS CYSTS

Sebaceous cysts develop frequently in the hair-bearing skin of the scrotum or the proximal shaft of the penis. Excision of these benign lesions is frequently performed either to prevent infection of the cyst, which may lead to abscess formation, or because the patient finds the swelling awkward or unsightly.

CARCINOMA OF THE SCROTAL SKIN

Carcinoma of the scrotum, which was once commonly caused by chronic exposure of the scrotum to soot, tar or oil, is now a rare malignancy.

Investigation
Clinical diagnostic indicators

Carcinoma of the scrotum usually begins as a painless unremarkable lump in the scrotal skin, but once it ulcerates it develops the **typical everted edge of a malignant ulcer** (see *Symptoms and Signs*).

The inguinal lymph nodes may be enlarged by secondary infection or metastatic spread.

Tissue biopsy

The diagnosis is made on the histological analysis of the excised lesion or a biopsy of it.

Management

Treatment is adequate **surgical excision**. The inguinal nodes should be treated in the same way as penile carcinoma (see above).

Adjuvant chemotherapy may be given if there is metastatic disease.

FOURNIER'S GANGRENE

Fournier's gangrene is a rapidly progressing **necrotizing fasciitis** (synergistic gangrene, see Chapter 3) of the scrotum and is a life-threatening surgical emergency with a poor prognosis. The pathogens are multiple and usually include both aerobic and anaerobic organisms, for example enteric Gram-negative organisms, Gram-positive streptococci or staphylococci and anaerobes.

The condition is more common in the diabetic or immunocompromised patient.

Investigation
Clinical diagnostic indicators

Early clinical diagnosis is vital. There are signs of acute inflammation with erythema, swelling and increased skin temperature. The presence of gas-forming bacteria is indicated if subcutaneous crepitus is found on gentle palpation. One or more black areas of skin necrosis will become evident. The patient is always extremely unwell with systemic signs of infection.

Imaging

A plain X-ray may demonstrate gas in the subcutaneous tissue (see Fig 3.2).

Management

Intravenous antimicrobial therapy must be given coupled with **immediate aggressive surgical excision of all involved tissue** – skin and subcutaneous tissue but rarely muscle (see Chapter 3).

An examination under anaesthetic with further excision as necessary should be performed every 24 hours until it is certain that all the necrotic tissue has been removed.

This inevitably leaves a large open wound. Although the scrotal skin has a remarkable ability to regenerate, **skin grafting** is sometimes necessary.

THE UNDESCENDED TESTIS

In 1 per cent of male infants a testicle fails to descend. Often the testis on the affected side is abnormal. Rarely, absence of the testicles is due to an endocrine or chromosomal abnormality. The risk of cancer is much higher in undescended testis. Fertility may be reduced and there is a higher risk of torsion. Clinical features are discussed in detail in *Symptoms and Signs*.

Investigation

Clinical diagnostic indicators

In addition to the obvious absence of the testis from the scrotum, the scrotum is usually undeveloped on the affected side. This does not occur with a retractile testis.

Differentiation between a **retractile testis**, which does not need surgical treatment, and the **truly undescended or ectopic testis**, which does, is usually made by clinical assessment alone.

Blood tests

If neither testis is present, **chromosome analysis** should be carried out to exclude a disorder of sexual differentiation. A **hormone profile** can be helpful in, for example, anorchia, where there will be high levels of leuteinizing hormone (LH) and follicle-stimulating hormone (FSH) but low testosterone.

Imaging

Ultrasound scanning is of little use in small children but may locate a missed abdominal testis in an adolescent or adult. **MRI scanning** may be useful in the rare patient with an intersex abnormality.

Laparoscopy

Laparoscopy is indicated when the testis cannot be palpated or located by ultrasound scanning. It may show that:

- the testis or testes are lying in the posterior abdominal wall
- the testis is congenitally absent (rare) with no vas or vessels entering the internal inguinal ring
- there is/are normal vas deferens and vessels entering the internal ring. In this event the testis is in the inguinal canal or has been destroyed by torsion.

Management

There is no place for hormone therapy, e.g. giving human chorionic gonadotrophin (HCG), as it is ineffective.

If the testis is truly undescended or ectopic, **surgery** should be performed as early as possible, as **there is evidence that future testicular function deteriorates with delay**. The safest time is between 6 and 12 months after birth.

An **orchidopexy** is performed **if the testicle is palpable**. The groin is explored, the testis and spermatic cord mobilized, the commonly associated indirect inguinal hernia sac separated and tied, and the testicle placed in the scrotum. The surgeon has to balance the benefit of extensive dissection to free a greater length of the cord and allow the testis to be placed in the scrotum more readily, against the risk of the dissection damaging the delicate testicular vessels with subsequent testicular atrophy. *It is essential to warn the parents of this possibility.*

Preliminary laparoscopy should be performed **if the testicle is impalpable**. If vas deferens and the testicular vessels are seen to be entering the inguinal canal, the groin is explored and either an orchidopexy or excision of an atrophic testicle is performed.

Management is difficult **if the testis is in the abdomen**. If the other testis is present in the scrotum the best option is probably to remove the abdominal testis. If both are in the abdomen, a bilateral staged mobilization may be attempted with additional manoeuvres such as sacrifice of the vas deferens to lengthen the cord.

The testicles may even be autotransplanted into the scrotum. These procedures leave little hope of fertility but there may be some endocrine function.

HYDROCELE

Hydrocele is a common condition in which there is a collection of fluid around the testis within the tunica vaginalis. The infantile hydrocele is a patent processus vaginalis and is in fact an indirect inguinal hernia (see *Symptoms and Signs*) and is treated as such.

Nearly all adult hydroceles are idiopathic and arise from an imbalance in the rate of production and resorption of fluid by the tunica vaginalis. Rarely, hydroceles are secondary to other conditions, usually trauma, infection, neoplasm or lymphatic obstruction.

Investigation

Clinical diagnostic indicators

The diagnosis may be made confidently on clinical grounds. Specifically, the hydrocele appears as a scrotal swelling which the examiner can 'get above'. The **testis cannot be palpated separately** within a hydrocele unless the fluid tension is low, something that may occur with a secondary hydrocele. Hydroceles transilluminate well, unless they are chronic and have developed a thick wall.

The condition never resolves spontaneously.

Microbiology

Any aspirated fluid should be cultured.

Blood tests

In cases secondary to advanced testicular cancer there may be **anaemia** or **abnormal liver function**.

Enlarged retroperitoneal lymph nodes may press on the ureters, leading to obstruction and renal impairment. Serological markers used in the diagnosis and staging of testicular tumours are discussed below.

Imaging

Ultrasound scanning of the scrotum is rapid, non-invasive and relatively inexpensive and consequently is used frequently in the diagnosis of scrotal masses. Benign fluid containing lesions such as hydroceles, epididymal cysts and varicoceles give characteristic appearances and testicular tumours are seen as solid lesions with a poor or heterogeneous echo pattern (Fig 21.2).

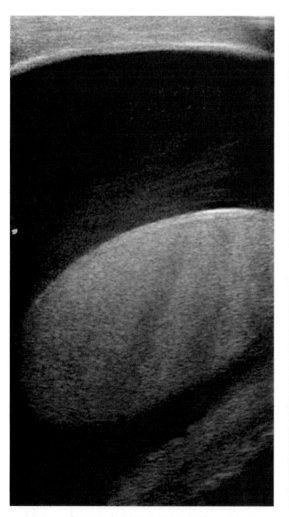

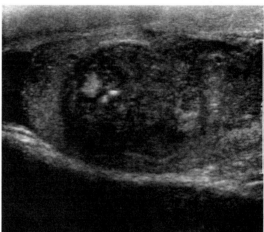

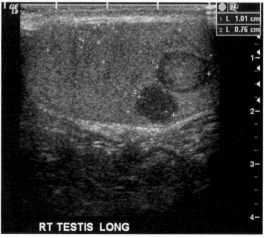

FIGURE 21.2 A panel of ultrasound images of scrotal masses

Management

Often, the patient only needs to be reassured that the condition is harmless. Treatment is offered when there is discomfort, the swelling is large and shows through the trousers, or the appearance is unacceptable.

Aspiration of fluid rarely gives long-term relief as the hydrocele quickly reaccumulates and there is risk of infection – the protein rich fluid in a hydrocele is an excellent bacterial culture medium.

Aspiration followed by the injection of a sclerosant material with the intention of obliterating the cavity has been tried, but has many complications and is best avoided.

Surgery is curative. The tunica is opened through a scrotal incision and the straw-coloured fluid evacuated. In the **Jaboulay operation** the tunica is turned inside out and sutured behind the testis. An alternative is **Lord's procedure**, where the sac is gathered up around the testis with a series of plicating sutures. In both the tunical vaginalis is not excised, but fluid secreted by it is presumably absorbed by scrotal lymphatics.

If the tunica vaginalis is thick and bulky, excision gives the best result.

Scrotal surgery may be complicated by postoperative swelling, infection and haematoma formation.

It is wise to give a single prophylactic perioperative dose of a broad-spectrum antibiotic.

EPIDIDYMAL CYST/SPERMATOCELE

Epididymal cysts are harmless scrotal swellings that transilluminate well. On palpation they are above and separate from the testis. **Ultrasound scanning** may assist in diagnosis.

Spermatoceles are retention cysts arising from the efferent ductules of the epididymis and contain cloudy fluid.

Management

Cysts that become large enough to be uncomfortable or unsightly may be **excised** surgically (Fig 21.3). This may require excision of some or all of the epididymis, and the patient should be warned that this is the equivalent of a unilateral vasectomy.

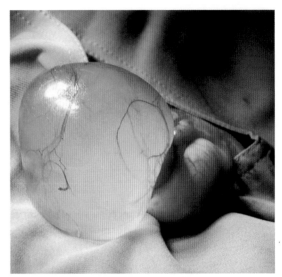

FIGURE 21.3   An epididymal cyst prior to excision

VARICOCELE

A varicocele is an abnormal tortuous dilated collection of the veins in the pampiniform plexus of the spermatic cord. It is possible that its presence impairs sperm production in the testis it drains.

Investigation

Clinical diagnostic indicators

Varicoceles are usually **symptomless** but may give rise to **aching discomfort** after long periods of standing.

The classical description is of a scrotal swelling that on palpation resembles a 'bag of worms', which can only be felt by careful palpation when the patient is standing. Most occur on the left side because the left testicular vein is longer that the right and drains into the left renal vein rather than directly into the inferior vena cava. The valves in the longer left vein are more likely to fail.

Rarely, a left varicocele is caused by a left-sided **renal tumour** occluding the left testicular vein.

Imaging

Scrotal **ultrasound scanning** and **colour Doppler blood flow** will confirm the diagnosis if necessary. **An ultrasound scan of the left kidney** is a wise precaution if the varicocele is on the left and has developed quickly.

Management

Surgical treatment is reserved for symptomatic varicoceles, although it is sometimes carried out with the small hope of improving a low sperm count.

The testicular vein must be interrupted above the varicocele. This may be done by **open ligation** through an inguinal or supra-inguinal incision, but an alternative approach is to **clip the vein**(s) where they lie on the posterior abdominal wall laparoscopically.

Embolization of the abnormal veins by retrograde phlebography is an alternative form of treatment that is preferred by some.

The condition tends to recur after all forms of treatment, as collateral veins quickly develop.

TORSION OF THE TESTIS

Torsion of the testis is a twisting of the testis around the vertical axis resulting in venous occlusion and then arterial occlusion with ischaemia and necrosis. There is a predisposing underlying congenital variation, known as the **bell-clapper deformity**, in which the testis and epididymis are unusually mobile within the tunica vaginalis (see *Symptoms and Signs*).

Patients with acute scrotal pain must be assessed urgently. Where testicular torsion cannot be excluded on clinical assessment, the patient should be taken immediately to the operating theatre for exploration.

Investigation

Clinical diagnostic indicators

Testicular torsion is a surgical emergency, requiring immediate recognition and intervention to prevent loss of the affected testis. The typical presentation is that of a young man with **rapid onset of excruciating hemiscrotal pain and swelling**, often with preceding poorly localized abdominal or loin pain, in contrast to the pain caused by infection, which tends to build up slowly.

It should be remembered that *some testicular cancers can present with acute pain and swelling*. Examination reveals swelling and exquisite tenderness, with the testis lying transversely and abnormally high in the scrotum.

There may be obvious swelling and erythema of the scrotal skin.

The appendices of the testis may also twist and present as an acutely swollen, painful scrotum, but the testis itself will lie in the correct position and orientation with the twisted appendage palpable as a tender nodule.

Urinalysis

The urine should be dipstick tested for the presence of **blood, nitrites or protein** to exclude epididymo-orchitis caused by an ascending urinary or sexually acquired infection.

Imaging

An **ultrasound scan**, particularly in combination with **Doppler flow studies**, can be useful in the assessment of acute scrotal pain. When there is torsion of the testis no blood flow will be seen on Doppler imaging. *However, never forget that if torsion is suspected there should be no delay waiting for investigation and the patient should go straight to the operating theatre.*

Blood flow may be abnormally high in epididymo-orchitis (hyperaemia).

Management

When torsion of the testis cannot be excluded on clinical examination, the patient *must* be taken directly to theatre for immediate **scrotal exploration**. There is no time for laboratory or radiological investigations, which may delay intervention and result in the testis failing to survive. The torted testicle is untwisted and fixed, unless it is clearly dead in which event it should be removed.

As the underlying anatomical variation is always bilateral, **the other side must always be fixed**.

Torsion of an appendage may be treated conservatively if the clinical diagnosis is certain or confirmed by ultrasound scanning. Spontaneous resolution is usual.

If there is any uncertainty about the diagnosis, the scrotum must be explored and the appendage removed.

EPIDIDYMITIS AND EPIDIDYMO-ORCHITIS

Infection or inflammation of the epididymis (epididymitis) or epididymis and testis (epididymo-orchitis) is a common problem. Bacteria gain access to the genitourinary tract either as a sexually transmitted infection (*Neisseria gonorrhoeae* or *Chlamydia trachomatis*) or from the lower urinary tract along the vas deferens, when *Escherischia coli* is a common infective organism. It is essential to take a detailed sexual history.

Occasionally orchitis can be caused by the **mumps virus** or may occur as part of a systemic infection such as **tuberculosis**.

Investigation

Clinical diagnostic indicators

The patient complains of severe pain and swelling in the affected side of the scrotum. Occasionally, the condition is bilateral. There may be dysuria and systemic symptoms of infection. Examination confirms a **red, swollen, hot, tender scrotum**.

Urinalysis

Urinalysis is often positive for blood, leucocytes or nitrites, indicating **infection**.

Bacteriology

An **MSU** for culture and sensitivity should be sent before starting antibiotics. Where a sexually acquired infection is suspected, **urethral swabs** should be taken.

Blood tests

A full blood count may reveal a **leucocytosis**.

Imaging

A scrotal **ultrasound scan** with **Doppler flow measurement** that shows the characteristic findings of a swollen, hypervascular testis or epididymis will confirm the diagnosis. An ultrasound study will also exclude other significant underlying pathology such as a testicular tumour. Abscesses are seen readily on ultrasound, if not diagnosed clinically.

Urinary tract studies

If the cause of the epididymo-orchitis is an ascending urinary infection, the lower urinary tract should be studied with measurements of urinary flow rate and post-micturition bladder volume, ultrasound of the urinary tract or cystoscopy once the acute episode has subsided.

Management

An **appropriate antibiotic** with a drug that penetrates into the epididymis such as **ciprofloxacin** is the first-line treatment.

Sexually transmitted infections require treatment with **doxycycline**. The patient's sexual partner(s) will also need treatment and sexual health advice.

Analgesia Epididymo-orchitis causes severe pain that is exacerbated by movement and relieved by rest. Although lying in a warm bath may relieve the pain best, these patients often need opiate analgesics.

MALIGNANT TUMOURS OF THE TESTIS

Testicular cancer is an uncommon malignancy accounting for 1–2 per cent of all male cancers with a peak age of incidence at 20–40 years. The disease is slightly more common on the right side and may occasionally be bilateral.

Nearly all are germ cell tumours, of which seminoma is the most common (35 per cent). Seminoma was formally classified as a carcinoma of the seminiferous tubules and is described as such in *Symptoms and Signs*.

The other (non-seminomatous) germ cell tumours include embryonal cell carcinoma, teratoma, choriocarcinoma and yolk sac tumours. Many tumours are of mixed cell type.

The only significant risk factor is testicular maldescent or cryptorchidism.

Testicular tumours may be staged using the TNM classification or into four simple levels:

- Stage 1 tumour confined to the testicle
- Stage 2 involvement of pelvic or other intra-abdominal lymph nodes
- Stage 3 lymph node involvement above the diaphragm
- Stage 4 metastases in other organs such as the lungs.

Investigation

Clinical diagnostic indicators

Patients usually present after noticing a **lump in the scrotum**. On palpation this is usually hard, heavy, non-tender and inseparable from the testis itself.

Alternatively, there may be more diffuse enlargement of the testis or associated tenderness, leading to a misdiagnosis of infection. A small proportion of patients will present with symptoms of metastatic disease.

Blood tests

In advanced disease there may be **anaemia or abnormal liver function** caused by metastases. Enlarged retroperitoneal lymph nodes may press on the ureters leading to obstruction and renal impairment.

Serum tumour markers

Three biochemical serum markers are of great importance in the diagnosis and management of testicular cancer (Table 21.5).

- **Alpha-fetoprotein** (AFP), which is produced specifically by the trophoblastic cells of embryonal carcinomas and yolk sac tumours, may be high in non-seminomatous germ cell tumours apart from pure choriocarcinoma but never in pure seminoma.
- **Human chorionic gonadotropin** (HCG) is elevated in all cases of choriocarcinoma, many embryonal carcinomas and a small proportion of pure seminomas.
- **Lactate dehydrogenase** (LDH) is a cellular enzyme. Levels are raised in metastatic disease, particularly with non-seminomatous germ cell tumours.

It should be noted that the levels of these markers will be normal in many cases of testicular cancer and so **normal values do not exclude the diagnosis**.

It is vitally important that these markers are measured preoperatively as they provide valuable staging information and allow monitoring of response to treatment.

Imaging

Testicular tumours have a characteristic appearance on **ultrasound scanning** (see Fig 21.2).

Chest X-ray and **CT scanning** are used as staging investigations to assess the abdominal lymph nodes and to look for pulmonary metastases.

Management

Radical orchidectomy is the primary treatment.

The inguinal canal is opened through a groin incision and the spermatic cord isolated and occluded with a soft clamp at the internal inguinal ring, to prevent intravenous dissemination of tumour cells due to manipulation. The testis is then delivered from the scrotum and inspected to confirm the presence of a tumour. The cord is then divided at the internal ring, so that the testis, all the cord structures and all the cord covering layers can be removed.

A direct biopsy of the testis through the overlying scrotal skin and the covering layers of the testis *is never done* because of the risk of seeding cancer cells into the wound.

Retroperitoneal lymph node dissection has an uncertain role. It is now mostly used to remove residual tumour after chemotherapy.

Radiotherapy Seminomas are very radiosensitive. Prophylactic radiotherapy to the pelvic and para-aortic lymph nodes is now routine for patients with a seminoma and no evidence of disseminated disease.

Chemotherapy Non-seminomatous tumours respond well to chemotherapy. A commonly employed combination is BEP (**bleomycin, etoposide** and **cisplatin**). It is effective even when there are widespread metastases and is also given as adjunctive treatment to those with Stage 1 disease.

Chemotherapy is also effective for seminoma patients with metastatic disease, and may be used as adjunctive treatment for those with Stage 1 tumours, commonly employing carboplatin.

Table 21.5
Tumour markers in testicular cancers

Marker	Elevated in
Alpha-fetoprotein	Many non-seminomatous germ cell tumours (apart from pure choriocarcinomas)
	Never high in pure seminomas
Human chorionic gonadotropin	All cases of choriocarcinoma
	Many embryonal carcinomas
	A small proportion of pure seminomas
Lactate dehydrogenase	Metastatic disease, particularly non-seminomatous germ cell tumours

Prognosis

Before the use of chemotherapy the 5-year survival of all patients with testicular cancer was only about 40 per cent, most of whom had a seminoma. The overall 5-year survival is now around 95 per cent, and is near to 100 per cent in Stage 1 tumours.

CONDITIONS SPECIFIC TO FEMALES

BARTHOLIN'S CYST AND ABSCESS

Bartholin's glands are paired structures that produce mucinous fluid. The ducts open between the labia minora and the hymen and may become blocked, with retention of secretions and formation of a cyst, which appears as a painless lump in the vulva. If the cyst becomes infected an abscess develops which gives rise to an exquisitely painful fluctuant swelling. The patient may be systemically unwell.

Investigation

The diagnosis is made on clinical examination alone. If a purulent discharge is evident or sexually transmitted infection is suspected, swabs should be taken. Any signs suggestive of a vulval malignancy indicate a biopsy.

Management

Bartholin's cysts and abscesses may rupture spontaneously, with relief of symptoms.

In the case of a **fluctuant abscess**, incision and drainage is required, with deroofing and gentle packing of the abscess cavity.

Marsupialization is used for an uninfected cyst. The cyst is opened and the wall sutured to the skin to leave an open pouch. To avoid dyspareunia drainage should be external and not into the lumen of the vagina.

If a sexually acquired infection is suspected (most commonly *Neisseria gonorrhoeae*), an appropriate course of antibiotics and sexual health counselling is required.

SYPHILITIC CHANCRE

Syphilitic chancres may be seen on the female external genitalia during the primary phase of the disease,

although they are more commonly located on the vaginal wall or cervix and only seen on speculum examination. Investigation and treatment is as for male disease.

URETHRAL CARUNCLE

A urethral caruncle is a friable out-pouching of urethral mucosa at the urethral meatus, occasionally seen in postmenopausal women. The everted mucosal surface may become sore and bleed. Rarely, it can disturb or even obstruct the flow of urine.

Investigation

Bacteriology

An **MSU or swab** should be taken if an associated infection is suspected.

Imaging

Cysto-urethroscopy may be useful to confirm that the proximal urethra is normal and exclude neoplasia.

Tissue biopsy

An excision biopsy is essential if the lesion cannot be readily distinguished from a urethral or vulval carcinoma.

Management

Caruncles are often symptomless, the patient only needing **reassurance**. Local symptoms may respond to topical **oestrogen cream**.

Surgical excision is rarely needed but is straightforward and effective. The caruncle is excised and the mucosal edge joined to the vaginal epithelium with absorbable sutures.

CARCINOMA OF THE VULVA

Carcinoma of the vulva is an uncommon condition that affects elderly women. Almost all are squamous cell carcinomata. It may present with local symptoms of vulval itching (pruritus vulvae), soreness or a lump. Examination of the genitalia will reveal an ulcerated lesion with an everted edge. Signs of metastatic disease (such as inguinal lymphadenopathy) may be present.

Invasive cancer may be preceded by pre-malignant vulval intraepithelial carcinoma (VIN). This condition is associated with infection with human papilloma virus (HPV).

Investigation

Imaging

Chest X-ray and cross-sectional imaging with **CT** or **MRI** are required for staging the disease.

Tissue biopsy

Diagnosis is made by histological examination of a biopsy.

Management

The treatment of invasive carcinoma of the vulva is adequate **surgical excision** of the primary lesion. For more advanced disease this may involve a **radical vulvectomy** (excision of the whole vulva).

The inguinal lymph nodes are managed in the same way as for a scrotal carcinoma (see page 518) with fine needle aspiration cytology followed by **inguinal node block dissection** if indicated.

Radiotherapy may be used to treat involved pelvic lymph nodes.

Appendix

Revision panel 1 (see page 15)
A routine for the examination of a plain chest X-ray

Check in turn:

The position of the patient
Is the view truly AP or PA or is the patient slightly rotated?
(*In the true PA or AP view the ends of the clavicles should be symmetrically related to the vertebral column.*)

The bones
Is the chest cage symmetrical?
Are all the ribs present? (*one missing suggests previous surgery*)
Is there an extra rib?
Are the ribs
    notched? (*coarctation*)
    eroded? (*metastic deposits*)
Are there any fractures?
Are the thoracic vertebrae intact and the spine straight?

The trachea
Is the trachea central or deviated? If deviated, is it being pushed or pulled out of line?
Is the trachea symmetrical, narrowed or compressed?
Is the carina widened. (*lymph node enlargement*)

The heart
Is the heart outline normal in size, shape and position?
Is there evidence of a pericardial effusion (large globular heart shadow)?
Is there left ventricular enlargement (boot-shaped heart) (*aortic incompetence, aortic stenosis, hypertension*)
Is the left atrium enlarged (convex swelling of the left border of the heart) (*mitral stenosis, mitral incompetence*) (left atrial enlargement can also be delineated by a right oblique view of a barium swallow)

The mediastinum
Is the aorta dilated or unfolded?
Are there any soft tissue shadows (*retrosternal goitre, enlarged thymus, lymph nodes*)
Are there any visible fluid levels apparent? (hiatus hernia, achalasia, mediastinal abscess)

The diaphragm
Is the outline of the diaphragm clear on both sides and of normal shape and position?
Are the cardiophrenic and costophrenic angles clear or is there an effusion?
Is there any free air under the diaphragm?

The lungs
Divide the lungs into three zones:
Upper zone: apex to anterior end of second costal cartilage
Mid zone: from anterior end of second costal cartilage to lower border of fourth costal cartilage
Lower zone: from lower border of fourth costal cartilage to the base
Are there any abnormal shadows?
Are size and positions of the hilar shadows normal?
Are the vascular markings more prominent (*pulmonary plethora*)?
Are the vascular markings inconspicuous (*pulmonary oligaemia*)?
Are any fissures visible? (the minor interlobar fissure on the right may sometimes be seen in a normal film)
Are there any Kerley B lines (engorged subpleural lymphatics at the lung bases caused by raised left atrial pressure)?
Is there any evidence of a pneumothorax?
Is one lung field more opaque than the other? (If so, an erect film may show a large effusion or haemothorax)

Soft tissue shadows
If the patient is female, are both breast shadows present and symmetrical? (*if one is missing the patient has had a mastectomy*)
Are there any other extrathoracic soft tissue swellings?

Revision panel 2 (see page 15)
A routine for the examination of a plain abdominal X-ray

Check in turn:

The position of the patient

Is the patient erect, supine or in a lateral decubitus position?

Check the flank stripes and the psoas shadows for symmetry and normal sharp interfaces.

The penetration of the film

Is it overpenetrated? This might indicate (*free peritoneal air, a large amount of gas in the gut, a very thin patient*).

Is it underpenetrated? This might indicate ascites, an obese patient, fluid-filled loops of gut, a soft tissue mass.

The bones

Are the lower ribs present? (*an absent twelfth rib may indicate previous renal surgery*)

Is the spine normal, or is there evidence of:

- scoliosis
- osteoarthritis with osteophyte formation
- ankylosing spondylitis
- secondary deposits and/or collapse?

Is the pelvis normal, or is there evidence of:

- Paget's disease
- secondary deposits
- osteoarthritis of the hips
- fractures?

The intestinal gas pattern

- Is it normal?
- Are there any fluid levels?

(More than the following three fluid levels – in the gastric fundus, the duodenal cap and the terminal ileum (rare) – is regarded as being abnormal but in children under 2 years, fluid levels in the small bowel are a normal occurrence)

- Are there any distended loops of bowel?
- Can the loops be identified by the gas pattern?
- In the *jejunum* the transverse folds of the valvulae conniventes extend across the whole width of the bowel giving a concertina appearance.
- In the *ileum* the gas has no characteristic outline.
- In the *caecum* the gas appears as a rounded blob.
- In the *colon* the gas is divided by the haustral folds which are spaced irregularly and do not traverse the complete width of the bowel

Is there any uncontained air?

- in the biliary tree (*pneumobilia*)
- under the liver or lateral to it
- under the diaphragm
- in abscess cavities
- in the bladder – (*pneumaturia*)

The soft tissue shadows

- Are any visible solid organs normal in size and shape? i.e. the splenic tip, the liver edge, the kidneys and the urinary bladder
- Are the psoas shadows present and normal?
- Are there any unexplained soft tissue shadows?

Is there any extraskeletal calcification?

- in rib cartilages
- in vessels
  especially aortic, iliac or splenic aneurysms phleboliths
- in the genitourinary tract (*calculi*)
- in the gallbladder (*gallstones*, only 10 per cent of all which are calcified)
- in the pancreas (*chronic pancreatitis*)
- in the mesenteric lymph nodes
- in abnormal structures, such as *dermoid cysts*

Revision panel 3 (see page 15)
A method for the examination of plain X-rays of the limbs and bones

Check in turn:

The orientation of the X-ray
Which bone and which side?
Are two views available, e.g. anteroposterior, lateral or oblique?
Are X-rays of both limbs available for comparison?
The patient's maturity (age and epiphyseal fusion)

The soft tissues
Are any foreign bodies visible?
Is there any extraosseus calcification?
(e.g. in an old haematoma (*myositis ossificans*), tendons or tendon sheaths (*pertendonitis calcarea*) or veins (*phleboliths*)
Are there any soft tissue swellings (*tumours* or *lipomata*)?

The structure of the bones
Their shape
Are they too wide? (*Paget's disease*)
Are they too narrow? (*osteogenesis imperfecta*)
Are they bent? (*Paget's disease, malunion, rickets*)
Are any fractured?
Their density
Is it increased? (*osteopetrosis – marble bones*)
Is it decreased? (*osteoporosis, osteomalacia*)
Is it uniform or irregular with loss of normal architecture? (*osteomyelitis, fibrous dysplasia, malignant deposits*)

The periosteum
Is the periostium visible? (if so, it is abnormal, except in infants)
Is the periostium lifted up by:
- *callus* from a fracture
- *scurvy*
- *syphilis*
- *osteogenic sarcoma*
- *hypertrophic pulmonary osteoarthropathy*
- *Caffrey's disease (infantile cortical hyperostosis).*

The cortex
Is the cortex thinner or eroded? (*cysts, tumours, aneurysms*)
Is the cortex thicker? (*Paget's disease*)

The medulla
Are there any rarefied areas in the medulla?
Are they single? (*solitary bone cyst, Brodie's abscess, chondroma, giant cell tumour, eosinophilic granuloma, osteogenic sarcoma*)
Are they multiple? (*fibrous dysplasia, storage diseases such as Gaucher's diseas and Hand–Schuller–Christian disease, sarcoidosis, primary and secondary malignant disease, multiple myeloma, leukaemia*)
Are there any areas of increased density in the medulla?
- single, as *in aseptic necrosis after trauma, septic necrosis (a sequestrum) and some tumours.*
- multiple, as in *some tumours, secondary deposits of prostatic carcinoma, Engelmann's disease.*

Joints
Check the joint's position
- Is it dislocated?
- Is it subluxed?
- Is it in a position of deformity?
Check the joint space
- Is it decreased? (*osteoarthritis, and rheumatoid arthritis*)
- Is it increased? (*osteochondritis, Perthe's, disease, effusion*)
Are there any intra-articular loose bodies?
Check the joint edge: is there *lipping* or *osteophyte* formation?
Check the joint's soft tissues
- Is there any soft tissue calcification, e.g. in a meniscus?
- Is there soft tissue swelling (*bursitis*)

Revision panel 4 (see page 295)
The management of haemoptysis

The term **massive haemoptysis** refers to a volume of blood lost into the bronchial tree that may threaten life, i.e. >600 mL in 24 hours. The problem such a degree of bleeding causes is one of asphyxiation (drowning in blood) rather than exsanguination.

Management

- Ensure the airway is protected (this may require intubation/rigid bronchoscopy)
- Restore the intravascular blood volume
- Identify the site of bleeding and its cause. This may require a chest X-ray or CT scan and bronchoscopy
- Stop the bleeding:
  Treat the cause (e.g. antibiotics, reversal of heparin/warfarin)
  Bronchial angiography and embolization
  Surgical resection if required
  Radiotherapy for inoperable lung cancer

Revision panel 5 (see page 339)
Three variations of triple assessment

For a palpable lump	History and examination Imaging with mammography or ultrasound Core biopsy or fine needle aspiration cytology
For nipple discharge of inversion	History and examination Imaging with mammography Cytology of nipple discharge
For changes in nipple skin	History and examination Imaging with mammography Punch biopsy of nipple skin

Revision panel 6 (see page 350)
Hormone manipulation for oestrogen receptor-positive breast cancer

Premenopausal	**Tamoxifen** If not tolerated, progestogen or LHRH inhibitor
Postmenopausal	**Aromatase inhibitor** If not tolerated, tamoxifen

Revision panel 7 (see page 354)
Management of breast cysts

First presentation – full triple assessment, aspiration for cytology or core biopsy will drain the cyst

Subsequent cysts – aspiration in primary care or by specialist nurse

If lump resolves the cyst fluid may be discarded

Residual swelling after aspiration or bloody fluid – full triple assessment

Index